Salmonella enterica Serovar Enteritidis in Humans and Animals

Salmonella enterica Serovar Enteritidis in Humans and Animals

EPIDEMIOLOGY, PATHOGENESIS, AND CONTROL

A.M. SAEED

EDITOR IN CHIEF

RICHARD K. GAST
MORRIS E. POTTER
PATRICK G. WALL

ASSOCIATE EDITORS

IOWA STATE UNIVERSITY PRESS / AMES

© 1999 Iowa State University Press, Ames, Iowa 50014
All rights reserved

Iowa State University Press
2121 South State Avenue, Ames, Iowa 50014

Orders: 1-800-862-6657
Office: 1-515-292-0140
Fax: 1-515-292-3348
Web site: www.isupress.edu

Chapter 28, C (British) Crown copyright 1999. Published with the permission of the Controller of Her (Britannic) Majesty's Stationary Office. The views expressed are those of the authors and do not reflect those of Her Majesty's Stationary Office or the Central Veterinary Laboratory or any other (British) government department.

Authorization to photocopy items for internal or personal use, or the internal or personal use of specific clients, is granted by Iowa State University Press, provided that the base fee of $.10 per copy is paid directly to the Copyright Clearance Center, 27 Congress Street, Salem, MA 01970. For those organizations that have been granted a photocopy license by CCC, a separate system of payments has been arranged. The fee code for users of the Transactional Reporting Service is 0-8138-2707-8/99 $.10.

Printed on acid-free paper in the United States of America

First edition, 1999

Library of Congress Cataloging-in-Publication Data
Salmonella enterica serovar Enteritidis in humans and animals:
    epidemiology, pathogenesis, and control / A.M. Saeed, editor-in-chief;
    associate editors, Richard K. Gast, Morris E. Potter, Patrick
    G. Wall.
        p.   cm.
    Includes bibliographical references and index.
    ISBN 0-8138-2707-8
    1. Salmonellosis.   2. Salmonellosis in animals.   3. Salmonella
enteritidis.   I. Saeed, A. M.   II. Gast, Richard K.   III. Potter,
Morris E.   IV. Wall, Patrick G.
    RA644.S15S23   1999
    615.9'529344—dc21   98-39318

The last digit is the print number: 9 8 7 6 5 4 3 2 1

About the Editors

Editor in Chief

A.M. Saeed, DVM, MS, PhD, MPH, Diplomate of the American College of Veterinary Preventive Medicine, is an associate professor of Epidemiology and Infectious Diseases at Purdue University School of Veterinary Medicine and professor of records for the public health and zoonoses and food animal epidemiology courses. For the past nine years, Dr. Saeed has been the university representative to several national food safety committees. He participated in the two National Spent Hen Surveys of 1991 and 1995 by processing samples from over 50,000 spent hens in his laboratory for the isolation of *Salmonella* Enteritidis and other salmonella serotypes. He is the recipient of the U.S. Department of Agriculture Certificate of Appreciation. Dr. Saeed is a member of several professional organizations such as the American Veterinary Medical Association, the American Society of Microbiologists, the Society of Epidemiologic Research, and the U.S. Animal Health Association. Dr. Saeed's research in epidemiology and infectious diseases spans two decades. In 1989, Dr. Saeed initiated a research program on *Salmonella* Enteritidis infections in humans and animals, which he conducts in collaboration with other universities, the U.S. Department of Agriculture, and the Centers for Disease Control and Prevention.

Associate Editors

Richard K. Gast, PhD, is a research microbiologist at the U.S. Department of Agriculture—Agricultural Research Service Southeast Poultry Research Laboratory in Athens, Georgia. He is also an adjunct faculty member in the Departments of Poultry Science and Avian Medicine at the University of Georgia. His research interests in recent years have focused on the very diverse issues involved in the detection, prevention, and control of *Salmonella* Enteritidis infections in chickens. He is the author of the chapter on paratyphoid *Salmonella* infections in the 10th edition of *Diseases of Poultry* published by Iowa State University Press.

Morris E. Potter, DVM, MSPH, is the assistant director for foodborne diseases in the Division of Bacterial and Mycotic Diseases, National Center of Infectious Diseases. He is also the chief of the Food Safety Initiative Activity and the director of the World Health Organization Collaborating Center for Foodborne Disease Surveillance. Dr. Potter presently administers national food safety initiative resources that come to the Centers for Disease Control and Prevention, coordinates foodborne disease prevention activities at the CDC, and integrates CDC activities into the national food safety program. He was a member of the U.S. delegation to the Codex Alimentarius Food Hygiene Committee, and he belongs to a number of professional organizations, including the American Association of Avian Pathologists and the U.S. Animal Health Association.

Patrick G. Wall, DVM, MD, was until 1998 the epidemiologist in charge of the Gastrointestinal Diseases Section of the Communicable Disease Surveillance Centre of the U.K. Public Health Laboratory Service. This section is responsible for national surveillance and is involved in the investigation of national and international outbreaks of food and waterborne disease. Dr. Wall is currently chief executive of the Food Safety Authority of Ireland, which is accountable to the Minister of Health. This body was established in 1998 after a succession of foodscares, from bovine spongiform encephalopathy, *E. coli* O157, and salmonella to agrochemical, therapeutic, and illegal residues in meat, had damaged consumer confidence throughout the European Union. The authority's mission is to protect consumers' health from illness related to the consumption of food by ensuring that the highest standards are observed throughout the foodchain and that there are no gaps in the continuum from farm to fork.

Contents

Foreword

SALMONELLA ENTERITIDIS: THE CONTINUING GLOBAL PUBLIC HEALTH CHALLENGE

In the last two decades, *Salmonella enterica* serovar Enteritidis has caused a growing worldwide pandemic. This pandemic makes *S.* Enteritidis the most common of the nontyphoidal serovars of salmonella in many countries and has lent new impetus to food-safety efforts everywhere. As a group, nontyphoid salmonella infections became important public health concerns in parallel with the modern intensification of animal rearing—in the 1920s in Western Europe, and in the 1950s and 1960s in North America. Since then, in most parts of the developed world, several different nontyphoidal salmonella serovars have increased, including the ubiquitous serovar Typhimurium, but few so dramatically or universally as *S.* Enteritidis. This serovar actually emerged in Europe as an important cause of human illness in the 1920s and 1930s, and was frequently associated with the consumption of duck eggs. Indeed, this earlier epidemic may have contributed to the disappearance of the European commercial duck-egg industry. More recently, by exploiting a specific niche in our industrialized food supply among intensively raised chickens, this salmonella serovar has proved remarkably adaptable to the modern era. Thus far, it has defied general control efforts and remains a greater public health challenge than ever. After a decade of focused research, this is a timely moment to review what is known and what still needs to be learned about this resourceful organism.

In many countries, awareness of the public health threat posed by *S.* Enteritidis is just beginning. It usually starts with an increase in observed cases, which is recognized because salmonella isolates from humans are routinely serotyped in a public health laboratory. The increase in *S.* Enteritidis infections may be heralded by a particularly dramatic outbreak. An epidemiological investigation into the source of the outbreak may reveal that it is related to consumption of undercooked eggs or chickens. When public health authorities turn to their agricultural colleagues for help, they may learn that because no parallel health problem has been recognized in chickens, it is often difficult for some in agriculture to believe that the source could be the hen that laid the egg or went to slaughter. After the fact of the reservoir in hens is documented and accepted, public health and agricultural scientists then begin to discuss what can be done, see solutions in the other's area of expertise, and slowly come to the realization that solving the problem will require their joint efforts.

In the United States, *S.* Enteritidis first began to increase in the late 1970s in the extreme northeastern part of the country. Although there were several outbreaks at the time, most cases were sporadic; that is, they were unconnected with each other or with other outbreaks. This growing problem did not register as a major public health concern until 1986, when a large multistate outbreak occurred. This outbreak, which affected an estimated 3300 persons in 7 states, was caused by a commercial stuffed-pasta product, filled with a stuffing containing raw eggs. To determine the origin of the *S.* Enteritidis, the epidemiologists traced the eggs back to a single source farm and succeeded in isolating *S.* Enteritidis from environmental swabs on the farm. Review and intensive investigation of other outbreaks rapidly documented that *S.* Enteritidis was much more likely to be associated with egg-containing foods than were other salmonella serovars, that the eggs involved were almost always U.S. grade-A commercial shell eggs, that they came from many different source farms, and that they were typically not fully cooked. The general problem was outlined in an article in the medical press published in 1988. At that time, it was possible to make general estimates of the magnitude of the problem, to document the regular association of *S.* Enteritidis with eggs, and to identify the groups at highest risk, namely, the nursing-home and hospitalized patient populations. With this information in hand, it was also possible to begin an initial public health prevention program. The first priority was to warn high-risk groups of the potential risk of exposure to raw eggs, and to promote the use of pasteurized eggs among the highest-risk populations. Similarly, restaurants and other institutions needed to be informed of the risk of pooling large numbers of shell eggs and of undercooking them. Finally, the egg industry, which was alert to the problem, encouraged avian researchers to find potential solutions to the problem on the farm. None of these measures turned out to be particularly easy in practice, and none have been fully applied.

In the 10 years since the pandemic of *S.* Enteritidis infections was first recognized in the United States, it has spread from an initial concentration in the extreme northeast to affect most of the country. The wave of cases that is spreading westward from the northeast is associated with phage types 8, 13a, and 14b. A second wave began in the west in 1994 and is now spreading eastward and is associated with phage type 4. This is also the phage type that predominates in Western Europe and parts of Latin America. In 1996, serovar Enteritidis represented 25% of all human salmonellosis reported in the United States. In many other countries, which have pursued a variety of different control strategies, the story is similar or even more challenging, and, in some, infection with *S.* Enteritidis has become almost synonymous with salmonellosis itself. This pandemic has proved very difficult to control. Although several countries may have thus far managed to exclude the problem, it is difficult to say that any country has successfully controlled it once it is established. Thus, after more than a decade of concentrated research, the problem of *S.* Enteritidis is a greater challenge to public health than ever.

The challenge posed by *S.* Enteritidis is related to the extraordinary biology of the infection in the avian host. It has now been clearly established that these strains can cause lifelong colonization of the peri-reproductive tissues of the hens, from which the contents of the egg can be colonized before the shell is formed. As an evolutionary strategy, the ability to invade the host, to colonize the reproductive tissues, and to pass to the embryo is brilliant. Because the next generation of hosts is infected from the beginning, the pathogen avoids selection by events taking place outside the host, and something close to bacteriologic immortality is achieved. It is perhaps no coincidence that *S.* Enteritidis shares major surface antigens with, and may be closely related to, other salmonella serovars (Gallinarum and Pullorum) that also transmit transovarially in the chicken from hen to egg, but that cause severe pathology in the hen. Similar vertical transmission of salmonellae has been documented for a number of different serovars in a number of different reptilian and avian hosts. Indeed, this characteristic is sufficiently widespread among salmonellae that we may speculate it arose early in the evolutionary history of the ancestral reptiles and birds, perhaps soon after they evolved the ability to lay eggs in shells on land. Thus, the current success of the organism in egg-laying flocks may be related to a far earlier success in the course of evolution. If this capacity has a long evolutionary history, we should not be surprised to find that it is complex, refined, and can occur without causing major pathology in the host.

The subtle interaction between *S.* Enteritidis and host chicken illustrates a larger issue. *Salmonella* Enteritidis is just one of a group of emerging foodborne zoonotic pathogens, which challenges the health of humans in many developed nations. This new group includes *Escherichia coli* O157:H7 and other Shiga-toxin-producing *E. coli, Campylobacter jejuni, Yersinia enterocolitica,* and *Vibrio vulnificus,* which have major reservoirs in cattle, poultry, swine, and oysters, respectively. These pathogens share a number of characteristics, which makes the lessons learned about one of potential relevance to the others. First, as a group, they are remarkably nonpathogenic toward their animal hosts. Just as *S.* Enteritidis causes lifelong infection of the reproductive tissues of the host chicken without interfering greatly with the productivity or efficiency of the infected bird, so, similarly, *E. coli* O157:H7 does not cause appreciable morbidity in bovines or other ruminants that

carry that major human pathogen. *Campylobacter jejuni* is present in many chicken flocks without causing any overt illness, *Y. enterocolitica* is a commensal inhabitant of the pig's oropharynx, and *V. vulnificus* is concentrated in the oyster without harming it. Perhaps this is because traditional disease-control measures in animal production have eliminated many of the animal pathogens, so only the selectively less pathogenic remain. However, this innocuous behavior in the host animal leads many to think erroneously that it is not a pathogen in any host and particularly in the human host. Similar concerns about other salmonella serovars were laid to rest in the 1950s by a definitive series of human volunteer feeding studies; any salmonella serovar should be considered pathogenic to humans.

Another important shared characteristic of this group of emerging foodborne zoonoses is that foods contaminated with them appear entirely normal. A hen's egg with *S.* Enteritidis on the yolk membrane looks and tastes entirely normal, as does a ground-beef patty with *E. coli* O157:H7 or an oyster with *V. vulnificus.* This means that visual inspection or screening can do little to detect the problem. In addition, these organisms are often not eliminated by standard methods of food preparation. Many traditional recipes are insufficient to kill the salmonellae in an egg-based hollandaise sauce, the *E. coli* O157:H7 in a rare hamburger, or the vibrios in a raw oyster. It is difficult to fault consumers who are following centuries of tradition in food preparation. Because of the presence of these foodborne pathogens, food preparation techniques that were once believed to be safe and even desirable now may be labeled a "food-handling error."

These emerging foodborne zoonoses are sustained in the food animals and their environments by a complex ecology. This is perhaps best understood for *S.* Enteritidis, but it is likely that similar complexity occurs for the others, perhaps as a result of substantial evolutionary adaptation. This complexity is usually discovered through attempts to eliminate the organism from a flock or herd. For example, when a flock of chickens with *S.* Enteritidis is identified, eliminated, and replaced as part of a disease-control effort, the new replacement flock often acquires the infection, indicating that transmission is not only vertical from parent to chick but also horizontal through the environment. Reinfection can occur following extensive disinfection of the immediate environment, including one heroic effort I am aware of, an attempt to literally heat treat a chicken house by bringing its internal temperature above 145°F. The failure of simple disinfection led to the appreciation of the potential importance of the rodent reservoir, and of the potential impact of basic principles of biosecurity and farm sanitation. Although simple flock replacement after a modicum of cleaning and disinfection has been insufficient, flock-control measures that are based on the new ecological understanding of *S.* Enteritidis may be having an important impact.

Finally, *S.* Enteritidis, like some other salmonella serovars, *E. coli* O157:H7, and *Y. enterocolitica,* has emerged in a global pandemic. How *S.* Enteritidis increased at about the same time in many different countries remains a central and unsolved mystery. It is made more complex by the tantalizing fact that the pandemic is polyclonal, composed of several different strains, defined by phage type and by molecular methods, so that different geographical regions harbor their own subtypes. This makes the pandemic difficult to explain as the spread of a single clone of the bacterium. If a bacterial clone is not spreading, then what is? A transmissible bacterial virulence element affecting different strains of S. Enteritidis? A selective susceptibility of modern chicken breeds to S. Enteritidis infection? Infected mice? Is it possible that an unsuspected practice or technology could select for this serovar?

A multidisciplinary approach to prevention will be the hallmark of efforts to control these new foodborne disease challenges. Our challenge is to interrupt the transmission of the organism through food to the human population. Standard control measures have failed. On the farm, disease-control measures are not effective, because there is little animal disease to trigger them. Once the eggs are laid, the egg-grading and sanitation programs that successfully reduced the threat of salmonellae on the outside of the eggshell can do little to reduce the risk of salmonellae on the inside. During distribution, there is no traditional requirement that eggs be refrigerated. In the kitchen, we educate chefs and consumers to beware raw, pooled, and undercooked eggs but can not expect them routinely and willingly to handle eggs they think are dangerous. This means that new control measures are needed. Because no single measure is the definitive "silver bullet," several protective steps are needed along the chain of production, from farm to table. Education of egg producers in good farm sanitation practices that minimize rodent infestations is one critical step. Requiring refrigeration of eggs between laying and cooking is a second. Requiring the use of liquid pasteurized egg product in nursing homes and hospitals for all pooled egg recipes is a third. In the future, new technologies may provide even better control. The ability to pasteurize an intact shell egg at a commercially viable price would be a dramatic step forward but would not obviate the need for other measures. Indeed, the combination of better farm sanitation and pasteurization would mirror the measures that successfully controlled milkborne infections. Other new technologies may also be available in the future, including the development of a breed of hens resistant to salmonella infection, flock vaccination with salmonellae that are avirulent to humans, and competitive exclusion products for young chicks that render their gut flora more resistant to colonization with salmonellae. Development and application of new strategies will require the collaboration of avian pathologists, food microbiologists, public health scientists, farm-management specialists, and, most important, of the industry itself.

To approach the epidemiology, microbiology, and ecology of S. Enteritidis is to open a window on coming foodborne-disease challenges. The many advances in our understanding, summarized in this volume, are a model for the future of food safety and food science. Some countries are poised to move forward with a new generation of sophisticated control measures. Other countries are just becoming aware that S. Enteritidis is an important public health problem. This volume can serve as a guide and reference to all.

Robert V. Tauxe, MD, MPH
Chief, Foodborne and Diarrheal Diseases Branch
Division of Bacterial and Mycotic Diseases
National Center for Infectious Diseases
Centers for Disease Control and Prevention
Atlanta, Georgia

Acknowledgments

This book is the result of the efforts of an international team of scholars and scientists. I thank all individuals who participated in the preparation of data that enabled contributors to write and submit their chapters for this book.

I also express my most sincere appreciation and thanks to several individuals who played a significant role in making this book's project possible. Special thanks go to Mr. Ian Fisher, Co-ordinating Scientific Secretary of the European Salm-Net Project. Mr. Fisher's kindness and generosity in providing adequate information about the European Salm-Net Project and his follow-up on the progress of the book were instrumental in making the project a success. I can not thank enough Dr. Ahmad M. Al-Majali, who during his stay at Purdue University, as my graduate student, helped immensely in typing, formatting, and converting the very many figures and tables of the book into a uniform style. Ahmad's role in this project was simply instrumental and based on pure enthusiasm for learning and keenness to help. Ms. Carol Koons, chief technician at my laboratory, played a substantial role in completing assigned research work in a timely manner and in maintenance of excellent records.

Many colleagues at Purdue University School of Veterinary Medicine provided substantial advice and encouragement during the project. Dean Alan H. Rebar provided valuable help and encouragement. Drs. H. Leon Thacker and Carl Lamar kindly accepted reviewing the book manuscript and made valuable suggestions. Drs. Keven Kazacos, Jim Freeman, and Raymond Morter have been excellent sources of wisdom and encouragement. Mr. Sam Royer from Medical Illustration was always kind and accommodating in providing skillful photographic work.

Dr. Eldon Ortman from Purdue Agricultural Research Programs (ARP) has been very supportive of the research on *Salmonella* Enteritidis and provided valuable input during several stages of the research surveys. Support and research funds from ARP were vital to the success of *S.* Enteritidis research in the U.S. Midwest.

During the long months of editing and formatting of the book's chapters, my wife, Khaola, and my children, Huda and Ali, were understanding and supportive. Without their support, my job would have been most difficult.

Finally, Carolyn Arnold, Lisa Holeman, Linda Hudson, and Barbara White, secretarial staff at the Department of Veterinary Pathobiology of Purdue University School of Veterinary Medicine, were very accommodating and helpful in handling countless tasks related to the book.

Contributors

Numbers in parentheses beside names refer to chapters.

Yvonne Anderson (26)
Swedish Institute of Infectious Disease Control
S-105 21 Stockholm, Sweden

Friderick J. Angulo (4)
Centers for Disease Control and Prevention
Atlanta, Georgia, U.S.A.

Elikplimi Asem (19)
Department of Basic Medical Sciences
School of Veterinary Medicine
Purdue University
West Lafayette, Indiana 47907, U.S.A.

Paul A. Barrow (17)
Institute for Animal Health
Compton Laboratory
Compton, Newbury, Berks RG20 7NN, U.K.

Andreas Baumgartner (9)
Swiss Federal Office of Public Health (SFOPH)
Division of Food Science
Bern, Switzerland

Charles E. Benson (20)
Department of Pathobiology
Laboratory of Microbiology
School of Veterinary Medicine
University of Pennsylvania
Kennett Square, Pennsylvania 10348, U.S.A.

P. Bouvet (5)
Centre National de Reference des Salmonella et
    Shigella Unite des Enterobacteries
Unite des Institute Pasteur
75724 Paris Cedex, France

D.J. Caldwell (38)
Department of Veterinary Pathobiology
College of Veterinary Medicine
Texas A&M University
College Station, Texas 77845, U.S.A.

Rosalind J. Carter (12)
Bureau of Laboratories
Bureau of Communicable Disease, and Office
    of AIDS Surveillance
New York City Department of Health
455 First Avenue
New York, New York 10016, U.S.A.

Elisabeth Chaslus-Dancla (14)
Institut National de la Recherche Agronomique
Station d'Aviare et Parasitologie
Centre de Tours-Nouzilly
37380 Monnaie, France

Donald E. Corrier (35)
Agricultural Research Service
U.S. Department of Agriculture
College Station, Texas 77845, U.S.A.

Roy Curtiss III (37)
Department of Biology
Washington University
St. Louis, Missouri 63130, U.S.A.

Robert H. Davies (28)
Central Veterinary Laboratory
New Haw, Addleston KT15 3NE, U.K.

J.-C. Desenclos (5)
Reseau National de Sante Publique
14 rue du Val d'Osne
94415 Saint-Maurice Cedex, France

Eric D. Ebel (31, 32)
U.S. Department of Agriculture
Agricultural Research Service
Boise, Idaho, U.S.A.

Anders Engvall (26)
Department of Epizootiology
National Veterinary Institute
S-750 07 Uppsala, Sweden

Sarah J. Evans (28)
Central Veterinary Laboratory
New Haw, Addleston KT15 3NE, U.K.

Kathy E. Ferris (29)
National Veterinary Service Laboratories
Ames, Iowa 50010, U.S.A.

Richard K. Gast (Associate Editor, 22)
U.S. Department of Agriculture
Agricultural Research Service
Southeast Poultry Research Laboratory
934 College Station Road
Athens, Georgia 30605, U.S.A.

B. Gericke (6)
National Veterinary Reference Laboratory (BgVV)
Robert Koch Institute
Burgstr. 37
D-38855 Wernigerode, Germany

Peter Gerner-Smidt (7)
Department of Gastrointestinal Infections
State Serum Institute
Artillerivej 5
DK-2300 Copenhagen S, Denmark

R.W.A. Girdwood (3)
Scottish Salmonella Reference Laboratory
Balornock Road
Glasgow, G21 3UW Scotland

F. Grimont (5)
Centre National de Reference pour le Typage
    Moleculaire Enterique
Unite des Institute Pasteur
75724 Paris Cedex, France

Patrick A.D. Grimont (5)
Centre National de Reference des Salmonella et
    Shigella Unite des Enterobacteries and Centre
    National de Reference pour le Typage
    Moleculaire Enterique
Unite des Institute Pasteur
75724 Paris Cedex, France

Ruben Gruenewald (12)
Bureau of Laboratories
Bureau of Communicable Disease, and Office
    of AIDS Surveillance
New York City Department of Health
455 First Avenue
New York, New York 10016, U.S.A.

Jean Guard-Petter (21)
U.S. Department of Agriculture
Agricultural Research Service
Southeast Poultry Research Laboratory
934 College Station Road
Athens, Georgia 30605, U.S.A.

Billy M. Hargis (38)
Department of Veterinary Pathobiology
College of Veterinary Medicine
Texas A&M University
College Station, Texas 77845, U.S.A.

Jubril O. Hassan (37)
Department of Biology
Washington University
St. Louis, Missouri 63130, U.S.A.

R. Helmuth (6)
National Veterinary Reference Laboratory (BgVV)
Robert Koch Institute
Burgstr. 37
D-38855 Wernigerode, Germany

David J. Henzler (30, 32)
Commonwealth of Pennsylvania
Department of Agriculture
Bureau of Animal Health and Diagnostic Services
2301 North Cameron Street
Harrisburg, Pennsylvania 17110, U.S.A.

Alan T. Hogue (31, 32)
U.S. Department of Agriculture
Food Safety and Inspection Service
Emerging Pathogens and Zoonotic Diseases
300 12th Street SW, Room 205
Washington, DC 20250, U.S.A.

Peter S. Holt (33)
U.S. Department of Agriculture
Agricultural Research Service
Southeast Poultry Research Laboratory
934 College Station Road
Athens, Georgia 30605, U.S.A.

Tom J. Humphrey (18)
Public Health Laboratory Service (PHLS)
PHLS Food Microbiology Research Unit
Church Lane
Heavitree, Exeter EX2 5AD, U.K.

Scott H. Hurd (32)
U.S. Department of Agriculture
Animal and Plant Health Inspection Service
Fort Collins, Colorado, U.S.A.

Linda H. Keller (20)
Bureau of Communicable Disease Control
Department of Public Health, Commonwealth
    of Massachusetts
Jamaica Plain, Massachusetts, U.S.A.

M.H. Kogut (38)
U.S. Department of Agriculture
Agricultural Research Service
Food and Feed Protection Research Laboratory
College Station, Texas 77845, U.S.A.

David Kradel (32)
Pennsylvania Poultry Federation
Harrisburg, Pennsylvania, U.S.A.

Elena Landeras (13)
Departmento de Biologia Functional
Area de Microbiologia, Universidad de Oviedo
Oviedo, Spain

Almut Liesegang (6)
National Veterinary Reference Laboratory (BgVV)
Robert Koch Institute
Burgstr. 37
D-38855 Wernigerode, Germany

Kevin A. Lindell (23)
Department of Pathobiology
School of Veterinary Medicine
Purdue University
West Lafayette, Indiana 47907, U.S.A.

John Mason (Part IV Introduction, 32)
Food Safety Consultants
301 East 64th Street
New York, New York 10021, U.S.A.

Robert M. McDowell (25)
U.S. Department of Agriculture
Animal and Plant Health Inspection Service
Washington, DC, U.S.A.

M. Carmen Mendoza (13)
Departmento de Biologia Functional
Area de Microbiologia
Universidad de Oviedo
Oviedo, Spain

Yves Millemann (14)
Ecole Nationale Veterinaire
Department des Productions Animales et des
    Science de l'Aliment
94704 Maisons-Alfort, France

Roberta A. Morales (25)
Department of Agricultural and Resource Economics
Patterson Hall
North Carolina State University
Raleigh, North Carolina 27695-8109, U.S.A.

Donald S. Munro (3)
Scottish Salmonella Reference Laboratory
Balornock Road
Glasgow, G21 3UW Scotland

Kukambi V. Nagaraja (36)
Department of Veterinary Pathobiology
College of Veterinary Medicine
University of Minnesota
Saint Paul, Minnesota, 55108, U.S.A.

U.S. Nair (16)
Los Alamos National Laboratory
Los Alamos, New Mexico, U.S.A.

Masayuki Nakamura (34)
School of Veterinary Medicine and Animal Sciences
Kitasato University 35-1
Higashi 23
Bancho, Towada-Shi, Amori 034, Japan

David J. Nisbet (35)
U.S. Department of Agriculture
Agricultural Research Service
College Station, Texas, 77845, U.S.A.

H. Mike Opitz (30)
Cooperative Extension and Department of Animal,
    Veterinary, and Aquatic Science
University of Maine
5735 Hitchner Hall
Orono, Maine 04469, U.S.A.

Cornelius Poppe (1)
Health of Animals Laboratory, Health Canada
110 Stone Road
West Guelph, Ontario, Canada N1G 3W4

Morris E. Potter (Associate Editor)
Centers for Disease Control and Prevention
Atlanta, Georgia, U.S.A.

Rita Prager (6)
National Veterinary Reference Laboratory (BgVV)
Robert Koch Institute
Burgstr. 37
D-38855 Wernigerode, Germany

W. Rabsch (6)
National Veterinary Reference Laboratory (BgVV)
Robert Koch Institute
Burgstr. 37
D-38855 Wernigerode, Germany

G. Rajashekara (36)
College of Veterinary Medicine
University of Minnesota
St. Paul, Minnesota 55108, U.S.A.

Alexander Ramon (12)
Bureau of Laboratories
Bureau of Communicable Disease, and Office
    of AIDS Surveillance
New York City Department of Health
455 First Avenue
New York, New York 10016, U.S.A.

W.J. Reilly (3)
Scottish Salmonella Reference Laboratory
Balornock Road
Glasgow, G21 3UW Scotland

Andy R. Rhorer (27)
U.S. Department of Agriculture
Animal and Plant Health Inspection Service,
    Veterinary Service
National Poultry Improvement Plan
1500 Klondike Road
Conyers, Georgia 30094, U.S.A.

A.M. Saeed (Editor in Chief, 16, 19, 23, 24)
Department of Pathobiology
School of Veterinary Medicine
Purdue University
West Lafayette, Indiana 47907, U.S.A.

Wayne D. Schlosser (31, 32)
U.S. Department of Agriculture
Animal and Plant Health Inspection Service,
    Food Safety Inspection Service
555 South Howes Street, Suite 200
Fort Collins, Colorado 80521, U.S.A.

Hans Schmid (9)
Swiss Federal Office of Public Health (SFOPH)
Division of Epidemiology and Infectious Diseases
CH-3003 Bern, Switzerland

Gabriella Scuderi (11)
Labarotorio di Epidemiologia e Biostatistica
Instituto Superiore di Sanita
Viale Regina Elena 299
00161 Rome, Italy

Larry Shipman (32)
U.S. Department of Agriculture
Animal and Plant Health Inspection Service
Indianapolis, Indiana, U.S.A.

Tejinder P. Singh (12)
Bureau of Laboratories
Bureau of Communicable Disease, and the Office of
    AIDS Surveillance
New York City Department of Health
455 First Avenue
New York, New York 10016, U.S.A.

William Sischo (32)
Pennsylvania State University
State College, Pennsylvania, U.S.A.

D.L. Swerdlow (4)
Centers for Disease Control and Prevention
Atlanta, Georgia, U.S.A.

Sarah Terry (12)
Bureau of Laboratories
Bureau of Communicable Disease, and the Office
    of AIDS Surveillance
New York City Department of Health
455 First Avenue
New York, New York 10016, U.S.A.

H. Leon Thacker (23, 24)
Department of Pathobiology
School of Veterinary Medicine
Purdue University
West Lafayette, Indiana 47907, U.S.A.

Dorirarajan Thiagarajan (19, 24)
Department of Pathobiology
School of Veterinary Medicine
Purdue University
West Lafayette, Indiana 47907, U.S.A.

Werner Thiel, Director (10)
National Salmonella Center
A-8010 Graz, Austria

Susan Trock (32)
U.S. Department of Agriculture
Animal and Plant Health Inspection Service
Syracuse, New York, U.S.A.

H. Tschäpe (6)
National Reference Centre for Salmonellae and Other
    Enterics (RKI)
Robert Koch Institute
Burgstr. 37
D-38855 Wernigerode, Germany

A.W. van de Giessen (8)
National Institute of Public Health and the
    Environment
Bilthoven, The Netherlands

B.A.M. van der Zeijst (15)
Faculty of Veterinary Medicine
Department of Bacteriology
Utrecht University
Yalelaan 1, PO Box 80.165
3508 TD Utrecht, The Netherlands

W. J. van Leeuwen (8)
National Institute of Public Health and the
    Environment
Bilthoven, TheNetherlands

Wilfrid van Pelt (8)
National Institute of Public Health and the
    Environment
Bilthoven, The Netherlands

Patrick G. Wall (Associate Editor, 2)
Public Health Laboratory Service (PHLS)
PHLS Communicable Disease Surveillance Centre
Gastrointestinal Disease Section
61 Colindale Avenue
London NW9 5EQ, U.K.

W. Douglas Waltman (39)
Georgia Poultry Laboratory
Oakwood, Georgia 30566, U.S.A.

L.R. Ward (2)
Public Health Laboratory Service (PHLS)
PHLS Laboratory of Enteric Pathogens Centre
Gastrointestinal Disease Section
61 Colindale Avenue
London NW9 5EQ, U.K.

Henrick C. Wegener (7)
Danish Zoonosis Centre
Danish Veterinary Laboratory
Bulowsvej 27
DK-1790 Copenhagen V, Denmark

George Williams (12)
Bureau of Laboratories
Bureau of Communicable Disease, and Office of AIDS
    Surveillance
New York City Department of Health
455 First Avenue
New York, New York 10016, U.S.A.

Clifford Wray (28)
Central Veterinary Laboratory
New Haw, Addleston KT15 3NE, U.K.

Y. Zhao (15)
Faculty of Veterinary Medicine
Department of Bacteriology
Utrecht University
Yalelaan 1, PO Box 80.165
3508 TD Utrecht, The Netherlands

Part I
Salmonella enterica Serovar Enteritidis Epidemiological and Public Health Considerations: A Global Prospective

Epidemiology of *Salmonella enterica* Serovar Enteritidis

C. Poppe

INTRODUCTION

Salmonella serovars can be divided into those that are more or less host adapted and others that are not (Buxton, 1957; McCoy, 1975; Clarke and Gyles, 1993). The serovars adapted for humans include *S. typhi,* causing typhoid fever, and the paratyphoid salmonellae (*S. paratyphi* A, *S. paratyphi* B, and *S. paratyphi* C), causing paratyphoid fever (Seeliger and Maya, 1964; Mandal, 1979). The nomenclature that is followed in this chapter is that described by Le Minor and Popoff (1987) on the taxonomy of the genus *Salmonella.* Based on this taxonomy, all members of the nontyphoidal salmonellae are designated as serovars of the *Salmonella* subspecies *enterica* and may be written as *S.* (italicized) followed by the serovar (nonitalicized). Thus, *Salmonella enterica* subspecies *enterica* serovar Enteritidis is written as *Salmonella* Enteritidis (*S.* Enteritidis).

Animal host-adapted salmonellae include *S.* Choleraesuis causing septicemia, pneumonia, and enterocolitis in pigs (Salmon and Smith, 1886; Schofield, 1944; Schwartz, 1990); *S.* Dublin causing mucohemorrhagic enteritis, septicemia, pneumonia, and abortion in cattle, and septicemia, necrotic enteritis, pneumonia, and mortality in calves (Wray and Sojka, 1977); *S. abortusequi* causing abortion in horses (Schofield, 1945); *S. abortusovis* causing abortion in sheep (Buxton, 1957); and *S.* Gallinarum and *S.* Pullorum, which cause fowl typhoid (Klein, 1889; Hewitt, 1928) and pullorum disease (Rettger, 1900, 1909), respectively, in chickens and turkeys. *Salmonella enterica* serovar Enteritidis (*S.* Enteritidis) belongs to the large number of more than 2300 non-host-adapted salmonella serovars (Le Minor and Popoff, 1992). The non-host-specific salmonella serovars cause salmonellosis in humans and a wide variety of animal hosts (Fey, 1964; Seeliger and Maya, 1964).

Salmonellae are important zoonotic pathogens (Edwards et al., 1948a,b; Bynoe and Yurack, 1964; Galton et al., 1964; Sickenga, 1964; Fox, 1974; McCoy, 1975; Payne and Scudamore, 1977). Salmonellae often cause an inapparent infection, but the infection may also, albeit less frequently, result in enteritis, septicemia, and other serious illnesses in animals and humans, especially in the young (Sadler et al., 1969; Turnbull, 1979). Excretion of the organism causes widespread contamination of the environment and of foods and feeds (McCoy, 1975; Edel et al., 1977; Wray and Sojka, 1977; Oosterom, 1991). Salmonellae are readily and frequently transferred from animals to animals and from animals to humans, especially by indirect but also by direct means (Schaaf, 1936; Edwards, 1956; Atkinson, 1964; Fey, 1964; Galton et al., 1964; Peluffo, 1964; Sickenga, 1964). Transfer from humans to humans is somewhat less common (Turnbull, 1979), and indirect spread from humans to animals has been reported occasionally (Johnston et al., 1981; Kinde et al., 1996b).

During the first 5–6 decades of the 1900s, the main issues with respect to salmonellosis were the occurrence of typhoid fever in humans, which declined dramatically during that period in Europe and North America (Ranta and Dolman, 1947; Edwards, 1958; Bynoe and Yurack, 1964; Nicolle, 1964; Seeliger and Maya, 1964; Sommers, 1980), and the widespread prevalence of pullorum disease and fowl typhoid in chickens and turkeys (Hinshaw and McNeil, 1940; Moore, 1946; Chase, 1947), which caused high mortalities in flocks worldwide and prevented the establishment and growth of the poultry industry until the development and widespread application of testing and control measures (Schaffer et al., 1931; Hinshaw and McNeil, 1940; Chase, 1947; McDermott, 1947; Bullis, 1977a; Pomeroy, 1984; Snoeyenbos, 1984). Since the 1940s, there has been a rapid increase in the isolation of the non-host-specific salmonella serovars from humans and animals (Galton et al., 1964; Guthrie, 1992). This was particularly the case with *Salmonella* Typhimurium, which, until more recently, has been the most prevalent serovar isolated from humans and animals (especially cattle) in many countries (Kelterborn, 1967; McCoy, 1975;

Bullis, 1977b; Wray, 1985; Lior, 1989; Ferris and Miller, 1990; Rodrigue et al., 1990; Kühn et al., 1993; Hargrett-Bean and Potter, 1995). Poultry and poultry products have been the main sources of non-host-specific salmonellae infecting humans (Schaaf, 1936; Edwards, 1958; Bynoe and Yurack, 1964; Galton et al., 1964; Seeliger and Maya, 1964; McCoy, 1975; Laszlo et al., 1985; Humphrey et al., 1988; St. Louis et al., 1988), but dairy products (Bezanson et al., 1985; Ryan et al., 1987; Hennessy et al., 1996), beef (Bryan, 1981; Parham, 1985; Bean and Griffin, 1990), and pork (Maguire et al., 1993) have also been associated with large outbreaks of salmonellosis.

HISTORY

Salmonella Enteritidis was the cause of the historic outbreak of meat "poisoning" in May 1888 in Frankenhausen, Thüringen, Germany, described by A. Gärtner. Gärtner isolated the causative agent, which he called *Bacillus enteritidis,* from the meat of a cow that had diarrhea and was slaughtered, and from the spleen of a 21-year-old man who had eaten about 800 g of raw meat from the cow and who died 1 day later [see Kelterborn (1967)]. An outbreak affecting more than 200 soldiers followed the consumption of insufficiently fried meat from a cow infected with *S.* Enteritidis (Glässer, 1937). Foods incorporating contaminated meats, such as sausages, minced meats, meat pies, and reheated meat preparations, have long been recognized as common sources of infection with *S.* Enteritidis (Buxton, 1957).

Until about 1970–80, *S.* Enteritidis was isolated at a medium to low frequency from humans and animals in most countries. In Western Germany and West Berlin, the isolation rates of *S.* Enteritidis from humans varied between 4.4% and 5.9% of all cases of salmonella infection during the years 1956–59, whereas for *S.* Typhimurium the rates were 34%–41% (Seeliger and Maya, 1964). During the period 1958–67, *S.* Enteritidis constituted 3.3% of all salmonella isolates from humans, 1.6% of all salmonella isolates from poultry, and 0.5% of all bovine isolates in England and Wales (McCoy, 1975). *Salmonella* Enteritidis accounted for 150 (9%) of 1744 salmonella isolates from poultry in England and Wales during the years 1968–73 (Sojka et al., 1975). Thereafter, *S.* Enteritidis accounted for only 74 (1.2%) of 6221 salmonella strains isolated from poultry in Great Britain between 1974 and 1983, and no *S.* Enteritidis were isolated from poultry in 1984 (McIllroy and McCracken, 1990). *Salmonella* Enteritidis was regularly isolated from cattle and calves in most of the European countries but not nearly as often as *S.* Typhimurium and *S.* Dublin (Seeliger and Maya, 1964; McCoy, 1975). In the 1950s, in North America, Europe, and other geographical areas, liquid egg, dried egg, egg-containing cake mixes, and other egg products both imported from other countries and produced at home were frequently (as often as 35%–45%) contaminated with salmonellae and a major source of foodborne salmonella infection. The products were mainly contaminated with serovars such as *S.* Bredeney, *S.* Heidelberg, *S.* Infantis, *S.* Typhimurium, *S.* Meleagridis, *S.* Oranienburg, *S.* Montevideo, *S.* Anatum, and rarely with *S.* Enteritidis (Butler and

Josephson, 1962; Bynoe and Yurack, 1964; Galton et al., 1964; McCoy, 1975). Pasteurization of all liquid egg products curtailed the infections (McCoy, 1975). Salmonella serovars, primarily *S.* Typhimurium, were commonly isolated from poultry meat in the 1940s–60s (Galton et al., 1964; McCoy, 1975).

In Eastern Europe, *S.* Enteritidis ranked as the second to fourth most common serovar in humans and animals during the 1945–60 period (Lachowicz, 1964). It was the fifth most common serovar (5.7%) isolated from humans during the period 1949–62 in Israel (Silberstein and Gerichter, 1964). In Central Africa, it ranked second (10.2%) in isolation from humans during the period 1946–60 (van Oye, 1964), but it was isolated rarely in the south of Africa (Brede, 1964). *Salmonella* Enteritidis was uncommonly isolated (2%) from humans and animals in Mexico during the years 1940–62 (Valera and Valera, 1964), and the same low percentage of isolation has been reported for *S.* Enteritidis isolation from animals and humans during the 1940s and 1950s in South America (Peluffo, 1964). It was the most common cause of foodborne salmonellosis in Japan in the 1950s and was isolated commonly from cattle, dogs, and rats but infrequently from chickens, pigs, and horses. A few isolations were also made from eggs (Fukumi, 1964). *Salmonella* Enteritidis was rarely isolated from humans and animals in Indochina and China (Le Minor, 1964) and Australia in the 1950s (Atkinson, 1964). Records of the 12 commonest serovars isolated during the years 1934–63 in the United States show that *S.* Enteritidis was the ninth most common salmonella serovar (3.1% of all isolates) in humans during the years 1939–55, and the fifth most common (8.7% of all isolates) from animals during the years 1947–58 (Galton et al., 1964). In Canada, the number of *S.* Enteritidis isolates from humans varied between 0.3% and 0.5% annually between 1953 and 1958 and varied between 1.3% and 2.5% during the years 1959–62 (Bynoe and Yurack, 1964).

SURVEILLANCE AND ITS LIMITATIONS

Most of the information regarding the prevalence of salmonellae has been based on passive laboratory salmonella surveillance (Faddoul and Fellows, 1966; Sojka et al., 1975). Often no distinction has been made between symptomatic and asymptomatic infection or chronic carriage. Such surveillance systems have inherent biases (Bynoe and Yurack, 1964; Galton et al., 1964). Many factors—including intensity of surveillance (Galton et al., 1964), submission for serotyping (Sojka et al., 1975), severity of illness and association with a recognized outbreak in the human population (Philbrook et al., 1960; Telzak et al., 1990; van de Giessen et al., 1992; Altekruse et al., 1993), and lack of a systematic method of reporting (Edwards, 1958)—affect whether an infection will be reported. Reporting of animal and human salmonellosis has been substantially underestimated. However, the surveillance data allow broad comparisons and identify trends, reservoirs, and routes of transmission of salmonella serovars.

PREVALENCE IN HUMANS

During the last 10–15 years, there has been a dramatic rise in the prevalence of *S.* Enteritidis infections in humans, commencing initially in the European countries and later reported worldwide (Laszlo et al., 1985; Rodrigue et al., 1990; Binkin et al., 1993; Kühn et al., 1993; Threlfall et al., 1993; Wong et al., 1994). During the 1985–95 period, 582 *S.* Enteritidis outbreaks were reported in the United States, which accounted for 24,058 cases of illness, 2290 hospitalizations, and 70 deaths [Centers for Disease Control (CDC), 1996]. In the process, *S.* Enteritidis replaced *S.* Typhimurium as the commonest serovar isolated from humans in many countries (Rodrigue et al., 1990; CDC, 1992; Kühn et al., 1993; Bean and Potter, 1994). The human infections were often associated with the consumption of eggs or food products containing eggs (Laszlo et al., 1985; Anon., 1988; St. Louis et al., 1988). Unlike the outbreaks and sporadic cases of eggborne salmonellosis in the past, which were caused by cracked and dirty eggs (Schaaf, 1936; Watt, 1945; Edwards, 1956), the more recent egg-associated *S.* Enteritidis infections were linked to contaminated, intact grade-A shell eggs (Anon., 1988; Lin et al., 1988; St. Louis et al., 1988; Hedberg et al., 1993). Shell eggs, scrambled eggs, food products containing raw or partly cooked eggs (including homemade mayonnaise, eggnog, milk shakes, mousse, and egg sandwiches), soft-boiled eggs, lightly cooked eggs, lightly cooked omelets, dishes containing raw egg white, ice cream containing uncooked eggs, and poultry meat have all been implicated in outbreaks (Anon., 1988; Coyle et al., 1988; Humphrey et al., 1988; Paul and Batchelor, 1988; Perales and Audicana, 1988; Cowden et al., 1989; Mawer et al., 1989; Stevens et al., 1989; Hennessy et al., 1996).

In Canada, the annual isolation rates of *S.* Enteritidis varied between 3.7% and 8.7% of all salmonella isolates from humans during the period 1976–82 (Khakhria et al., 1991). During the 12-year period 1983–94, *S.* Enteritidis ranked mostly as the third or fourth most common isolated salmonella serovar, except in 1991 and 1994, when it ranked second, and in 1993, when it ranked first, and the isolation rate of *S.* Enteritidis was slightly higher than of *S.* Typhimurium (Fig. 1.1). The percentage of *S.* Enteritidis of all salmonella isolates from human sources during the 12-year period 1983–94 increased from a low of 2.7% in 1984 to 16.9% in 1994 (Khakhria et al., 1994, 1995, 1997). During the 1976–89 period, phage type 8 was the most common phage type (PT) (Ward et al., 1987) among *S.* Enteritidis strains that were phage typed from human sources in Canada, followed by PT4, PT13, and PT13a. During this period, a large foodborne outbreak of *S.* Enteritidis PT8 affecting 104 laboratory-confirmed cases occurred in Ontario, Canada. It was associated with the consumption of contaminated cake. PT13 was identified in a large outbreak involving 36 laboratory-confirmed cases in people who had consumed cream-filled cakes sold by two bakeries in British Columbia, Canada (Khakhria et al., 1991). The isolation rates of *S.* Enteritidis PT4 from human sources increased gradually during the period 1990–94, and PT4 became the most frequent *S.* Enteritidis phage type in 1992 (Khakhria et al., 1991, 1997). Until 1993, many of

the human cases of infection with PT4 were acquired while traveling abroad (Khakhria et al., 1991, 1994). More recently, however, an egg-associated outbreak of human infection with *S.* Enteritidis PT4 affecting 170 people occurred in Northern Ontario and Québec, Canada. The flocks producing the contaminated eggs were destroyed.

Large nosocomial infections have rarely occurred in Canada. A notable exception is an outbreak of 95 laboratory-confirmed cases of infection with *S.* Enteritidis PT13 that occurred among patients and staff of a regional hospital in Ontario, Canada. A difficult-to-clean vertical mixer used to blend raw shelled eggs, minced ham, and sandwich fillings was the most likely vehicle of transmission (Anon., 1992). A large nosocomial infection in which a more direct relation between outbreak, eggs, and flocks producing the eggs was established occurred in 1987 in a New York City acute-care and long-term-care hospital where 404 (42%) of 965 patients were affected and 9 patients died. Pooled batches of eggs from the hospital kitchen tested positive for *S.* Enteritidis PT8, as did 383 (69%) of 555 ovaries from hens at the farm from which the eggs were obtained. The eggs had been used to prepare mayonnaise that was used in turn to prepare a tuna-macaroni salad (Telzak et al., 1990).

Salmonella Enteritidis infection in humans is not only eggborne but may also be caused by the consumption of meat (Humphrey et al., 1988; Reilly et al., 1988) or raw milk contaminated with this serovar (Wood et al., 1991). Over a 5-year period, two adults and six children at a farm in Alberta, Canada, experienced clinical salmonellosis, and *S.* Enteritidis PT8 was isolated from the farm family and repeatedly from one-quarter of the udder of a cow at the farm (Wood et al., 1991).

Serovars other than *S.* Enteritidis have also been identified as a cause of foodborne infections associated with the consumption of insufficiently cooked or raw eggs, egg white or yolk, or food products containing such ingredients. An outbreak involving 104 cases and six fatalities caused by *S.* Typhimurium occurred in an institution for the treatment of mental disease in Massachusetts. Eggnog was the vehicle of transmission. The same phage type of *S.* Typhimurium was found in the flock of hens that supplied the eggs and was cultured from some of the eggs (Philbrook et al., 1960). In another egg-associated outbreak, *S.* Heidelberg affected 91 of a total of about 1000 persons who attended a convention in New Mexico and consumed fried eggs; the eggs appeared to be "runny" and insufficiently cooked (Weisse et al., 1986).

SYMPTOMS OF SALMONELLOSIS IN HUMANS

The incubation period varies from a few hours to 72 h and the duration of illness varies from 4 to 10 days. Symptoms commonly observed are diarrhea, headache, abdominal pain, nausea, chills, fever, and vomiting (Steinert et al., 1990; CDC, 1992). In patients with underlying disease, septicemia is not uncommon and, in healthy subjects, there may be a wide range of sequelae, including pericarditis,

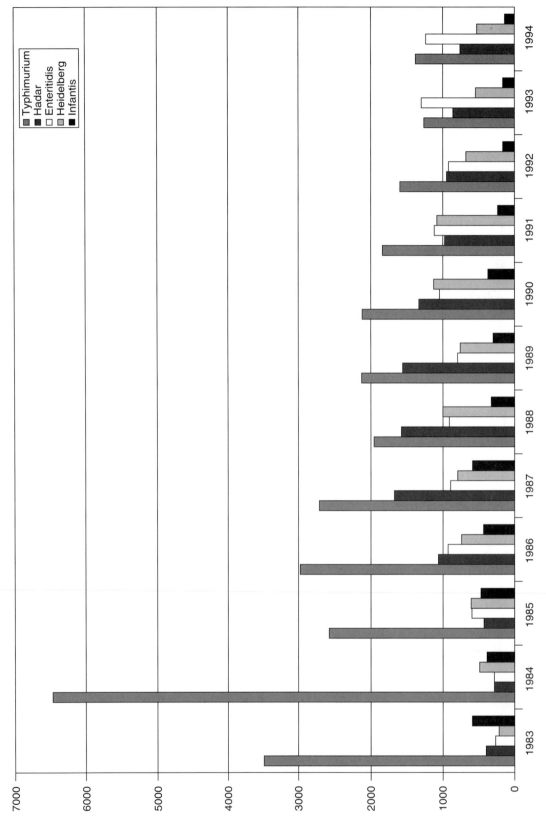

FIGURE 1.1 The five most commonly isolated salmonella serovars from human sources in Canada, 1983–94.

neurological and neuromuscular diseases, reactive arthritis, ankylosing spondylitis, and osteomyelitis. Damage to the mucous membrane of the small intestine and colon may occur that may lead to malabsorption and nutrient loss (Baird-Parker, 1990). Severe dehydration, bloody diarrhea, and hematogenous spread of *S.* Enteritidis to bone, the meninges, and soft tissues have occurred in infants (Cross et al., 1989). The carrier stage can last for weeks to months. Antibiotic treatment is likely to prolong the carrier state and is therefore not recommended in cases with no complications (Dixon, 1965; Aserkoff and Bennett, 1969).

SUSCEPTIBILITY OF THE HUMAN HOST TO THE INFECTION

Susceptibility to and severity of salmonella infection in people depends on factors including the dose of the pathogen (Taylor et al., 1984), the type of food, and the age of the host (Steinert et al., 1990), and factors known to affect the immune status of the host, such as infection with the human immunodeficiency virus (HIV) (Levine et al., 1991; Wong et al., 1994), leukemia, and/or the use of immunosuppressive drugs. Other host-associated factors are diabetes (Telzak et al., 1991), partial gastrectomy, and the low gastric acidity (Mandal and Brennand, 1989; Penman, 1989) associated with these conditions. Prior use of antimicrobial agents to which the infecting salmonellae are resistant may aggravate the disease (Holmberg et al., 1984; Pavia et al., 1990).

A relationship between size of the infecting dose and severity of the resulting disease has been reported not only for *S.* Enteritidis, but also for infections due to *S.* Typhimurium, *S.* Infantis, *S.* Newport, and *S.* Thompson (Glynn and Bradley, 1992; Hedberg et al., 1993). In an outbreak of *S.* Enteritidis affecting 169 persons who ate hollandaise sauce made from grade-A shell eggs, it was noted that as the dose increased, the medium incubation period decreased and a greater proportion of the patients reported body aches, vomiting, weight loss, maximum daily number of stools, increased illness severity, and an increased number of days of confinement to bed (Mintz et al., 1994). Sometimes the infecting dose is large, as in a family outbreak when two sisters suffered gastroenteritis after consuming homemade ice cream containing approximately 10^5 *S.* Enteritidis PT4, probably due to contamination by an infected shell egg containing between 10^5 and 10^8 organisms (Morgan et al., 1994). Although the dose of *S.* Enteritidis in eggborne salmonellosis may often be small (Hennessy et al., 1996), infection still occurs because the high fat content of egg yolk (Mawer et al., 1989) allows the salmonellae to survive the acidic milieu in the stomach before passing into the intestines and penetrating the enterocytes of the intestinal mucosa. This is reminiscent of the small number of salmonellae required to infect people after consumption of other salmonella-containing high-fat foods such as cheese and chocolate (Craven et al., 1975; D'Aoust, 1985).

Salmonella Enteritidis PT4 infections may be life-threatening when contracted by infants younger than 3 months of age (Cross et al., 1989). Rates of reported salmonella isolations were highest for 1- to 4-month-old infants, decreased abruptly among early childhood age groups, showed a small increase in the 20–29 age group, gradually declined in the 30–65 age group, and increased thereafter (Hargrett-Bean et al., 1988). *Salmonella* Enteritidis bacteria were less invasive in humans than were *S. typhi, S. sendai, S. paratyphi* A, and *S.* Choleraesuis, but as invasive as *S.* Typhimurium (Wong et al., 1994). The latter finding agrees with the observation that increased blood-isolate percentages of *S.* Enteritidis, *S.* Typhimurium, and *S.* Dublin, but not of *S.* Heidelberg, were found among AIDS patients (Levine et al., 1991).

PREVENTION OF THE INFECTION IN HUMANS

Outbreaks of *S.* Enteritidis infections due to consumption of contaminated eggs, or foods containing such eggs, have led to several recommendations to eliminate or curtail salmonellosis in humans. Health-care facilities have been directed to eliminate raw or undercooked eggs from the diets of persons who are institutionalized, elderly, and/or immunocompromised. It has been recommended to pasteurize eggs for use in nursing homes, and other institutional settings, and commercial foods that may not be adequately cooked before eating (Telzak et al., 1990; Hedberg et al., 1993). Consumers have been advised to avoid eating raw or undercooked eggs, as well as foods that contain raw eggs, such as homemade Caesar salad, homemade eggnog, homemade mayonnaise, and homemade ice cream (Steinert et al., 1990; Buckner et al., 1994). Cooking the eggs at a sufficiently high temperature and for a sufficient period of time appears to prevent infections. During a study of sporadic cases of *S.* Enteritidis and *S.* Typhimurium infections in adults in Minnesota, it was observed that the extent to which eggs were cooked was inversely related with illness (Hedberg et al., 1993). Boiling the eggs for 7–8 min is sufficient to destroy *S.* Typhimurium (Schaaf, 1936; Baker et al., 1983; Humphrey et al., 1989b). Even though *S.* Enteritidis was shown to be somewhat more resistant to heat than some other common egg-associated salmonellae, it did not survive in liquid egg at the pasteurization temperature of 64°C for 1 min (Humphrey et al., 1990).

Consumers have been advised to refrigerate eggs. It has been found that several *S.* Enteritidis phage types, *S.* Typhimurium, and other salmonella serovars did not grow in the egg or egg yolk when stored below 10°C (Rizk et al., 1966; Kim et al., 1989; Humphrey, 1990; Saeed and Koons, 1993). Other recommendations are not to microwave dishes containing raw egg (Evans et al., 1995); to prevent cross-contamination from raw egg or raw-egg-containing food products; to wash hands, cooking utensils, and food-preparation surfaces with soap and water after contact with raw egg; not to sample food products containing raw egg, such as cookie batter; and to refrigerate foods containing egg promptly (Humphrey et al., 1994; CDC, 1996). Whenever an outbreak of human infection occurs, efforts should be made to trace it to the flock of laying hens (Telzak et al., 1990; Altekruse et al., 1993) and from there to the multiplier and primary breeder flocks so that control measures may be instituted (McIllroy et al., 1989).

ASSOCIATION OF HUMAN INFECTION WITH THE CONSUMPTION OF EGGS OR POULTRY MEAT

Many of the human S. Enteritidis infections have been traced to contaminated eggs and to the laying hens at the farm that supplied the eggs (Telzak et al., 1990; van de Giessen, 1992; CDC, 1992; Altekruse et al., 1993; Henzler et al., 1994). People may also become infected with S. Enteritidis as a result of infected broiler breeder flocks and broiler rearing flocks and contamination of broilers at slaughter (McIllroy et al., 1989; Roberts, 1991; Corkish et al., 1994; Plummer et al., 1995). Broilers may exhibit a pericarditis due to S. Enteritidis infection, and pure cultures of S. Enteritidis have been obtained from such infections (O'Brien, 1988; Rampling et al., 1989). However, this route of infection and subsequent contamination of poultry meat appears to be a lesser cause of S. Enteritidis infection in humans than contaminated eggs.

PREVALENCE IN POULTRY

The number of S. Enteritidis isolations from poultry has risen dramatically during the last 10–15 years and may have reached its peak in certain countries. In England and Wales, the percentage of S. Enteritidis isolates from poultry rose from 3.3% of all salmonella serovars in 1985 to 48.3% in 1989. The most frequently reported phage type was PT4, which accounted for 71% of the isolates in poultry in 1988. Concurrent with the increased isolation of S. Enteritidis in poultry, a dramatic increase in the number of cases of human infection with S. Enteritidis (mainly PT4) occurred (McIllroy and McCracken, 1990). A significant reduction in the number of incidents and isolations of S. Enteritidis in domestic fowl occurred during the years 1993 and 1994 in the United Kingdom. The decline was largely due to fewer isolations and incidents of S. Enteritidis PT4 (Anon., 1995). A survey to estimate the prevalence of S. Enteritidis in 1991 in U.S. commercial egg-production flocks showed that 24% of 23,431 pooled cecal samples collected from 406 layer houses contained salmonella of any serovar and that 3% of the samples contained S. Enteritidis. The estimated prevalence of S. Enteritidis–positive poultry houses (that is, at least one positive sample found in a house) for the northern, southeastern, and central/ western regions was 45%, 3%, and 17%, respectively.

Overall, the prevalence of salmonella-positive houses was 86% (Ebel et al., 1992).

The three most common salmonella serovars isolated from animals, foods of animal origin, and environmental sources in Canada during the 12-year period 1983–94 are shown in Figure 1.2. Other serovars occurred at a much lower frequency. The number of S. Enteritidis isolations accounted for 0.8% in 1984 to 8.6% in 1990 (average, 3.0%) of all the salmonella serovars, and S. Enteritidis was the eighth most common serovar during the 1983–92 period (Khakhria et al., 1997). In 1993 and 1994, the percentage of S. Enteritidis of all salmonella serovars from animals, foods, and environmental sources was 1.4% and 1.5%, respectively, and S. Enteritidis no longer ranked among the 10 most common salmonella serovars from these sources.

A Canada-wide survey to estimate the prevalence of S. Enteritidis and other salmonella serovars in 295 commercial layer flocks and their environment showed that environmental samples of 2.7% of the flocks were positive for S. Enteritidis. PT8 was isolated from five flocks, PT13a from two flocks, and PT13 from one flock (Poppe et al., 1991a). Follow-up culture of tissues from 580 hens from seven of the eight environmentally (feces, dust, and scrapings from the egg belts) positive flocks detected 26 S. Enteritidis–infected hens (4.5%) from two flocks. In one flock, two of 150 hens were infected with S. Enteritidis PT8, which was confined to the ceca, and no salmonella serovars were isolated from 2520 eggs (1 day's lay). In the second flock, where 24 of 150 hens were infected with S. Enteritidis PT13, extraintestinal infection was found in nine hens and involved the ovaries and/or oviduct in two. Salmonella Enteritidis PT13 was isolated from one sample of egg contents and from one sample of cracked shells from among 14,040 eggs (1 day's lay) from this flock (Poppe et al., 1992). A similar nationwide survey of 294 broiler flocks showed that 3% of environmental samples were contaminated with S. Enteritidis. PT8 was isolated from seven flocks, and PT13a was isolated from two flocks (Poppe et al., 1991b). No S. Enteritidis was isolated from any environmental samples taken from 274 turkey flocks in another Canada-wide study (Irwin et al., 1994). In Canada, S. Enteritidis is infrequently isolated from animal sources other than poultry. Only four of 81 S. Enteritidis strains that belonged to three of 42 independent submissions were derived from animal sources other than poultry and their environment, and consisted of three bovine strains and one strain from a lynx (Poppe, 1994).

CONTAMINATION OF EGGS

Contamination of the egg contents may occur by direct transmission from an infected ovary and/or oviduct, or by contamination of the eggshell with feces in a laying bird excreting salmonellae (Schaaf, 1936; Stokes et al., 1956; Williams et al., 1968; Borland, 1975; Timoney et al., 1989). For an oophoritis or an oviductitis to occur, the bird must have experienced a systemic infection. Contamination of

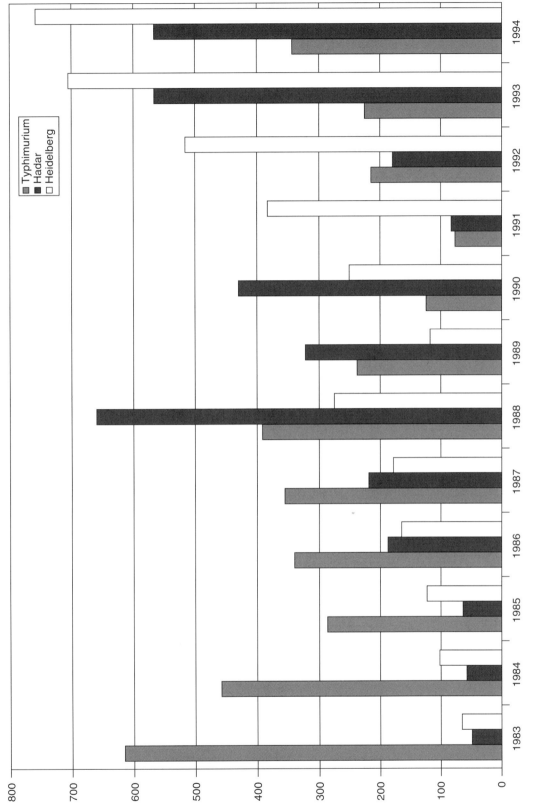

FIGURE 1.2 The three most commonly isolated salmonella serovars from animal, food, and environmental sources in Canada, 1983–94.

egg contents may also occur in a bird that had only an enteric infection. The salmonellae present in the feces may penetrate the eggshell pores as the egg cools (Stokes et al., 1956; Williams et al., 1968). After the shell has been formed, salmonella bacteria from contaminated feces may enter the egg (Forsythe et al., 1967) before the establishment on its surface of the proteinaceous cuticular barrier that is considered to be the primary method of preventing bacterial invasion of the egg contents (Board, 1966). Alternatively, fecal matter adherent to the shell may contaminate the egg contents when the eggs have cracks, or when the eggs are broken out for the preparation of food products (Borland, 1975). Contamination of the egg contents subsequent to ovarian infection has been called transovarian infection or transmission. Salmonella serovars that have been reported to infect the ovaries and cause a transovarian transmission include *S.* Pullorum and *S.* Gallinarum, the salmonella serovars host specific for poultry (Pomeroy, 1984; Snoeyenbos, 1984), *S.* Enteritidis, *S.* Typhimurium, *S.* Heidelberg, and a few other salmonella serovars (Schaaf, 1936; Gordon and Tucker, 1965; Snoeyenbos et al., 1969; Hopper and Mawer, 1988; Cooper et al., 1989; Timoney et al., 1989; Barnhart et al., 1991). During the last decade, many of the outbreaks of *S.* Enteritidis affecting humans involved grade-A table eggs. This would suggest that these outbreaks were not the result of dirty, soiled, or cracked eggs but due to internal contamination of eggs because of an oophoritis of the laying hens. Infection of the ovaries with *S.* Enteritidis has been reported on many occasions (Schaaf, 1936; Gordon and Tucker, 1965; Faddoul and Fellows, 1966; Snoeyenbos et al., 1969; Hopper and Mawer, 1988; Cooper et al., 1989; Timoney et al., 1989).

Salmonella Enteritidis, like *S.* Pullorum and *S.* Gallinarum, may have a predilection for colonizing the reproductive tract. Ovarian infection, congestion of ovules, misshapen ovules, and egg peritonitis were found in hens from a laying flock infected with *S.* Enteritidis PT4. The organism was isolated from the affected tissues (Hopper and Mawer, 1988). A diffuse yellow fibrinous peritonitis, internal laying of soft-shelled eggs, clots of inspissated yolk in the peritoneal cavity and/or the oviduct, and shrunken thick-walled congested follicles containing coagulated yolk were observed in hens of a layer flock infected with *S.* Enteritidis PT4 (Read et al., 1994).

Many organs may be colonized in a *S.* Enteritidis infection. Inoculation into the crop of adult hens with approximately 10^6 *S.* Enteritidis organisms caused a bacteremia with infection of many body sites, including the peritoneum, ovules, and oviduct in the majority of the hens (Timoney et al., 1989). The organisms were present in the yolk or albumen of eggs of about 10% of the hens shortly after infection and again 10 days later, which is evidence for egg or transovarian transmission of the infection. The finding that the albumen, but not yolk samples, of some of the eggs was positive suggests that some eggs became infected in the oviduct (Timoney et al., 1989). Albumen has markedly better antibacterial properties than yolk, which is an excellent growth medium for bacteria, including salmonellae (Board, 1966; Timoney et al., 1989).

Through chelation of iron, ovotransferrin in the albumen is the major growth inhibitor of gram-negative bacteria (Clay and Board, 1991). When adult laying hens were inoculated orally with 10^8 *S.* Enteritidis organisms, *S.* Enteritidis was detected 2 days later from the spleen, liver, heart, gallbladder, and intestinal tissues, and from various sections of the ovary and oviduct (Keller et al., 1995). Detection of organisms by immunohistochemical staining was rare for most tissues despite their culture-positive status, but they could be detected in oviduct tissues associated with forming eggs, indicating a heavier colonization in the egg during its development. Forming eggs taken from the oviduct were culture positive at a rate of about 30%, whereas freshly laid eggs in the same experiment were positive at a rate of less than 0.6%, suggesting that forming eggs are colonized in the reproductive tract, but that factors within the eggs significantly control the pathogen before the eggs are laid. When the cloacal tissues were heavily contaminated with *S.* Enteritidis the eggs were culture positive, whereas if these tissues had a low rate of infection the eggs were culture negative. Thus, prior to eggshell deposition, forming eggs are subject to descending infections from colonized ovarian tissue, lateral infection from colonized upper-oviduct tissues, and ascending infections from colonized vaginal and cloacal tissues (Keller et al., 1995).

The number of infected hens, the number of eggs containing *S.* Enteritidis laid by infected flocks, and the number of salmonella bacteria per egg may vary considerably, but are often low (Cooper et al., 1989; Humphrey et al., 1989a, 1991c; Perales and Audicana, 1989). In one study of two naturally infected small flocks of 35 hens, 10 of the hens produced eggs containing *S.* Enteritidis PT4 in a clustered, though intermittent, manner. Of 1119 eggs, 11 were positive for *S.* Enteritidis, and positive eggs contained fewer than 10 salmonella bacteria each (Humphrey et al., 1989a). In another study of over 5700 hens, eggs from 15 flocks naturally infected with *S.* Enteritidis, 32 (0.6%) of the eggs contained the bacteria in the contents. The levels of contamination were low (<100 bacteria); however, three of the eggs contained more than 100, 1.5×10^4, and 1.2×10^5 bacteria, respectively. Examination of both the shell and contents of 1952 eggs from naturally infected flocks resulted in the isolation of *S.* Enteritidis from the shell of 21 eggs (1.1%) and the contents of 18 eggs (0.9%) (Humphrey et al., 1991c). In a Canadian study, naturally infected hens were found in only two of 295 flocks of laying hens, and the overall prevalence of *S.* Enteritidis-contaminated eggs from the two flocks was less than 0.06% (Poppe et al., 1992).

The age of the hens at the time of infection with *S.* Enteritidis influenced intestinal colonization of the hens, egg production, and isolation rates of *S.* Enteritidis from eggshells and from the egg albumen. Hens of 62 weeks of age inoculated orally with 10^9 *S.* Enteritidis of a PT13a strain were more often intestinally colonized, produced fewer eggs, and produced a higher percentage of eggs with contamination of the eggshells and the egg albumen than hens of 37 and 27 weeks of age (Gast and Beard, 1990).

The clustered, though intermittent, production of contaminated eggs may be related to stress, such as food or water deprivation and molting. A short-term exposure to environmental stress resulted in a rapid increase in the shedding rate of *S.* Enteritidis for a brief time (Nakamura et al., 1994). Significantly more molted hens shed detectable intestinal *S.* Enteritidis than did unmolted hens, the intestinal pilocarpine-induced levels of *S.* Enteritidis were increased 100- to 1000-fold in molted hens compared with unmolted hens, and many of the molted hens exhibited bloody alimentary secretions (Holt and Porter, 1992). There appears to be a link between shedding high numbers of *S.* Enteritidis bacteria and contamination of eggs (Keller et al., 1995). Others observed a relationship between the oral dose and the period of shedding by the hens. The period during which specific pathogen-free hens, infected by direct introduction into the crop of either 10^3, 10^6, or 10^8 cells of *S.* Enteritidis PT4, excreted the organism in feces was closely related to the size of the inoculum, with the birds excreting for mean periods of 3, 16, and 37 days, respectively (Humphrey et al., 1991a).

SYMPTOMS OF THE DISEASE IN POULTRY

Symptoms of disease in poultry infected with *S.* Enteritidis PT4 are mostly seen in young chicks. In one report, they consisted of a mortality rate of 2% in broilers during the first 48 h of life, a cumulative mortality of 6% at 5 days of age, and a morbidity rate of 20% at the same age (McIllroy et al., 1989). Young chicks affected by salmonellosis caused by *S.* Enteritidis or *S.* Typhimurium may exhibit symptoms including anorexia, adipsia, depression, ruffled feathers, huddling together in groups, reluctance to move, drowsiness, somnolence, dehydration, white diarrhea, and stained or pasted vents (Marthedal, 1977; McIllroy et al., 1989). During the second week of life, the chicks may fail to grow and may have a stunted appearance (O'Brien, 1988). At postmortem examination, an unresorbed or poorly resorbed yolk sac, infection of the yolk sac and necrotic debris in the yolk sac, dehydration, emaciation, splenomegaly, hepatomegaly, necrotic foci and petechiae in the liver and spleen, pseudomembranous perihepatitis and peritonitis, enteritis, typhlitis with or without cecal cores, mild to severe mucopurulent or fibrinous pericarditis, and dilation of the pericardial sac by a thin bloodstained or a thick purulent fluid have been observed (Schaaf, 1936; Turnbull and Snoeyenbos, 1973; Marthedal, 1977; O'Brien, 1988; McIllroy et al., 1989; Rampling et al., 1989; Cooper et al., 1994; Gorham et al., 1994). Morbidity and mortality within the first 24 h of life and no identification of any possible common route for the lateral introduction of infection may suggest transmission by the vertical route. Parent flocks are often clinically normal despite the isolation of *S.* Enteritidis from cecal droppings, dust, and litter (McIllroy et al., 1989).

ROUTES OF INFECTION IN POULTRY

Flocks of laying hens may be infected with salmonellae by various routes. Flocks of laying hens are derived from multiplier breeding flocks that in turn are derived from breeding flocks composed of progeny of a primary breeding flock. Primary breeding flocks are composed of one or more generations that are maintained for the purpose of establishing, continuing, or improving parent lines. As a result of this breeding system to produce pullets for layer flocks, one pair of the primary breeding flock may have an offspring numbering hundreds of thousands of birds (McCoy, 1977; Hunter and Izsak, 1990). Thus, if one or a few of the hens in the primary flock were infected with *S.* Enteritidis and transmitted the infection by transovarian transmission, many of the offspring could be infected. Prevention and eradication of infection at the level of the (primary) breeding flocks would therefore be of utmost importance (McIllroy et al., 1989; O'Brien, 1989; Wierup et al., 1995). However, eggborne transmission is not the only source of infection, since environmental sources, separate from the primary breeder, are involved in the infection of chickens (Borland, 1975). Therefore, prevention and eradication at the primary breeder must be followed by control measures in breeding and multiplier flocks (Laszlo et al., 1985) and flocks of laying hens (Nakamura et al., 1994). Infection of many other chicks by one or a few infected hatching chicks in the hatcher, via equipment, vaccinations or other procedures applied in the hatchery, by personnel, during shipment, on arrival at the farm, or during the growing and rearing period should be avoided. A study on the lateral or horizontal transmission of *S.* Enteritidis and the effect of stress on shedding in laying hens showed that previously uninfected hens became rapidly infected through contaminated drinking water (Nakamura et al., 1994). Other sources of lateral transmission include mice (Henzler and Opitz, 1992; Davies and Wray, 1996) and other animal species, transmission through the feed (Hinton et al., 1989; McIllroy et al., 1989), transmission by airborne droplets or dust particles (Baskerville et al., 1992), transmission by exposure to human sewage via rodents (Kinde et al., 1996a,b), and transmission by contact with other fomites.

VIRULENCE OF *SALMONELLA* ENTERITIDIS FOR POULTRY

The invasive ability of *S.* Enteritidis is perhaps not phage type but strain related (Timoney et al., 1989; Poppe et al., 1993a; Gast and Benson, 1996). Major differences in invasive ability for adult hens were seen among *S.* Enteritidis PT8 strains (Timoney et al., 1989). One PT8 strain behaved like an invasive PT4 strain originally isolated from the pericardial fluid of a chicken, whereas other strains were shed in the feces but did not cause invasive infections

(Timoney et al., 1989). Similarly, inoculation of groups of 5-day-old leghorn chicks with a range of oral doses of three PT4 isolates and isolates from three other PTs showed that, whereas some significant differences were observed among *S.* Enteritidis PT4 strains in the frequencies at which they colonized the intestinal tracts and invaded to reach the spleens of the chicks, no consistent overall pattern differentiated PT4 isolates from isolates of other PTs (Gast and Benson, 1996). Others reported that colonies of *S.* Enteritidis PT13a with an unusual wrinkled morphology were the result of the production of lipopolysaccharide (LPS) with a high-molecular-weight O antigen and an elevated ratio of O antigen to core (O/C) ratio, and that bacteria producing such colonies were more virulent for intraperitoneally inoculated 5-day-old chicks in that they yielded higher numbers per gram of spleen 3 days after inoculation and caused a higher percentage of contaminated eggs after intravenous inoculation of laying hens than did nonwrinkled colonies with a lower O/C ratio (Petter, 1993; Guard-Petter et al., 1995). An *S.* Enteritidis PT4 strain producing colonies with a wrinkled appearance (Cox, 1996) was more invasive for the reproductive and other tissues of laying hens, and more tolerant to heat, acid, and hydrogen peroxide than were nonwrinkled colonies (Humphrey et al., 1996).

However, others claim that virulence is phage type related and reported that strains of *S.* Enteritidis PT4 were more invasive for young chicks than were strains of PT7, 8, and 13a, and suggested that the increased invasiveness of PT4 may be one of the factors that contributed to the establishment of *S.* Enteritidis PT4 in the United Kingdom (Hinton et al., 1990a). The same authors also found that more recent isolates of *S.* Enteritidis PT4 were more invasive than strains isolated in previous years and suggested that recent isolates of PT4 may have enhanced virulence for chickens, which was shown for one pair of strains to be independent of the possession of the 38-MDa virulence-associated plasmid (Hinton et al., 1990b). Cox and Woolcock (1994) examined the LPS of 54 Australian isolates of *S.* Enteritidis PT4, 14, and 26 and found that they all expressed long-chain LPS, but that only the PT4 strains produced a lethal infection in Balb/c mice.

Salmonella Enteritidis PT4 has the propensity to infect a large number of poultry flocks, and human infections with PT4 are the most numerous and widespread (McIllroy and McCracken, 1990; Rodrigue et al., 1990). A possible reason for the widespread occurrence of PT4 in poultry would perhaps be the presence of a higher percentage of more invasive and virulent strains among the PT4 strains than among strains of other phage types of *S.* Enteritidis. Another explanation could be the establishment of *S.* Enteritidis PT4 in primary layer breeder flocks as happened in broiler breeder flocks in Northern Ireland (McIllroy et al., 1989). Infection of primary breeder flocks may result in spread to many countries by shipment of day-old chicks or hatching eggs (Wierup et al., 1995). Introduction to poultry via human sewage has occurred also (Kinde et al., 1996b). In Canada, human infections with *S.* Enteritidis PT4 occurred increasingly before it was isolated from poultry or

other animal sources. International travel undoubtedly played a significant role in the acquisition of these infections (Tauxe et al., 1987).

PLASMID PROFILES

Characterization of *S.* Enteritidis by determination of the plasmid profiles has shown that plasmid-profile typing is not as sensitive as phage typing for the primary subdivision of *S.* Enteritidis. Examination of 534 British isolates of 27 phage types identified 11 plasmid-profile patterns. Nine profile patterns were found among PT4 strains. Of 247 PT4 strains, however, 193 (78%) possessed a single 38-MDa plasmid. Plasmid-profile typing was considered an effective adjunct to phage typing for the subdivision of *S.* Enteritidis (Threlfall et al., 1989, 1994; Rodrigue et al., 1992; Poppe et al., 1993b). However, phage typing and plasmid profile may be decreasingly sufficient to discriminate between cultures of a predominant strain isolated from many samples in one geographical area (Morris et al., 1992).

A study of 318 *S.* Enteritidis strains isolated mainly from poultry and their environment in Canada showed that the strains belonged to 15 different plasmid profiles and 12 phage types. However, a 36-MDa plasmid was found in 97% of the strains, and in 88% of the strains this was the only plasmid present. Phage typing was more discriminatory than determination of plasmid profiles, biotyping, hybridization with a probe for the salmonella plasmid virulence (*spv*) genes, size of outer membrane proteins, length of LPS, and resistance to antimicrobial agents. Phage types 8, 13, and 13a rated first, second, and third in percentage of unrelated submissions (56%, 25%, and 4%, respectively) (Poppe et al., 1993b). Only the 36-MDa plasmid hybridized with the probe for the Spv genes (Gulig and Curtiss, 1988; Poppe et al., 1989, 1993b). Strains of PT13 often possessed a small plasmid of 2.6–5.0 MDa in addition to the 36-MDa plasmid (Singer et al., 1992; Poppe et al., 1993b). More diverse patterns of plasmid profiles have been seen in strains isolated from poultry than among those isolated from humans (Altekruse et al., 1993; Threlfall et al., 1994).

RESISTANCE TO ANTIMICROBIAL AGENTS

Most strains of *S.* Enteritidis are drug sensitive (Frost et al., 1989; Threlfall et al., 1989; Pohl et al., 1991; Singer et al., 1992; Poppe et al., 1993b). Not all phage types of *S.* Enteritidis are equally sensitive to antimicrobial agents. It was shown that *S.* Enteritidis PT4 strains that acquired plasmids belonging to the IncN incompatibility group encoding resistance to a range of antimicrobials, among which resistance to ampicillin, streptomycin, and tetracycline (AST) was most common, had converted to PT24. However, the PT24 strains were only a small percentage of the total number of *S.* Enteritidis strains (Frost et al., 1989). A study of 318 *S.* Enteritidis strains isolated from poultry in Canada showed that 54 strains (17%) were resistant to one or more of the 15 antimicrobial agents employed in the drug-testing panel. Resistance to sulfisoxazole was most common (23 strains), followed by resistance to nitrofurantoin (15 strains). Ten of the strains showed resistance to one or more antibiotics, primarily to ampicillin and carbenicillin, both derivatives of 6-aminopenicillanic acid. All of the strains were sensitive to ciprofloxacin, cotrimoxazole, and kanamycin at all levels employed (Poppe et al., 1993b).

REFERENCES

Altekruse, S., Koehler, J., Hickman-Brenner, R., Tauxe, R.V., and Ferris, K. 1993. A comparison of *Salmonella enteritidis* phage types from egg-associated outbreaks and implicated laying flocks. Epidemiol. Infect. 110:17–22.

Anonymous. 1988. *Salmonella enteritidis* phage type 4: chicken and egg. Lancet 2:720–722.

Anonymous. 1992. Hospital outbreak of *S. enteritidis* infection: Ontario. Can. Commun. Dis. Rep. 18:57–60.

Anonymous. 1995. *Salmonella* in animal and poultry production. Glasgow: Ministry of Agriculture, Fisheries and Food; Welsh Office, Agriculture Department; Scottish Office, Agriculture and Fisheries Department, pp. 7–35.

Aserkoff, B., and Bennett, J.V. 1969. Effect of antibiotic therapy in acute salmonellosis on the fecal excretion of salmonellae. N. Engl. J. Med. 281:636–640.

Atkinson, N. 1964. Salmonellosis in Australia. In: van Oye, E., ed. The world problem of salmonellosis. The Hague: Dr. W. Junk, pp. 539–589.

Baird-Parker, A.C. 1990. Foodborne salmonellosis. Lancet 336:1231–1235.

Baker, R.C., Hogarty, S., Poon, W., and Vadehra, D.V. 1983. Survival of *Salmonella typhimurium* and *Staphylococcus aureus* in eggs cooked by different methods. Poult. Sci. 62:1211–1216.

Barnhart, H.M., Dreesen, D.W., Bastien, R., and Pancorbo, O.C. 1991. Prevalence of *Salmonella enteritidis* and other serovars in ovaries of layer hens at time of slaughter. J. Food Prot. 54:488–491.

Baskerville, A., Humphrey, T.J., Fitzgeorge, R.B., Cook, R.W., Chart, H., Rowe, B., and Whitehead, A. 1992. Airborne infection of laying hens with *Salmonella enteritidis* phage type 4. Vet. Rec. 130:395–398.

Bean, N.H., and Griffin, P.M. 1990. Foodborne disease outbreaks in the United States, 1973–1987: pathogens, vehicles, and trends. J. Food Prot. 53:804–817.

Bean, N.H., and Potter, M.E. 1994. *Salmonella* serotypes from human sources, January 1992 through December 1992. In: Proceedings of the 98th annual meeting of the United States Animal Health Association. Richmond, VA: Promiter Communications and Spectrum, pp. 439–442.

Bezanson, G.S., Khakhria, R., Duck, D., and Lior, H. 1985. Molecular analysis confirms food source and simultaneous involvement of two distinct but related subgroups of *Salmonella typhimurium* bacteriophage type 10 in major interprovincial *Salmonella* outbreak. Appl. Environ. Microbiol. 50:1279–1284.

Binkin, N., Scuderi, G., Novaco, F., Giovanardi, G.L., Paganelli, G., Ferrari, G., Cappelli, O., Ravaglia, L., Zilioli, F., Amadei, V., Magliani, W., Viani, E., Ricco, D., Borrini, B., Magri, M., Alessandrini, A., Bursi, G., Barigazzi, G., Fantasia, M., Filetici, E., and Salmaso, S. 1993. Egg-related *Salmonella enteritidis*, Italy, 1991. Epidemiol. Infect. 110:227–237.

Board, R.G. 1966. The course of microbial infection of the hen's eggs. J. Appl. Bacteriol. 29:319–341.

Borland, E.D. 1975. *Salmonella* infection in poultry. Vet. Rec. 97:406–408.

Brede, H.D. 1964. Les salmonelloses au sud de l'Afrique. In: van Oye, E., ed. The world problem of salmonellosis. The Hague: Dr. W. Junk, pp. 379–393.

Bryan, F.L. 1981. Current trends in foodborne salmonellosis in the United States and Canada. J. Food Prot. 44:394–402.

Buckner, P., Ferguson, D., Anzalone, F., Anzalone, D., Taylor, J., Hlady, W.G., and Hopkins, R.S. 1994. Outbreak of *Salmonella enteritidis* associated with homemade ice cream: Florida, 1993. MMWR 43:669–671.

Bullis, K.L. 1977a. The history of avian medicine in the US. II. Pullorum disease and fowl typhoid. Avian Dis. 21:422–429.

Bullis, K.L. 1977b. The history of avian medicine in the US. III. Salmonellosis. Avian Dis. 21:430–435.

Butler, R.W., and Josephson, J.E. 1962. Egg-containing cake-mixes as a source of *Salmonella*. Can. J. Public Health 53:478–482.

Buxton, A. 1957. Salmonellosis in animals: a review. Review Series 5. Farnham Royal, Bucks, England: Commonwealth Agricultural Bureaux, 209 pp.

Bynoe, E.T., and Yurack, J.A. 1964. Salmonellosis in Canada. In: van Oye, E., ed. The world problem of salmonellosis. The Hague: Dr. W. Junk, pp. 397–420.

Centers for Disease Control. 1992. Outbreak of *Salmonella enteritidis* infection associated with consumption of raw shell eggs, 1991. MMWR 41:369–372.

Centers for Disease Control. 1996. Outbreaks of *Salmonella* serotype Enteritidis infection associated with consumption of raw shell egg: United States, 1994–1995. MMWR 45:737–742.

Chase, F.E. 1947. *Salmonella* studies in fowl. Can. J. Public Health 38:82–83.

Clarke, R.C., and Gyles, C.L. 1993. *Salmonella*. In: Gyles, C.L., and Thoens, C.O., eds. Pathogenesis of bacterial infections in animals. Ames: Iowa State University Press, pp. 133–153.

Clay, C.E., and Board, R.G. 1991. Growth of *Salmonella enteritidis* in artificially contaminated hens' shell eggs. Epidemiol. Infect. 106:271–281.

Cooper, G.L., Nicholas, R.A., and Bracewell, C.D. 1989. Serological and bacteriological investigations of chickens from flocks naturally infected with *Salmonella enteritidis*. Vet. Rec. 125:567–572.

Cooper, G.L., Venables, L.M., Woodward, M.J., and Hormaeche, C.E. 1994. Invasiveness and persistence of *Salmonella enteritidis*, *Salmonella typhimurium* and a genetically defined *S. enteritidis aroA* strain in young chickens. Infect. Immun. 62:4739–4746.

Corkish, J.D., Davies, R.H., Wray, C., and Nicholas, R.A.J. 1994. Observations on a broiler breeder flock naturally infected with *Salmonella enteritidis* phage type 4. Vet. Rec. 134:591–594.

Cowden, J.D., Chisholm, D., O'Mahony, M., Lynch, D., Mawer, S.L., Spain, G.E., Ward, L., and Rowe, B. 1989. Two outbreaks of *Salmonella enteritidis* phage type 4 infection associated with the consumption of fresh shell-egg products. Epidemiol. Infect. 103:47–52.

Cox, J.M. 1996. What makes *Salmonella enteritidis* stick in chickens? World Poult. Misset May:22–23.

Cox, J.M., and Woolcock, J.B. 1994. Lipopolysaccharide expression and virulence in mice of Australian isolates of *Salmonella enteritidis*. Lett. Appl. Microbiol. 19:95–98.

Coyle, E.F., Palmer, S.R., Ribeiro, C.D., Jones, H.I., Howard, A.J., Ward, L., and Rowe, B. 1988. *Salmonella enteritidis* phage type 4 infection: association with hens' eggs. Lancet 2:1295–1297.

Craven, P.C., Mackel, D.C., Baine, W.B., Barker, W.H., and Gangarosa, E.J. 1975. International outbreak of *Salmonella eastbourne* infection traced to contaminated chocolate. Lancet 1:788–792.

Cross, J.H., George, R.H., Booth, I.W., and Mayne, A.J. 1989. Life-threatening *Salmonella enteritidis* phage type 4 gastroenteritis in infancy. Lancet 1:625–626.

D'Aoust, J.-Y. 1985. Infective dose of *Salmonella typhimurium* in cheddar cheese. Am. J. Epidemiol. 122:717–720.

Davies, R.H., and Wray, C. 1996. Studies of contamination of three broiler breeder houses with *Salmonella enteritidis* before and after cleansing and disinfection. Avian Dis. 40:626–633.

Dixon, J.M.S. 1965. Effect of antibiotic treatment on duration of excretion of *Salmonella typhimurium* by children. BMJ 2:1343–1345.

Ebel, E.D., David, M.J., and Mason, J. 1992. Occurrence of *Salmonella enteritidis* in the US commercial egg industry: report on a national spent hen survey. Avian Dis. 36:646–654.

Edel, W., van Schothorst, M., and Kampelmacher, E.H. 1977. Salmonella and salmonellosis: the present situation. In: Barnum, D.A., ed. Proceedings of the international symposium on salmonella and prospects for control. Guelph, Canada: University of Guelph, pp. 1–26.

Edwards, P.R. 1956. Salmonella and salmonellosis. Ann. N.Y. Acad. Sci. 66:44–53.

Edwards, P.R. 1958. Salmonellosis: observations on incidence and control. Ann. N.Y. Acad. Sci. 70:598–613.

Edwards, P.R., Bruner, D.W., and Moran, A.B. 1948a. The genus *Salmonella*: its occurrence and distribution in the United States. Ky. Agric. Exp. Stn. Bull. 525.

Edwards, P.R., Bruner, D.W., and Moran, A.B. 1948b. Further studies on the occurrence and distribution of salmonella types in the United States. J. Infect. Dis. 83:220–231.

Evans, M.R., Parry, S.M., and Ribeiro, C.D. 1995. Salmonella outbreak from microwave cooked food. Epidemiol. Infect. 115:227–230.

Faddoul, G.P., and Fellows, G.W. 1966. A five-year survey of the incidence of salmonellae in avian species. Avian Dis. 10:296–304.

Ferris, K.E., and Miller, D.A. 1990. *Salmonella* serotypes from animals and related sources reported during July 1988–June 1989. In: Proceedings of the 93rd annual meeting of the United States Animal Health Association. Richmond, VA: Carter, pp. 521–538.

Fey, H. 1964. Die Salmonellosen der Haustiere und ihre Epidemiologische Bedeutung. In: van Oye, E., ed. The world problem of salmonellosis. The Hague: Dr. W. Junk, pp. 171–204.

Forsythe, R.H., Ross, W.J., and Ayres, J.C. 1967. *Salmonella* recovery following gastro-intestinal and ovarian inoculation in the domestic fowl. Poult. Sci. 46:849–855.

Fox, M.D. 1974. Recent trends in salmonellosis epidemiology. J. Am. Vet. Med. Assoc. 165:990–993.

Frost, J.A., Ward, L.R., and Rowe, B. 1989. Acquisition of a drug resistance plasmid converts *Salmonella enteritidis* phage type 4 to phage type 24. Epidemiol. Infect. 103:243–248.

Fukumi, H. 1964. Salmonelloses in Japan. In: van Oye, E., ed. The world problem of salmonellosis. The Hague: Dr. W. Junk, pp. 507–529.

Galton, M.M., Steele, J.H., and Newell, K.W. 1964. Epidemiology of salmonellosis in the United States. In: van Oye, E., ed. The world problem of salmonellosis. The Hague: Dr. W. Junk, pp. 421–444.

Gast, R.K., and Beard, C.W. 1990. Production of *Salmonella enteritidis*-contaminated eggs by experimentally infected hens. Avian Dis. 34:438–446.

Gast, R.K., and Benson, S.T. 1996. Intestinal colonization and organ invasion in chicks experimentally infected with *Salmonella enteritidis* phage type 4 and other phage types isolated from poultry in the United States. Avian Dis. 40:853–857.

Glässer. 1937. Beobachtungen bei einer Fleischvergiftung, bedingt durch den Paratyphusbazillus B (Schottmüller). DTW (Dtsch Tieraerztl Wochenschr) 45:7–9.

Glynn, J.R., and Bradley, D.J. 1992. The relationship between infecting dose and severity of disease in reported outbreaks of salmonella infections. Epidemiol. Infect. 109:371–388.

Gordon, R.F., and Tucker, J.F. 1965. The epizootiology of *Salmonella menston* infection of fowls and the effect of feeding poultry food artificially infected with *Salmonella*. Br. Poult. Sci. 6:251–264.

Gorham, S.L., Kadavil, K., Vaughan, E., Lambert, H., Abel, J., and Pert, B. 1994. Gross and microscopic lesions in young chickens experimentally infected with *Salmonella enteritidis*. Avian Dis. 38:816–821.

Guard-Petter, J., Lakshmi, B., Carlson, R., and Ingram, K. 1995. Characterization of lipopolysaccharide heterogeneity in *Salmonella enteritidis* by an improved gel electrophoresis method. Appl. Environ. Microbiol. 61:2845–2851.

Gulig, P.A., and Curtiss III, R. 1988. Cloning and transposon insertion mutagenesis of virulence genes of the 100-kilobase plasmid of *Salmonella typhimurium*. Infect. Immun. 56:3262–3271.

Guthrie, R.K. 1992. Salmonella. Boca Raton, FL: CRC, pp. 1–20.

Hargrett-Bean, N.T., Pavia, A.T., and Tauxe, R.V. 1988. *Salmonella* isolates from humans in the United States, 1984–1986. MMWR 37:25–31.

Hargrett-Bean, N.T., and Potter, M.E. 1995. *Salmonella* serotypes from human sources, January 1992 through December 1992. In: Proceedings of the 98th annual meeting of the United States Animal Health Association, Grand Rapids, Michigan, Oct. 29–Nov. 4, 1994. Richmond, VA: Promiter Communications and Spectrum, pp. 439–442.

Hedberg, C.W., David, M.J., White, K.E., MacDonald, K.L., and Osterholm, M.T. 1993. Role of egg consumption in sporadic *Salmonella enteritidis* and *Salmonella typhimurium* infections in Minnesota. J. Infect. Dis. 167:107–111.

Hennessy, T.W., Hedberg, C.W., Slutsker, L., White, K.E., Besser-Wiek, J.M., Moen, M.E., Feldman, J., Coleman, W.W., Edmonson, L.M., MacDonald, K.L., Osterholm, M.T., and the investigation team. 1996. A national outbreak of *Salmonella enteritidis* infections from ice cream. N. Engl. J. Med. 334:1281–1286.

Henzler, D.J., Ebel, E., Sanders, J., Kradel, D., and Mason, J. 1994. *Salmonella enteritidis* in eggs from commercial chicken layer flocks implicated in human outbreaks. Avian Dis. 38:37–43.

Henzler, D.J., and Opitz, H.M. 1992. The role of mice in the epizootiology of *Salmonella enteritidis* infection on chicken layer farms. Avian Dis. 36:625–631.

Hewitt, E.A. 1928. Bacillary white diarrhea in baby turkeys. Cornell Vet. 18:272–276.

Hinshaw, W.R., and McNeil, E. 1940. Eradication of pullorum disease from turkey flocks. In: Proceedings of the 44th annual meeting of the US Livestock Sanitary Association, Dec. 4–6, 1940, Chicago, Illinois, pp. 178–194.

Hinton, M., Pearson, G.R., Threlfall, E.J., Rowe, B., Woodward, M., and Wray, C. 1989. Experimental *Salmonella enteritidis* infection in chicks. Vet. Rec. 124:223.

Hinton, M., Threlfall, E.J., and Rowe, B. 1990a. The invasive potential of *Salmonella enteritidis* phage types for young chickens. Lett. Appl. Microbiol. 10:237–239.

Hinton, M., Threlfall, E.J., and Rowe, B. 1990b. The invasiveness of different strains of *Salmonella enteritidis* phage type 4 for young chickens. FEMS Microbiol. Lett. 70:193–196.

Holmberg, S.D., Wells, J.G., and Cohen, M.L. 1984. Animal-to-man transmission of antimicrobial-resistant *Salmonella*: investigations of US outbreaks, 1971–1983. Science 226:833–836.

Holt, P.S., and Porter, R.E. 1992. Microbiological and histopathological effects of an induced-molt fasting procedure on a *Salmonella enteritidis* infection in chickens. Avian Dis. 36:610–618.

Hopper, S.A., and Mawer, S. 1988. *Salmonella enteritidis* in a commercial layer flock. Vet. Rec. 123:351.

Humphrey, T.J. 1990. Growth of salmonellas in intact shell eggs: influence of storage temperature. Vet. Rec. 126:292.

Humphrey, T.J., Mead, G.C., and Rowe, B. 1988. Poultry meat as a source of human salmonellosis in England and Wales. Epidemiol. Infect. 100:175–184.

Humphrey, T.J., Baskerville, A., Mawer, S., Rowe, B., and Hopper, S. 1989a. *Salmonella enteritidis* phage type 4 from the contents of intact eggs: a study involving naturally infected hens. Epidemiol. Infect. 103:415–423.

Humphrey, T.J., Greenwood, M., Gilbert, R.J., Rowe, B., and Chapman, P.A. 1989b. The survival of salmonellas in shell eggs cooked under simulated domestic conditions. Epidemiol. Infect. 103:35–45.

Humphrey, T.J., Chapman, P.A., Rowe, B., and Gilbert, R.J. 1990. A comparative study of the heat resistance of salmonellas in homogenized whole egg, egg yolk or albumen. Epidemiol. Infect. 104:237–241.

Humphrey, T.J., Baskerville, A., Chart, H., Rowe, B., and Whitehead, A. 1991a. *Salmonella enteritidis* PT4 infection in specific pathogen free hens: influence of infecting dose. Vet. Rec. 129:482–485.

Humphrey, T.J., Chart, H., Baskerville, A., and Rowe, B. 1991b. The influence of age on the response of SPF hens to infection with *Salmonella enteritidis* PT4. Epidemiol. Infect. 106:33–43.

Humphrey, T.J., Whitehead, A., Gawler, A.H.L., Henley, A., and Rowe, B. 1991c. Numbers of *Salmonella enteritidis* in the contents of naturally contaminated hens' eggs. Epidemiol. Infect. 106:489–498.

Humphrey, T.J., Martin, K.W., and Whitehead, A. 1994. Contamination of hands and work surfaces with *Salmonella enteritidis* PT4 during the preparation of egg dishes. Epidemiol. Infect. 113:403–409.

Humphrey, T.J., Williams, A., McAlpine, K., Lever, M.S., Guard-Petter, J., and Cox, J.M. 1996. Isolates of *Salmonella enterica* Enteritidis PT4 with enhanced heat and acid tolerance are more virulent in mice and more invasive in chickens. Epidemiol. Infect. 117:79–88.

Hunter, P.R., and Izsak, J. 1990. Diversity studies of salmonella incidents in some domestic livestock and their potential relevance as indicators of niche width. Epidemiol. Infect. 105:501–510.

Irwin, R.J., Poppe, C., Messier, S., Finley, G.G., and Oggel, J. 1994. A national survey to estimate the prevalence of *Salmonella* species among Canadian registered commercial turkey flocks. Can. J. Vet. Res. 58:263–267.

Johnston, W.S., Munro, D., Reilly, W.J., and Sharp, J.C.M. 1981. An unusual sequel to imported *Salmonella zanzibar.* J. Hyg. Camb. 87:525–528.

Keller, L.H., Benson, C.E., Krotec, K., and Eckroade, R.J. 1995. *Salmonella enteritidis* colonization of the reproductive tract and forming and freshly laid eggs of chickens. Infect. Immun. 63:2443–2449.

Kelterborn, E. 1967. *Salmonella* species: first isolations, names, and occurrence. The Hague: Dr. W. Junk, pp. 20, 140–141, 377–379.

Khakhria, R., Duck, D., and Lior, H. 1991. Distribution of *Salmonella enteritidis* phage types in Canada. Epidemiol. Infect. 106:25–32.

Khakhria, R., Johnson, W., and Lior, H. 1994. Canada's most common *Salmonella* serotypes and *Salmonella enteritidis* phage types (1992–1993). Safety Watch 33:4.

Khakhria, R., Woodward, D., and Johnson, W. 1995. Salmonellae, shigellae, pathogenic *E. coli,* campylobacters and *Aeromonas*: annual summary 1994. Guelph, Canada: Health Canada.

Khakhria, R., Woodward, D., Johnson, W.M., and Poppe, C. 1997. Salmonella isolated from humans, animals and other sources in Canada, 1983–92. Epidemiol. Infect. 119:15–23.

Kim, C.J., Emery, D.A., Rinke, H., Nagaraja, K.V., and Halvorson, D.A. 1989. Effect of time and temperature on growth of *Salmonella enteritidis* in experimentally inoculated eggs. Avian Dis. 33:735–742.

Kinde, H., Read, D.H., Ardans, A., Breitmeyer, R.E., Willoughby, D., Little, H.E., Kerr, D., Gireesh, R., and Nagaraja, K.V. 1996a. Sewage effluent: likely source of *Salmonella enteritidis,* phage type 4 infection in a commercial chicken layer flock in Southern California. Avian Dis. 40:672–676.

Kinde, H., Read, D.H., Chin, R.P., Bickford, A.A., Walker, R.L., Ardans, A., Breitmeyer, R.E., Willoughby, D., Little, H.E., Kerr, D., and Gardner, I.A. 1996b. *Salmonella enteritidis,* phage type 4 infection in a commercial layer flock in Southern California: bacteriologic and epidemiologic findings. Avian Dis. 40:665–671.

Klein, E. 1889. Ueber eine epidemische Krankheit der Hühner, verursacht durch einen Bacillus: Bacillus Gallinarum. Zentralbl. Bakteriol. Parasitenkd. 5:689–693.

Kühn, H., Rabsch, W., Gericke, B., and Reissbrodt, R. 1993. Infektionsepidemiologische Analysen von Salmonellosen, Shigellosen und anderen Enterobacteriaceae-Infektionen. Bundesgesundheitsblatt 36:324–333.

Lachowicz, K. 1964. *Salmonella* infections in East Europe. In: van Oye, E., ed. The world problem of salmonellosis. The Hague: Dr. W. Junk, pp. 295–334.

Laszlo, V.G., Csorian, E.S., and Paszti, J. 1985. Phage types and epidemiological significance of *Salmonella enteritidis* strains in Hungary between 1976 and 1983. Acta Microbiol. Hung. 32:321–340.

Le Minor, L. 1964. Les salmonelloses en Indochine et en Chine. In: van Oye, E., ed. The world problem of salmonellosis. The Hague: Dr. W. Junk, pp. 530–538.

Le Minor, L., and Popoff, M.Y. 1987. Designation of *Salmonella* enterica sp. nov., nom. rev., as the type and only species of the genus *Salmonella.* Int. J. Syst. Bacteriol. 37:465–468.

Le Minor, L., and Popoff, M.Y. 1992. Antigenic formulas of the *Salmonella* serovars, 6th ed. Paris: World Health Organisation Collaborating Centre for Reference and Research on Salmonella, pp. 1–145.

Levine, W.C., Buehler, J.W., Bean, N.H., and Tauxe, R.V. 1991. Epidemiology of nontyphoidal *Salmonella* bacteraemia during the human immunodeficiency virus epidemic. J. Infect. Dis. 164:81–87.

Lin, F.-Y.C., Morris, J.G., Trump, D., Tilghman, D., Wood, P.K., Jackman, N., Israel, E., and Libonati, J.P. 1988. Investigation of an outbreak of *Salmonella enteritidis* gastroenteritis associated with consumption of eggs in a restaurant chain in Maryland. Am. J. Epidemiol. 128:839–844.

Lior, H. 1989. Isolations of enteric pathogens from people in Canada. Safety Watch 14:3.

Maguire, H.C.F., Codd, A.A., Mackay, V.E., Rowe, B., and Mitchell, E. 1993. A large outbreak of human salmonellosis traced to a local pig farm. Epidemiol. Infect. 110:239–246.

Mandal, B.K. 1979. Typhoid and paratyphoid fever. Clin. Gastroenterol. 8:715–735.

Mandal, B.K., and Brennand, J. 1988. Bacteraemia in salmonellosis: a 15-year retrospective study from a regional infectious diseases unit. BMJ 297:1242–1243.

Marthedal, H.E. 1977. The occurrence of salmonellosis in poultry in Denmark 1935–75, and the controlling programme established. In: Barnum, D.A., ed. Proceedings of the international symposium on salmonella and prospects for control. Guelph, Canada: University of Guelph, pp. 78–94.

Mawer, S.L., Spain, G.E., and Rowe, B. 1989. *Salmonella enteritidis* phage type 4 and hens' eggs. Lancet 1:280–281.

McCoy, J.H. 1975. Trends in salmonella food poisoning in England and Wales 1941–72. J. Hyg. Camb. 74:271–282.

McCoy, J.H. 1977. Human salmonellosis: the poultry reservoir. In: Barnum, D.A., ed. Proceedings of the international symposium on salmonella and prospects for control. Guelph, Canada: University of Guelph, pp. 27–40.

McDermott, L.A. 1947. The K formula stained antigen in the detection of standard and Younie types of *Salmonella pullorum* infection. Can. J. Public Health 38:83–84.

McIllroy, S.G., and McCracken, R.M. 1990. The current status of the *Salmonella enteritidis* control programme in the United Kingdom. In: Proceedings of the 94th annual meeting of the United States Animal Health Association. Richmond, VA: Carter, pp. 450–462.

McIllroy, S.G., McCracken, R.M., Neill, S.D., and O'Brien, J.J. 1989. Control, prevention and eradication of *Salmonella enteritidis* infection in broiler and broiler breeder flocks. Vet. Rec. 125:545–548.

Mintz, E.D., Carter, M.L., Hadler, J.L., Wassell, J.T., Zingeser, J.A., and Tauxe, R.V. 1994. Dose-response effect in an outbreak of *Salmonella enteritidis.* Epidemiol. Infect. 112:13–23.

Moore, E.N. 1946. The occurrence of fowl typhoid. Circular 19. Newark: University of Delaware, pp. 1–20.

Morgan, D., Mawer, S.L., and Harman, P.L. 1994. The role of home-made ice cream as a vehicle of *Salmonella enteritidis* phage type 4 infection from fresh shell eggs. Epidemiol. Infect. 113:21–29.

Morris, J.G., Dwyer, D.M., Hoge, C.W., Stubbs, A.D., Tilghman, D., Groves, C., Israel, E., and Libonati, J.P. 1992. Changing clonal patterns of *Salmonella enteritidis* in Maryland: evaluation of strains isolated between 1985 and 1990. J. Clin. Microbiol. 30:1301–1303.

Nakamura, M., Nagamine, N., Takahashi, T., Suzuki, S., Kijima, M., Tamura, Y., and Sato, S. 1994. Horizontal transmission of *Salmonella enteritidis* and effect of stress on shedding in laying hens. Avian Dis. 38:282–288.

Nicolle, P. 1964. La lysotypie de *Salmonella typhi:* son principe, sa technique, son application l'épidémiologie de la fi vre typho de. In: van Oye, E., ed. The world problem of salmonellosis. The Hague: Dr. W. Junk, pp. 67–88.

O'Brien, J.D.P. 1988. *Salmonella enteritidis* infection in broiler chickens. Vet. Rec. 122:214.

O'Brien, J.D.P. 1989. Control of *Salmonella enteritidis* in poultry. Vet. Rec. 125:333–334.

Oosterom, J. 1991. Epidemiological studies and proposed preventive measures in the fight against human salmonellosis. Int. J. Food Microbiol. 12:41–52.

Parham, G.L. 1985. Salmonellae in cooked beef products. In: Snoeyenbos, G.H., ed. Proceedings of the international symposium on *Salmonella,* New Orleans, Louisiana, USA, July 19–20, 1984. Kennett Square, PA: American Association of Avian Pathologists, pp. 275–280.

Paul, J., and Batchelor, B. 1988. *Salmonella enteritidis* phage type 4 and hens' eggs. Lancet 2:1421.

Pavia, A.T., Shipman, L.D., Wells, J.G., Puhr, N.D., Smith, J.D., McKinley, T.W., and Tauxe, R.V. 1990. Epidemiologic evidence that prior antimicrobial exposure decreases resistance to infection by antimicrobial-sensitive *Salmonella.* J. Infect. Dis. 161:255–260.

Payne, D.J.H., and Scudamore, J.M. 1977. Outbreaks of *Salmonella* food-poisoning over a period of eight years from a common source. Lancet 1:1249–1251.

Peluffo, C.A. 1964. Salmonellosis in South America. In: van Oye, E., ed. The world problem of salmonellosis. The Hague: Dr. W. Junk, pp. 476–506.

Penman, H.G. 1989. Bacteraemia in salmonellosis. BMJ 298:323.

Perales, I., and Audicana, A. 1988. *Salmonella enteritidis* and eggs. Lancet 2:1133.

Perales, I., and Audicana, A. 1989. The role of hens' eggs in outbreaks of salmonellosis in north Spain. Int. J. Food Microbiol. 8:175–180.

Petter, J.G. 1993. Detection of two smooth colony phenotypes in a *Salmonella enteritidis* isolate which vary in their ability to contaminate eggs. Appl. Environ. Microbiol. 59:2884–2890.

Philbrook, F.R., MacCready, R.A., Van Roekel, H., Anderson, E.S., and Smyser, C.F. 1960. Sanen, avian source. N. Engl. J. Med. 263:713–718.

Plummer, R.A.S., Blissett, S.J., and Dodd, C.E.R. 1995. *Salmonella* contamination of retail chicken products sold in the UK. J. Food Prot. 58:843–846.

Pohl, P., Lintermans, P., Marin, M., and Couturier, M. 1991. Epidemiological study of *Salmonella enteritidis* strains of animal origin in Belgium. Epidemiol. Infect. 106:11–16.

Pomeroy, B.S. 1984. Fowl typhoid. In: Hofstad, M.S., Barnes, H.J., Calnek, B.W., Reid, W.M., and Yoder, H.W., eds. Diseases of poultry, 8th ed. Ames: Iowa State University Press, pp. 79–91.

Poppe, C. 1994. *Salmonella enteritidis* in Canada. Int. J. Food Microbiol. 21:1–5.

Poppe, C., Curtiss III, R., Gulig, P.A., and Gyles, C.L. 1989. Hybridization studies with a DNA probe derived from the virulence region of the 60 Mdal plasmid of *Salmonella typhimurium*. Can. J. Vet. Res. 53:387–384.

Poppe, C., Irwin, R.J., Forsberg, C.M., Clarke, R.C., and Oggel, J. 1991a. The prevalence of *Salmonella enteritidis* and other *Salmonella* spp. among Canadian registered commercial layer flocks. Epidemiol. Infect. 106:259–270.

Poppe, C., Irwin, R.J., Messier, S., Finley, G.G., and Oggel, J. 1991b. The prevalence of *Salmonella enteritidis* and other *Salmonella* spp. among Canadian registered commercial chicken broiler flocks. Epidemiol. Infect. 107:201–211.

Poppe, C., Johnson, R.P., Forsberg, C.M., and Irwin, R.J. 1992. *Salmonella enteritidis* and other *Salmonella* in laying hens and eggs from flocks with *Salmonella* in their environment. Can. J. Vet. Res. 56:226–232.

Poppe, C., Demczuk, W., McFadden, K., and Johnson, R.P. 1993a. Virulence of *Salmonella enteritidis* phage types 4, 8, and 13 and other *Salmonella* spp. for day-old chicks, hens and mice. Can. J. Vet. Res. 57.

Poppe, C., McFadden, K.A., Brouwer, A.M., and Demczuk, W. 1993b. Characterization of *Salmonella enteritidis* strains. Can. J. Vet. Res. 57:176–184.

Rampling, A., Anderson, J.R., Upson, R., Peters, E., Ward, L.R., and Rowe, B. 1989. *Salmonella enteritidis* phage type 4 infection of broiler chickens: a hazard to public health. Lancet 2:436–438.

Ranta, L.E., and Dolman, C.E. 1947. Experience with salmonella typing in Canada. Can. J. Public Health 38:286–294.

Read, D.H., Kinde, H., and Daft, B.M. 1994. Pathology of *Salmonella enteritidis* phage type 4 infection in commercial layer chickens in southern California. In: Proceedings of the 44th meeting of the Western Poultry Disease Conference, Sacramento, California, March 5–7, 1995, pp. 76–78.

Reilly, W.J., Forbes, G.I., Sharp, J.C.M., Oboegbulem, S.I., Collier, P.W., and Paterson, G.M. 1988. Poultry-borne salmonellosis in Scotland. Epidemiol. Infect. 101:115–122.

Rettger, L.F. 1900. Fatal septicaemia among young chicks. N.Y. Med. J. 71:803–805.

Rettger, L.F. 1909. Further studies on fatal septicaemia in young chicken, or "white diarrhea." J. Med. Res. 21:115–123.

Rizk, S.S., Ayres, J.C., and Kraft, A.A. 1966. Effect of holding condition on the development of *Salmonellae* in artificially inoculated hens' eggs. Poult. Sci. 45:825–829.

Roberts, D. 1991. *Salmonella* in chilled and frozen chicken. Lancet 337:984–985.

Rodrigue, D.C., Cameron, D.N., Puhr, N.D., Brenner, F.W., St. Louis, M.E., Wachsmuth, I.K., and Tauxe, R.V. 1992. Comparison of plasmid profiles, phage types, and antimicrobial resistance patterns of *Salmonella enteritidis* isolates in the United States. J. Clin. Microbiol. 30:854–857.

Rodrigue, D.C., Tauxe, R.V., and Rowe, B. 1990. International increase in *Salmonella enteritidis*: a new pandemic? Epidemiol. Infect. 105:21–27.

Ryan, C.A., Nickels, M.K., Hargrett-Bean, N.T., Potter, M.E., Endo, T., Mayer, L., Langkop, C.W., Gibson, C., McDonald, R.C., Kenney, R.T., Puhr, N.D., McDonnell, P.J., Martin, R.J., Cohen, M.L., and Blake, P.A. 1987. Massive outbreak of antimicrobial-resistant salmonellosis traced to pasteurized milk. JAMA 258:3269–3274.

Sadler, W.W., Brownell, J.R., and Fanelli, M.J. 1969. Influence of age and inoculum level on shed pattern of *Salmonella typhimurium* in chickens. Avian Dis. 13:793–803.

Saeed, A.M., and Koons, C.W. 1993. Growth and heat resistance of *Salmonella enteritidis* in refrigerated and abused eggs. J. Food Prot. 56:927–931.

Salmon, D.E., and Smith, T. 1886. Investigations in swine plague. In: Second annual report of the bureau of animal industry for the year 1885. Washington, DC: US Department of Agriculture, Government Printing Office, pp. 184–246.

Schaaf, J. 1936. Die Salmonellose (infektiöse Enteritis, Paratyphose) des Geflügels, ihre Bedeutung und Bekämpfung. Z. Infektionskr. Parasitaere Krankheiten Hyg. Haustiere 49:322–332.

Schaffer, J.M., MacDonald, A.G., Hall, W.J., and Bunyea, H. 1931. A stained antigen for the rapid whole blood test for pullorum disease. J. Am. Vet. Med. Assoc. 79:236–240.

Schofield, F.W. 1944. Salmonellosis in swine: a field and laboratory study of four outbreaks. Can. J. Comp. Med. 8:273–280.

Schofield, F.W. 1945. *Salmonella* infections of the domestic animals: their relationship to salmonellosis (food infection) in man. Can. J. Comp. Med. 9:62–68.

Schwartz, K.J. 1990. Salmonellosis in Midwestern swine. In: Proceedings of the 94th annual meeting of the United States Animal Health Association. Richmond, VA: Carter, pp. 443–449.

Seeliger, H.P.R., and Maya, A.E. 1964. Epidemiologie der Salmonellosen in Europa 1950–1960. In: van Oye, E., ed. The world problem of salmonellosis. The Hague: Dr. W. Junk, pp. 245–294.

Sickenga, F.N. 1964. Transmission of salmonellae and pathogenesis of salmonellosis in man. In: van Oye, E., ed. The world problem of salmonellosis. The Hague: Dr. W. Junk, pp. 205–232.

Silberstein, W., and Gerichter, Ch.B. 1964. Salmonellosis in Israel. In: van Oye, E., ed. The world problem of salmonellosis. The Hague: Dr. W. Junk, pp. 335–352.

Singer, J.T., Opitz, H.M., Gershman, M., Hall, M.M., Muniz, I.G., and Rao, S.V. 1992. Molecular characterization of *Salmonella enteritidis* isolates from Maine poultry and poultry farm environments. Avian Dis. 36:324–333.

Snoeyenbos, G.H. 1984. Pullorum disease. In: Hofstad, M.S., Barnes, H.J., Calnek, B.W., Reid, W.M., and Yoder, H.W., eds. Diseases of poultry, 8th ed. Ames: Iowa State University Press, pp. 66–79.

Snoeyenbos, G.H., Smyser, C.F., and Van Roekel, H. 1969. *Salmonella* infection of the ovary and peritoneum of chickens. Avian Dis. 13:668–670.

Sojka, W.J., Wray, C., Hudson, E.B., and Benson, J.A. 1975. Incidence of salmonella infection in animals in England and Wales, 1968–73. Vet. Rec. 96:280–287.

Sommers, H.M. 1980. Infectious diarrhoea. In: Youmans, G.P., Paterson, P.Y., and Sommers, H.M., eds. The biologic and clinical basis of infectious diseases. Philadelphia: W.B. Saunders, pp. 525–553.

Steinert, L., Virgil, D., Bellemore, E., Williamson, B., Dinda, E., Harris, D., Scheider, D., Fanella, L., Bogacki, V., Liska, F., Birkhead, G.S., Guzewich, J.J., Fudala, J.K., Kondracki, S.F., Shayegani, M., Morse, D.L., Dennis, D.T., Healey, B., Tavris, D.R., Duffy, M., and Drinnen, K. 1990. Update: *Salmonella enteritidis* infections and grade A shell eggs: United States, 1989. MMWR 38:877–880.

Stevens, A., Joseph, C., Bruce, H., Fenton, D., O'Mahony, M., Cunningham, D., O'Connor, B., and Rowe, B. 1989. A large outbreak of *Salmonella enteritidis* phage type 4 associated with eggs from overseas. Epidemiol. Infect. 103:425–433.

St. Louis, M.E., Morse, D.L., Potter, M.E., DeMelfi, T.M., Guzewich, J.J., Tauxe, R.V., Blake, P.A., and the *Salmonella enteritidis* Working Group. 1988. The emergence of grade A eggs as a major source of *Salmonella enteritidis* infections. JAMA 259:2103–2107.

Stokes, J.L., Osborne, W.W., and Bayne, H.G. 1956. Penetration and growth of *Salmonella* in shell eggs. Food Res. 21:510–518.

Tauxe, R.V., Tormey, M.P., Mascola, L., Hargrett-Bean, N.T., and Blake, P.A. 1987. Salmonellosis outbreak on transatlantic flights: foodborne illness on aircraft—1947–1984. Am. J. Epidemiol. 125:150–157.

Taylor, D.N., Bopp, C.A., Birkness, K., and Cohen, M.L. 1984. An outbreak of *Salmonella* associated with a fatality in a healthy child: a large dose and severe illness. Am. J. Epidemiol. 119:907–912.

Telzak, E.E., Budnick, L.D., Zweig Greenberg, M.S., Blum, S., Shayegani, M., Benson, C.E., and Schultz, S. 1990. A nosocomial outbreak of *Salmonella enteritidis* infection due to the consumption of raw eggs. N. Engl. J. Med. 323:394–397.

Telzak, E.E., Zweig Greenberg, M.S., Budnick, L.D., Singh, T., and Blum, S. 1991. Diabetes mellitus: a newly described risk factor for infection from *Salmonella enteritidis*. J. Infect. Dis. 164:538–541.

Threlfall, E.J., Chart, H., Ward, L.R., de Sa, J.D.H., and Rowe, B. 1993. Interrelationships between strains of *Salmonella enteritidis* belonging to phage types 4, 7, 7a, 8, 13, 13a, 23, 24 and 30. J. Appl. Bacteriol. 75:43–48.

Threlfall, E.J., Hampton, M.D., Chart, H., and Rowe, B. 1994. Use of plasmid profile typing for surveillance of *Salmonella enteritidis* phage 4 from humans, poultry and eggs. Epidemiol. Infect. 112:25–31.

Threlfall, E.J., Rowe, B., and Ward, L.R. 1989. Subdivision of *Salmonella enteritidis* phage types by plasmid profile typing. Epidemiol. Infect. 102:459–465.

Timoney, J.F., Shivaprasad, H.L., Baker, R.C., and Rowe, B. 1989. Egg transmission after infection of hens with *Salmonella enteritidis* phage type 4. Vet. Rec. 125:600–601.

Turnbull, P.B.C. 1979. Food poisoning with special reference to *Salmonella*: its epidemiology, pathogenesis and control. Clin. Gastroenterol. 8:663–714.

Turnbull, P.C.B., and Snoeyenbos, G.H. 1973. Experimental salmonellosis in the chicken. I. Fate and host response in alimentary canal, liver, and spleen. Avian Dis. 18:153–177.

Valera, J.O., and Valera, G. 1964. In: van Oye, E., ed. The world problem of salmonellosis. The Hague: Dr. W. Junk, pp. 445–475.

van de Giessen, A.W., Dufrenne, J.B., Ritmeester, W.S., Berkers, P.A.T.A., van Leeuwen, W.J., and Notermans, S.H.W. 1992. The identification of *Salmonella enteritidis*-infected poultry flocks associated with an outbreak of human salmonellosis. Epidemiol. Infect. 109:405–411.

van Oye, E. 1964. Les salmonelloses en Afrique Centrale. In: van Oye, E., ed. The world problem of salmonellosis. The Hague: Dr. W. Junk, pp. 354–365.

Ward, L.R., de Sa, J.D.H., and Rowe, B. 1987. A phage-typing scheme for *Salmonella enteritidis*. Epidemiol. Infect. 99:291–294.

Watt, J. 1945. An outbreak of *Salmonella* infection in man from infected chicken eggs. Public Health Rep. US 60:835–839.

Weisse, P., Libbey, E., Nims, L., Gutierrez, P., Madrid, T., Weber, N., Voorhees, C., Crocco, V., Hules, C., Hill, S., Ray, T.M., Gurule, R., Ortiz, F., Eidson, M., Sewell, C.M., Castle, S., Hayes, P., and Hull, H.F. 1986. *Salmonella heidelberg* outbreak at a convention: New Mexico. MMWR 35:91.

Wierup, M., Engström, B., Engvall, A., and Wahlström, H. 1995. Control of *Salmonella enteritidis* in Sweden. Int. J. Food Microbiol. 25:219–226.

Williams, J.E., Dillard, L.H., and Hall, G.O. 1968. The penetration patterns of *Salmonella typhimurium* through the outer structures of chicken eggs. Avian Dis. 12:445–466.

Wong, S.S.Y., Yuen, K.Y., Yam, W.C., Lee, T.Y., and Chau, P.Y. 1994. Changing epidemiology of human salmonellosis in Hong Kong, 1982–93. Epidemiol. Infect. 113:425–434.

Wood, J.D., Chalmers, G.A., Fenton, R.A., Pritchard, J., Schoonderwoerd, M., and Lichtenberger, W.L. 1991. Persistent shedding of *Salmonella enteritidis* from the udder of a cow. Can. Vet. J. 32:738–741.

Wray, C. 1985. Is salmonellosis still a serious problem in veterinary practice? Vet. Rec. 116:485–489.

Wray, C., and Sojka, W.J. 1977. Reviews of the progress of dairy science: bovine salmonellosis. J. Dairy Sci. 44:383–425.

2

Epidemiology of *Salmonella enterica* Serovar Enteritidis Phage Type 4 in England and Wales

P.G. Wall and L.R. Ward

INTRODUCTION

Salmonella food poisoning has long been a common cause of human illness in England and Wales. Since 1986, however, the incidence has increased markedly, and a particular subtype of one of the many serovars, *Salmonella enterica* serovar Enteritidis (*S.* Enteritidis) phage type 4 (PT4), has been identified as responsible for the majority of infections (Fig. 2.1). The evidence collectively shows that this *S.* Enteritidis epidemic is primarily due to infection in chickens, not only from surface contamination of carcasses and eggs but also from the contents of intact eggs (Coyle et al., 1988; Cowden et al., 1989; Mawer et al., 1989; Harrison et al., 1992). The proportion of eggs infected internally is very low, but because very large numbers of eggs are consumed daily, the number of human cases of infection nationally is large and represents an important challenge to public health. This was recognized in August 1988 when the Chief Medical Officer of the Department of Health in the United Kingdom issued advice to the public warning them of the risks associated with consuming raw or undercooked eggs.

SURVEILLANCE

The surveillance of human salmonellosis in England and Wales is undertaken by the Public Health Laboratory Service (PHLS). Most initial human isolates are sent to the national reference laboratory—the PHLS Laboratory of Enteric Pathogens (LEP)—for confirmation and definitive typing. The phage-typing scheme for *S.* Enteritidis, now adopted in many countries, was developed in this laboratory (Ward et al., 1994). There are over 2200 different salmonella serovars, but only about 200 occur in any 1 year in people in England and Wales. In 1981, the LEP identified 10,251 strains of various serovars from human infections. In 1993, the number had increased to 30,650. Phage typing of *S.* Enteritidis shows that almost all the increase is due to PT4 (Table 2.1; Fig. 2.2), which in 1981 accounted for 4% of all Salmonella isolates and peaked at 56% of the isolates in 1993. This represents approximately a 44-fold increase in *S.* Enteritidis PT4 (from 395 to 17,257). During this period, the number of salmonella serovar cases increased slightly (from 3992 to 4778) and the number of infections due to other serovars has remained relatively unchanged (from 5172 to 5618).

Salmonella isolates referred to the LEP represent only a proportion of all infections, because not all patients consult a doctor and not all will have a fecal or other culture taken (Feldman and Banatvala, 1994). In England and Wales, about 1% of human salmonella isolations identified by the LEP (excluding *S. typhi* and *S. paratyphi*) are from blood (bacteremia). The number of *S.* Enteritidis PT4 isolations from blood has increased over the years, but the percentage remains close to 1%, suggesting that this organism is not more invasive in humans than the other food-poisoning salmonellas (Table 2.2). Patients with severe infections are more likely to be investigated and also to have a blood culture than are patients with mild infections who may not even consult a doctor. Therefore, the true proportion of salmonella cases developing bacteremia is likely to be lower than 1%.

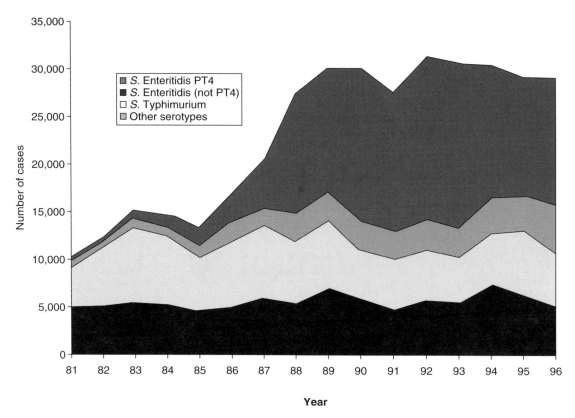

FIGURE 2.1   Salmonella serovars in England and Wales, 1981–96, PT4, phage type 4.

TABLE 2.1   Salmonella in humans: England and Wales

Year	*Salmonella* Typhimurium (%)	*Salmonella* Enteritidis		Other serotypes (%)	Total
		All (%)	PT4 (%)		
1981	3992 (39)	1087 (11)	395 (4)	5172 (50)	10,251
1982	6089 (49)	1101 (9)	413 (3)	5132 (42)	12,322
1983	7785 (51)	1774 (12)	823 (5)	5596 (37)	15,155
1984	7264 (49)	2071 (14)	1362 (9)	5392 (37)	14,727
1985	5478 (41)	3095 (23)	1771 (13)	4757 (36)	13,330
1986	7094 (42)	4771 (28)	2971 (18)	5111 (30)	16,976
1987	7660 (37)	6858 (33)	4962 (24)	6014 (30)	20,532
1988	6444 (23)	15,427 (56)	12,522 (46)	5607 (20)	27,478
1989	7306 (24)	15,773 (53)	12,931 (43)	6919 (23)	29,998
1990	5451 (18)	18,840 (63)	16,151 (54)	5821 (19)	30,112
1991	5331 (19)	17,460 (63)	14,693 (53)	4902 (18)	27,693
1992	5401 (17)	20,094 (64)	16,987 (54)	5860 (19)	31,355
1993	4778 (16)	20,254 (66)	17,257 (56)	5618 (18)	30,650
1994	5522 (18)	17,371 (57)	13,782 (45)	7518 (25)	30,411
1995	6743 (23)	16,044 (54)	12,482 (42)	6527 (22)	29,314
1996	5573 (19)	18,296 (62)	13,184 (45)	5242 (18)	29,111

PT4, phage type 4.
Source: Laboratory of Enteric Pathogens (formerly DEP) data: 1981–91. The PHLS Salmonella dataset: 1992 to 1996 provisional data; last update, 2 May 1997.

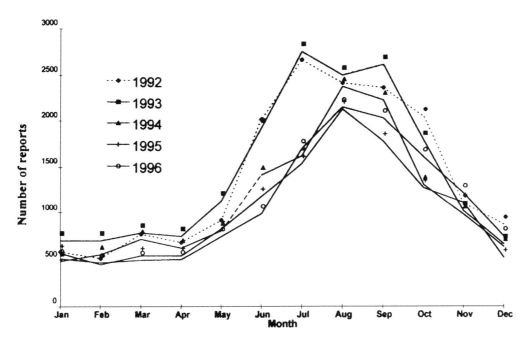

FIGURE 2.2   *Salmonella* Enteritidis phage type 4 in England and Wales, 1992–96: all laboratory reports by month of the report.

TABLE 2.2   Total human isolations and those from blood

	Salmonella Enteritidis PT4	
Year	Total	Blood (%)
1981	392	4 (1.0)
1982	413	5 (1.2)
1983	823	6 (0.7)
1984	1362	7 (0.5)
1985	1771	11 (0.6)
1986	2979	45 (1.5)
1987	4962	57 (1.1)
1988	12,522	163 (1.3)
1989	12,931	126 (1.0)
1990	16,151	125 (0.8)
1991	14,693	129 (0.9)
1992	16,987	211 (1.2)
1993	17,257	204 (1.2)
1994	13,782	174 (0.7)
1995	12,482	165 (1.3)
1996	13,184	159 (1.2)

PT4, phage type 4.
Source: Laboratory of Enteric Pathogens.

AGE-SPECIFIC AND SEX-SPECIFIC INCIDENCE

Incidence rates of infection are highest in children under age 10, with the highest rates in children under age 1 year (Table 2.3). This may reflect increased susceptibility, but a proportion of the increase is likely to be due to these young children being brought to medical care and having specimens submitted for examination.

SEASONALITY

Salmonella Enteritidis PT4 infections peak in the summer months (Fig. 2.3). This may result from the warm weather enabling salmonellas to multiply in conditions where food-hygiene practices are poor—egg cross-contamination or inadequate refrigeration or cooking. In addition, people's eating habits are different in the summer months, with more cold food consumed, more buffets where food is left for long periods before consumption, and more barbecues.

TRAVEL

Salmonella Enteritidis PT4 cases are also associated with foreign travel; for example, 950 (8%) of 12,482 patients in 1995 and 754 (6%) of 13,184 patients in 1996 acquired their infection abroad. Most tourist destinations are involved, and because *S.* Enteritidis PT4 is a global problem, the number of cases is usually related to the volume of tourists traveling to the destination. Those countries with warmer climates pose the greatest risk, because the margin of safety is reduced when food-hygiene standards are poor. Also, people eat out more on holidays and are therefore not in control of their own food preparation.

GENERAL OUTBREAKS

Although a large number of cases of salmonellosis are reported annually, most of our information linking food to illness comes from outbreak data. A surveillance system exists in England and Wales for general outbreaks, which

TABLE 2.3 *Salmonella* **Enteritidis phage type 4: age-specific and sex-specific incidence rates per 100,000 population in England and Wales, 1992–96**

				Age group			
Year/sex	<1 y	1–4 y	5–9 y	10–14 y	15–44 y	45–64 y	>65 y
1992							
Female	109	74	30	19	28	26	18
Male	122	76	31	23	29	22	15
1993							
Female	114	77	31	20	29	26	18
Male	98	78	31	23	30	24	17
1994							
Female	88	61	24	17	23	22	15
Male	93	58	24	19	25	19	14
1995							
Female	78	52	23	17	20	20	14
Male	83	49	28	18	21	18	14
1996							
Female	80	51	25	16	22	22	17
Male	76	51	27	20	23	21	16

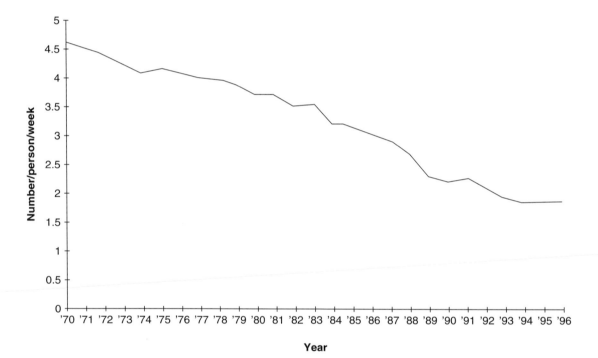

FIGURE 2.3   Household consumption of shell eggs: number per person per week and yearly average (1970–96).
Source: British Egg Information Service.

are defined as "outbreaks affecting members of more than one private residence or residents of an institution" (Cowden et al., 1995). A minimum set of data is collected on all outbreaks, including details of the setting in which the outbreak occurred, mode of transmission, causative pathogen, and details of laboratory and epidemiological investigations. Between 1992 and 1996, there were 73,692 reports of *S.* Enteritidis PT4 in England and Wales, of which 5165 (7%) arose from 393 general outbreaks.

Reports not linked to identified general outbreaks may be genuine sporadic cases, arise from family outbreaks, or be associated with unrecognized or unreported outbreaks.

Between 1989 and 1996, a total of 590 general outbreaks were reported to Communicable Disease Surveillance Center from England and Wales. At least 8800 people were affected: 362 were hospitalized and 27 died. The number of general outbreaks increased from 56 in 1989 to a peak of 108 in 1993 before decreasing again to 56 in

1996. Table 2.4 shows the food vehicles implicated in outbreaks of *S.* Enteritidis PT4. Food vehicles are pinpointed on the basis of microbiological evidence (the pathogen is isolated from the food), a statistically significant association between the consumption of food and illness (case-control or cohort study), or strong circumstantial evidence. Poultry and eggs remain common vehicles of infection for *S.* Enteritidis PT4, and eggs probably contribute to many outbreaks associated with sauces and desserts. In addition, many of the foods, such as quiches, classified under miscellaneous, may contain eggs (Holtby et al., 1995). This suggests that, despite the Department of Health's advice, raw eggs are still being used in foodstuffs that are not subjected to sufficient heat to kill salmonellas.

TABLE 2.4   Suspected food vehicles reported in outbreaks of *Salmonella* Enteritidis phage type 4 in England and Wales, 1989–96

Food vehicle implicated	Number of outbreaks
Eggs and egg dishes	103
Desserts	98
Poultry	75
Red meat/meat products	39
Fish/shellfish	18
Salads/vegetables/fruit	17
Sauces	12
Milk/milk products	9
Miscellaneous food	130

SALMONELLAS IN RAW CHICKEN

The consumption of poultry meat has increased dramatically in the United Kingdom from 16 kg per head in 1985 to 27.9 in 1996 (Fig. 2.4). A combination of factors has contributed to the increase, one being the decreasing price of poultry meat relative to other meat. A second factor resulted from the epidemic of bovine spongiform encephalopathy in British cattle, which caused a decrease in the consumption of beef and a switch to other meats, including poultry (Fig. 2.4).

Table 2.5 shows the results of PHLS surveys of the prevalence of salmonellas in U.K. chickens on retail sale. These results suggest that there has been a moderate decline in salmonella contamination of U.K.-produced retail raw chicken. The 1994 survey revealed that giblets tended to be more frequently contaminated than skin or carcass samples, and that chicken carcasses that contained a bag of giblets tended to be more frequently positive for *S.* Enteritidis PT4 than those that did not [Advisory Committee on the Microbiological Safety of Food (ACMSF), 1996].

SALMONELLAS IN EGGS

The ACMSF in its report on salmonellas in eggs (1993) recommended that regular surveys be carried out on the incidence of *S.* Enteritidis in eggs on retail sale. Table 2.6 shows the results of several PHLS studies of retail eggs.

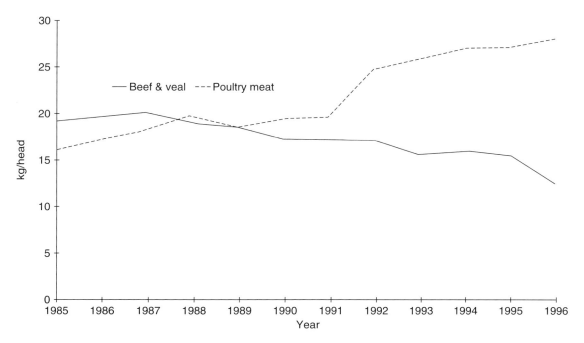

FIGURE 2.4   Estimated kilograms (kg) per capita meat consumption in the United Kingdom, 1985–96: total supplies of meat moving into human consumption divided by U.K. midyear population.
Source: British Meat and Livestock Commission.

TABLE 2.5 **Prevalence of salmonella species in raw chicken: Public Health Laboratory Service surveys, 1979–94**

Survey date	Source and type	No. of chickens	No. (%) with Salmonella spp.	No. (%) with S. Enteritidis PT4
1979/1980	U.K., frozen	100	79 (79)	0 (0)
1987	U.K., frozen	101	65 (64)	20 (20)
1990	U.K., frozen	143	77 (54)	33 (23)
1994	U.K., frozen	281	114 (41)	55 (20)
1987	U.K., chilled	103	56 (54)	10 (10)
1990	U.K., chilled	143	58 (41)	29 (20)
1994	U.K., chilled	281	93 (33)	33 (12)

Note: The frequency of contamination with *S.* Enteritidis phage type 4 (PT4) increased until 1990 and has decreased in the 1994 study.

TABLE 2.6 **Prevalence of salmonella species and *Salmonella* Enteritidis in shell eggs**

Date	Source	No. of (six egg) samples	No. (%) of samples containing		
			Salmonellas	S. Enteritidis	S. Enteritidis PT4
1991	U.K.	7045	65 (0.9)	47 (0.7)	33 (0.5)
1991	EC non-U.K.	8630	138 (1.6)	19 (0.2)	16 (0.2)
1992–93	U.K. (prolonged)	7730	17 (0.2)	16 (0.2)	13 (0.2)
1995–96	U.K.	13,970	138 (0.99)	119 (0.85)	82 (0.6)

PT4, phage type 4. From De Louvois (1997).

The conclusions of the 1995–96 study (De Louvois, 1997) are that, since the first study that was completed in 1991, there has been no significant change in the prevalence of contamination of *S.* Enteritidis PT4, other *S.* Enteritidis phage types, and other salmonellas in U.K.–produced retail eggs. Most of the salmonellas were isolated from the shell, but in 18 of 138 positive samples the salmonellas were isolated from the contents of the eggs: 16 of the 18 were *S.* Enteritidis, of which 13 were PT4. The studies did not attempt to quantify the number of *S.* Enteritidis present within the contaminated eggs. It may be that in most cases the number of organisms is low and therefore not sufficient to be a risk unless the eggs undergo prolonged storage at ambient temperature or are used to prepare foods that are eaten uncooked (Humphrey et al., 1991). In many of the reported outbreaks of *S.* Enteritidis PT4 infection, there is evidence of inadequate heat treatment or storage of egg dishes (Cowden et al., 1995).

CONTROL OF *SALMONELLA* ENTERITIDIS PHAGE TYPE 4

Salmonella Enteritidis PT4 is a zoonosis and will be effectively controlled if only it is tackled at the level of the poultry reservoir. Concern over the rising incidence of *S.* Enteritidis PT4 infections led to the 1989 Zoonoses Order, which required that isolations of salmonellas from poultry had to be reported to the Ministry of Agriculture, Fisheries, and

Food. In addition, laying flocks were subject to compulsory testing and all infected flocks were slaughtered. Between March 1989 (when the order came into effect) and February 1993 (when compulsory slaughter ceased), 386 flocks in Great Britain were found to be infected with either *S.* Enteritidis (334 or 87%) or salmonella serovars (52). *Salmonella* Enteritidis infection alone led to the compulsory slaughter of nearly 2 million birds over this period. The policy was motivated by public concern over salmonellas in eggs and poultry. Other measures aimed at controlling the spread of salmonellas focused on reducing contamination of animal/poultry feeds (via the 1989 Processed Animal Protein Order and the Code of Practice for the Control of Salmonella in Animal Feeding Stuffs). Infection rates among commercial flocks have declined in recent years, although it is impossible to evaluate the relative contributions of the feed and slaughter policies to this decline. The slaughter policy was criticized by parts of the industry as being unnecessarily drastic.

Flocks of breeding fowl in the United Kingdom are currently subject to a statutory program of testing under the Poultry Breeding Flocks and Hatcheries Order of 1993. In addition to the statutory scheme, a number of commercial companies operate voluntary testing schemes. Therefore, in contrast to other species, a significant number of reports of salmonellas from poultry are the result of examinations made under testing programs rather than as the result of clinical disease. If the incidence of *S.* Enteritidis PT4 in humans is to be reduced, the pathogen will have to be controlled in the poultry reservoir. Eradication is not easy, because the poultry industry is complex, there is a complex relationship between infection, excretion, and environmental contamination, and the pattern of infection on different premises shows considerable variation (Corkish et al., 1994). Control is made difficult by the ability of *S.* Enteritidis to survive in dust and bird droppings in the environment of poultry units and in poultry feed for prolonged periods (Davies and Wray, 1996). In addition, wild rodents can act as a reservoir for maintaining infection in poultry units (Davies and Wray, 1995). Because the ovaries and oviducts of poultry can be infected with *S.* Enteritidis PT4, vertical transmission of infection is recognized as important in the epidemiology and control of this pathogen (Humphrey et al., 1989; Humphrey, 1994). If *S.* Enteritidis is to be controlled, the elite birds at the top of the pyramid of poultry production must be salmonella free. Sweden has succeeded in keeping *S.* Enteritidis out of its poultry flock by importing only broiler and layer grandparent birds certified as originating from salmonella-free parents and keeping these birds in quarantine for 15 weeks after arrival in Sweden, during which time they are regularly tested for salmonellas (Wierup et al., 1995). In addition to testing imported birds, imported ingredients for poultry feed are tested in Sweden, and most of the feed for layers and broilers is heat treated.

The poultry flock is much larger, and the costs of production are kept low to provide cheaper chicken for the consumers in the United Kingdom compared with those in Sweden. In the United Kingdom, rigid biosecurity and cleaning regimens are being applied to reduce the incidence of salmonellas in poultry flocks. Further improvements may result from the use of vaccination or competitive exclusion (the feeding of probiotics that compete with the pathogens), which may have a role to play in reducing the rate of salmonella infections and symptomless excretors (Mead and Barrow, 1990).

REFERENCES

Advisory Committee on the Microbiological Safety of Food. 1993. Report on salmonella in eggs. London: HMSO.

Advisory Committee on the Microbiological Safety of Food. 1996. Report on poultry meat. London: HMSO.

Corkish, J.D., Davies, R.H., Wray, C., and Nicholas, R.A.J. 1994. Observations on a broiler breeder flock naturally infected with *Salmonella enteritidis* phage type 4. Vet. Rec. 134:591–594.

Cowden, J., Lynch, D., Joseph, C.A., O'Mahoney M., Mawer, S.L., Rowe, B., and Bartlett, C.L.R. 1989. Case control study of infections with *Salmonella enteritidis* PT4 in England. BMJ 299:771–773.

Cowden, J.M., Wall, P.G., Adak, G., Evans, H., Le Baigue, S., and Ross, D. 1995. Outbreaks of foodborne infectious intestinal disease in England and Wales: 1992–1993. Communicable Dis. Rep. 5:R109–R117.

Coyle, E., Palmer, S., Ribeiro, C., Howard, A.J., Palmer, S.R., Jones, H.I., Ward, L., and Rowe, B. 1988. *Salmonella enteritidis* phage type 4 infection: association with hens' eggs. Lancet 2:1295–1296.

Davies, R.H., and Wray, C. 1995. Mice as carriers of *S.* Enteritidis in persistently infected poultry units. Vet. Rec. 137:337–341.

Davies, R.H., and Wray, C. 1996. Persistence of *Salmonella enteritidis* in poultry units and poultry food. Br. Poult. Sci. 37:589–596.

De Louvois, J. 1997. Report of a study into *Salmonella* contamination of UK produced retail eggs 1995/1996. London: Department of Health.

Feldman, R.A., and Banatvala, N. 1994. The frequency of culturing stools from adults with diarrhoea in Great Britain. Epidemiol. Infect. 113:41–44.

Harrison, C., Quigley, C., Kaczmarski, E., and Devlin, E. 1992. An outbreak of gastro-intestinal illness caused by eggs containing *Salmonella enteritidis* phage type 4. J. Infect. 24:207–210.

Holtby, I., Tebbutt, G.M., Harrison, R., and Kett, J. 1995. Outbreak of *Salmonella enteritidis* phage type 4 infection associated with cheese and onion quiche. Communicable Dis. Rep. 5:R118–R119.

Humphrey, T.J. 1994. Contamination of egg shells and contents with *Salmonella enteritidis*: a review. Int. J. Food Microbiol. 21:31–40.

Humphrey, T.J., Baskerville, A., Mawer, S., Rowe, B., and Hopper, S. 1989. *Salmonella enteritidis* phage type 4 from the contents of intact eggs: a study involving naturally infected hens. Epidemiol. Infect. 103:415–423.

Humphrey, T.J., Whitehead, A., Gawler, A.H.L., Henley, A., and Rowe, B. 1991. Numbers of *Salmonella enteritidis* in the contents of naturally contaminated hens eggs. Epidemiol. Infect. 106:489–496.

Mawer, S.L., Spain, G.E., and Rowe, B. 1989. *Salmonella enteritidis* phage type 4 and hens' eggs [Letter]. Lancet 1:281.

Mead, G.C., and Barrow, P.A. 1990. A review: salmonella control in poultry by "competitive exclusion" or immunisation. Lett. Appl. Microbiol. 10:221–227.

Ward, L.R., de Sa, J.D.H., and Rowe, B. 1994. A phage typing scheme for *Salmonella enteritidis*. Epidemiol. Infect. 112:25–31.

Wierup, M., Engstrom, B., Engvall, A., and Wahlstrom, H. 1995. Control of *Salmonella enteritidis* in Sweden. Int. J. Food Microbiol. 25:219–226.

3

Salmonella enterica Serovar Enteritidis in Scotland

D.S. Munro, R.W.A. Girdwood, and W.J. Reilly

The Scottish Salmonella Reference Laboratory (SSRL) provides an integrated service to medical and veterinary laboratories in Scotland from a base at Stobhill General Hospital, in Glasgow, Scotland. The Scottish Centre for Infection and Environmental Health (SCIEH) is the national surveillance unit for Scotland. The SSRL has always maintained a close working relationship with the SCIEH and provides the laboratory information on which the national data set is based. These data are supplemented by additional epidemiological information obtained from medical and environmental health colleagues on health boards and local authorities, respectively (Fig. 3.1).

At the time of its formation in 1960, the SSRL focused primarily on the needs of hospital laboratories, serving a population of some 5 million. Throughput grew with time from the initial 179 submissions in 1960 to 650 isolates in 1965. In the early years, isolates of *Salmonella enterica* serovar Enteritidis (*S.* Enteritidis) were few, with phage type 8 (PT8) predominating (Table 3.1).

From the mid-1960s, veterinary laboratories also made submissions to the SSRL. Again the numbers increased annually, and by 1970, submissions of isolates from animal sources were greater than those from cases of human infection. This increase in activity may have been driven by an increasing awareness of the role of farm animals in human disease and the concerns expressed in the Swann Report in 1969 arising from the perceived relationship between the use of antibiotics in animal feed, as growth enhancers, and the development of bacterial antibiotic resistance.

In the early 1970s, an increase (albeit small) in the numbers of *S.* Enteritidis from animals was seen. Isolates were reported from a wide range of species (for example, monkey, mink, and lion cub, as well as the more usual domestic animals). This included the first isolates from chicken in 1970 and again in 1974 and duck specimens in 1971.

Throughout the 1970s, the numbers of animal isolates of *S.* Enteritidis remained low whereas the incidence of human infection increased with no obvious sources identified. No further poultry isolates of *S.* Enteritidis were made until 1981 and 1985.

A phage-typing service for the SSRL was initially provided by the Public Health Laboratory Service (PHLS) of England and Wales. In 1989, the SSRL began phage typing of *S.* Enteritidis in using the typing scheme developed and generously supplied by the PHLS.

In the 1970s, a restricted range of phage types of *S.* Enteritidis was seen: PT2, PT4, PT5, PT8, PT11, PT13, and PT15. Not all isolates were submitted for phage typing during this period, but, of those that were, PT8 was the most common. Anecdotal evidence suggested a link between the consumption of chicken at barbecues and isolations of this phage type, but no statistically significant association was ever established. Although the incidence of human infection with salmonellae had been increasing, the most common serovar associated with the consumption of poultry at that time was *S.* Typhimurium. Between 1980 and 1990, the incidence of *S.* Enteritidis in the human population continued to increase, with a gradual substitution of the initially more common *S.* Typhimurium by *S.* Enteritidis without any overall increase in the numbers of salmonellae reported (Fig. 3.2).

In 1987, submissions of *S.* Enteritidis from human sources overtook those of *S.* Typhimurium for the first time. The majority of the *S.* Enteritidis isolates were PT4, which by 1993 represented 84% of all isolates of *S.* Enteritidis and 52% of all salmonellae isolated from humans.

This increasing incidence of human infection was not, however, paralleled by an increase in isolations reported in poultry, which remained low. Since most salmonellae rarely cause clinical disease in poultry, and routine monitoring of

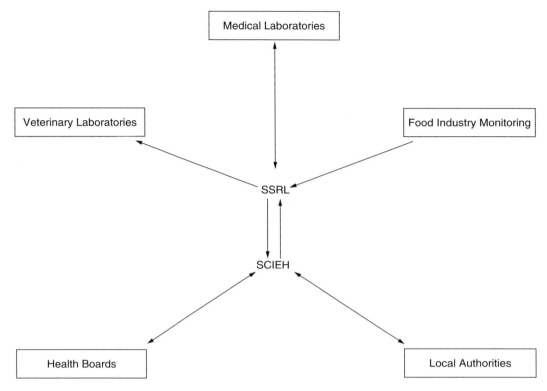

FIGURE 3.1 Salmonella surveillance in Scotland.

TABLE 3.1 Isolates of salmonellae typed by SSRL 1960–65

Year	Total salmonellae	Total *S. Enteritidis*
1960	179	4
1961	205	16
1962	311	9
1963	389	15
1964	616	3
1965	650	8

laboratory returns usually reflects disease problems being investigated, it may not be a good indicator of what is present in the poultry population. There was no evidence, however, that poultry companies were not submitting for typing any salmonella isolates made during their own routine product-sampling programs. The evidence is therefore unclear with regard to the presence of *S. Enteritidis* in poultry during this period.

The first indications of a significant increase in the level of infection in poultry occurred in 1988, when the numbers of *S. Enteritidis* isolates increased to 33, followed by a further rise to 138 in 1989 (Fig. 3.3).

Samples submitted by commercial companies for typing confirmed the presence of *S. Enteritidis* in poultry flocks. By 1988, this was the most commonly found salmonella in commercial flocks and continued to be so until 1990. During 1991–93, *S. Enteritidis* became the second most common isolate and has declined further since then.

Two surveys during the 1980s (Girdwood et al., 1985; Reilly et al., 1991) further demonstrated what was happening with *S. Enteritidis* in birds. Between 1982 and 1984, in a study of wild gulls, 5888 were trapped and tested for salmonellae. Of these, 459 (7.8%) were infected with salmonellae, but only once was *S. Enteritidis* isolated. In 1988–89, in a study to examine food exposures and salmonella carriage in patients in a long-stay hospital, raw chicken delivered to the kitchen was routinely sampled. Of 477 carcasses tested, 214 (44.8%) had salmonellae, of which 51 (23.8%) were *S. Enteritidis*, all but three of which were PT4.

The incidence of human infection with *S. Enteritidis* continued to increase until 1993, when 1797 isolates were reported, of which 1512 (84.1%) were PT4. This increase had been paralleled elsewhere in Europe though the relative rates of increase had varied. Molecular studies undertaken at the SSRL demonstrated that the PT4 seen in Scotland was the same as that seen elsewhere in Europe.

In 1994, reported human isolates fell slightly from 1797 to 1703, and a reduction was also seen in the percentage of the total *S. Enteritidis* isolates that were PT4 to 80% (1364). While in 1995 the overall numbers of *S. Enteritidis* increased slightly to 1724, the number of reports of PT4 fell to 1269. At the same time, reported rates of infection were falling in England and Wales and also elsewhere in Europe, although the rate of decline appeared not to be as great in Scotland as was reported elsewhere. One explanation for the more gradual decline in Scotland may be that the substitution of *S. Typhimurium* by *S. Enteritidis* in Scotland occurred later and more gradually than elsewhere.

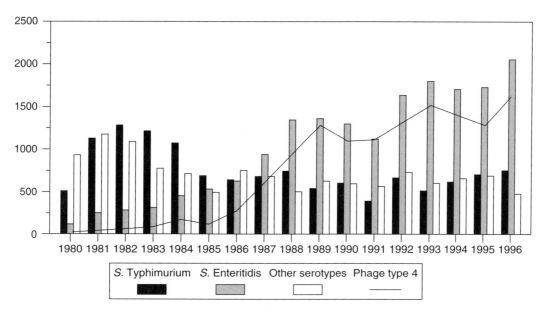

FIGURE 3.2 *Salmonella* Typhimurium and *Salmonella* Enteritidis isolates in Scotland, 1980–96.

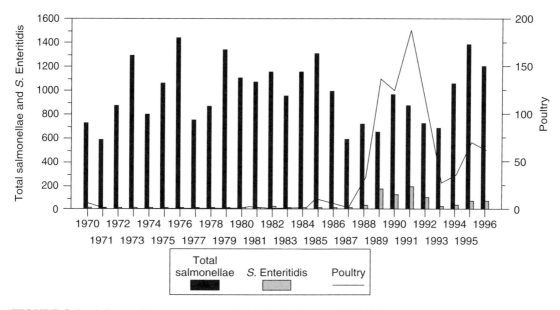

FIGURE 3.3 Salmonella serovars in animals in Scotland, 1980–96.

The continued decline in human isolates seen through 1995 was accompanied by a decline in statutory reporting of *S.* Enteritidis in poultry under the provision of the Zoonoses Order of 1989, and this continued through 1996–97.

Against the background of an apparent peaking in 1993, it was unexpected that a dramatic increase in the incidence of human infection occurred in 1996. The reported incidence increased by 19% to an all time high of 2057 isolates of *S.* Enteritidis, of which 1608 (78.2%) were PT4. This gave an overall rate of infection in Scotland of 40.04 per 100,000, which varied from nil in the Shetland islands to 55.35 in the Grampian Health Board (Fig. 3.4A). This is not significantly different from the distribution of all salmonellae (Fig. 3.4B).

Of the 2057 isolates, 177 (9.4%) were reported as imported infections primarily in persons returning from holiday, and 24 were reported as resistant to three or more antibiotics.

This increase continued into 1997, in the first 6 months of which isolates of *S.* Enteritidis increased by 42% over the same period in 1996 and PT4 increased by 17%. Other phage types

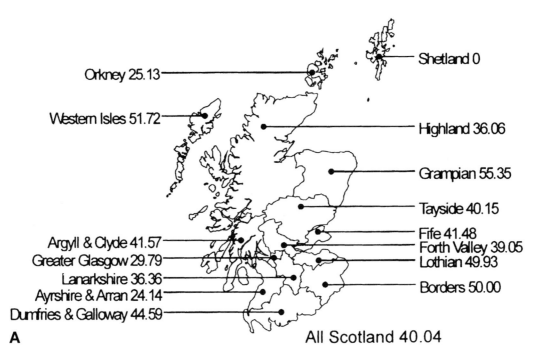

FIGURE 3.4A   Rates per 100,000 of *Salmonella* Enteritidis in Scotland: health board of reporting laboratory, 1996.

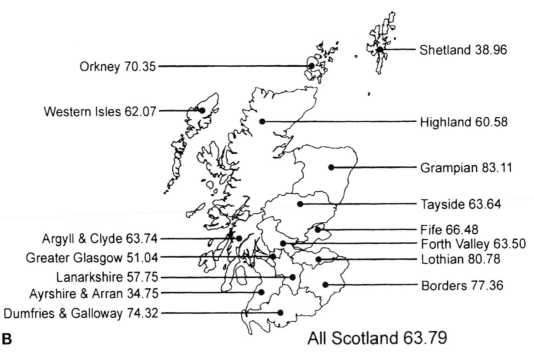

FIGURE 3.4B   Rates per 100,000 of all salmonella serovars in Scotland by health board of reporting laboratory, 1996.

such as PT1, PT6, PT6a, and PT14b also appeared in greater numbers. There is no obvious explanation for this increase.

During the period 1995–97, a diversification of phage types was seen, and work done at the SSRL demonstrated how phage types could be derived one from another (Rankin and Platt, 1995). This followed on the work by Stanley et al.

(1991), Threlfall et al. (1993), and Olsen et al. (1994), which showed that *S.* Enteritidis has distinct clonal lines.

This diversification has been accompanied by the gradual acquisition of resistance to a range of antibiotics, although less so than has been observed in other salmonellae, such as *S.* Typhimurium PT104. The resistance seen has

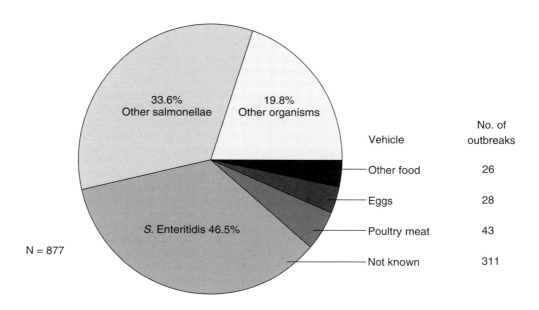

FIGURE 3.5 Outbreaks of foodborne infection in Scotland, 1990–94.

been predominantly plasmid mediated, with the exception of a single strain in 1996 resistant to ciprofloxacin where this resistance is chromosomally mediated.

Much of the increase in human infection with PT4 in England and Wales has been attributed to the consumption of eggs and egg products (PHLS Microbiology Digest, 1989) as in the case in the United States, which coincidentally experienced a similar epidemic of infection with *S.* Enteritidis, although a different phage type (PT8).

Investigation of outbreaks of foodborne infection coordinated by the SCIEH as part of the World Health Organization surveillance program for control of foodborne infections and intoxications in Europe during 1990–94 demonstrated the importance of *S.* Enteritidis and, in particular, PT4 (Fig. 3.5).

During this study period, *S.* Enteritidis accounted for 408 of the 877 outbreaks reported, of which 347 were PT4. In the majority of the investigations, no foodstuff was identified. Of the 97 outbreaks where a specific food was implicated, the majority were caused by poultry meat or eggs. Much of the evidence to associate a food with an outbreak was circumstantial, and in only a few outbreaks was the organism isolated from food or was there statistically significant evidence to confirm the vehicle of infection. In many outbreaks, it was reported that there had been a failure to maintain a satisfactory temperature-controlled and hygienic food chain.

Since 1960, when there has been comprehensive surveillance of salmonellae in Scotland, no single salmonella has behaved in such a manner as *S.* Enteritidis, particularly PT4. Others such as *S.* Agona, *S.* Hadar, and *S.* Typhimurium definitive type 204c have risen in importance and subsequently declined. None have endured as well nor reached the same numbers as *S.* Enteritidis. In recent years, different phage types have emerged, yet while increasing in numbers, they are still a long way from causing a problem of the same order as that caused by PT4.

Despite the declines recorded after 1993, the subsequent increases in 1996 and 1997 to record levels illustrate that this is a particularly successful pathogen, which has behaved differently than most salmonellae.

REFERENCES

Girdwood, R.W.A., Fricker, C.R., Munro, D., Shedden, C.B., and Monaghan, P. 1985. The incidence and significance of salmonella carriage by gulls (*Larus* spp.) in Scotland. J. Hyg. Camb. 95:229–241.

Olsen, J.E., Skov, M.N., Threlfall, E.J., and Brown, D.J. 1994. Clonal lines of *Salmonella enterica* serotype Enteritidis documented by IS200-, ribo-, pulsed-field gel electrophoresis and RFLP typing. J. Med. Microbiol. 40:15–22.

PHLS Microbiology Digest. 1989. Memorandum of evidence to the Agriculture Committee inquiry on salmonella in eggs. PHLS Microbiol. Digest no. 1.

Rankin, S., and Platt, D.J. 1995. Phage conversion in *Salmonella enterica* serotype Enteritidis: implications for epidemiology. Epidemiol. Infect. 114:227–236.

Reilly, W.J., Oboegbulem, S.I., Munro, D.S., and Forbes, G.I. 1991. The epidemiological relationship between salmonella isolated from poultry meat and sewage effluents at a long-stay hospital. Epidemiol. Infect. 106:1–10.

Stanley, J., Jones, C.S., and Threlfall, E.J. 1991. Evolutionary lines among *Salmonella enteritidis* phage types are identified by insertion sequence IS200 distribution. FEMS Microbiol. Lett. 82:83–90.

Threlfall, E.J., Chart, H., Ward, L.R., de Sa, J.D.H., and Rowe, B. 1993. Interrelationships between strains of *Salmonella enteritidis* belonging to phage types 4, 7, 7a, 8, 13, 23, 24 and 30. J. Appl. Bacteriol. 75:43–48.

4

Epidemiology of Human *Salmonella enterica* Serovar Enteritidis Infections in the United States

F.J. Angulo and D.L. Swerdlow

INTRODUCTION

Salmonellosis is both one of the most common foodborne diseases and one of the most commonly reported bacterial infections. There are an estimated 800,000 to 4 million human salmonella infections (300 to 1500 cases per 100,000 persons) each year in the United States (Chalker and Blaser, 1988; Council for Agricultural Science and Technology,1994). Most salmonella infections result in a mild,self-limiting illness characterized by diarrhea, fever, and abdominal cramps. However, the infection can spread to the bloodstream, bone marrow, or meningeal linings of the brain, leading to a severe and occasionally fatal illness. Each year, an estimated 500 to 1000 persons die of salmonella infections in the United States (Cohen and Tauxe, 1986; Council for Agricultural Science and Technology, 1994).

National surveillance for salmonella infections is based on serovar-specific laboratory-confirmed cases (Hargrett-Bean et al., 1988). However, only a small proportion of the many persons with salmonellosis are reported to the Centers for Disease Control and Prevention (CDC), because a complex chain of events must occur before a case is reported, and a break at any linkage along the chain will result in the case not being reported (Fig. 4.1). For a salmonella infection to be reported to the CDC, a person usually must become ill, this ill person usually must go to a physician or other health-care provider, the health-care provider must order the collection of a stool culture or other specimen, the specimen must be appropriately collected and forwarded to a clinical microbiology laboratory, and the laboratory must culture the specimen for salmonellae and report the isolation of salmonellae to the appropriate local or state health department, who must report the case to the CDC. In addition, because serotyping of salmonellae is an essential subtyping procedure for public health surveillance of salmonella infections, the salmonella isolate must also be serotyped; the clinical laboratory usually forwards the isolate to the public health laboratory for serotyping.

Fortunately, the activities that occur at several of the steps in this reporting process are relatively comprehensive, resulting in few unreported cases. Almost all clinical microbiology laboratories in the United States appropriately test all stool specimens for salmonellae that are submitted to their laboratory. Most laboratories, as legally required in most states, also report salmonella isolations to public health authorities. In addition, many clinical laboratories, as legally required in many states, forward salmonella isolates to public health laboratories for serotyping.

Largely because many salmonella infections are relatively mild, however, only a fraction of the persons with salmonella infections seek medical care. Of the estimated 800,000 to 4 million persons with salmonellosis each year in the United States, only an estimated 18,000 are hospitalized (Cohen and Tauxe, 1986). In addition, perhaps because of the perception that the specimen result would not influence the patient's medical treatment, specimens are not routinely collected and submitted. Of those persons with salmonella infections who seek medical care, approximately 40,000 each year (15 cases per 100,000 persons) have a stool sample collected and submitted to a clinical laboratory that isolates salmonellae and reports the isolation to the CDC through the local and state health departments. More than 97% of reported culture-confirmed cases are serotyped.

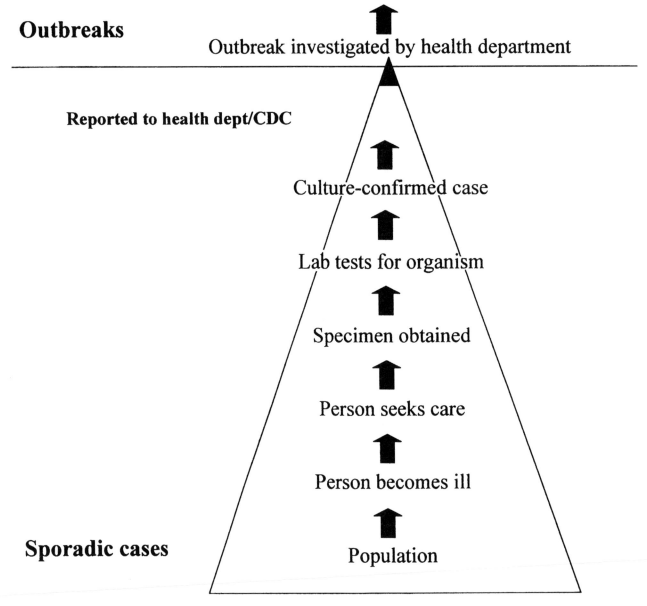

Outbreaks

Outbreak investigated by health department

Reported to health dept/CDC

Culture-confirmed case

Lab tests for organism

Specimen obtained

Person seeks care

Person becomes ill

Sporadic cases   Population

FIGURE 4.1   Pyramid of chain of events required for reporting culture-confirmed salmonella cases to the Centers for Disease Control and Prevention (CDC).

During the past 3 decades, the number of culture-confirmed salmonella infections in the United States reported to the CDC has steadily increased (Fig. 4.2). There were 39,032 reported cases in 1996 compared with 26,326 in 1972, a 47% increase during this 26-year period. Much of the increase in salmonella isolations has been due to the increase in isolates of *Salmonella enterica* serovar Enteritidis. *Salmonella* Enteritidis isolates increased by 459% during this period, while all other serovars increased by only 18%; among other common serovars, *S.* Typhimurium increased by 46% and *S.* Heidelberg by 36% (Fig. 4.3).

SALMONELLA ENTERITIDIS INFECTIONS IN HUMANS

Salmonella Enteritidis (*S.* Enteritidis) is the prototypic emerging pathogen (Altekruse and Swerdlow, 1996). Prior to the 1980s, *S.* Enteritidis was a relatively infrequent cause of human illness. In the late 1980s, the reported number of *S.* Enteritidis cases increased dramatically. By 1990, *S.* Enteritidis had emerged as the most common serovar in the United States and remained the most common serovar from 1993 to 1996. The emergence of *S.* Enteritidis is demonstrated clearly

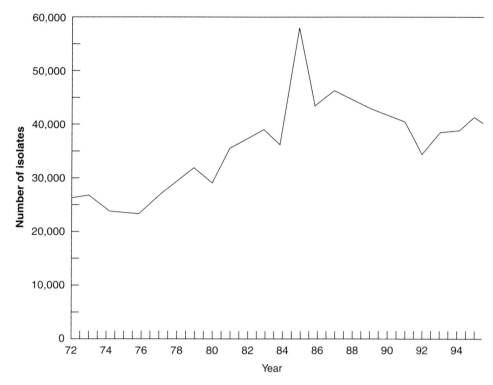

FIGURE 4.2 Salmonella isolations from human sources reported to the CDC, by year, 1972–96.

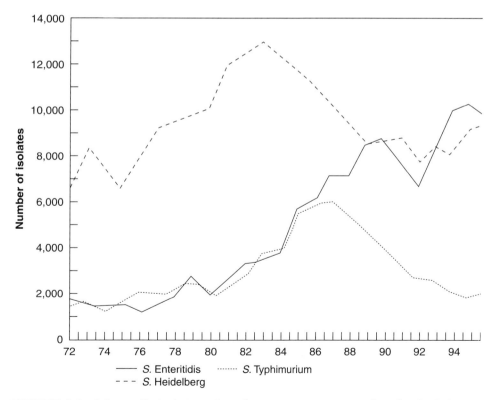

FIGURE 4.3 Salmonella isolations from human sources reported to the CDC, by serovar and year, 1972–96.

when compared with the total number of salmonella isolates reported for each year; *S.* Enteritidis represented only 6% of the reported salmonella isolates in 1972, compared with 25% of the culture-confirmed cases in 1996 (Fig. 4.4).

Salmonella Enteritidis in the United States initially emerged in the New England region in 1979, the mid-Atlantic region beginning in 1984, and most recently in the Pacific region in 1993 (Fig. 4.5). In these regions, *S.* Enteritidis is often more frequently reported than any other serovar and represents more than 50% of all salmonellae reported in some states (Fig. 4.6). The increase in *S.* Enteritidis, which began in California in 1993, has been particularly dramatic; in 1990, *S.* Enteritidis accounted for only 11% of salmonella isolates in that state compared with 37.6% in 1994. In 1996, more than 25% of all *S.* Enteritidis isolates in the United States were from California.

Nationwide, 9552 cases of *S.* Enteritidis (1.5 cases per 100,000 population) were reported in 1996. Since each year there are an estimated 800,000 to 4 million cases of salmonellosis, resulting in up to 1000 deaths, these data suggest that there were 200,000 to 1 million cases of *S.* Enteritidis infections, resulting in up to 250 deaths in 1996. Of the reported *S.* Enteritidis isolates in 1996, 53% were from females. *Salmonella* Enteritidis infections were most commonly reported among persons at the extremes of age, especially children younger than age 5 (Fig. 4.7). Most isolates in 1996 were from stool specimens, but 6% were collected from normally sterile sites (blood, cerebral spinal fluid, bone, or joints).

SOURCES OF *SALMONELLA* ENTERITIDIS IN HUMANS

Eggs are the dominant source of *S.* Enteritidis infections in humans (St. Louis et al., 1988). Investigations of outbreaks and sporadic cases have shown repeatedly that the most common source is grade-A shell eggs, usually consumed undercooked or raw. The silent spread and emergence of *S.* Enteritidis in the United States (and globally) reflects the perhaps recent phenomenon of eggs being internally contaminated with *S.* Enteritidis as a result of infection in the hen's ovaries and oviducts (Humphrey et al., 1989; Rodrigue et al., 1990; Thiagarajan et al., 1994). The unusual ability of *S.* Enteritidis to infect the hen's ovary enables the bacterium to contaminate the contents of intact eggs sold to consumers.

Outbreaks of *S.* Enteritidis infection are investigated by state and local health departments and reported to the CDC through the foodborne disease outbreak surveillance system (Bean et al., 1996). An outbreak of *S.* Enteritidis infection was defined as two or fewer cases of laboratory-confirmed *S.* Enteritidis infection in persons who shared a common exposure. A food vehicle was considered to be confirmed if it was implicated epidemiologically or if *S.* Enteritidis was isolated from remaining food samples. From 1985 to 1996, a total of 660 outbreaks of *S.* Enteritidis were reported to the CDC (Table 4.1). The outbreaks involved at least 25,935 cases, 2508 hospitalizations

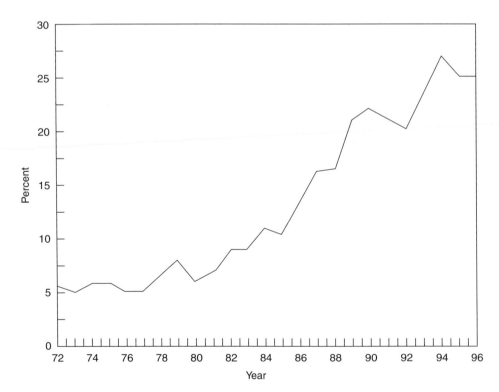

FIGURE 4.4   Proportion of salmonella isolations from human sources reported to the CDC that were *Salmonella* Enteritidis, by year, 1972–96.

(10%), and 77 deaths (0.3%). Reported outbreaks occurred most frequently in restaurants and other commercial food establishments but also occurred in hospitals, nursing homes, schools, camps, and prisons, as well as private gatherings, including at homes (Mishu et al., 1994). Most of those who died were in hospitals and nursing homes (Levine et al., 1991). Eggs alone or egg-containing foods were implicated in 233 (79%) of the 293 outbreaks with known vehicles. Many of these egg-associated outbreaks were traced back to their farm of origin and have demonstrated that infected hens were the source of the outbreak. For example, during 1990 and 1991, in 18 outbreaks in which eggs were implicated as the source, the predominant human outbreak phage type was also recovered from the environment in 100% and from internal organs in 88% of implicated flocks.

Further evidence that many human *S.* Enteritidis infections are caused by contaminated shell eggs is provided from investigations of persons with *S.* Enteritidis infections that were not recognized as belonging to an outbreak. Case-control studies of sporadic cases of *S.* Enteritidis were conducted in Minnesota in 1989–90 (Hedberg et al., 1993), in New York in 1989 (Morse et al., 1994), and in California in 1994 (Passaro et al., 1996). Each study found that eating raw or undercooked eggs was the most important risk factor for acquiring *S.* Enteritidis infections. In addition, in Minnesota the extent to which eggs were undercooked was directly associated with the likelihood of becoming infected.

EMERGENCE AND SPREAD OF *SALMONELLA* ENTERITIDIS PHAGE TYPE 4

Perhaps the most alarming recent development in the epidemiology of *S.* Enteritidis in the United States is the emergence and spread of phage type 4 (PT4). Although PT4 is apparently similar to other phage types that cause little or no mortality in poultry, PT4 is remarkable in its ability, once it is introduced into poultry, to cause marked increases in human illness. *Salmonella* Enteritidis PT4 caused tremendous increases in human salmonella infections in Europe, increasing illness rates by fivefold in some countries (Rodrigue et al., 1990). In many countries, PT4 has replaced all other phage types in poultry populations, but the reasons for the marked increased human illness are not fully understood.

The phage types most commonly associated with human outbreaks in the United States are PT8, PT13a, and PT13 (Altekruse et al., 1993; Mishu et al., 1994). The first recognized outbreaks of *S.* Enteritidis PT4 in the United States not associated with foreign travel occurred in Texas in 1993 (Boyce et al., 1996). The outbreaks were caused by contaminated shell eggs. The source of the eggs was not established, but they may have originated in Mexico. In 1994, *S.* Enteritidis PT4 was also isolated from a poultry farm in southern California, the first time PT4 was isolated

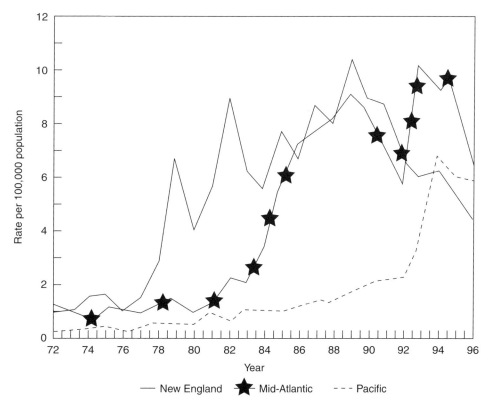

FIGURE 4.5   Isolation rate for *Salmonella* Enteritidis from human sources (per 100,000 population) reported to the CDC, by region and year, 1972–96.

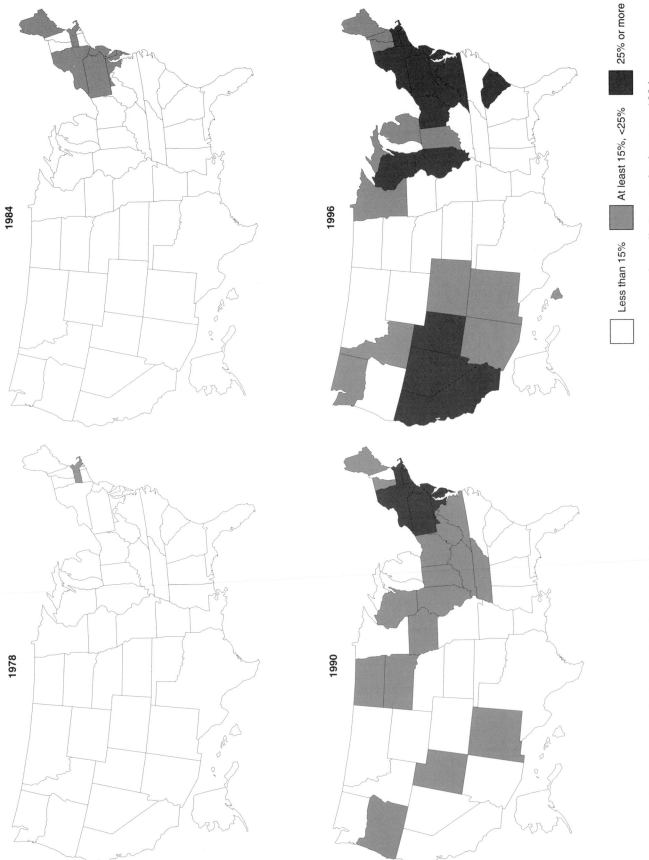

FIGURE 4.6 Proportion of salmonella isolations from human sources reported to the CDC that were *Salmonella* Enteritidis, by state, 1996.

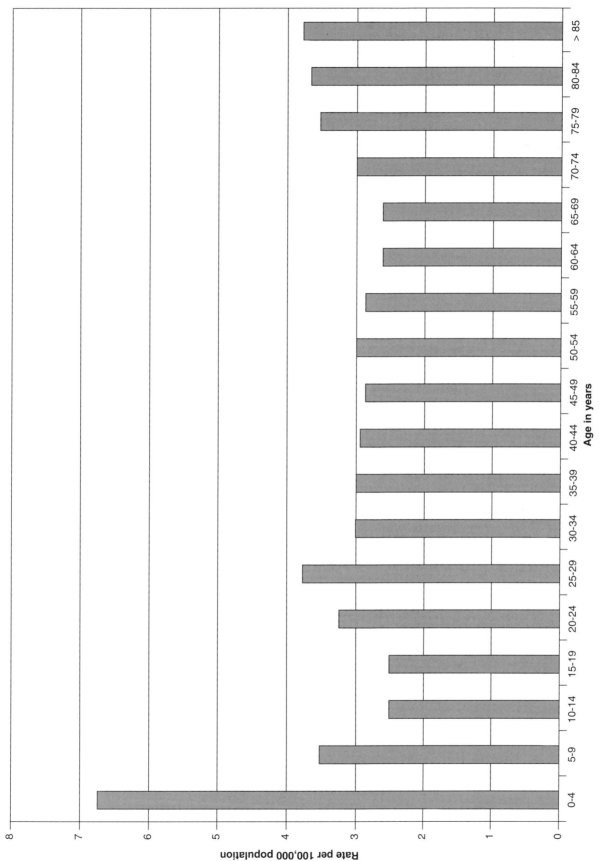

FIGURE 4.7 Salmonella isolations from human sources by age, reported to the CDC, 1996.

TABLE 4.1 *Salmonella* **Enteritidis outbreaks, United States, 1985–96**

Year	No. of outbreaks	No. of patients	No. hospitalized	No. of deaths
1985	26	1159	144	1
1986	47	1444	107	6
1987	53	2511	544	15
1988	42	995	145	11
1989	77	2467	179	14
1990	70	2327	295	3
1991	68	2398	158	5
1992	59	2438	232	4
1993	63	2217	214	6
1994	47	5198	215	2
1995	57	1320	118	8
1996	51	1461	157	2
Total	660	25,935	2508	77

from poultry in the United States (Passaro et al., 1996). Since then, PT4 has caused large increases in human illness in California. PT4 has recently also been reported from Arizona and Nevada, and emerged in Utah in 1995 and Hawaii 1996, where again it has caused marked, fourfold to fivefold, increases in human illness. The documentation of epidemic increases of *S.* Enteritidis PT4 in several western states associated with people eating shell eggs, and the isolation of this strain from poultry in the United States, suggest that this major public health problem will persist and may spread to other regions of the country.

SUMMARY

In recent years, human illness caused by *S.* Enteritidis has increased dramatically in the United States and throughout the world. Consumption of undercooked or raw shell eggs is the dominant source of *S.* Enteritidis infections involved in both outbreaks and sporadic cases. Emergence of *S.* Enteritidis appears to be primarily due to the acquired ability of *S.* Enteritidis to infect the hen's ovary and thereby infect intact shell egg. Recent increases in human illness, particularly in the western United States, are associated with the introduction and spread of *S.* Enteritidis PT4. Consumers can reduce their risk of becoming infected with *S.* Enteritidis by not eating undercooked or raw eggs. Control of *S.* Enteritidis, however, will require preventing infections in the chickens, egg-laying and broilers, themselves.

REFERENCES

Altekruse, S., Koehler, J., Hickman-Brenner, F., Tauxe, R.V., and Ferris, K. 1993. A comparison of *Salmonella enteritidis* phage types from egg-associated outbreaks and implicated laying flocks. Epidemiol. Infect. 110:17–22.

Altekruse, S.F., and Swerdlow, D.L. 1996. The changing epidemiology of foodborne diseases. Am. J. Med. Sci. 311:23–29.

Bean, N.H., Goulding, J.S., Lao, C., and Angulo, F.J. 1996. Surveillance for foodborne disease outbreaks: United States, 1993–1996. MMWR Surveill. Summ. 45:1–67.

Boyce, T.G., Koo, D., Swerdlow, D.L., Gomez, T.M., Serrano, B., Nickey, L.N., Hickman-Brenner, F.W., Malcom, G.B., and Griffin, P.M. 1996. Recurrent outbreaks of *Salmonella* Enteritidis infections in a Texas restaurant: phage type 4 arrives in the United States. Epidemiol. Infect. 117:29–34.

Chalker, R.B., and Blaser, M.J. 1988. A review of human salmonellosis. III. Magnitude of *Salmonella* infection in the United States. Rev. Infect. Dis. 9:111–124.

Cohen, M.L., and Tauxe, R.V. 1986. Drug-resistant *Salmonella* in the United States: an epidemiologic perspective. Science 234:964–969.

Council for Agricultural Science and Technology. 1994. Foodborne pathogens: risks and consequences. Task Force Report 122. Ames: Iowa State University Press.

Hargrett-Bean, N.T., Pavia, A.T., and Tauxe, R.V. 1988. *Salmonella* isolates from humans in the United States, 1984–1986. MMWR Surveill. Summ. 37(SS-2):25–31.

Hedberg, C.W., David, M.J., White, K.E., MacDonald, K.L., and Osterholm, M.T. 1993. Role of egg consumption in sporadic *Salmonella enteritidis* and *Salmonella typhimurium* infections in Minnesota. J. Infect. Dis. 167:107–111.

Humphrey, T.J., Baskerville, A., Mawer, S.L., Rowe, B., and Hopper, S. 1989. *Salmonella enteritidis* PT4 from the contents of intact eggs: a study involving naturally infected hens. Epidemiol. Infect. 103:415–423.

Levine, W.C., Smart, J.F., Archer, D.L., Bean, N.H., and Tauxe, R.V. 1991. Foodborne disease outbreaks in nursing homes, 1975 through 1987. JAMA 266:2105–2109.

Mishu, B., Koehler, J., Lee, L.A., Rodrigue, D., Brenner, F.H., Blake, P., and Tauxe, R.V. 1994. Outbreaks of *Salmonella enteritidis* infections in the United States, 1985–1991. J. Infect. Dis. 169:547–552.

Morse, D.L., Birkhead, G.S., Guardino, J., Kondracki, S.F., and Guzewich, J.J. 1994. Outbreak and sporadic egg-associated cases of *Salmonella enteritidis*: New York experience. Am. J. Public Health 84:859–860.

Passaro, D.J., Reporter, R., Mascola, L., Kilman, L., Malcolm, G.B., Rolka, J., Werner, S.B., and Vugia, D.J. 1996. Epidemic *Salmonella enteritidis* infection in Los Angeles County, California: the predominance of phage type 4. West. J. Med. 165:126–130.

Rodrigue, D.C., Tauxe, R.V., and Rowe, B. 1990. International increase in *Salmonella enteritidis*: a new pandemic? Epidemiol. Infect. 105:21–27.

St. Louis, M.E., Morse, D.L., Potter, M.E., DeMelfi, T.M., Guzewich, J.J., Tauxe, R.V., Blake, P.A., and the *Salmonella enteritidis* Working Group. 1988. The emergence of grade A eggs as a major source of *Salmonella enteritidis* infections: new implications for control of salmonellosis. JAMA 259:2103–2107.

Thiagarajan, D., Saeed, A.M., and Asem, E.K. 1994. Mechanism of transovarian transmission of *Salmonella enteritidis* in laying hens. Poult. Sci. 73:89–98.

5

Salmonella enterica Serovar Enteritidis in France: Epidemiology, Prevention, and Control

P.A.D. Grimont, P. Bouvet, F. Grimont, and J.-C. Desenclos

INTRODUCTION

France is a founding member of the European Union, and its population is about 58.3 million. The lowest administrative subdivision is the commune (city, town, or village). Communes are grouped in 96 districts called *departments*, which are grouped in 22 *regions*. In addition, there are four overseas departments and four overseas *territories*. In epidemiological studies, overseas departments and territories are usually treated separately from mainland France. They are not considered in this chapter. Corsica is included in mainland France. The most useful administrative subdivision as far as public health is concerned is the department.

Within the European Union (EU), food is exchanged on a large scale by several multinational companies, which commercialize the same food in many different states of the EU. However, cultural differences in Europe explain different patterns of food choice and cooking habits. This is obvious regarding beverage type, cheese type, vegetables, fruits, and seasoning or cooking-oil type. Meat consumption may vary in some aspects (for example, horse or rabbit meat, and degree of meat cooking) and not in others (for example, chicken and other poultry consumption, or eggs and egg-containing products). Since the large pandemics of *Salmonella enterica* serovar Enteritidis were associated with chicken and eggs, very few epidemiological differences are to be expected among European states in relation to food sources. Surveillance systems and preven-

tive measures, however, differ among states and may result in some epidemiological differences.

The bacterial nomenclature used in this chapter follows the recommendations of Le Minor and Popoff (1987), which considers all named salmonella serovars to belong to *Salmonella enterica* subspecies *enterica*. Therefore, *Salmonella enterica* serovar Enteritidis is referred to as *Salmonella* Enteritidis.

HISTORY OF *SALMONELLA* ENTERITIDIS EMERGENCE IN FRANCE

Salmonella Enteritidis (*S.* Enteritidis) isolates have been recovered from human specimens with about the same frequency from 1978 (earliest computerized data) to 1986, with the exception of 1984, when school foodborne outbreaks in the outskirts of Paris were traced to a single caterer. For example, in 1985, *S.* Enteritidis ranked 17th (in order of decreasing frequency), with 215 isolates, while all serovars accounted for 10,068 isolates.

During the summer of 1987, the French National Reference Center for Salmonella informed the health authorities of an increase in *S.* Enteritidis isolations. A total of 998 isolates were reported for 1987, with 65.5% recovered between August and November. Epidemiological investigation by the

Board of Health (Direction Générale de la Santé or DGS) indicated that, between August and November, more than 1064 cases were from outbreaks (40 family outbreaks and 8 outbreaks associated with school or company canteens or cafeterias). Suspected foods contained eggs (for example, eggs, cream, ice cream, pastries, and mayonnaise) and their mode of preparation lacked sufficient heating to kill salmonellae. Departments of health and veterinary authorities were asked to cooperate in the investigation of food production process whenever a particular food was involved in a salmonella outbreak. The isolation rate decreased in December 1987, only to raise again in April 1988, and reached unprecedented levels in the summer. Attention was called to egg products (Olivarås and Hubert, 1988).

In 1988, more than 30 outbreaks were reported, the most serious one occurring in Seine-et-Marne Department, where 80 people developed diarrhea, 23 were hospitalized, and one died, among 100 people who had attended a wedding lunch. Among the suspected food, a cream pastry was proven to be contaminated. The pastry had been made in a shop in Meaux, where employees had also been infected (Hubert, 1988). Other outbreaks involved mayonnaise and other egg products. Three factors likely to make the epidemic durable were (a) that eggs were contaminated by transovarian route (in contrast to the usual cracked-shell route), (b) that hens showed little or no clinical signs (in contrast to serovar Gallinarum infection), and that (c) egg contamination was at a low level and at random, making bacteriological detection more difficult. Health authorities considered the situation to be serious (Hubert, 1988).

EPIDEMIOLOGY OF *SALMONELLA* ENTERITIDIS INFECTIONS IN FRANCE: SURVEILLANCE SYSTEMS

Surveillance objectives are (a) to document occurrence and trends of serovars across time and space; (b) to detect local, regional, or national outbreaks; (c) to suggest preventive action; (d) to evaluate the impact of preventive actions; and (e) to be aware of any antibiotic resistance (Desenclos et al., 1996).

Surveillance of salmonella infections in France relies on the cooperation of the following agencies:

The National Reference Centers Located at the Pasteur Institute in Paris

The Pasteur Institute is a private, nonprofit research institute that hosts about half of the 30 French National Reference Centers (NRCs). Besides research, public health activities of the Pasteur Institute are supported in part by the French Ministry of Health. The NRC for Salmonella receives 10,000–15,000 isolates yearly from about 1500 hospital and private laboratories (about one-third of all French clinical laboratories). Referring isolates to the NRC is voluntary. Isolates

must be accompanied by a form on which the following epidemiological information should be provided: date received, patient's name, laboratory name and address, patient's age group, specimen type, date the specimen was taken, patient status (diseased, carrier, or unknown), recent travel history, and epidemiological context, such as isolated case or school, hospital, recreational, day-care, or occupational outbreak. In the case of an outbreak, the suspected food and the approximate number of cases should be indicated.

Full serotyping is performed at the NRC, where all sera are available. The serotyping service is free of charge, provided that some criteria are met: Isolates should be pure cultures of salmonellae recovered from a human clinical specimen or from any specimen (for example, food or environment) in the process of an epidemiological investigation and accompanied by epidemiological information. In addition, the sending laboratory should have attempted agglutination with anti-O:4,5; anti-O:9; and anti-O:6,7,8 sera. These rules are aimed at minimizing reception of inadequate cultures, and about 90% of the cultures received are currently serotyped at no charge. In addition, clinical laboratories are encouraged to send completed epidemiological information forms for those isolates they could completely serotype (for example, serovar Typhimurium). Thus, information on about 15,000 or more salmonella isolates is received at the NRC for *Salmonella* per year.

Output from the NRC for *Salmonella* includes (a) serovar identification returned to the referring clinical laboratory, (b) a daily message to the National Public Health Network (Réseau National de Santé Publique or RNSP) and DGS listing any outbreak mentioned by clinical laboratories, (c) monthly alert statistics indicating numbers of isolates identified with the 60 most frequent serovars (and comparison with the data from the preceding month and preceding year) and sent to the RNSP and DGS, and (d) yearly statistics showing the distribution of about 30,000 isolates (studied at the NRC or at the clinical laboratory level) by serovar and, for each serovar, the distribution by specimen and other sources. This latter document is sent together with the annual report to health authorities and collaborating institutions. Upon request from local or national health authorities or from any clinical laboratory, similar statistics limited to isolates recovered from a French department can be produced.

The NRC for Molecular Typing of Enterics uses several subtyping methods, such as phage typing, ribotyping, IS200 typing, flagellar gene typing, and pulsed-field gel electrophoresis. Typing for epidemiological investigations is free.

A phage-typing system was designed by Vieu et al. (1990) for serovar Dublin and extended to type *S.* Enteritidis. This system consists of 14 bacteriophages that recognize 85 phage types for *S.* Enteritidis and 101 phage types for Dublin. In this system, French phage type (FTP) 33 corresponds to British phage type (BPT) 4.

Réseau National de Santé Publique

The RNSP coordinates nationally the surveillance of infectious diseases and outbreak investigations. The mission of the RNSP is to provide, through these activities, timely epidemiological data for health authorities at the national or department level to guide control-and-prevention activities. It works closely with the national and district health authorities (see below) and the NRC.

In the field of salmonellae, the RNSP centralizes and analyzes mandatory reports of foodborne outbreaks, of which 70% are caused by salmonellae. By law, any physician must notify the health department authorities of the communicable diseases that are listed as notifiable. Each outbreak, particularly foodborne outbreaks, should be investigated by the department health authority and then reported to the RNSP. The RNSP also coordinates epidemiological investigations of community outbreaks occurring over a large geographical area. The RNSP is usually notified by the NRCs about salmonella outbreaks and then leads a descriptive study and an investigation aimed at generating hypotheses about possible sources and vehicles of infection. Case-control studies are then designed to test the hypotheses.

Direction Générale de la Santé of the Ministry of Health and Its Decentralized Services

The DGS is responsible for decision making in the area of disease control and prevention. In each department, the missions of the DGS are implemented by a decentralized public health service under its authority, the Departmental Board of Health and Social Services (Direction Départementale de l'Action Sanitaire et Sociale or DDASS). The public health officers and the sanitary engineers of each DDASS are responsible for the investigation and control of foodborne outbreaks and for forwarding epidemiological information on each outbreak to the RNSP. For salmonella control and prevention in humans, decisions at the national level are based on the data forwarded by the RNSP and the NRC. For the control of salmonella infection in humans, the DGS works closely with the Food and Drug Administration (Direction Générale de l'Alimentation or DGAL) of the Ministry of Agriculture and the Ministry of Consumption and Fraud Control (Direction Générale de la Concurrence et de la Répression des Fraudes or DGCCRF) of the Ministry of Finance and their respective decentralized services in each department (see below).

Direction Générale de l'Alimentation of the Ministry of Agriculture and Its Decentralized Services

This central administration of the Ministry of Agriculture is responsible for the veterinary control of foods (meat, fish, vegetables, and so on) from production to distribution (for example, farms, slaughterhouses, and wholesalers). At the department level, the policy of the DGAL is implemented by decentralized services of the Ministry of Agriculture: the Departmental Board of Veterinary Services (Direction Départementale des Services Vétérinaires or DDSV), which is under the authority of the DGAL (one in

each department). The public health veterinarians of the DDSV collaborate with the public health officers of the DDASS in the investigation of foodborne outbreaks (veterinary investigation). The prevention and control of salmonellosis caused by *S.* Enteritidis in the poultry industry is under the responsibility of the DGAL and the DDSV.

Direction Générale de la Consommation de la Concurrence et de la Répression des Fraudes and Its Decentralized Services

This administration of the Ministry of Finance has responsibility for the control of quality and labeling of goods (including foods) that are marketed to the public (shops, groceries, supermarkets, and restaurants). This administration is represented by its own services in each department and participates in the control and prevention of *S.* Enteritidis infection, although to a lesser extent than the DGAL and DGS.

Centre National d'Études Vétérinaires et Alimentaires

The National Center for Veterinary Sciences (Centre National d'Études Vétérinaires et Alimentaires or CNEVA) serotypes salmonella isolates recovered from diseased animals or systematic samples, food, or equipment and animal/food environment (for example, a slaughterhouse or farm). Serotyping is done either at the request of authorities (regarding, for instance, investigations and seized food) or agro-industries in the framework of quality assurance.

At the European level, the French NRC for Salmonella and RNSP participate in Salm-Net, a concerted action supported by Directorate General XII of the EU. Epidemiological data on salmonellae obtained from NRCs are pooled and used to document epidemiological trends and detect interstate outbreaks. Messages are frequently exchanged by fax or the Internet about travel-associated salmonellosis or cases linked to imported food.

DEMOGRAPHIC CHARACTERISTICS OF AFFECTED POPULATIONS

Yearly Variations

The evolution of reporting *S.* Enteritidis and other salmonella serotypes to the NRC (isolates studied at the NRC and notification of isolates identified in local laboratories) is shown in Figure 5.1 for the decade 1986–96. Obviously, in spite of all actions taken by health authorities, *S.* Enteritidis occurred in France much more often in 1996 than in 1986.

Most isolates probably represent a single strain. Phage typing of 710 isolates recovered from 1993 to 1996 showed that 88.6% of isolates belong to FPT33, 1.8% belong to FPT32, 1.4% belong to FPT45, 1.1% belong to

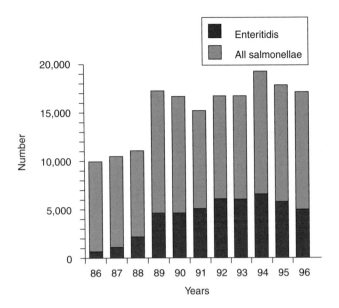

FIGURE 5.1   Annual occurrence of salmonellae and *Salmonella* Enteritidis in France, 1986–96.

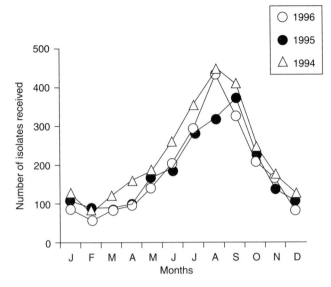

FIGURE 5.2   Seasonal distribution of *Salmonella* Enteritidis in France, 1994–96 (isolates studied at national reference centers).

FPT30, and 0.8% belong to FPT35. Other phage types were represented by less than 0.5% of isolates. Unpublished correlation studies between the British and French phage-typing systems showed FPT33 and FPT32 to correspond to BPT4 and FPT35 to correspond to BPT8.

In our hands, molecular typing systems have not been very successful in subtyping FPT33. Six isolates from human and animal sources showed one restriction pattern of the 38-MDa virulence plasmid. For FPT32, two isolates showed different plasmid restriction patterns and 10 isolates had no plasmid (F. Grimont, unpublished).

Seasonal Variations

Salmonella infections have a strong seasonal variation in France, with a low level from January to May and a peak from July to November (maximum in August–September). The peak height is usually two or three times the value of the lowest level (Fig. 5.2).

Geographical Distribution

The *S.* Enteritidis to all serovars ratio (pooled data, 1994–96) varies widely from one department to another (Fig. 5.3). Understanding these variations would require a study on the implantation of major food-store chains and their buying policies (that is, local or national choice of suppliers, diversity of suppliers, and so on) in addition to consumers' preferences (farm products or brand names).

Male–Female Ratio

The gender of patients has only been recorded since 1 January 1996. In 1996, the male–female ratio was 0.98 for *S.* Enteritidis infections (for 8.7%, the gender was not recorded) and 1.1 for serovar Typhimurium infections (for 9.0%, the gender was not recorded).

Affected Age Groups

The percentage distributions of patients infected by serovars Typhimurium and Enteritidis and the general French population among age groups are indicated in Figure 5.4. The incidence per million population was much higher for children younger than age 5 than for older people. The male–female ratio (for both Enteritidis and Typhimurium) was examined by age groups (data for 1996): younger than age 1 (ratios of 1.17 and 1.24, respectively), ages 1–5 (1.32 and 1.08), 6–14 (1.14 and 1.29), 15–64 (0.97 and 1.08), and older than age 64 (0.53 and 0.81). These variations are still unexplained.

Commonly Incriminated Food Sources

Foodborne outbreaks of diarrhea caused by *S.* Enteritidis were associated with the consumption of raw or undercooked eggs or egg products, particularly those bought at farms (Lepoutre et al., 1994). An investigation of four outbreaks in Haute-Vienne Department incriminated "Chantilly" cream, cream for pastry, and mayonnaise. *Salmonella* Enteritidis FPT33 was found in eggs. A search for salmonellae at the farms that had provided the eggs recovered *S.* Enteritidis from 10 of 45 eggs (white, yolk, or shell), from cloacae of 3 of 38 hens, and from internal organs of 13 of 35 hens that were killed. No lesion was significantly associated with the presence of *S.* Enteritidis. Hens were thus the carriers (Nicolas et al., 1991).

To understand sporadic cases in young children, a national case-control study was conducted in France among young children (age 5 years or younger) in 1995 (Delarocque-Astagneau et al., 1997). The study showed that consumption of raw, undercooked eggs or food containing raw or lightly cooked eggs (for example, homemade mayonnaise or chocolate mousse) was a risk factor.

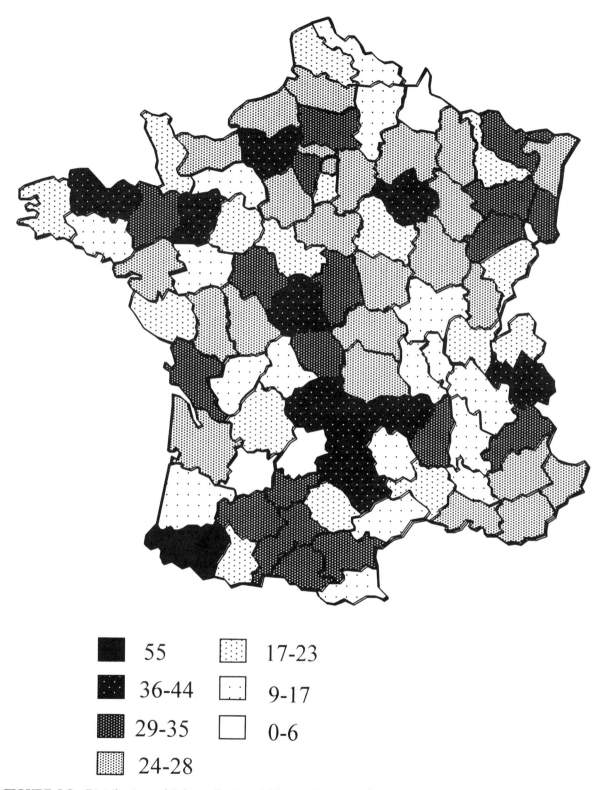

■	55	▦	17-23
■	36-44	⬚	9-17
▦	29-35	☐	0-6
▦	24-28		

FIGURE 5.3 Distribution of *Salmonella* Enteritidis to all salmonella serovars among the French Departments, 1994–96. Rates are given in percentage. Corsica had a rate of 24%–28%.

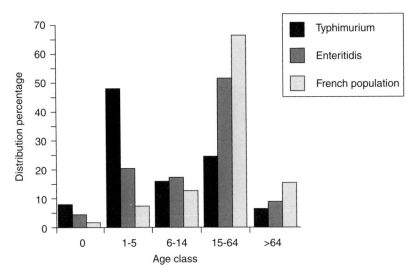

FIGURE 5.4 Percentage distribution of infected patient age classes (serovars *Salmonella* Typhimurium and *S.* Enteritidis) compared with the general French population.

The study also documented the hazard of prolonged egg storage, particularly during the summer. Parents' consumption of ready-to-eat chicken was also a risk factor for infection in children. This finding may suggest within-home contamination (Delarocque-Astagneau et al., 1997).

Salmonella Enteritidis isolates identified by the CNEVA in 1994–95 were often recovered from chicken or egg products (Brisabois et al., 1996). Of 938 *S.* Enteritidis isolates from animals, 70.6% were from chicken and eggs, 11.3% from duck, and 6.3% from turkey. Of 1056 *S.* Enteritidis isolates from food, 56.6% were from chicken (meat and offal), 6.9% from prepared food containing chicken or eggs, 3.7% from pastry, and 20.0% from egg products. Of 917 environmental *S.* Enteritidis isolates, 88.5% were from henhouses and 6.9% from hatcheries (Brisabois et al., 1996). *Salmonella* Enteritidis represented 19.9% of all 4340 salmonella isolates from poultry and 27.3% of all 2426 salmonella isolates from chicken. This serovar represented 12.6% of 4748 isolates from poultry meat, carcasses, and offal, and 17% of chicken meat, carcasses, and offal. This serovar represented 50.9% of 511 salmonella isolates from eggs and egg-containing food (Brisabois et al., 1996).

The CNEVA has tested salmonella isolates for susceptibility to ampicillin, streptomycin, gentamycin, tobramycin, amikacin, kanamycin, neomycin, chloramphenicol, tetracycline, trimethoprim-sulfamethoxazole, nalidixic acid, and flumequine. *Salmonella* Enteritidis isolated from animals, foods, and the environment were mostly (94.5%) susceptible to all of the aforementioned antibiotics (Brisabois et al., 1996).

When the estimated annual number of cases of salmonellosis (30,000 to 150,000) is compared with the annual number of eggs eaten in France (14 billion), the maximum risk is about 1 per 100,000 eggs.

PREVENTION

Egg Production Level

A working group has been assembled by the Ministry of Agriculture with representatives from different branches of the egg production industry, Ministry of Health, and Ministry of Consumption and Fraud Control. A convention was signed between government representatives and egg producers, whereby the state would compensate the producers for the eradication of infected flocks and would reimburse associated laboratory costs. This working group produced a "code of good practice" for the egg production industry: selection of breeder flocks, egg production flocks, animal food, and egg products (Hubert 1988; Hubert et al., 1989). This included the following recommendations:

Increased controls on animal foods and raw products

For French selection-breeder flocks (80% of the market), an official hygienic and sanitary control program aimed at preventing serovar Gallinarum had been working for more than 20 years. This program included general sanitary measures and the serological control of all animals. For imported fertilized eggs or 1-day chicks, bacteriological and serological controls have to be done during quarantine. All these controls now extended to include *S.* Enteritidis were increased and enforced. Contaminated flocks must be destroyed.

For layer flocks, a follow-up protocol was set up. This concerned chicken coop and layer henhouse and included general sanitary protection and hygiene measures, bacteriological screening at regular intervals, and destruction of contaminated flocks. Since May 1989, eggs from flocks found to be infected have been diverted to pasteurization plants or the flock has been destroyed (Watier et al., 1993). In 1989, for example, eggs were diverted to pasteurization plants for six flocks while three flocks were destroyed.

For the egg-product industry: systematic examination of imported eggs and egg products, extension of pasteurization.

About 20% of eggs are from family layer farms and these might escape the above-mentioned regulations.

Collective Eating-Place Level

In 1989, the DGAL sent the following recommendations to directors of commercial catering outlets:

—Eggs should be traceable to registered packing plants;
—Eggs should be stored in a cold room;
—Egg shell should show no cracks and be clean: shells should be washed before storage;
—Egg-containing preparations that cannot be cooked (mayonnaise, cream) should be prepared a short time before use. Leftovers should be discarded;
—Industrial mayonnaise, pasteurized egg products and egg powders should be used when possible;
—Preparations that can be heated but not boiled (cream, gravy) should be kept at a temperature above 70°C.

Consumer Level

The media provided consumers with advice similar to that which was given to commercial catering outlets. Recommendations to the public also insisted on the storage of risk food (for example, mayonnaise and pastry) in a refrigerator.

To prevent emergence of *S.* Enteritidis and reduce the number of infected birds, a working group composed of health officials and egg producers was set up. Specific recommendations concerning hygiene and poultry health checks were made in 1990 (Watier et al., 1993). Watier et al. (1993), using a deterministic mathematical model with 1989 and 1990 data, showed a limited impact of the measures undertaken to reduce the acceleration of contamination.

An EU regulation (1992) included in the council directive concerning measures for protection against specified zoonoses prescribes control measures aimed at the eradication of both serovars, Enteritidis and Typhimurium. The member states should therefore implement control and prevention measures all along the food chain and must report to the European Commission on a yearly basis the number of infections related to both serovars among humans and animals and in food specimens.

REFERENCES

Brisabois, A., Fremy, S., Moury, F., Oudart, C., Piquet, C., and Pires Gomes, C. 1996. Inventaire des *Salmonella* 1994–1995. Maisons-Alfort, France: Editions CNEVA.

Delarocque-Astagneau, E., Bouvet, P., Grimont, P.A.D., and Desenclos, J.-C. 1997. How young children get *Salmonella* Enteritidis infection in France: a national case-control study. Epidemiol. Infect. (in press).

Desenclos, J.-C., Bouvet, P., Pierre, V., Brisabois, A., Fremy, S., Lahellec, C., Grimont, F., and Grimont, P.A.D. 1996. Epidemiologie des infections à *Salmonella*: tendances recentes en France et en Europe. Bull. Soc. Fr. Microbiol. 11:209–215.

European Union. 1992. Council directive concerning measures for protection against specified zoonoses and specified zoonotic agents in animals and products of animal origin in order to prevent outbreaks of food-borne infections and intoxications. Council Directive 92/117/EEC. Brussels: Commission of the European Communities.

Hubert, B., Maillot, E., Quenum, B., and Massenot, C. 1989. Les infections à *Salmonella enteritidis*. Bull. Epidemiol. Hebdomadaire 16:66–67.

Hubert, J.-C. 1988. Mise au point sur l'Epidemie d'infections à *Salmonella enteritidis*. Bull. Epidemiol. Hebdomadaire 38:151.

Le Minor, L., and Popoff, M.Y. 1987. Request for an opinion: designation of *Salmonella enterica* sp. nov., nom. rev. as the type and only species of the genus *Salmonella*. Int. J. Syst. Bacteriol. 37:465–468.

Lepoutre, A., Salomon, J., Charley, C., and Le Querrec, F. 1994. Les toxi-infections alimentaires collectives en 1993. Bull. Epidemiol. Hebdomadaire 52:245–247.

Nicolas, J.-A., Champagnol, M.-P., Ferial, M.-L., and Mauratille, M. 1991. Toxi-infections alimentaires familiales à *Salmonella enteritidis* en region Limousin. Bull. Epidemiol. Hebdomadaire 16:64–65.

Olivaräs, R., and Hubert, J.-C. 1988. Les infections à *Salmonella enteritidis* en 1987. Bull. Epidemiol. Hebdomadaire 26:101.

Vieu, J.F., Jeanjean, S., Tournier, B., and Klein, B. 1990. Application d'une serie unique de bacteriophages à la lysotypie de *Salmonella* serotype Dublin et de *Salmonella* serotype Enteritidis. Med. Mal. Infect. 20:229–233.

Watier, L., Richardson, S., and Hubert, B. 1993. *Salmonella enteritidis* infections in France and the United States: characterization by a deterministic model. Am. J. Public Health 83:1694–1700.

6

Ups and Downs of *Salmonella enterica* Serovar Enteritidis in Germany

H. Tschäpe, A. Liesegang, B. Gericke, R. Prager, W. Rabsch, and R. Helmuth

INTRODUCTION AND HISTORY

Prior to 1984, strains of *Salmonella enterica* serovar Enteritidis (*S.* Enteritidis) occurred only rarely and sporadically among people in Germany. Beef and pork were found to be the most frequent source of infection, and occasionally poultry was implicated. In 1972, an increase in the incidence of *S.* Enteritidis was recorded. These *S.* Enteritidis isolates originated in calves and were transmitted via beef to consumers. Since 1972, a rapid increase in *Salmonella typhimurium* (*S. enterica* serovar Typhimurium) had also been registered, and the overall percentage of *S.* Enteritidis remained low. In contrast to serovar Typhimurium strains, which increased continuously with the incidence of salmonellosis, serovar Enteritidis strains began disappearing from the "salmonella landscape" in 1973 and continued to be a clinical and epidemiological rarity in Germany until 1984 (Fig. 6.1). At that time, *S.* Enteritidis was not further subtyped or characterized by phage typing, genotyping, or electrotyping, although occasionally subtyped by antibiogram, plasmid profile, or distinct fermentative properties.

Suddenly, in 1984, outbreaks and sporadic cases of salmonellosis caused by strains of *S.* Enteritidis were recorded with increasing frequency in Germany. Strains of this serovar rose to about 2×10^5 reported cases per year in 1992 and continues to remain the main causative agent of salmonellosis in Germany. Since 1992, the number of cases has been decreasing (Fig. 6.1). Taking into consideration that only approximately 10% of salmonellosis cases are reported to public health authorities, the true number of *S.* Enteritidis infections must rank between 1 and 2 million cases per year in Germany. The decreasing tendency shown in Figure 6.1 together with other findings help to predict that, within the next couple of years, *S.* Enteritidis will probably decline to its former level. Such a sudden increase and the currently observed decrease in the incidence of a distinct salmonella serovar unregistered before in Germany (exceptions might come from serovar Typhimurium) has forced intensive investigations into the epidemiological and microbiological nature of this process [see Kühn and Tschäpe (1996)].

PROPERTIES AND CLONAL NATURE OF *SALMONELLA* ENTERITIDIS DURING THE NATIONAL EPIDEMIC IN GERMANY

Between 1984 and the present, when strains of *S.* Enteritidis became the leading serovar in Germany, more than 50,000 isolates of *S.* Enteritidis were definitively typed in both the National Reference Center (NRC) and the National Veterinary Reference Laboratory by phage typing, genotyping, electrotyping, and antibiograms. Whereas all 50,000 of the isolates were phage typed, only a representative number of about 2500 were genotyped and electrotyped. As predicted epidemiologically, *S.* Enteritidis isolates from this epidemic were mainly identified as one clone (Table 6.1). In particular, phage type 4 (PT4), according to the Ward system (Ward

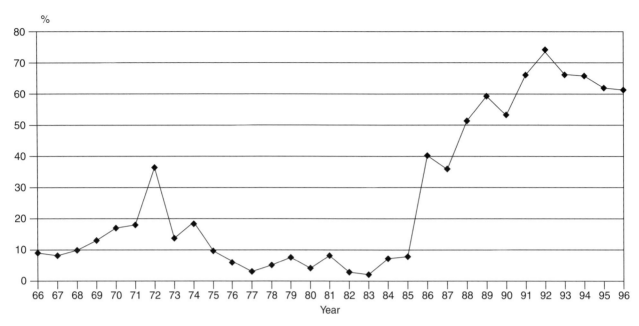

FIGURE 6.1   Incidence of *Salmonella* Enteritidis in Germany, 1966–96.

et al., 1994), was found in an overwhelming majority of cases (Table 6.2), revealing the same restriction fragment length polymorphism (RFLP) genotype of the chromosome as well as IS*200*, enterobacterial repetitive intergenic consensus (ERIC), and ribotype (Table 6.1; Figs. 6.2–6.4). A minority of other phage types, but without a tendency to increase (such as PT6, PT1, PT8, PT21, and PT34; see Table 6.2), have been occurring since 1988. However, genotyping and electrotyping of the non-PT4 strains revealed (with the exception of the PT8, PT13, PT11, and PT34 strains) an identical pattern of RFLP type of chromosome, IS*200*, ERIC, and ribotype, in addition to multilocus enzyme electrophoresis (MLEE) and outer-membrane protein (OMP) type as found among PT4 isolates (Table 6.1; Figs. 6.2–6.4). These phage-type variations (conversions) of the PT4 epidemic clone indicated that temperate phages had spread among PT4 strains and that, in turn, phage-type conversions had occasionally taken place. PT8 and PT13 strains isolated in Germany revealed variations in RFLP (Table 6.1; Fig. 6.2, lane 5) and IS*200* pattern (data not shown), which can be explained as indications of another genotype and another epidemic clone. It is interesting to note that these genotypically different patterns of PT8 and PT13 isolates from Germany were identical to such isolates from the United States and England (Stanley et al., 1992; Mishu et al., 1994; Olsen et al., 1994), which indicates that both are spread worldwide (for epidemiological considerations, see below).

As just mentioned and as shown in Figure 6.1, epidemic *S.* Enteritidis had already been observed in 1972. It was of evolutionary and genetic interest to determine whether the strains that caused the epidemics in 1972–73 and from 1984 to 1997 differed clonally. Surprisingly, the 1972–73 epidemic was caused by *S.* Enteritidis strains of PT4 but with different patterns in chromosomal RFLP (Table 6.1;

Fig. 6.2, lane 1; Fig. 6.3, lane 1; Fig. 6.4, lane 1) and MLEE (Table 6.1). On the one hand, this teaches us that the strains isolated in 1972–73 did not persist and that a new *S.* Enteritidis genotype (clone) carrying the phage pattern typically for PT4 developed that was the causative agent in the epidemic beginning in 1984 (Schroeter et al., 1994; Kühn and Tschäpe, 1996). On the other hand, a phage type such as PT4 can occur in various genotypes, because of the horizontal spread of distinct temperate phages.

Obviously, PT4 is the most frequent phage pattern among *S.* Enteritidis. However, PT4 isolates with different genotypes have not been identified in the national epidemic in Germany. Moreover, isolates with a non-PT4 pattern (for example, PT1, PT21, PT14b, and PT6) have not increased during the national epidemic in Germany (Table 6.2). In addition, a prevailing epidemic spread of PT4 vs non-PT4 strains was found among outbreaks as well as among sporadic cases (discussed later), and PT4 isolates have been the most common type found among various livestock (in particular, poultry), food products (in particular, hens' eggs), and environmental samples. There is no preference of distinct phage types among the non-PT4 strains for distinct epidemic or environmental sources (Table 6.3).

The epidemiologically important role of the epidemic PT4 clone marked with a distinct genotype (see Table 6.1; Figs. 6.2–6.4) points to its probable outstanding virulent makeup (epidemic virulence), which might enable the clone to maintain a continuous long-term epidemic process. Also, the increasing rate of fatal outcome of salmonellosis registered during this national epidemic (Fig. 6.5) might support the hypothesis that the *S.* Enteritidis clone has a distinct epidemic virulence. Investigations into the presence of virulence properties of PT4 strains have not revealed any outstanding features different from

TABLE 6.1 Clonal properties of *Salmonella* Enteritidis in Germany

Phage type/year of isolation/source	PFGE pattern (Fig. 6.2)	ERIC pattern (Fig. 6.3)	IS*200* pattern[a]	Ribotype pattern (Fig. 6.4)	MLEE pattern	OMP pattern
PT4/1984/human	1	1	1	1	1	1
PT4/1988 human	1	1	1	1	1	1
PT4/1992/human	1	1	1	1	1	1
PT4/1996/human	1	1	1	1	1	1
PT4/1988/egg	1	1	1	1	1	1
PT4/1986/chicken	1	1	1	1	1	1
PT4/1996/egg	1	1	1	1	1	1
PT4/1996/human	1	1	1	1	1	1
PT4/1973/human	3	1	1	1	2	1
PT4/1973/human	3	1	1	1	2	1
PT4/1973/calf	3	1	1	1	2	1
PT4/1992/calf	1	1	1	1	1	1
PT4/1992/pig	1	1	1	1	1	1
PT1/1995/human	1	1	1	1	1	1
PT1/1993/egg	1	1	1	1	1	1
PT8/1996/human	2	1	2	1	1	1
PT8/1996/calf	2	1	2	1	1	1
PT13a/1996/human	2	1	2	1	1	1
PT34/1995[b]	5	1	1	1	1	1
PT21/1993/human	1	1	1	1	1	1
PT14b/1995/chicken	1	1	1	1	1	1
PT14b/1996/human	1	1	1	1	1	1
PT14b/1995/chicken	1	1	1	1	1	1
PT6/1990/human	1	1	1	1	1	1
PT6/1990/human	1	1	1	1	1	1
PT6/1990/pig	1	1	1	1	1	1
PT6a/1996/human	1	1	1	1	1	1
PT25/1993/chicken	1	1	1	1	1	1
PT7/1990/human	1	1	1	1	1	1
PT11/1990[b,c]	4	1	3	2	2	1
PT11/1995/dog	4	1	3	2	2	1
PT11/1996/pig	4	1	3	2	2	1

ERIC, enterobacterial repetitive intergenic consensus; MLEE, multilocus enzyme electrophoresis; OMP, outer-membrane protein; PFGE, pulsed-field gel electrophoresis.
[a]Data not shown.
[b]Reference strains from PHLS, London Colindale.
[c]To date, not found in human beings.

TABLE 6.2 Percentage of *Salmonella* Enteritidis PT4 isolates in Germany in relation to other phage types

Phage type (total number of strains)	Occurrence (%)						
	1991	1992	1993	1994	1995	1996	Total
PT4 (15852)	79.8	84.1	77.2	78.4	72.8	70.8	78.0
PT1 (451)	2.3	2.0	3.8	1.0	1.3	2.7	2.2
PT8 (1007)	8.8	2.7	7.4	4.5	3.9	3.2	5.0
PT6 (492)	0.7	1.4	1.8	2.3	5.1	4.6	2.4
PT21 (172)	0.1	0.1	0.0	2.2	0.8	2.6	0.8
PT14b (163)	0.0	0.0	0.0	0.0	4.0	1.9	0.8
PT7 (284)	0.1	0.0	1.1	1.8	2.7	4.1	1.4
PT25 (605)	5.4	3.5	1.6	2.1	1.6	2.5	3.0
Other PTs[a] (1295)	3.2	5.3	7.0	7.7	7.8	7.6	6.4

[a]The number of other phage types, such as PT34, PT13, and PT36, increased from 1991 to 1996 in the following manner: 20 phage types in 1991, 28 phage types in 1992, 33 phage types in 1993, 36 phage types in 1994, 32 phage types in 1995, and 28 phage types in 1996.

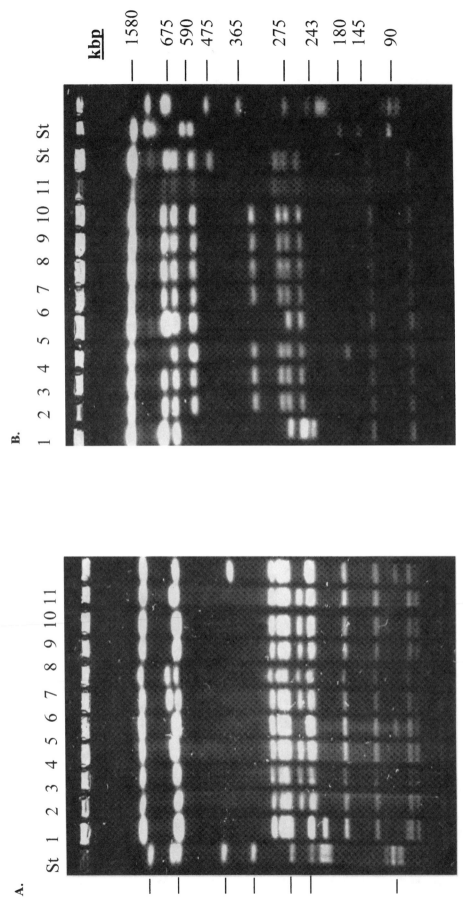

FIGURE 6.2 Restriction fragment length polymorphism of chromosomal DNA from *Salmonella* Enteritidis isolates. **A.** DNA digested with *XbaI*; **B.** DNA digested with *BlnI*.

54

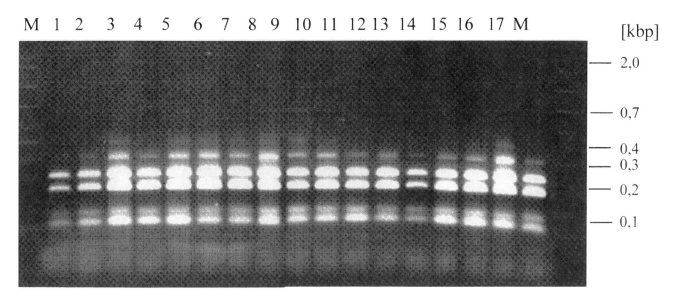

FIGURE 6.3 Enterobacterial repetitive intergenic consensus (ERIC) PCR pattern of *Salmonella* Enteritidis isolates.

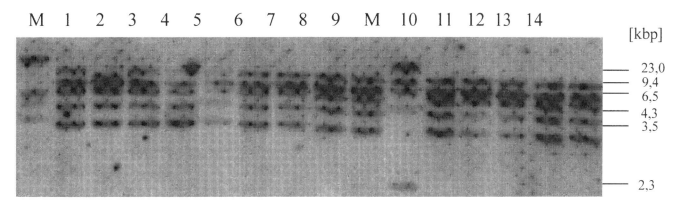

FIGURE 6.4 Ribotype of *Salmonella* Enteritidis isolates.

those of other *S.* Enteritidis strains or other respective serovars, such as Typhimurium. The PT4 clone reveals a relatively high production of salmonella enterotoxin, which is common among epidemic strains, and it contains determinants for both *Sef* and *Pef* fimbriae (Bäumler et al., 1997). Whether the joint presence of *Pef* and *Sef* fimbria among the epidemic clone will characterize its outstanding epidemic virulence remains unresolved for the time being. Further studies are needed, in particular among *S.* Typhimurium epidemic strains.

With regard to antibiotic resistance, it is remarkable that drug-resistant isolates have rarely occurred among the epidemic clone of *S.* Enteritidis in Germany irrespective of the various phage types. Most of the *S.* Enteritidis strains remain sensitive or resistant to only a single antimicrobial agent, such as sulfonamide (about 12%), streptomycin (about 15%), or ampicillin (about 8%) (Fig. 6.6). Multiple drug resistance of the epidemic clone (2%–5% without increasing frequency between 1990 and now) was found mostly to be associated with the occurrence of transferable

plasmids, such as members of the I1, Z, H1, and FII incompatibility groups. A representative number of plasmids encoding the most common drug-resistance patterns among *S.* Enteritidis isolates (PT4, PT1, PT6, and so on) observed in Germany are summarized in Table 6.4.

In summary, the national *S.* Enteritidis epidemic in Germany was caused by the spread of a distinct epidemic clone (defined by the pattern of properties presented in Table 6.1) that occurs in many European countries and most probably those throughout the countries of the northern hemisphere.

SOURCES AND EPIDEMIC SPREAD OF *SALMONELLA* ENTERITIDIS IN GERMANY

As just described and as presented in Figure 6.1, strains of *S.* Enteritidis were without epidemiological significance

TABLE 6.3 Frequency and sources of PT4 isolates in Germany[a]

Phage type	Year	Human	Cattle	Pig	Chicken	Hen's egg	Waterfowl	Other animals	Food (egg containing)	Meat/sausage	Total	%
4	1991	2726	14	0	179	24	7	16	13	7	2993	79.8
	1992	3492	46	10	239	100	30	42	136	47	4195	84.1
	1993	1748	48	17	179	75	29	39	112	119	2423	77.2
	1994	1337	83	6	198	109	33	34	125	190	2193	78.4
	1995	963	67	3	343	118	149	48	27	26	1809	73.2
	1996	997	74	27	510	138	145	38	40	37	2054	71.7
25	1991	190	0	0	7	5	0	0	2	0	204	5.4
	1992	144	2	1	13	4	0	3	3	1	173	3.5
	1993	30	0	0	8	2	1	0	5	3	51	1.6
	1994	32	0	0	20	3	0	0	0	2	58	2.1
	1995	23	0	0	3	2	0	1	5	2	42	1.7
	1996	31	0	0	22	12	0	0	1	5	73	2.5
8	1991	257	30	3	6	1	0	4	11	1	314	8.4
	1992	93	28	2	6	1	1	2	1	2	136	2.7
	1993	150	7	3	28	11	0	7	2	11	232	7.4
	1994	58	25	1	12	4	6	15	2	2	127	4.5
	1995	47	18	0	7	4	3	9	1	3	97	3.9
	1996	40	5	2	29	4	6	0	0	1	88	3.1
1	1991	79	0	0	1	1	0	7	0	0	88	2.3
	1992	88	0	2	3	0	1	0	6	1	102	2.0
	1993	108	4	1	2	0	0	0	0	1	118	3.8
	1994	18	2	1	0	0	0	2	3	2	28	1.0
	1995	12	0	0	12	3	0	0	1	1	31	1.3
	1996	51	0	0	23	1	0	7	0	2	84	2.9
6	1991	28	0	0	0	0	0	0	0	0	28	0.7
	1992	63	0	1	0	1	0	1	3	0	70	1.4
	1993	46	1	0	4	1	0	0	1	4	58	1.8
	1994	54	0	0	0	3	0	0	3	2	63	2.3
	1995	65	5	0	27	5	8	1	2	1	121	4.9
	1996	58	1	2	52	5	7	3	4	1	133	4.6

[a]As communicated to both the National Reference Center and the National Veterinary Reference Laboratory.

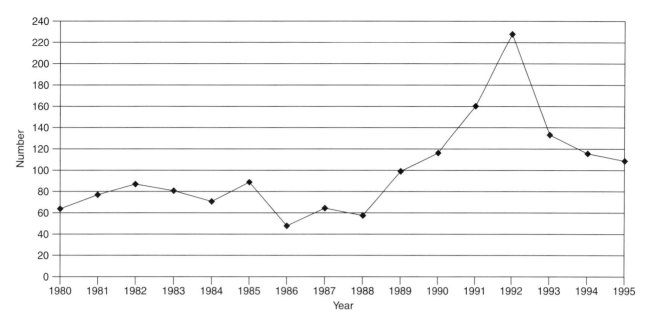

FIGURE 6.5   Fatal outcome of *Salmonella* Enteritidis infections in Germany, 1980–95.

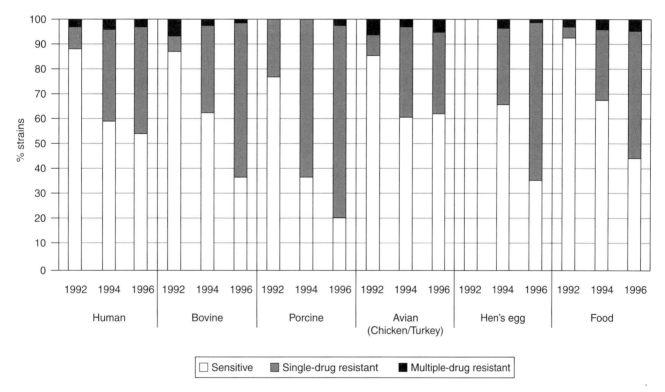

FIGURE 6.6   Antibiotic resistance patterns among *Salmonella* Enteritidis isolates, 1990–96.

before 1984. At the end of 1984, however, about 65 cases of *S.* Enteritidis occurred in Wandersleben, a little town in the German state of Thuringia, among people who shared a canteen meal of scrambled eggs. These eggs were traced back to a large egg-producing farm in the area. From this farm, eggs contaminated with *S.* Enteritidis were readily identified, and some of the eggs had to be destroyed. Some weeks later, though, an outbreak of *S.* Enteritidis again occurred among children who had consumed eggs originating from the same farm. This was surprising since, up to that time, *S.* Enteritidis had not occurred via hens' eggs, and the finding of *S.* Enteritidis at the egg-producing

TABLE 6.4   Drug-resistance plasmids of *Salmonella* Enteritidis in Germany

Designation	Inc group	Size (MDa)	Resistance pattern	Source
pIE812	H1	120	ACSSuT	PT4, calf, 1990
pIE1002	FI	75	ACSSuT	PT4, human, 1992
pIE1026	I1	75	ASSuT	PT6, human, 1992
pIE740	I2	58	SSuTp	PT4, chicken, 1993
pIE745	Z	80	CSSuTp	PT1, human, 1995
pIE301	FII	65	T	PT4, human, 1992
pIE302	I1	75	T	PT6, chicken, 1990
pIE303	I1	75	SSuT	PT6, human, 1990
pIE420	X	45	AS	PT4, human, 1996
pIE1027	I1	75	ASSuT	PT8, human, 1992

Inc, incompatibility; MDa, mega-Dalton; A, resistance to ampicillin; C, resistance to chloramphenicol; G, resistance to gentamicin; S, resistance to streptomycin; Su, resistance to sulfonamides; T, resistance to tetracyclines; Tp, resistance to trimethoprim.

farm indicated a massive contamination of the flock. The management decided to destroy more than 1 million eggs and to eradicate the flock. When the freshly installed flock and freshly laid eggs were inspected, it became obvious that the multiplier breeding flock itself was grossly infected. There were, however, no clinical signs or symptoms. Moreover, when other outbreaks of *S.* Enteritidis that were associated with eggs, mayonnaise, ice cream, cooked eggs, and the like occurred at the same time, it turned out that many of the egg-farm flocks had been infected with *S.* Enteritidis.

The public was alarmed when the outbreaks were reported on television or in the newspapers and when politicians and other VIPs were involved. During a religious meditation in the Maria Laach Benedictine monastery (in the Eifel Mountains in Germany), 15 top politicians together with 30 monks in the holy order fell ill with *S.* Enteritidis PT4 after eating pizza prepared with egg yolk. Two elderly monks died, and some of the politicians suffered severe gastroenteritis, including cardiovascular problems or systemic disorders and abdominal cramps. At the same time, in a Veterans Administration Hospital, 100 seniors fell ill with *S.* Enteritidis (PT21) after eating cream pudding prepared with raw egg yolk. As 15 persons died, the outbreak received media attention. Also, the increasing lethality of salmonellosis observed at this time (Fig. 6.5) raised the public awareness of *S.* Enteritidis problems in Germany.

However, outbreaks and other sensational events receiving public attention constituted only 15% of all cases of salmonellosis in Germany. The overwhelming majority of cases were sporadic. Typing and clonal analysis of the isolates from sporadic cases revealed an identical clonal pattern to that of the outbreak strains. Since there was no clonal or phage-type diversity among strains causing outbreaks compared with sporadic cases (as mentioned previously) and since *S.* Enteritidis strains of PT4 were found to be dominant both in outbreaks and in sporadic cases, it was assumed that gross contamination of food (see Tables 6.3, 6.5) with *S.* Enteritidis is the causative event of the current epidemic peak. In turn, individual mistakes in proper and skillful hygienic handling of

food in private kitchens have turned out to be the most common contributing factor in infections.

Since the food chain is the single route of *S.* Enteritidis infections in humans, the high risk of *S.* Enteritidis contamination of chickens, eggs, and other food products in Germany required that this food had to be handled carefully and under specific hygienic conditions. As a consequence of such high risks due to contaminated eggs (Table 6.5), a governmental regulation on the use of eggs in the food industry and in large kitchens was issued, and the consumption of eggs decreased from about 300 to about 200 per head and year (see below).

Beginning in 1988, however, not only eggs but also beef and pork were found to be major sources of human infections, obviously due to cross-contamination. Table 6.3 summarizes the source of *S.* Enteritidis during the past 6 years and, in turn, the large-scale distribution of *S.* Enteritidis in Germany. The epidemic spread of the *S.* Enteritidis clone PT4 was obviously facilitated not only by its persistence among poultry and hens' eggs and the widespread consumption of eggs (Table 6.5) but also by the fact that the healthy human population lacked anti–*S.* Enteritidis antibodies. Figure 6.7 shows that only about 6% of healthy people had anti–*S.* Enteritidis antibodies in 1984, whereas about 35% had antibodies against *Salmonella* serovar Typhimurium. In contrast, 38% of the healthy population had anti–*S.* Enteritidis antibodies in 1995, whereas antibodies to serovar Typhimurium could be detected among only 2%. These findings are in accord with the epidemiological situation presented in Figure 6.1 and with the rather short life span of antisalmonella antibodies. These data also suggest that *S.* Enteritidis will probably decline within the coming years and be replaced by an upcoming epidemic strain, such as *Salmonella* serovar Typhimurium DT104.

The sharply rising incidence of salmonellosis in Germany since 1985 seems to parallel what is happening in other European countries (including Russia) as well as overseas (for example, in the United States, Israel, and Canada). Whereas PT4 strains are occurring mainly in Western and Middle Europe and PT1 strains mainly in Eastern European countries and in Israel, PT8 strains have

TABLE 6.5   Consumption of eggs and risks calculation for *Salmonella* Enteritidis infection in Germany

Consumption	22×10^6 eggs per day in industry
	33×10^6 per day in private households
Number of contaminated eggs	2 per 10^3
Risk calculation	1.1×10^4 per day in industry
	1.7×10^4 per day in private households
Number of exposed people per year	8×10^6
Number of recorded salmonella isolates	$1.0–1.5 \times 10^5$
Number of cases of salmonellosis per year including number of unreported cases	2×10^6

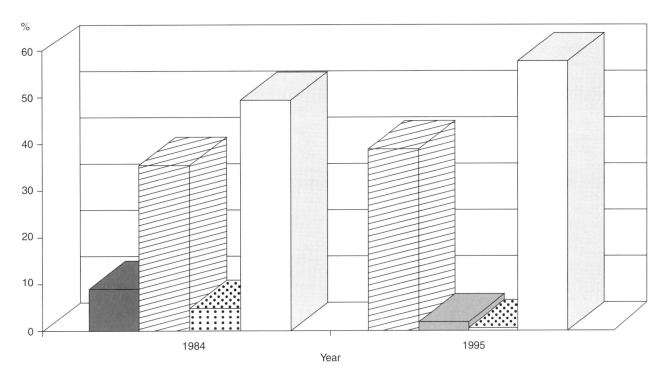

FIGURE 6.7   Prevalence (titers between 1:50 and 1:1000 were taken as positive as measured by ELISA) of antisalmonella antibodies among the healthy human population in Germany, 1984 versus 1995: *white bars,* no relevant antisalmonella antibodies; *black bars,* anti-*Salmonella* Enteritidis (anti-O9/d) antibodies; *lined bars,* anti-*S.* Typhimurium (O4/5) antibodies; and *dotted bars,* antibodies other than *S.* Enteritidis and *S.* Typhimurium.

been distributed mainly in the United States (70%). As indicated by Table 6.1 and Figures 6.2–6.4, the PT8 strains isolated in Germany are of the identical genotype as the U.S. isolates but genotypically different from the PT4 strains in Europe, which, together with epidemiological evidence, speaks in favor of a direct transfer of PT8 strains to Europe (for example, the transfer of *S.* Enteritidis PT8 via turkeys to the Czech Republic).

It is of genetic interest that the other common phage types in the United States (PT13 and PT34) also belong to other genotypes that are different from the European types but very similar to each other. *Salmonella* Enteritidis is most probably disseminated among the various countries

through the transport (import/export) of the chickens themselves. Such an import of *S.* Enteritidis via breeding chickens was directly observed in 1993 when a German layer-flock farm attempted to substitute its *S.* Enteritidis PT4-contaminated flocks with a noncontaminated multiplier breeding flock from South Africa. When the layer flocks were established and began to produce eggs, *S.* Enteritidis PT32 strains were isolated, a phage type that is uncommon in Germany (about 0.03% between 1990 and 1997). This demonstrated that the import/export of multiplier breeding flocks is one of the main epidemic routes of the worldwide spread of *S.* Enteritidis and of the presently rising human incidence of salmonellosis.

TRIALS OF PUBLIC HEALTH CONTROL MEASURES AND OUTLOOK

The epidemiological and laboratory-based evidence about the *S.* Enteritidis epidemics (from 1984 until now) just summarized speaks in favor of a European-wide spread of a distinct *S.* Enteritidis clone: PT4. A minority of other strains carry non-PT4 patterns but an identical genotype and electrotype that originated from poultry and eggs of commercial layer flocks, too. Whereas in Eastern Europe and Israel PT1 strains are the most common phage type but genetically identical to PT4 strains, *S.* Enteritidis isolates carrying the PT8 (or PT13) marker have turned out to reveal another genotype and have been found mainly in the United States. Epidemics caused by PT1 and PT8 strains have also been associated with poultry and egg farming in Israel and the United States, respectively.

In Germany, the overwhelming majority of outbreaks and sporadic cases of *S.* Enteritidis have been associated with the consumption of contaminated hens' eggs. Therefore, antiepidemic measures should be directed at eliminating this source. The evidence of *S.* Enteritidis–contaminated eggs and flocks on egg-layer farms pressed public health authorities and the Federal Ministry of Health to issue regulations for the commercial use of eggs in the food industry and for the distribution of eggs for private use [the decree on hygienic standards on egg-containing products (1993), and the decree on handling and commercial distribution of eggs and egg-containing food products (1994)].

Moreover, programs to educate and train public health officers, physicians, and the general public were established in order to increase the awareness of the risk of consuming raw products (Table 6.5; compare the high rate of egg consumption in Germany). Furthermore, a salmonellosis information sheet for the scientific community was issued by the NRC. However, governmental regulations were not issued prior to 1993–94, when the incidence of *S.* Enteritidis had already begun to decrease (beginning in 1992; see Fig. 6.1). Nevertheless, these regulations might have reinforced the continuing decrease together with a 30% decline in egg consumption by Germans. According to the viewpoint of the NRC, the most striking reason for the continuing decrease in the incidence of *S.* Enteritidis infections in Germany has been the continuing increase in anti–*S.* Enteritidis antibodies among the healthy human population to about 40% (Fig. 6.7). These antibody levels suggest a quite higher contamination rate with *S.* Enteritidis than is indicated by the recorded cases of *S.* Enteritidis infection. The increasing number of anti–*S.* Enteritidis antibodies implies that the spread of *S.* Enteritidis will fail to cause illness because it will face an increasingly immune population.

Since the poultry industry is considered the source of *S.* Enteritidis outbreaks and sporadic cases in Germany, antiepidemic activities can be undertaken on farms to prevent and eliminate *S.* Enteritidis infection in breeding and commercial egg-layer flocks. Vaccination (using living vaccine, such as Zoosaloral) together with hygienic control measures successfully eradicated *S.* Enteritidis from a layer flock in Germany (Meyer and Methner, 1992).

In summary, a number of measures and regulations in Germany, including eradicating *S.* Enteritidis from layer flocks, helped to decrease the incidence of *S.* Enteritidis nationally:

- Better food handling in the home and in food-service establishments
- Improved refrigeration of raw food (in particular, eggs)
- Increased use of pasteurized eggs in institutions
- A program of gradual elimination of the *S.* Enteritidis–infected birds by the replacement of infected flocks with clean pullets, and an effective vaccination of the flocks as well as application of *S.* Enteritidis–free feed and effective rodent and fly control, because mice are a significant risk factor for the spread of *S.* Enteritidis in a flock.

Whereas *S.* Enteritidis infections have decreased in Germany since 1992 and their ongoing decrease within the next couple of years can be predicted, new epidemic salmonella strains are emerging: for example, *S. enterica* serovar Typhimurium phage type DT104, carrying multiple drug resistance. This clone originated among cattle and has been spreading in Germany since 1992 (Liesegang et al., 1997).

REFERENCES

Bäumler, A.J., Gilde, A.J., Tsolis, R.M., van der Velden, A.W.M., Ahmer, B.M.M., and Heffron, F. 1997. A contribution of horizontal gene transfer and deletion events to development of distinctive patterns of fimbrial operons during evolution of *Salmonella* serotypes. J. Bacteriol. 179:317–322.

Kühn, H., and Tschäpe, H., eds. 1996. Salmonellosen des Menschen—Epidemiologische und ätiologische Aspekte. RKI-Schriften, 3/95. Munich: MMV, Medizin-Verlag, 204 pp.

Liesegang, A., Prager, R., Streckel, W., Rabsch, W., Gericke, B., Seltmann, G., Helmuth, R., and Tschäpe, H. 1997. Wird der *Salmonella* enterica-Stamm DT 104 des Serovars Typhimurium der neue führende Epidemietyp in Deutschland? Infektionsepidemiol. Forsch. 1:6–10.

Meyer, H., and Methner, U. 1992. Zur Senkung des Salmonellavorkommens in Tierbeständen mit Hilfe von Immunisierungsmaßnahmen. In: Proceedings of the Third World Congress on Foodborne Infections and Intoxications, 16–19 June 1992, vol. 2, 1011–1015. Berlin: Institute of Medicine–Robert von Ostertag Institute (FAO/WHO Collaborating Center for Research and Training in Food Hygiene and Zoonoses).

Mishu, B., Koehler, J., Lee, L.A., Rodrigue, D., Hickman-Brennert, F., Blake, P., and Tauxe, R.V. 1994. Outbreaks of *Salmonella enteritidis* infections in the United States, 1985–1991. J. Infect. Dis. 169:547–552.

Olsen, J.E., Skov, M.N., Threlfall, E.J., and Brown, D.J. 1994. Clonal lines of *Salmonella enterica* serotype Enteritidis documented by IS*200*-, ribo-, pulsed-field gel electrophoresis and RFLP typing. J. Med. Microbiol. 40:15–22.

Schroeter, A., Ward, L.R., Rowe, B., Protz, D., Hartung, M., and Helmuth, R. 1994. *Salmonella enteritidis* phage types in Germany. Eur. J. Epidemiol. 10:645–648.

Stanley, J., Goldsworthy, M., and Threlfall, E.J. 1992. Molecular phylogenetic typing of pandemic isolates of *Salmonella enteritidis*. FEMS Microbiol. Lett. 90:153–160.

Verordnung über die hygienischen Anforderungen an das Behandeln und Inverkehrbringen vo Hühnereiern und roheihaltigen Lebensmitteln (Hühnerei-Verordnung) v. 05.07.1994, Bundesanzeiger Nr. 124, geändert durch Verordnung v. 16.12.1994. Bundesgesetzblatt I/1994:3837.

Verordnung über die hygienischen Anforderungen an Eiprodukte (Eiprodukt-Verordnung) v. 17.12.1993. Bundesgesetzblatt I/1993:2288–2301.

Ward, L.R., de Sa, J.D.H., and Rowe, B. 1994. A phage typing scheme for *Salmonella enteritidis*. Epidemiol. Infect. 112:25–31.

7

Salmonella enterica Serovar Enteritidis in Denmark

P. Gerner-Smidt and H.C. Wegener

SURVEILLANCE

Human Surveillance System

Salmonellosis is not an individually reportable disease in Denmark, and before 1980 no systematic statistics on its prevalence were available. The first national surveillance report on the prevalence of bacterial enteric zoonoses was made in 1980 and has been published ever since by the Statens Serum Institut. At that time, all stool cultures for enteric pathogens were made at this institute, and the reports included data on all sporadic and epidemic cases. Since then, stool culturing has been partially decentralized to the clinical microbiological laboratories at the hospitals, but the completeness of the statistics had first been secured through a voluntary notification system. Since 1994, however, a mandatory laboratory notification system through the National Board of Health was established.

Based on this system, quarterly reporting on the number of diagnosed cases of salmonellosis and other enteric zoonoses is obtained. Clinical information is not reportable. Information on patients' international travel is available only from patients diagnosed at the Statens Serum Institut and only to the extent that the information has been stated on the clinical information sheet following a patient's specimen sampling. The reporting system does not include a mandatory centralized characterization of strains, either. Only isolates of less common serovars that can not be identified locally, and during outbreaks also common serovars, are sent in to the Danish reference center at Statens Serum Institut for further examination. Thus, information on sporadic salmonellosis caused by *Salmonella enterica* serovar Enteritidis (*S.* Enteritidis) has mostly originated from patient specimens processed at the institute. Today, approximately 75% of all stool cultures are still processed centrally. In 1996, a voluntary strain collection system was established in order to secure a survey reflecting the geographical distribution of the isolates.

Invasive salmonellosis is reported through the same laboratory notification system as for enteric disease, but systematic statistics on systemic disease have not been compiled until now.

Surveillance of Salmonella in Animal and Food Production

Broiler and layer flocks are investigated 2–3 weeks prior to slaughter by culturing of 60 fecal samples per flock, thereby enabling the slaughterhouse to deal with flocks according to their salmonella status. After slaughter, each flock is controlled by the culture of 50 neck-skin samples that are taken from each flock

From 1992 to 1996, flocks of layers were monitored by the culture of 100 cloacal-swab samples a few weeks prior to termination of the laying period (Table 7.1). Since January 1997, flocks of layers have also been monitored by serological analysis of 60 eggs and by culture of 60 fecal samples at approximately 10 and 30 weeks of production and 7–10 weeks prior to termination. Eggs are not systematically cultured in the surveillance system.

TABLE 7.1 Salmonella serovars in Danish layer flocks tested by 100 cloacal-swab samples per flock

	Year			
	1992	1993	1994	1995
No. of flocks tested	320	294	332	339
S. Enteritidis	1	0	8	5
S. Typhimurium	1	4	3	3
Other serovars	6	2	13	10
Total % positive	2.5	2.0	7.2	5.3

The surveillance of salmonellae in pigs and pork is based on a serological test for salmonella-specific antibodies in blood or meat-juice samples and the culture of cuts of fresh pork and offal. Approximately 800,000 samples of meat juice of slaughtered pigs are analyzed serologically per year. Breeding and multiplier herds are tested by 20 monthly blood samples collected at random from animals 4–6 months of age. Slaughter-pig herds are tested by samples of meat juice collected at the slaughterhouse. A central computer system containing the relevant data on all herds determines the number of animals to be tested per quarter for each herd, based on the number of pigs produced by that herd. At the slaughterhouses, a total of 2500 samples of end products of meat and offal are cultured each month according to a specific plan.

Herds of cattle are only investigated for salmonellae on clinical indications. At the slaughterhouses, a total of approximately 250 samples are collected at random each month from a representative sample of the beef cuts and offal.

The Danish Zoonosis Center

The Danish Zoonosis Center is an epidemiological surveillance and research unit that serves as a coordinating body for all institutions involved in research or control of salmonellae and salmonellosis in Denmark. The corresponding administrative boards are affiliated with the center. The surveillance data from the participants are collected and analyzed on a regular basis to prepare a full and collective survey of the incidence of salmonellae and salmonellosis. Based on the conclusions reached, measures to control salmonellosis are proposed or modifications to the existing control programs are suggested.

HUMAN SALMONELLOSIS

Before 1980, S. Enteritidis was the second most prevalent serovar after S. Typhimurium. After 1980, and especially after 1984, a steady increase in the incidence of human salmonellosis has been observed, reaching a maximum of more than 4200 diagnosed cases in 1994 (82.3 cases per 100,000 inhabitants) (Fig. 7.1). Although the total number of diagnosed salmonellosis cases decreased in 1995, S. Enteritidis peaked with 2058 registered cases (41.2 cases per 100,000 inhabitants). In 1996, salmonellosis was still the most common zoonosis, followed closely by campylobacteriosis.

As in other countries, the predominant clinical presentation of salmonellosis, including illness due to S. Enteritidis, is a self-limiting gastroenteritis. Around 5% of salmonellosis cases are extraintestinal, with bacteremia alone accounting for two-thirds of these. The seasonal distribution of S. Enteritidis in Denmark is the same as for most other zoonotic enteric pathogens, that is, low levels in the winter and spring, and more than a doubling of the incidence in the late summer and autumn. Small peaks are seen following all heat waves during the spring and summer, probably reflecting the Danes' predilection for a special cold soup made from buttermilk and raw eggs when the weather is hot. Men and women are affected at an almost equal rate. The age distribution of patients with diagnosed disease due to S. Enteritidis is shown in Figure 7.2.

Larger general outbreaks occur from time to time. In 1996, an outbreak occurred in a small town, with more than 100 people falling ill. This outbreak was unusual in that person-to-person contact seemed to be the main route of transmission. At least three transmission chains were identified. This route of transmission is very uncommon in Denmark. The usual mode of transmission is through ingestion of contaminated food.

SALMONELLAE IN ANIMALS AND FOOD

In 1996, salmonellae were found in 7.6% of 3963 flocks of broilers investigated. However, S. Enteritidis was found in only 0.1%. In layers, salmonellae were detected in 13 (3.1%) of 422 flocks investigated (Table 7.1). Ten of the flocks harbored S. Enteritidis. In 1995, a screening for salmonellae, including 14,800 eggs, found that 1 per 1000 Danish eggs was contaminated, mostly on the shell. Salmonella Enteritidis was the most frequent serovar, and it was the only serovar isolated from the contents of the eggs. The prevalence of salmonellae in Danish pork was 1.3% in 1996, but S. Enteritidis was not detected. Similarly, salmonellae were detected in 0.7% of all beef samples, with no isolations of S. Enteritidis.

PHAGE TYPES

All S. Enteritidis isolated from veterinary and food sources in the surveillance programs are phage typed. Human isolates had been typed irregularly until 1995, when it was decided to type a sample of 25% or at least a monthly number of 25 of all human isolates. The Colindale system is used. The percentage distribution of phage types observed in Danish patients overall and those reporting on international travel is presented in Table 7.2. The predominant phage types 4, 6, and 8 were detected only in layers and eggs in the veterinary and food-control system.

ANTIBIOTIC RESISTANCE

Antibiotic resistance is not a problem in Danish clinical S. Enteritidis isolates. Of 400 human strains investigated in 1995 and 1996, only 23 (6%) showed resistance to at least one of 16 antibiotics tested: ampicillin (A), amoxicillin–clavulanate, mecillinam, cephalothin, streptomycin (S), gentamicin, spectinomycin (Sp), neomycin, apramycin, nalidixic acid, ciprofloxacin, sulfonamides (Su), trimethoprim (Tr), chloramphenicol (C), polymyxins, and tetracycline (T). Multiresistance as defined as resistance to four or more antibiotics was seen in only two strains: one ASSpSuTrCT

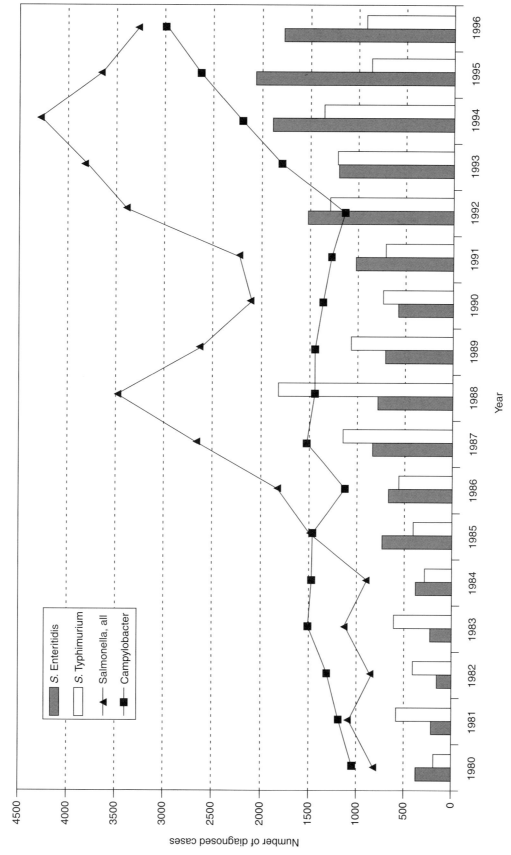

FIGURE 7.1 Human salmonellosis and campylobacteriosis in Denmark, 1980–96.

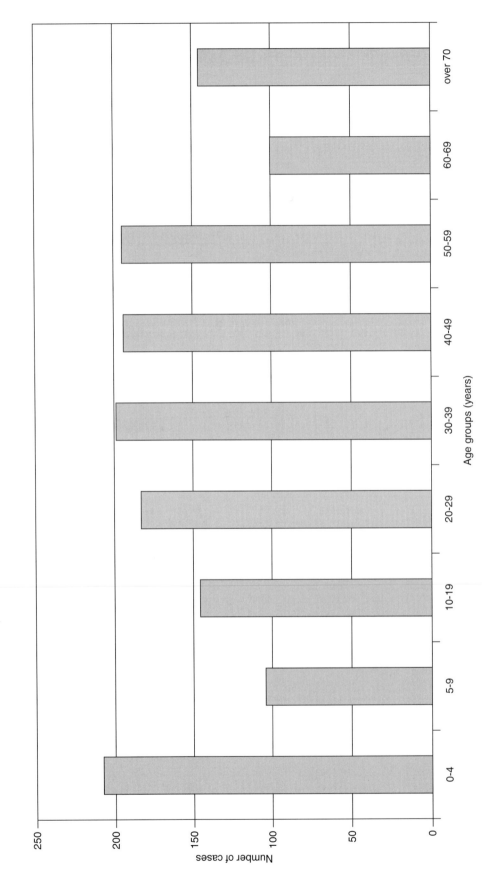

FIGURE 7.2 Age distribution of diagnosed *Salmonella* Enteritidis gastroenteritis in Denmark in 1996.

TABLE 7.2   Distribution of the most common phage types of *Salmonella* Enteritidis in humans in general and in human reporting on international travel in Denmark

Phage type	All patients (%)	Travel (%)
1	3.2	5.5
4	23.0	51.8
6	51.1	24.5
8	15.1	8.2
25	2.4	1.8
No. typed	531	110

and one ASSuTr. Quinolone resistance was seen in only one strain, and this strain was resistant to nalidixic acid but susceptible to ciprofloxacin.

Antimicrobial resistance is also uncommon in Danish poultry isolates of *S.* Enteritidis. Among 29 isolates recovered during 1996, 3% were resistant to ampicillin and 3% were resistant to tetracycline. All isolates were susceptible to amoxycillin–clavulanate, polymyxins, enrofloxacin, gentamicin, neomycin, spectinomycin, streptomycin, and trimethoprim–sulfamethizole.

SOURCES OF HUMAN SALMONELLOSIS

The phage types found predominantly in Danish patients also predominate in Danish layer flocks. *Salmonella* Enteritidis is practically absent from Danish pork and beef. Therefore, raw eggs are assumed to be the main source of human disease caused by *S.* Enteritidis. This assumption is also supported by data from outbreaks. In 28 household outbreaks and 15 general outbreaks investigated in 1996, most cases were associated with ingestion of food products containing raw unpasteurized eggs. Around 400,000 eggs are consumed daily in Denmark. In addition to this, at least 15% of all Danish cases have a history of recent international travel. It is suggested that nearly all cases of *S.* Enteritidis infection in Denmark are associated with the consumption of eggs, domestically or abroad. This means that approximately half of the human cases of salmonellosis in Denmark have eggs as the most likely primary source. In this light, the increased effort to control salmonellae in layer flocks in this country is extremely justified.

CONTROL OF SALMONELLOSIS IN DENMARK

The principles of the salmonella-control program in broiler and layer production are a top-down approach with eradication of parent and grandparent flocks infected with

S. Enteritidis or *S.* Typhimurium. All parent and breeder flocks are monitored closely by combinations of serological and culture methods. Furthermore, environmental samples from all hatcheries are collected and analyzed weekly. The program is shown schematically in Table 7.3. Vaccines or antimicrobials are not approved for the control of salmonellae in Danish poultry production, partly because of a lack of evidence for their efficacy. Broiler flocks that at antemortem controls are positive for salmonellae are slaughtered after the salmonella-free flocks, thereby reducing the risk of cross-contamination. Since its implementation in 1989, the control system has greatly reduced the prevalence of salmonellae in Danish broiler flocks (Fig. 7.3). There has been a close association between the number of positive broiler flocks and the number of flocks found to be contaminated after slaughter, suggesting that preharvest control is the most important means of controlling salmonellae in broiler products.

If *S.* Typhimurium or *S.* Enteritidis is detected in a layer flock in a surveillance culture, production will be terminated, the flock destroyed, and the products heat treated.

The salmonella-control system in pork production is primarily based on serological monitoring of the herds. Based on the number of seropositive samples, each herd is classified into one of three groups. Herds in group 1 are salmonella free, and groups 2 and 3 are herds with low-grade infection and high-grade infection, respectively. Mandatory action is taken to reduce salmonellae in group-2 and group-3 herds and, furthermore, group-3 herds are slaughtered under special hygiene precautions with heat treatment or salting of all meat. This has reduced the prevalence of salmonellosis due to *S.* Typhimurium since 1994.

Because cattle are only a minor source of human salmonellosis in Denmark, no control program exists for this production.

THE FUTURE AND CONCLUSIONS

With plans aimed at controlling salmonellae in pork, broiler, and layer production, the incidence of human disease caused by *S.* Enteritidis is expected to decrease. However, to confirm the indirect evidence of the sources of human salmonellosis and to identify sources not revealed by the typing and the outbreak data, a case-control study on sporadic *S.* Enteritidis disease is in progress and will be terminated in 1998. Preliminary results point to consumption of food containing raw eggs as the major risk factor for *S.* Enteritidis infection.

We are convinced that *S.* Enteritidis can be effectively controlled in layer flocks. The successful control of salmonellae in broilers in this country has shown that it is possible. Preharvest control programs are the key to reducing the number of human infections caused by this organism. Because foodstuffs increasingly are crossing borders as a consequence of trade, international collaboration between the food industry, the medical and veterinary communities, and official bodies is a prerequisite for controlling *S.* Enteritidis not only in Denmark but worldwide.

TABLE 7.3   Sampling scheme of the Danish *Salmonella* control program in parent flocks and flocks of commercial layers: detection of *S.* Enteritidis or *S.* Typhimurium leads to destruction of the infected flock

Age/time	Sampling	Samples[a]
Rearing (parent)		
Day old	Per delivery	10 crates and 20 chicks[b]
Week 1	Per unit	40 chicks
Week 2	Per unit	20 chicks
Week 3	Per unit	30 chicks + 60 feces samples[b]
Two weeks before movement	Per unit	60 feces samples + 60 blood samples[b]
Production of hatching eggs		
Every 2nd week	Per flock	50 chicks or meconium from 250 chicks sampled in the hatchery[b]
Every 4th week	Per unit	60 feces samples + 60 blood samples or eggs
Hatchery		
Every week	Each hatcher	Wet dust
Rearing (layers)		
Day old	Per delivery	10 crates and 20 chicks
Week 3	Per flock	60 feces samples
From week 12 up to 2 weeks before moving	Per flock	60 feces samples + 60 blood samples
Consumer egg production for authorized egg-packing/product business		
24–30 weeks	Per flock	60 feces samples + 60 eggs
45–50 weeks	Per flock	60 feces samples + 60 eggs
7–10 weeks before slaughter	Per flock	60 feces samples + 60 eggs
Consumer egg production for barnyard sale		
Twice per year	Per flock	60 feces samples + 60 eggs

[a]Eggs and blood samples are analyzed serologically; all others by culture.
[b]Requirements of the European Union Zoonoses Directive (92/117/EEC).

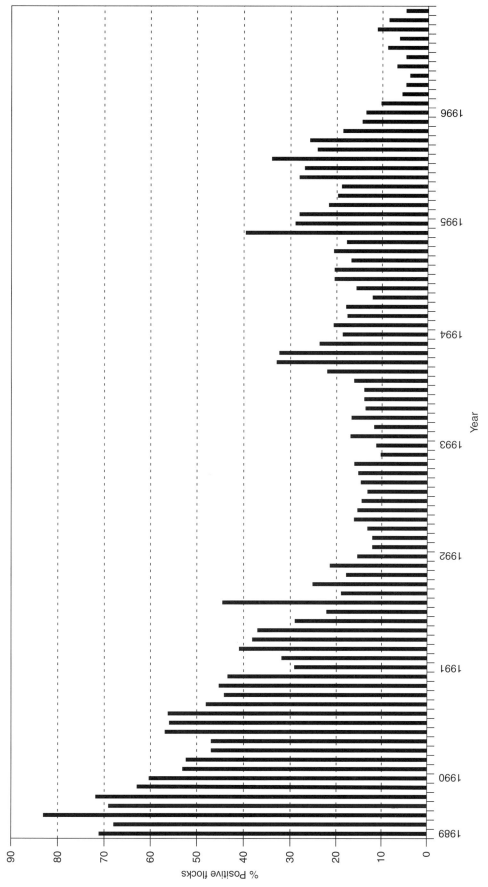

FIGURE 7.3 Salmonellae in Danish broilers by month, starting in July 1989 to December 1996.

8

Salmonella enterica Serovar Enteritidis in the Netherlands: Epidemiology, Prevention, and Control

A.W. van de Giessen, W.J. van Leeuwen, and W. van Pelt

INCIDENCE IN HUMANS

In the Netherlands, a sentinel study conducted at the general-practice level from 1987 to 1991 yielded an annual incidence of salmonella infection of about 75 cases per 100,000 persons (Hoogenboom-Verdegaal et al., 1994). In this study, salmonella serovars were isolated from 5% of diarrheal stools (n = 3653). As a follow-up, a sentinel study was conducted among about 1% of the Dutch general practices in 1992 and 1993. This study yielded an estimated annual incidence of salmonella infection of 22 cases per 100,000 persons (Goosen et al., 1995a), which is of the same order as the preliminary figure obtained in the 1996–97 sentinel study in progress. The discrepancy between the estimated incidences is probably due to differences in population and methodology. The estimated incidences imply that in the Netherlands each year approximately 3000–10,000 persons with salmonella infection consult physicians. However, the true incidence of salmonellosis in the general population is likely to be much higher, because only a small proportion of persons with gastrointestinal complaints consult physicians (Hoogenboom-Verdegaal et al., 1992; de Wit et al., 1996). Based on a population study in 1991, the annual incidence of *Salmonella enterica* serovar Enteritidis (S. Enteritidis) in the general population in the Netherlands is estimated to be approximately 700 cases per 100,000 persons, some 100,000 cases per year (de Wit et al., 1996). Although knowledge about outbreaks of salmonellosis due to S. Enter-

itidis in the Netherlands is incomplete, most incidents have proven to be sporadic cases. A few outbreaks have been described (Vliegenthart and van de Giessen, 1994; Goosen et al., 1995b). In 1992, salmonellosis was indicated as the primary cause of 14 deaths and as a secondary cause of another seven; in 1993, it was the primary cause of 12 deaths [Central Bureau for Statistics (CBS), 1992, 1993]. Hence, mortality as a result of salmonellosis is about 0.3%, a figure that is most probably an underestimation.

Since 1960, all first salmonella isolates obtained from patients at regional public health laboratories in the Netherlands are serotyped at the Dutch National Salmonella Center. Careful study at the community level of the coverage of these laboratories between 1984 and 1996 revealed a consistent overall coverage of 55% of the Dutch population (Esveld et al., 1996). This allows the estimation of the incidence of salmonellosis among the general population of those patients who consulted physicians and whose cases were considered worthy of microbiological study (Fig. 8.1). Trends in the estimated incidence figures at the national level (Fig. 8.1) are in good accord with those found for the individual laboratories and are not very sensitive to the degree of coverage of these laboratories. Incidence figures obtained in this way agree quite well with those from the sentinel studies but differ much less between years, probably due to the much larger sample size and less variable selection bias over the years.

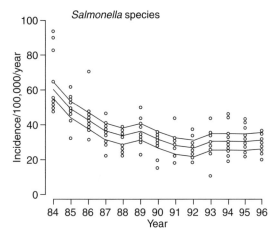

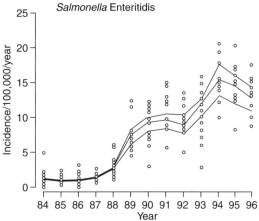

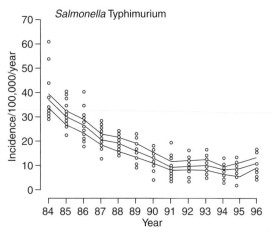

FIGURE 8.1 Change in estimated incidences of typed human salmonella isolates in the Netherlands between 1984 and 1996. Isolates are obtained at regional public health laboratories and serotyped at the Dutch National Salmonella Center. Markers indicate the incidence of the individual contributing laboratories. Communities not belonging to the regular coverage of the laboratories were removed: The resulting coverage is 55%. Upper boundaries correspond to a hypothetical coverage of 40%, and the lower one to 70% (Esveld et al., 1996).

Serotyping shows the dramatic increase of *S.* Enteritidis since 1988 (Fig. 8.1). Since the start of surveillance in 1960 until 1987, *S.* Enteritidis always constituted less than 1% of the isolates received. In 1994, almost twice as many human *S.* Enteritidis isolates were obtained as *S.* Typhimurium isolates. This proportion varies considerably throughout the year, because the seasonal peak is much more pronounced for *S.* Enteritidis than for *S.* Typhimurium (Figs. 8.2, 8.3).

GEOGRAPHICAL DISTRIBUTION

The sudden increase in *S.* Enteritidis among human salmonella isolates started at the local level in the southern and eastern regions of the Netherlands and has been the most abundant salmonella serovar in the urban western regions since 1993 (Fig. 8.2).

In contrast to *S.* Enteritidis, *S.* Typhimurium decreased between 1984 and 1991 (Fig. 8.1) and geographically it now predominates only in the rural northeastern regions (Fig. 8.2). The same pattern of geographical spread as between 1984 and 1996 repeats itself seasonally. The tropism of *S.* Enteritidis to poultry and of *S.* Typhimurium to pigs, cattle, and, to a lesser extent, to poultry, and the regional distribution of their respective industries, consumers, and changes therein, are the basis of the dynamics of the trends in geographical distribution and must be studied further.

DEMOGRAPHY

Isolates of *S.* Enteritidis and *S.* Typhimurium are much more common among children between 0 and 5 years of age relative to the proportion of Dutch children found in this age category in the general population (Fig. 8.4). Further comparison shows that twice as many isolates of *S.* Typhimurium are found among the youngest children between 0 and 5 years of age, compared with *S.* Enteritidis; the reverse holds for ages 16–60 (Fig. 8.4). This might be an indication of differences in severity of the manifestation of the salmonellosis between the two serovars. However, other circumstantial evidence, such as the number of registered complaints or the fraction of isolates from blood, is not significantly different and does not support this notion.

Quite remarkably, in the period before and during the increase in *S.* Enteritidis, isolates of this serovar were obtained much more frequently from boys younger than age 5 than from girls of the same age (Fig. 8.5); the same development, but in reverse order, held for the patients 16–60 years of age. In recent years, it has been about the same for *S.* Enteritidis as for *S.* Typhimurium and most other salmonellas.

RESERVOIRS

In the Netherlands, poultry constitutes the principal reservoir of *S.* Enteritidis (Table 8.1). *Salmonella* Enteritidis has occasionally been isolated from other animal species,

S. Enteritidis

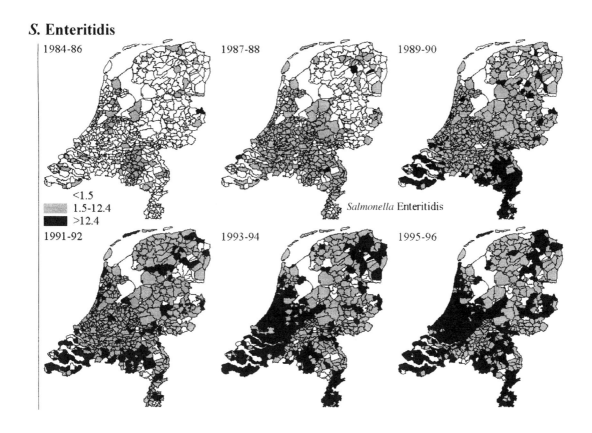

S. Typhimurium

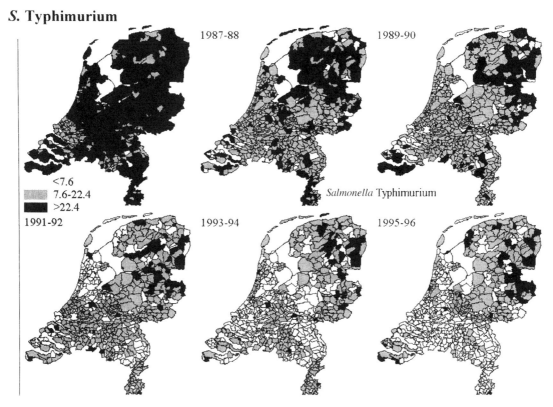

FIGURE 8.2 Regional distribution of *Salmonella* Enteritidis and *Salmonella* Typhimurium isolates in the Netherlands. Shaded bar-legends correspond to incidences per 100,000 (compare with Fig. 8.1).

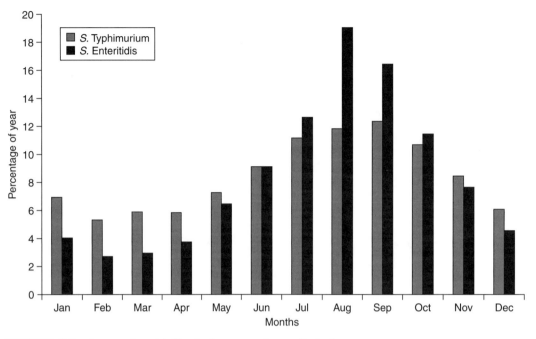

FIGURE 8.3   Seasonal variability in human salmonella isolates.

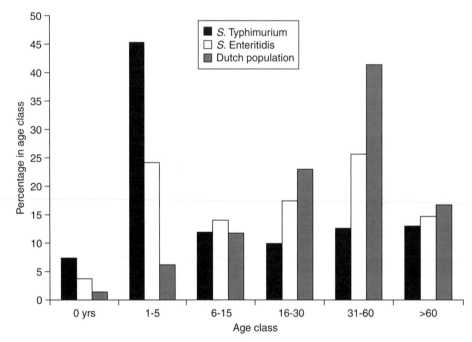

FIGURE 8.4   Age distribution of the general population and of patients with *Salmonella* Enteritidis and *Salmonella* Typhimurium infections.

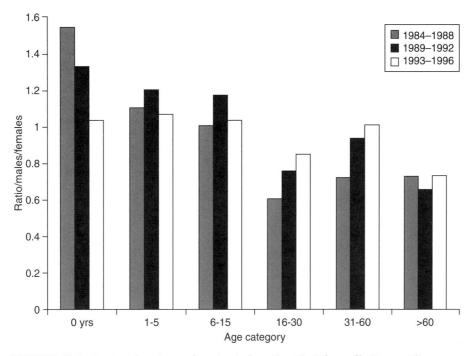

FIGURE 8.5   Ratio of males to females infected with *Salmonella* Enteritidis.

TABLE 8.1   Occurrence of *Salmonella* Enteritidis (SE) between 1984 and 1996 and phage types between 1989 and 1996 according to the Dutch phage-typing system, received at the Dutch Salmonella Center from human and nonhuman sources (cf. Fig. 8.7)

Source (1984–96)	SE isolates/ *Salmonella* spp. isolates	Years out of 13	Common phage types	Sporadic phage types
Human	11,214/54,445	13	1, 12, 2, 6, 3, 8, 20, 16, 18	4, 19, 11, 15, 7, 10, 17
Poultry	4078/39,388	13	1, 12, 16, 2, 20	18, 8, 11, 17, 7, 15, 10
Pigs	24/7173	7	1	16
Cattle	75/8913	12	1, 12	2, 6, 18, 16, 15
Calves	10/2468	8	1	
Horses	16/421	7	1	12, 20
Sheep	5/61	4	1	
Goats	0/22			
Ducks	21/103	8	1, 11, 12	
Turkeys	3/844	3		1, 12
Dogs	10/248	6	1	12
Cats	10/96	4	1	20
Rodents	1/82	1		1
Furbearers	0/94			
Pigeons	2/944	2		1
Reptiles	5/967	5		1, 2
Amphibians	0/24			
Meat products	847/6868	12	1, 12, 16	3, 8, 4, 2, 6, 18, 19, 11, 7, 17
Eggs (products)	2018/4256	13	1, 12, 16, 3, 6, 4	8, 20, 2, 11, 19, 15
Animal feed	34/3070	8	1	12, 2, 6
Surface water	6/173	2	1	

including pigs, cattle, sheep, horses, dogs, cats, birds, rodents, and reptiles, as well as from environmental samples, such as surface water; it comprises only about 1% of the isolates from animal feed (Table 8.1). Analysis of isolation frequencies of *S.* Enteritidis in poultry, pigs, and cattle over the past 13 years reveals a dramatic increase of this serovar in poultry since 1988, whereas the isolation frequencies of *S.* Enteritidis in pigs and cattle have remained low. Although the results in poultry are likely to be biased toward *S.* Enteritidis due to selective forwarding of isolates, the emergence of *S.* Enteritidis in poultry since 1988, which coincides with the dramatic increase of this serovar in humans, provides additional evidence that poultry is the principal source of human *S.* Enteritidis infection. This is illustrated in Figure 8.6 for different reservoirs, relative to the occurrence of *S.* Typhimurium. Indeed, the spectrum and abundance of *S.* Enteritidis phage types occurring in poultry and humans, as well as the degree of resistance (Table 8.1; Figs. 8.7, 8.8), strongly coincide.

Between 1989 and 1996, the majority of the human and nonhuman *S.* Enteritidis isolates belonged, according to the Dutch phage-typing system, to phage type 1 (DPT1, corresponding to PT4 in the Colindale system), followed by DPT12 (Fig. 8.7). The occurrence of the most important phage types in humans and in chickens and eggs between 1989 and 1996 evolves in a parallel way and shows a continuously changing spectrum of *S.* Enteritidis phage types in the Netherlands, with only the consistent occurrence of DPT1. For example, DPT20 occurred only in 1995; DPT2 occurred predominantly in 1989 and has not appeared in recent years; DPT6 peaked in 1991 and is now decreasing, whereas DPT3, DPT8, DPT12, and DPT16 are still increasing. A comparison of the Dutch phage-typing system with the English one is now in progress and will even-

tually enable the comparison of these trends with those in other countries.

RESISTANCE

The pattern of development of resistance in human and nonhuman isolates from *S.* Enteritidis (mainly poultry; see Table 8.1) before, during, and after the enormous increase of this serovar is depicted in Figure 8.8. There is a clear relationship between the development and the degree of antibiotic resistance in isolates from both sources. This is most strongly true for furazolidone, which is widely used nowadays against infections with *Eimeria* serovars in poultry flocks. Resistance to furazolidone has increased in the last few years and is now 15% in both human and nonhuman isolates (Fig. 8.8). Since 1993, infected broiler parent flocks have been treated with fluoroquinolones, and sensitivity to it has been tested. Resistance to fluoroquinolones is still very low in isolates from *S.* Enteritidis.

PREVALENCE IN POULTRY FLOCKS

Chickens frequently harbor salmonella serovars, and, since the mid-1980s, *S.* Enteritidis has emerged as a major serovar in many countries [World Health Organization (WHO), 1989; Salm-Net reports, 1994–96]. In the Netherlands, in 1989, van de Giessen et al. (1991) isolated *S.* Enteritidis from 18% of the commercial layer flocks and from 8% of the broiler flocks examined. In a follow-up study, in 1990, this serovar was detected in 7% and 8% of the layer and broiler flocks exam-

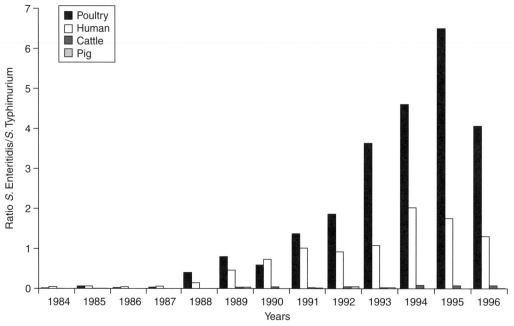

FIGURE 8.6 Ratio of occurrence of *Salmonella* Enteritidis to *Salmonella* Typhimurium.

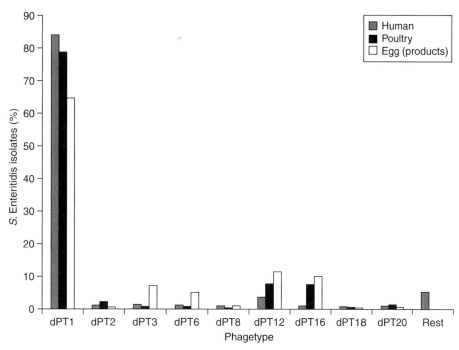

FIGURE 8.7   Abundance of Dutch *Salmonella* Enteritidis phage types, 1984–96. Phage types correspond to the Dutch phage-typing system (DPT).

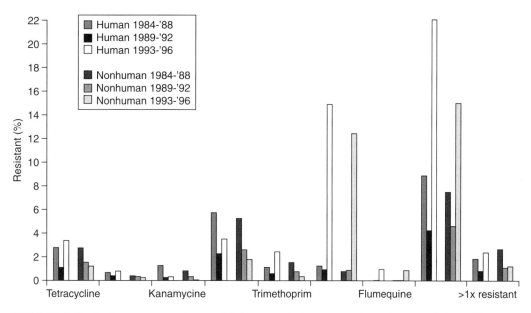

FIGURE 8.8   Resistance to antimocrobial agents in human and nonhuman *Salmonella* Enteritidis isolates.

ined, respectively (B.J. Hartog, personal communication on TNO nutrition and food research, Zeist, 1991; A.W. van de Giessen, unpublished data). In 1995, *S.* Enteritidis was isolated from 6% of 2656 broiler flocks constituting a representative sample of the Dutch broiler stock (W.J. van Leeuwen, unpublished data). Since 1990, no bacteriological studies on the occurrence of *S.* Enteritidis in Dutch commercial layer flocks have been reported, but the results of an immunological sur-

vey conducted in 1993 indicated that approximately 10%–15% of the Dutch layer flocks tested were infected with *S.* Enteritidis (A.W. van de Giessen, unpublished data). In 1995, the salmonella serovars most frequently isolated from Dutch poultry flocks included *S.* Hadar, *S.* Enteritidis, *S.* Heidelberg, *S.* Livingstone, *S.* Agona, *S.* Infantis, and *S.* Schwarzengrund. The predominant *S.* Enteritidis phage types in poultry were DPT1 and DPT12 (see Table 8.1; Fig. 8.7).

PREVALENCE IN POULTRY MEAT

During slaughter and processing of broilers, the presence of salmonella serovars, including *S.* Enteritidis, in the intestinal contents and on the feathers and skin of the birds inevitably results in the contamination of poultry meat (Bryan and Doyle, 1995). In a Dutch survey conducted in 1995, *S.* Enteritidis was isolated from 6.8% of 1359 samples of fresh chicken products from retail stores, and 34.2% of these samples were found to be salmonella positive (van der Zee and de Boer, 1996).

PREVALENCE IN COMMERCIAL SHELL EGGS AND EGG PRODUCTS

In the Netherlands, in 1988 and 1991, a total of 5100 eggs obtained from farms on which *S.* Enteritidis had previously been detected in layer flocks, and 5660 eggs obtained from retail outlets, were examined for salmonella serovars but no internally infected eggs were found (de Boer, 1991). However, *S.* Enteritidis was isolated from one of 14 eggs (de Boer, 1991) and one of 10 eggs (Vliegenthart and van de Giessen, 1994), respectively, that were examined in association with two outbreaks of *S.* Enteritidis infection. In another Dutch survey, conducted during 1991–93, *S.* Enteritidis was isolated from approximately 50% of samples of raw-egg material and from 2%–6% of samples of pasteurized egg products from the egg-product industry (van der Zee and de Boer, 1994).

CONTROL MEASURES IN THE EGG PRODUCTION CHAIN

As a result of the international increase of human *S.* Enteritidis infections and the epidemiological link with poultry, national programs of salmonella control, and especially *S.* Enteritidis control, have been implemented in many countries (WHO, 1992, 1994). In the Netherlands, a national *S.* Enteritidis eradication program in poultry breeder flocks was implemented in March 1989 by a joint effort of the government and the poultry industry. The objective of this program is to eradicate *S.* Enteritidis from the breeder stock in order to deliver chicks free of *S.* Enteritidis to the commercial layer and broiler farms, while maintaining good hygiene standards throughout the poultry industry. This strategy, which is known as the top-down approach, should lead to an elimination of *S.* Enteritidis from the top of the poultry production chain to the bottom. The program includes the screening of all breeder flocks (approximately 2300) at regular intervals as well as the examination of hatcheries and imported material.

During the first 3 years of the program, the breeder flocks were screened by bacteriological examination of cecal droppings, and *S.* Enteritidis–infected flocks were slaughtered. Thereafter, from April 1992 onward, serological screening with the double-antibody sandwich (GM-DAS) blocking enzyme-linked immunosorbent assay (ELISA) (van Zijderveld et al., 1992) and bacteriological confirmation of positive screening results were carried out. More recently, as a consequence of the European Union zoonoses order (European Union, 1992), which prescribes control measures aimed at eradicating both *S.* Enteritidis and *S.* Typhimurium from poultry breeder flocks, an indirect group-B/D lipopolysaccharide ELISA has come into use in the Dutch program as a prescreening test, followed by the testing of positive samples more specifically for antibodies to *S.* Enteritidis or *S.* Typhimurium by a GM-DAS-blocking ELISA.

As far as the layer breeder stock is concerned, the control program has been successful: in 1996, no more positive flocks were found (T.S. de Vries, personal communication about the Animal Health Service, Deventer, 1997). As a consequence, vertical transmission of *S.* Enteritidis from parent flocks to commercial layer flocks via eggs is minimal. However, the *S.* Enteritidis control program in layer breeder flocks did not reduce *S.* Enteritidis–infected commercial layer flocks. Epidemiological studies have revealed that these flocks become infected with *S.* Enteritidis mainly from the direct farm environment (van de Giessen et al., 1994). Therefore, additional control measures were recently implemented in the commercial layer stock.

In July 1996, cleaning and disinfection of poultry houses, followed by a bacteriological check on hygiene before restocking, became mandatory for all commercial layer farms. Moreover, since then, layer rearing flocks are serologically screened at 2 weeks before transfer to layer farms, and *S.* Enteritidis–infected and *S.* Typhimurium–infected flocks are treated as described for the broiler parent flocks. Additionally, an *S.* Gallinarum (attenuated) live vaccine is currently being tested in a selected group of commercial layer flocks (T.S. de Vries, personal communication about the Animal Health Service, Deventer, 1997). This vaccine is expected to provide cross-protection against *S.* Enteritidis infection due to possession of common somatic antigens (O1, O9, and O12) with *S.* Enteritidis. The vaccine is applied only in rearing flocks that will be transferred to commercial layer farms associated with an increased risk of *S.* Enteritidis infection (especially farms with a recent history of *S.* Enteritidis infection).

CONTROL MEASURES IN THE POULTRY MEAT PRODUCTION CHAIN

Until 1 April 1992, *S.* Enteritidis–positive broiler breeder flocks were slaughtered. However, because this was an expensive way of eradicating *S.* Enteritidis from flocks, from that date onward, *S.* Enteritidis–infected broiler parent flocks were treated with antibiotics (Baytril, enrofloxacin, or flumequine)

TABLE 8.2 Incidence of *Salmonella* Enteritidis (SE) in breeder flocks in the Netherlands, in 1989–96[a]

Year	Egg sector: no. of flocks		Poultry meat sector: no. of flocks	
	SE-positive/examined	%	SE-positive/examined	%
1989	9/316	2.8	18/1.045	1.7
1990	4/284	1.4	22/2.017	1.1
1991	0/292	0.0	15/1.997	0.8
1992	2/351	0.6	22/1.922	1.1
1993	15/348	4.3	27/2.752	1.0
1994	4/326	1.2	27/2.410	1.1
1995	3/379	0.8	36/2.040	1.8
1996	0/213	0.0	35/1727	2.0

[a]Data 1989–92 from Edel (1994); data 1993–96 from Animal Health Service, personal communication.

for 10 days, followed by treatment with a "competitive exclusion"–inducing microflora, instead of being slaughtered (Edel, 1994). As a result of the *S.* Enteritidis control program, *S.* Enteritidis contamination in broiler breeder flocks initially decreased from 1.7% of the flocks in 1989 to 0.8% in 1991. In the succeeding years, however, a contamination level of about 1% persisted, and, in 1995, 1.8% (36 of 2040) of the broiler breeder flocks examined were found to be *S.* Enteritidis positive (Table 8.2). Of these flocks, 24 were parent flocks that were found to be positive during the production period (T.S. de Vries, personal communication about the Animal Health Service, Deventer, 1997). Infection from environmental sources by horizontal pathways was suspected in 30 of the 36 cases, whereas infection was attributed to vertical transmission of the organism in six cases.

The failure to eradicate *S.* Enteritidis in the broiler breeder stock has been attributed to extensive environmental contamination and lack of preventive hygiene in this sector (Fris and van den Bos, 1995; Edel et al., 1996). Moreover, the treatment of *S.* Enteritidis–positive broiler breeder (parent) flocks with antibiotics (Baytril, enrofloxacin, or flumequine) and competitive-exclusion flora to eliminate and prevent *S.* Enteritidis infection turned out to be only partially (approximately 75%) successful (Goren, 1994). At present, three vaccines are being tested in a field trial in broiler parent flocks: (a) an *S.* Typhimurium (attenuated) live vaccine (TAD Salmonella vac T), (b) an *S.* Enteritidis inactivated vaccine (TAD Talovac 109 SE), and (c) another *S.* Enteritidis inactivated vaccine (Hoechst Salenvac). The use of vaccination is restricted to rearing flocks that will be transferred to breeder farms associated with an increased risk of *S.* Enteritidis infection. Furthermore, gradual extension of the national control program to cover all salmonellas according to the top-down approach is being considered.

REFERENCES

Boer, E. de. 1991. Onderzoek van kippeëieren op de aanwezigheid van *Salmonella* Enteritidis. Voedingsmiddelentechnologie 19:18–19.

Bryan, F.L., and Doyle, M.P. 1995. Health risks and consequences of *Salmonella* and *Campylobacter jejuni* in raw poultry. J. Food Prot. 58:326–344.

CBS. 1992, 1993. Overledenen naar doodsoorzaak. Central Bureau for Statistics.

Edel, W. 1994. *Salmonella* Enteritidis eradication programme in poultry breeder flocks in the Netherlands. Int. J. Food Microbiol. 21:171–178.

Edel, W., Smak, J.A., de Vries, T.S., and Westendorp, M.C. 1996. *Salmonella enteritidis* en *Salmonella typhimurium* onderzoek en bestrijding bij reproduktie pluimvee. VHI Ber. 4:1–8.

Esveld, M., Pelt, W. van, Leeuwen, W.J. van, and Banffer, J.R.J. 1996. Laboratorium surveillance infectieziekten: 1989–1995. RIVM report 068902002. Bilthoven, The Netherlands: National Institute of Public Health and Environmental Protection.

European Union. 1992. Council directive concerning measures for protection against specified zoonoses and specified zoonotic agents in animals and products of animal origin in order to prevent outbreaks of food-borne infections and intoxications. Council Directive 92/117-/EEC. Brussels: Commission of the European Communities.

Fris, C., and van den Bos, J. 1995. A retrospective case-control study of risk factors associated with *Salmonella enterica* subsp. *enterica* serovar Enteritidis infections on Dutch broiler breeder farms. Avian Pathol. 24:255–272.

Giessen, A.W. van de, Ament, A.J.H.A., and Notermans, S.H.W. 1994. Intervention strategies for *Salmonella* Enteritidis in poultry flocks: a basic approach. Int. J. Food Microbiol. 21:145–154.

Giessen, A.W. van de, Peters, R., Berkers, P.A.T.A., Jansen, W.H., and Notermans, S.H.W. 1991. *Salmonella* contamination of poultry flocks in the Netherlands. Vet. Q. 13:41–46.

Goosen, E.S.M., Hoogenboom-Verdegaal, A.M.M., Bartelds, A.I.M., Sprenger, M.J.W., and Borgdorff, M.W. 1995a. Incidentie van gastroenteritis in huisartsenpeilstations in Nederland, 1992–1993. RIVM report 149101012. Bilthoven, The Netherlands: National Institute of Public Health and Environmental Protection.

Goosen, E.S.M., Sprenger, M.J.W., and Borgdorff, M.W. 1995b. Meldingen van voedselinfecties en voedselvergiftigingen bij

Inspecties Gezondheidsbescherming/Keuringsdienten van Waren in de periode 1991–1994. RIVM report 149101013. Bilthoven, The Netherlands: National Institute of Public Health and Environmental Protection.

Goren, E. 1994. In: Report of the WHO–FEDESA–FEP workshop on competitive exclusion, vaccination and antimicrobials in *Salmonella* control in poultry. WHO report WHO/CDS/VPH/94.1-34. Geneva: World Health Organization.

Hoogenboom-Verdegaal, A.M.M., During, M., and Engels, G.B. 1992. Een bevolkin gsonderzoek naar maag/darmklachten in vier regio's van Nederland uitgevoerd in 1991. Deel 1. Onderzoeksmethodiek en incidentieberekening gastroenteritis. RIVM report 149101001. Bilthoven, The Netherlands: National Institute of Public Health and Environmental Protection.

Hoogenboom-Verdegaal, A.M.M., Goosen, E.S.M., During, M., Engels, G.B., Klokman-Houweing, J.M., and van de Laar, M.J.W. 1994. Epidemiologisch en microbiologisch onderzoek met betrek-king tot acute gastroenteritis in huisartsenpeil stations in Amsterdam en Helmond, 1987–1991. RIVM report 149101011. Bilthoven, The Netherlands: National Institute of Public Health and Environmental Protection.

Salm-Net Quarterly Report (94/1-96/4). 1994–96. Coordinating Scientific Secretary: I. Fisher. London: PHLS Communicable Disease Surveillance Centre.

Vliegenthart, J.S., and van de Giessen, A.W. 1994. Een explosie van een voedselinfectie na het eten van bavaroise die bereid was met rauwe eieren. Infectieziekten Bull. 9:164–168.

Wit, M.A.S. de, Hoogenboom-Verdegaal, A.M.M., Goosen, E.S.M., Sprenger, M.J.W., and Borgdorff, M.W. 1996. Een bevolkingsonderzoek in vier regio's in Nederland naar de incidentie en ziektelast van gastroenteritis en van *Campylobacter*—en *Salmonella*—infectie. RIVM report 149101014. Bilthoven, The Netherlands: National Institute of Public Health and Environmental Protection.

World Health Organization (WHO). 1989. Report by WHO on epidemiological emergency in poultry and egg salmonellosis. WHO report WHO/CDS/VPH/89.82. Geneva: WHO.

World Health Organization (WHO). 1992. WHO consultation on national and local schemes of *Salmonella* control in poultry. WHO report WHO/CDS/VPH/92.110. Geneva: WHO.

World Health Organization (WHO). 1994. Report of a WHO consultation on strategies for detection and monitoring of *Salmonella* infected poultry flocks. WHO report WHO/Zoon/94.173. Wray, C., and Davies, R.H., eds. Geneva: WHO.

Zee, H. van der, and de Boer, E. 1994. *Salmonella* spp. en *Salmonella enteritidis* in eiprodukten en rauwe grondstoffen voor eiprodukten in Nederland in 1991–1993. Ware(n) Chem. 24:86–90.

Zee, H. van der, and de Boer, E. 1996. Monitoring pathogenen in kip en kipprodukten, 1991 t/m 1995. Amsterdam: Inspectie Gezondheidsbescherming Amsterdam/Zutphen.

Zijderveld, F.G. van, Zijderveld-van Bemmel, A.M. van, and Anakotta, J. 1992. Comparison of four different enzyme-linked immunosorbent assays for serological diagnosis of *Salmonella enteritidis* infections in experimentally infected chickens. J. Clin. Microbiol. 30:2560–2566.

9

Salmonella enterica Serovar Enteritidis in Switzerland: Recognition, Development, and Control of the Epidemic

H. Schmid and A. Baumgartner

CHRONOLOGY OF PROBLEM ANALYSIS

From 1976 to 1986, a marked increase in human infections with *Salmonella enterica* serovar Enteritidis (*S.* Enteritidis) was registered in the United States (St. Louis et al., 1988). Furthermore, outbreaks of *S.* Enteritidis were significantly more frequently associated with the consumption of raw or undercooked eggs or egg dishes. In the mid-1980s, a similar trend was observed in Switzerland and some other European countries (Perales and Audicana, 1988; Baird-Parker, 1990; Baumgartner, 1990a). It was evident that the *S.* Enteritidis situation in Switzerland reflected a global phenomenon (Rodrigue et al., 1990).

In 1988, the Swiss Federal Office of Public Health (SFOPH) raised and discussed the *S.* Enteritidis topic for the first time in its weekly bulletin (Anon., 1988). The official statement included guidelines for the safe handling of eggs in the kitchen. The problem was subsequently taken up by the media. The result was a feeling of insecurity among consumers, followed by a strong fall in egg sales. With regard to the phenomenon of transovarian transmission, the poultry industry and veterinarians responded with skepticism and refused to believe that *S.* Enteritidis was isolated from the contents of eggs. Therefore, the SFOPH and the cantonal (district) health authorities made efforts to make a firmer epidemiological connection between eggs and *S.* Enteritidis infections. To achieve this, a sample of 8872 market eggs were bacteriologically analyzed. As a result, *S.* Enteritidis was isolated on the shells of two eggs imported from Poland and Germany. Phage

typing showed that the two *S.* Enteritidis strains belonged to phage type 4 (PT4) and PT7 (Baumgartner, 1990b).

At the time of this study, there was only a general detection method available and not a procedure specifically adapted to the problem. The percentage of positive results was probably therefore small, and no salmonellae could be identified in the contents of the eggs. However, the high number of local outbreaks showed that the increase in *S.* Enteritidis infections was not only a phenomenon due to imported, contaminated eggs. In the years from 1988 to 1990, the cantonal laboratories of food control investigated numerous outbreaks caused by *S.* Enteritidis and traced some of them back to egg-producing farms. Within the scope of these activities, 32 hens from two infected flocks were examined pathologically, bacteriologically, and serologically. *Salmonella* Enteritidis was found in 12 animals. In eight hens, the infection was located in the ovary and/or oviduct (Hoop and Keller, 1991). This study clearly showed that the phenomenon of transovarian transmission existed in Swiss flocks of layer hens and that *S.* Enteritidis must be expected in the contents of eggs.

MEASURES OF CONTROL AND SANITATION

Activities of the Food-Control Authorities

In Switzerland, the control of foodstuffs of animal origin is the responsibility of two authorities: the Swiss Federal

Veterinary Office and the associated cantonal veterinary authorities are responsible for problems associated with the primary production. As soon as the products are in the processing chain or on the market, the responsibility switches to the SFOPH and the cantonal laboratories of food control. The latter execute the legal provisions on foodstuffs. As the investigations of foodborne outbreaks are within the scope of duties of the cantonal laboratories, they studied various outbreaks caused by *S. Enteritidis*. In cases where infected flocks were traced, it was always decreed that the eggs be pasteurized. It was, however, evident that these measures were insufficient and that the root of the problem had to be addressed.

It was furthermore noted that a cheap and simple diagnostic instrument to screen eggs or chickens for *S. Enteritidis* should be available. The SFOPH decided to develop an enzyme-linked immunosorbent assay (ELISA) for the detection of *S. Enteritidis*-specific antibodies from chicken serum or egg yolk. The test, designed for flock screening, was commercialized in 1992 under the name Checkit *S. enteritidis*A (Furrer et al., 1993). A field study validated the ELISA more extensively. In this context, it was important to know whether there is a relationship between the seroprevalence and the presence of active infections in a flock. Our investigations have shown that the percentage of seropositive eggs is always high (47%–100%) in cases where *S. Enteritidis* is isolated from an egg sample taken in a suspected flock. In two flocks, the seroprevalence in egg samples was found to be 30% and 10%. In these cases, *S. Enteritidis* could be isolated from environmental samples but not from the egg contents. Based on these results, it was concluded that the probability of an active infection is very low in flocks with a seroprevalence of less than 10% and that, in this case, the bacteriological search for *S. Enteritidis* in eggs is not promising (Baumgartner et al., 1993).

For the detection of *S. Enteritidis* in eggs, the cantonal laboratories applied the finding that iron ions, added to an enrichment broth, stimulate the growth of the target microorganisms (Gast and Holt, 1995). Furthermore, the combination of iron-enriched media with immunomagnetic beads (Dynabeads) was shown to be a useful diagnostic instrument (data not published). In Switzerland, a polymerase chain reaction was also developed for the detection of *S. Enteritidis* in eggs (Burkhalter et al., 1995). However, this approach has not been introduced as a routine testing method in official laboratories, because not all laboratories are sufficiently equipped to perform it.

Activities in the Legislative Field

During the first outbreak investigations, public health authorities became aware that the *S. Enteritidis* problem could be effectively resolved only by taking measures at the root of the problem. This necessitated the adaptation of various legal norms, including the revision of the Ordinance for the Control and Eradication of Epizootic Diseases (Swiss Federal Council, 1993) having priority. Because infections of laying hens with *S. Enteritidis* did not correspond to the typical picture of a livestock epidemic, the revision project was considerably delayed and the vet-

erinary authorities had no legal instrument to eliminate infected flocks. Finally, in 1993, the necessary legal provisions were enforced. The most important measures for the elimination of *S. Enteritidis* are

- Flocks used for the production of hatching eggs and eggs for consumption with more than 50 animals have to be monitored for *S. Enteritidis*.
- Poultry keepers have to take samples for analysis as follows: (a) from breeders, periodically during lay, and (b) from laying hens, in week 30 and during lay at 6-month intervals.
- Among breeders, the official veterinary officer has to take samples for analysis at the following stages: from 1-day-old chicks between the days 1 and 3, at the age of 5 weeks, at the age of 15–20 weeks, and 2 weeks before the animals are transferred to a production unit. This regulation is also valid for future laying hens.
- In hatcheries with more than 1000 egg places and where broiler chicks are not exclusively produced, samples have to be taken from every hatch for analysis.
- Infection in a flock is suspected if (a) *S. Enteritidis* can be isolated from environmental samples, (b) blood or eggs are found to be seropositive for *S. Enteritidis*, or (c) human infections with *S. Enteritidis* can be traced to the flock.
- In case of suspicion, the cantonal veterinary officer takes samples as quickly as possible and orders a bacteriological analysis for *S. Enteritidis*.
- A flock is considered to be infected if *S. Enteritidis* is detected in eggs or animals. In this case, the animals cannot be sold and the eggs cannot be used for hatching purposes. Hatched eggs have to be disposed of as hazardous animal waste.
- In case of infection, the veterinary authorities order the elimination of the affected flock. This measure can be suspended if the flock is medically treated. Flocks that had contact with infected animals, directly or indirectly, have to be examined.
- Vaccines are authorized only if they do not detract from the measures laid down in the ordinance.
- Sampling and analyses have to be performed by officially recognized laboratories and according to technical directives established by the federal veterinary authorities.

In 1995, a completely revised Ordinance on Foodstuffs was introduced (Swiss Federal Council, 1995) that contained provisions for the storage and the marketing of eggs. As to the storage of eggs, the most recent knowledge on the biological behavior of *S. Enteritidis* was taken into consideration. The central innovations are

- From the day of laying, eggs have to be stored at temperatures of 20°C or less and in places that are well aerated, dry (free from condensed water), and protected from direct solar radiation.
- Eggs on sale that are more than 20 days old have to be cooled down to 5°C or less. The coolness chain may not be interrupted until delivery of the eggs.

Eggs must be stored in dry and well-aerated places. This regulation also applies if eggs are voluntarily refrigerated before day 21.

- The date of sale on the package has to state (a) until what date the eggs can be sold without refrigeration, and (b) that eggs which are refrigerated for sale should be kept at 5°C or less by the consumer.
- Egg products intended to be used as admixtures have to be pasteurized when there is no heat treatment after the admixing step.
- After pasteurization, egg products have to be immediately cooled down to 5°C or less and stored at this temperature until use.

The revised Ordinance on the Hygienic-Microbiological Standards on Foods, Utility Articles, Premises, Facilities, and Personnel (Federal Department of the Interior, 1995) should contribute to an improved hygienic situation regarding eggs and salmonellosis as well. This ordinance decrees that all food handlers have to establish a food safety concept in their business. This obliges food handlers to identify hygienically critical points and to keep them under surveillance.

Furthermore, the SFOPH has provided consumers with detailed information on the safe handling of eggs in the kitchen in its weekly bulletin, and an information sheet on kitchen hygiene published by the World Health Organization was translated into German, French, and Italian and distributed to the general public (Schwab, 1995).

EPIDEMIOLOGICAL ASPECTS

Characteristics of the *Salmonella* Enteritidis Epidemic in Switzerland

The Swiss Reporting System legally requires that federally registered laboratories report salmonella isolates from humans to the SFOPH. The laboratory reports contain information on age, sex, patient residence, date of diagnosis, infectious agent, and the material from which the isolation was made. These reports provide time trends and insights into the relative importance and the characteristics of salmonella serovars. However, it has to be assumed that an unknown fraction of the true number of salmonella infections are diagnosed.

Between 1984 and 1990, a more than eightfold increase in isolations of *S.* Enteritidis was observed (Fig. 9.1). During this period, the incidence rate rose from 7 to 55 isolations per 100,000 inhabitants per year, dropped in 1991, and then increased again to reach the peak of the epidemic in 1992 (79 cases per 100,000 inhabitants). The importance of *S.* Enteritidis relative to other salmonella serovars also increased considerably. In 1986, *S.* Enteritidis exceeded *S.* Typhimurium as the most frequently isolated serovar. The percentage of salmonella isolates identified as *S.* Enteritidis was 23% in 1984 and 67% in 1992. Since then, annual reports of *S.* Enteritidis have declined. Less than half the number of *S.* Enteritidis isolates were reported in 1996 compared with 1992. This trend coin-

cides with observations in other Western European countries (Fisher, 1997).

Epidemiologic characteristics of *S.* Enteritidis infections such as seasonality and age and sex distribution have remained constant over the years. The incidence of *S.* Enteritidis shows a distinct seasonal pattern, with a peak in late summer (Fig. 9.2). The highest incidence rates are observed in children under age 5 (Fig. 9.3). Males and females seem to be equally affected by infections, as the percentages of isolates from both sexes differ only slightly (for 1992, 49.4% of isolates from males, 50.0% from females, and 0.6% with missing information).

From the laboratory reports of *S.* Enteritidis, it can be concluded that about 15% of the overall caseload in recent years was associated with family clusters. Outbreaks of illness due to *S.* Enteritidis that involved persons from different households (general outbreaks) accounted for less than 10% of the total number of cases. This is a very crude estimate, since stool samples are not available for all persons involved in outbreaks. In addition, outbreaks are probably underreported. Despite these limitations, it can be concluded that the majority of reported isolations of *S.* Enteritidis come from sporadic cases.

Outbreak Investigations

Outbreaks of foodborne diseases are investigated by cantonal health authorities, occasionally with federal support. For the small fraction of laboratory reports that are implicated in outbreaks, these investigations provide information on sources of infection and places where infections occurred.

The majority of outbreak-associated infections reported in the period between 1988 and 1996 were caused by *S.* Enteritidis: namely, 63% among those of which the causative agent was identified (Table 9.1). The true percentage might be higher because nonserotyped *Salmonella* belonging to group D (probably also *S.* Enteritidis) was implicated in 12 more outbreaks (5%). The number of *S.* Enteritidis outbreaks was highest in the year of peak incidence of reported isolations (29 in 1992) and then decreased markedly (to 6 in 1996), concomitant with the decline in laboratory reports.

Salmonella Enteritidis outbreaks involved a few to about 400 persons. In most cases, the infections occurred in places of collective catering, such as hotels, restaurants, canteens, hospitals, nursing homes, psychiatric clinics, residences for the elderly, schools, kindergartens, scout camps, military quarters, monasteries, private parties, and in one case—the largest outbreak of all—at a public festival with many food stalls. Six outbreaks affected consumers in different households after they had eaten eggs from the same farm or a pastry product from the same bakery.

Almost all *S.* Enteritidis outbreaks were related to the consumption of eggs (Table 9.1). In the majority of investigations, epidemiological and/or microbiological evidence has pointed to dishes that contain raw or lightly cooked eggs. In Switzerland, these are predominantly desserts such as tiramisu or chocolate mousse. In other cases, the most likely sources

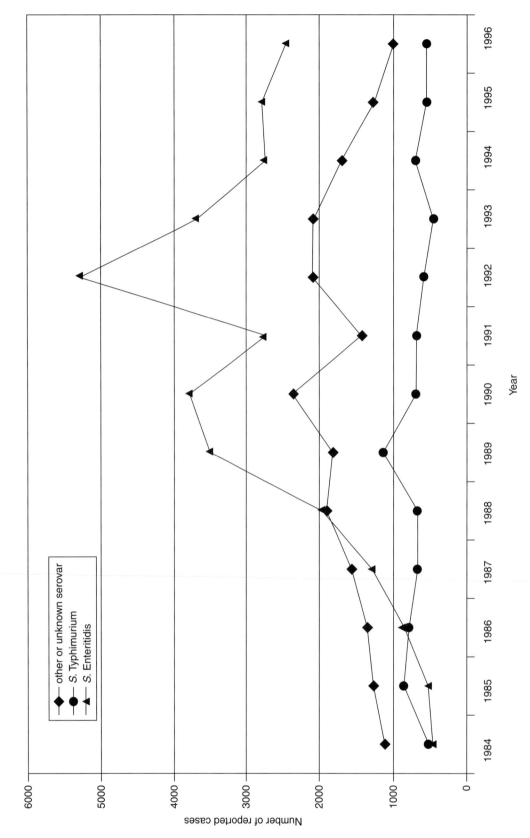

FIGURE 9.1 Reported cases of salmonellosis in Switzerland, 1984–96.

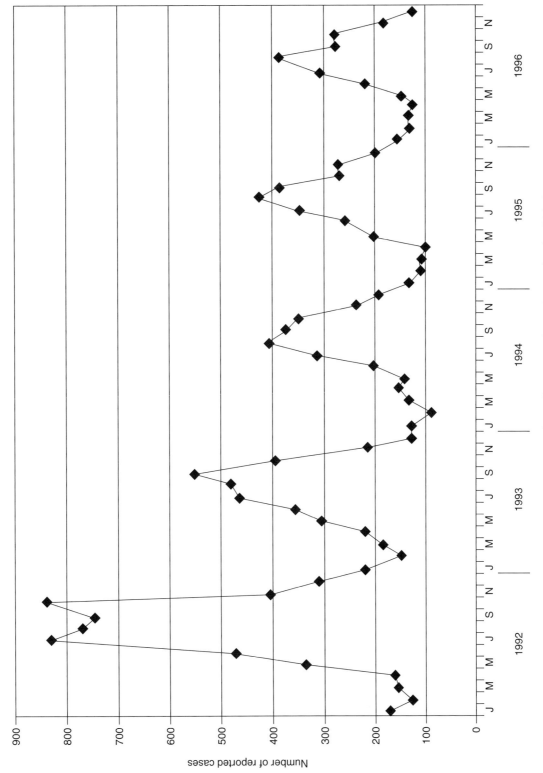

FIGURE 9.2 Seasonal patterns of reported isolations of *Salmonella* Enteritidis in Switzerland, 1992–96.

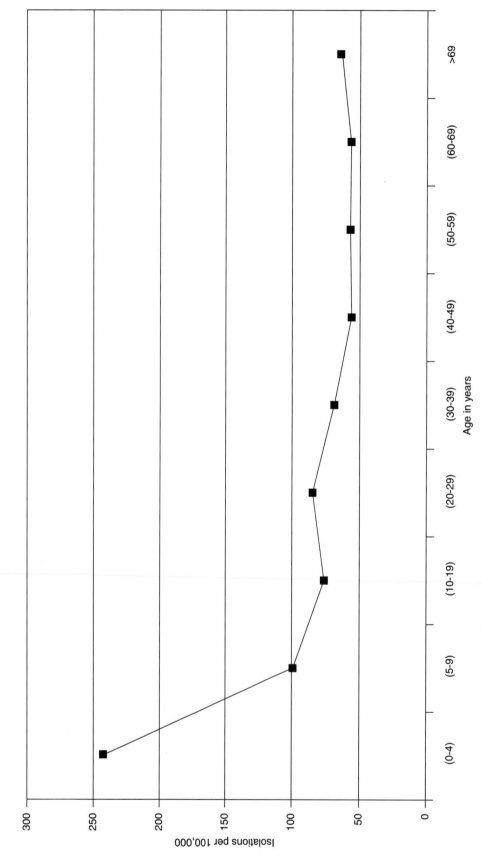

FIGURE 9.3 Isolation rate of *Salmonella* Enteritidis in Switzerland by age group, 1992.

TABLE 9.1 Reported *Salmonella* Enteritidis outbreaks in Switzerland, 1988–96

Year	Foodborne outbreaks with identified agent	S. Enteritidis outbreaks	S. Enteritidis outbreaks with known etiology	Egg-related S. Enteritidis outbreaks
		Number of outbreaks reported		
1988	21	18	6	5
1989	40	27	11	9
1990	32	16	11	9
1991	22	12	9	9
1992	40	29	26	23
1993	34	22	16	15
1994	21	11	8	8
1995	14	6	4	4
1996	18	6	5	5

of infection were fried eggs or other egg-containing dishes or food items: raw meat dishes, pasta sauce, mayonnaise, or pastry (eggs used for filling or glaze). Some of these egg-associated outbreaks were traced back to a particular flock of laying hens. This is highlighted by a series of related outbreaks in the summer of 1992 (Jaeggi et al., 1992): eggs from a farm with 7000 laying hens caused outbreaks at three different places. Five adults and 19 children in a vacation camp suffered from gastrointestinal symptoms after having eaten chocolate mousse and mayonnaise: 14 eggs had been used for the preparation of both food items. Some weeks later, three members of a family who had consumed fried eggs fell ill, and four persons in another family were affected because they had tasted the pastry of a cake before it was baked. In addition to these outbreaks, several sporadic cases were reported, all of which were associated with the consumption of fried eggs. *Salmonella* Enteritidis was isolated from the chocolate mousse and from eggs, and was found in environmental samples taken from the stall of the infected flock.

Only two *S.* Enteritidis outbreaks were traced to poultry meat. This observation is consistent with the findings of a study that compared salmonella isolates from broiler carcasses with those isolated from human cases of salmonellosis (Baumgartner et al., 1992). The frequency distribution of serovars found on chicken-neck skin samples were completely different from those of human isolates. Whereas *S.* Enteritidis was the most frequent serovar in human isolates, serovars other than *S.* Enteritidis dominated on broiler carcasses. These results indicate that broilers are not a major source of human salmonellosis in Switzerland.

On three occasions, there was evidence to suggest that an infected food handler had been the source of an *S.* Enteritidis outbreak. In all of them, the food handler continued to prepare food while suffering from symptoms of gastroenteritis. In other cases, when food-handling personnel were found to be *S.* Enteritidis positive, these persons became infected most probably from tasting contaminated food during preparation of a meal or from eating leftover food. They were therefore victims rather than sources of the outbreaks. Previous analyses in the U.K. concluded that asymptomatic food handlers are rarely responsible for initiating outbreaks of gastrointestinal outbreaks and that simply proper food hygiene eliminates the risk of transmitting illness (Pether and Scott, 1982; Roberts, 1982; Cruickshank and Humphrey, 1987).

Risk Factors for Sporadic Cases

Food items implicated in outbreaks of salmonellosis are not necessarily representative of sporadic cases. Therefore, a case-control study was conducted to identify determinants for the acquisition of sporadic salmonella infection in Switzerland (Schmid et al., 1996). Over a 1-year period, 223 case-control pairs were enrolled in the study and risk factors were assessed by means of self-administered questionnaires.

About 75% of the isolates were identified as *S.* Enteritidis, most of which belonged to PT4. The proportion of PT4 among the *S.* Enteritidis isolates was very similar to that reported in the U.K. (Baird-Parker, 1990) and Germany (Schroeter et al., 1994). There were distinct differences in risk factors between *S.* Enteritidis infections and other salmonella serovars. In both groups, travel abroad within the 3 days preceding illness was positively associated with illness. However, this association was more pronounced for infections with serovars other than *S.* Enteritidis: 22 different salmonella serovars were isolated from 55% of cases in the non-Enteritidis group who had acquired their infection abroad, compared with 20% of cases infected with *S.* Enteritidis. Among the presumably imported infections, *S.* Enteritidis was acquired mostly in other European countries, whereas other serovars were mostly acquired in countries outside of Europe. This finding concurs with reports from many of these countries, which showed that *S.* Enteritidis is the most common serovar in human salmonellosis (Gerigk, 1992).

The only food items associated with an increased risk of *S.* Enteritidis infection were undercooked eggs or desserts made with raw eggs, thereby confirming the findings regarding outbreak-related cases. Desserts made with raw eggs were more strongly associated with disease than was consumption of soft-boiled eggs (whose yolk was still liquid) or fried eggs, suggesting that the risk of infection depended on the extent to which eggs were cooked. Egg consumption was not associated with infections with serovars other than *S.* Enteritidis. This indicates that the mode of transmission of *S.* Enteritidis differs from that of other serovars.

CONCLUDING REMARKS

The *S.* Enteritidis situation in Switzerland has been a part of a European-wide *S.* Enteritidis PT4 epidemic. Results from different investigations suggest that sporadic as well as outbreak cases of *S.* Enteritidis infections are most often transmitted by eggs. Findings by several investigators support the hypothesis that a possible mode of transmission is from infected ovaries of laying hens to the contents of the eggs. *Salmonella* Enteritidis PT4 is known to cause an invasive infection of poultry (Hoop and Pospischil, 1993; Humphrey, 1994).

The decrease in laboratory reports for this salmonella serovar since 1992 indicates that the epidemic is declining. It is fair to assume that the epidemiological, legislative, and information activities have contributed to the continuous decrease in *S.* Enteritidis infections. The egg production chain has been improved at different levels. The specific recommendations for improvements in food and kitchen hygiene issued by the SFOPH and their subsequent dissemination by means of the media may have had a certain preventive impact. Increased awareness of the risk has led to greater care in the handling of eggs, especially in the catering industry (for example, the use of pasteurized eggs for egg dessert dishes).

Despite the encouraging decrease in reported *S.* Enteritidis infections, further surveillance and continued efforts in prevention are still necessary. A laboratory-based surveillance scheme for human salmonellosis on an international basis was established by the European Union–funded Salm-Net project. Switzerland, represented by the SFOPH and the National Reference Laboratory for Foodborne Diseases, is one of the 14 countries that participate in this European network. A common database has been created that enables the monitoring and comparison of salmonella serovars in Europe, so that outbreaks with international implications can be detected.

REFERENCES

Anonymous. 1988. Salmonella-Infektionen, verursacht durch rohe oder ungenhgend erhitzte Eier und Eierspeisen. Bull. Bundesamt Gesundheitswes. 46:589.

Baird-Parker, A.C. 1990. Foodborne salmonellosis. Lancet 336:1231–1235.

Baumgartner, A. 1990a. *Salmonella enteritidis* in Schaleneiern-Situation in der Schweiz und im Ausland. Mitt. Geb. Lebensmittelunters. Hyg. 87:180–193.

Baumgartner, A. 1990b. Salmonellosen in der Schweiz 1984–1989. Hospitalis 61:88–93.

Baumgartner, A., Heimann, P., Schmid, H., Liniger, M., and Simmen, A. 1992. *Salmonella* contamination of poultry carcasses and human salmonellosis. Arch. Lebensmittelhyg. 43:121–148.

Baumgartner, A., Simmen, A., Grand, M., Böttcher, J., Jäggi, N., Rudin, C., and Vetterli, J. 1993. Evaluation einer serologischen Methode (ELISA) zur Ueberwachung von Legebetrieben auf *Salmonella enteritidis.* Arch. Lebensmittelhyg. 44:143–146.

Burkhalter, P.W., Müller, C., Lüthy, J., and Candrian, U. 1995. Detection of *Salmonella* spp. in eggs: DNA analyses, culture techniques, and serology. J. AOAC Int. 78:1531–1537.

Cruickshank, J.G., and Humphrey, T.J. 1987. The carrier food handler and non-typhoid salmonellosis. Epidemiol. Infect. 98:223–230.

Federal Department of the Interior. 1995. Ordinance on the hygienic-microbiological standards on foods, utility articles, premises, facilities, and personnel. SR 817.051 (German, French, and English versions available).

Fisher, I.S.T., on behalf of the Salm-Net participants. 1997. *Salmonella enteritidis* and *S. typhimurium* in Western Europe for 1993–1995. Eurosurveillance 2:4–6.

Furrer, B., Baumgartner, A., and Bommeli, W. 1993. Enzyme-linked immunosorbent assay (ELISA) for the detection of antibodies against *Salmonella enteritidis* in chicken blood and egg yolk. Zentralbl. Bakteriol. 279:191–200.

Gast, R.K., and Holt, P.S. 1995. Iron supplementum to enhance the recovery of *Salmonella enteritidis* from pools of egg contents. J. Food Prot. 58:268–272.

Gerigk, K. 1992. WHO surveillance programme for control of foodborne infections and intoxications in Europe. In: Proceedings of the third world congress on foodborne infections and intoxications, vol. 1. Berlin: Institute of Veterinary Medicine, Robert von Ostertag Institute, pp. 20–25.

Hoop, R.K., and Keller, B. 1991. Pathologisch-anatomische, bakteriologische und serologische Befunde bei Legehennen aus Nebenerwerbshühnerhaltung mit *Salmonella enteritidis* Phagentyp 4-Infektionen. Schweiz. Arch. Tierheilkd. 133:83–88.

Hoop, R.K., and Pospischil, A. 1993. Bacteriological, serological, histological and immunohistochemical findings in laying hens with naturally acquired *Salmonella enteritidis* phage type 4 infection. Vet. Rec. 133:391–393.

Humphrey, T.J. 1994. Contamination of egg shell and contents with *Salmonella enteritidis*: a review. Int. J. Food Microbiol. 21:31–40.

Jaeggi, N., Hunziker, H.R., and Baumgartner, A. 1992. Case report: Einzel- und Gruppenerkrankungen mit *Salmonella enteritidis* ausgehend von einem verseuchten Legebetrieb. Bull. Bundesamt Gesundheitswes. 40:660–663.

Perales, I., and Audicana, A. 1988. *Salmonella enteritidis* and eggs. Lancet 2:1133.

Pether, J.V.S., and Scott, R.J.D. 1982. *Salmonella* carriers: are they dangerous? A study to identify finger contamination. J. Infect. 5:81–88.

Roberts, D. 1982. Factors contributing to outbreaks of food poisoning in England and Wales 1970–1979. J. Hyg. 89:491–498.

Rodrigue, D.C., Tauxe, R.V., and Rowe, B. 1990. International increase in *Salmonella enteritidis:* a new pandemic? Epidemiol. Infect. 105:21–27.

Schmid, H., Burnens, A.P., Baumgartner, A., and Oberreich, J. 1996. Risk factors for sporadic salmonellosis in Switzerland. Eur. J. Clin. Microbiol. Infect. Dis. 15:725–732.

Schroeter, A., Ward, L.R., Rowe, B., Protz, D., Hartung, M., and Helmuth, R. 1994. *Salmonella enteritidis* phage types in Germany. Eur. J. Epidemiol. 10:645–648.

Schwab, H. 1995. Hygiene im Alltag. Bull. Bundesamt Gesundheitswes. 20:23–25.

St. Louis, M.E., Morse, D.L., Potter, M.E., De Melfi, T.M., Gunzewich, J.J., Tauxe, R.V., Blake, P.A., and the *Salmonella enteritidis* working group. 1988. The emergence of grade A eggs as a major source of *Salmonella enteritidis* infections. JAMA 259:2103–2107.

Swiss Federal Council. 1993. Ordinance for the control and eradication of epizootic diseases. SR 916.401 (available only in German and French).

Swiss Federal Council. 1995. Ordinance on foodstuffs. SR 817.02 (available only in German and French).

10

Salmonella enterica Serovar Enteritidis Phage Types in Austria: From Understanding to Intervention

W. Thiel

INTRODUCTION

In Europe, epidemiological investigations of the ongoing epidemic of *Salmonella enterica* serovar Enteritidis (*S.* Enteritidis) implicated shell eggs and poultry as major vehicles of infection. This is in accord with data from Austria [World Health Organization (WHO), 1995a]. Besides a few case-control studies (Cowden et al., 1989; Kist, 1995), however, which also may have their limitations (Cowden, 1996), little is known about the mode of transmission and kinetics of the vast majority of the so-called sporadic and family-related cases; this is largely because of the traditionally existing gap between human and nonhuman salmonella data, especially in terms of timeliness, epidemiological linkage, and proper intervention.

The Austrian National Salmonella Center (NSC) is fortunate in having a well-established and stable reporting system with centralized data from human and nonhuman strains over decades, which enable day-to-day surveillance.

SOURCES OF *SALMONELLA* ENTERITIDIS ISOLATES

Human Sources

The NSC receives salmonella strains from human sources under the following categories:

- Case: clinical illness, either sporadic, family related, or part of a notified general outbreak.

- Surroundings: with or without symptoms, family related or part of a notified general outbreak; initiated by local health authorities (LHAs) or doctors.
- Food handlers: in general, healthy adults, who are screened once a year for salmonella excretion.

It should be noted that the different terms may not always be used consistently; for example, depending on diagnostic impetus, a sporadic case can become part of a family outbreak. Therefore, it seems reasonable to take these two categories as a preliminary entity at the serovar level, but with more benchwork and additional information to try to diminish this epidemiologically boring mass of undefined infections. On the other hand, strains from food handlers usually reflect an infection in the recent past and may help to show what is going on in the community (Table 10.1). Figures 10.1–10.5 include all of the aforementioned categories, whereas the general outbreaks are excluded from Figures 10.6 and 10.7.

Nonhuman Sources

Nonhuman sources include isolates from food, feed, animals, and the environment. Data presented are limited to select strains from poultry and eggs. In the early 1980s, *Salmonella* Typhimurium was the main isolate in Austria, but in 1985 it was second to *S.* Enteritidis. Since 1988, *S.* Enteritidis has increased to epidemic proportions, with a peak in 1992. After a gradual decrease from 1993 to 1995, a stable situation at a high level has taken place (Fig. 10.8). A similar epidemic curve of *S.* Enteritidis is drawn for the isolates from food handlers (Fig. 10.9).

TABLE 10.1 *Salmonella* Enteritidis isolates from human and nonhuman sources in Austria, 1989–96

Year	Total S. Enteritidis		S. Enteritidis in humans (%)		
	Nonhuman	Human	Sporadic cases + family outbreaks	Food handler	General outbreaks
1989	432	3820	84.8	9.4	5.8
1990	644	8752	80.1	10.1	9.8
1991	1339	9234	88.1	9.3	2.6
1992	1140	11,615	88.6	7.7	3.7
1993	1955	8726	90.8	6.2	3.0
1994	1353	7753	89.1	9.6	1.3
1995	1213	7763	91.0	7.6	1.4
1996	1294	7800	89.0	7.4	3.6
1989–96	9370	65,463	87.9	8.3	3.8

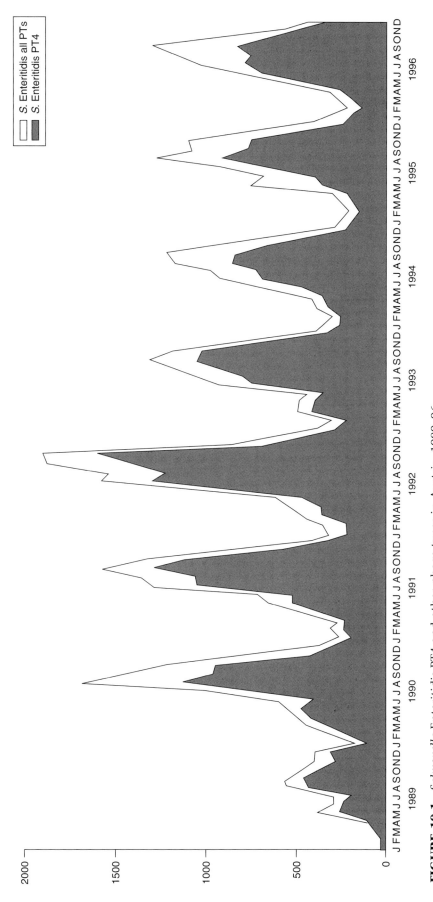

FIGURE 10.1 *Salmonella* Enteritidis PT4 and other phage types in Austria, 1989–96.

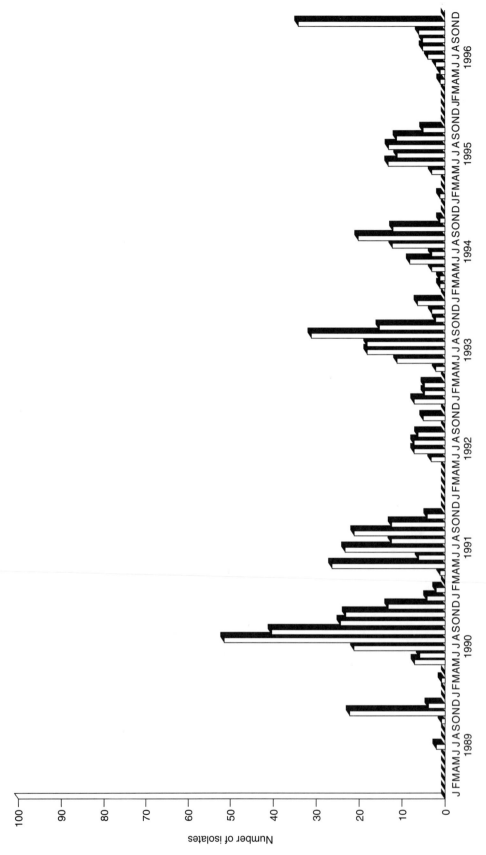

FIGURE 10.2 *Salmonella* Enteritidis PT14b isolates in Austria, 1989–96.

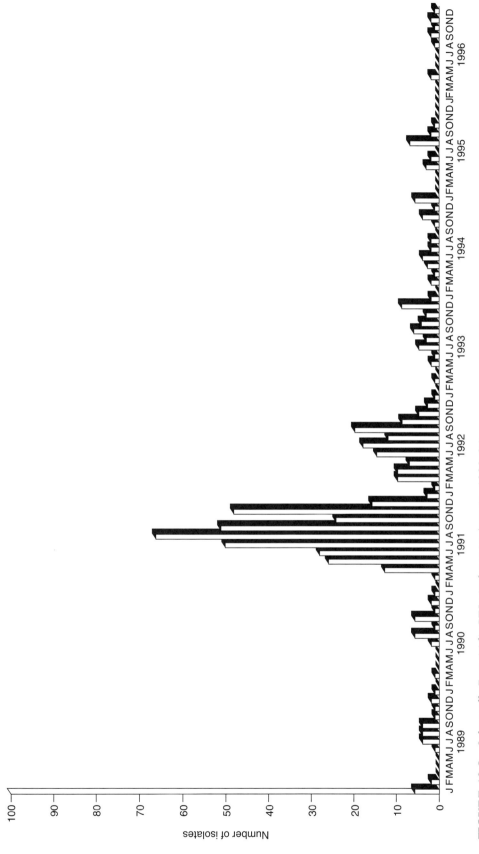

FIGURE 10.3 *Salmonella* Enteritidis PT5a isolates in Austria, 1989–96.

95

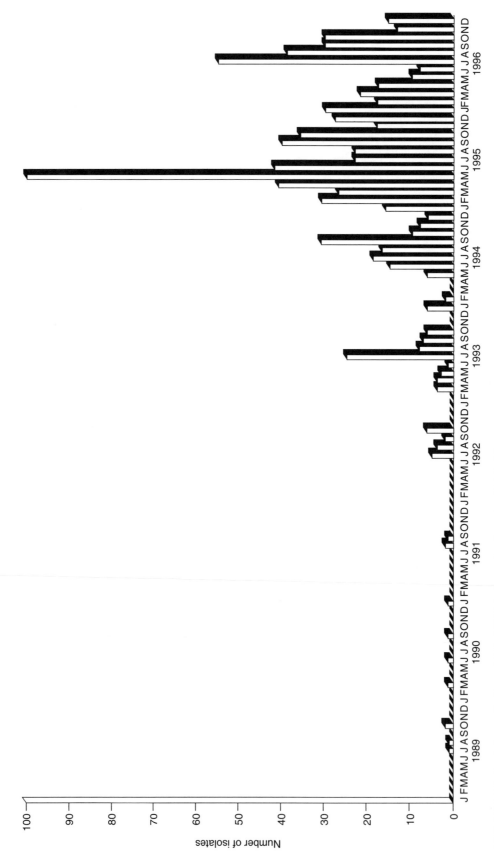

FIGURE 10.4 *Salmonella* Enteritidis PT21 isolates in Austria, 1989–96.

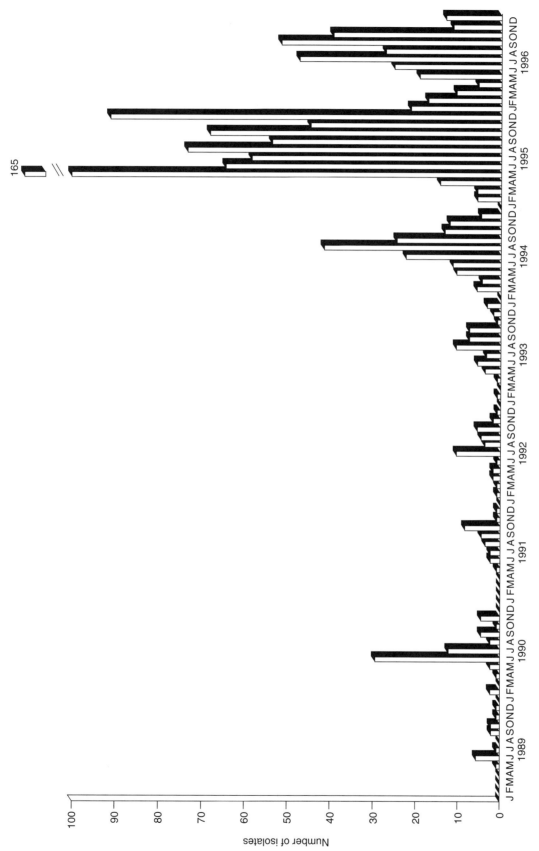

FIGURE 10.5 *Salmonella* Enteritidis PT6 isolates in Austria, 1989–96.

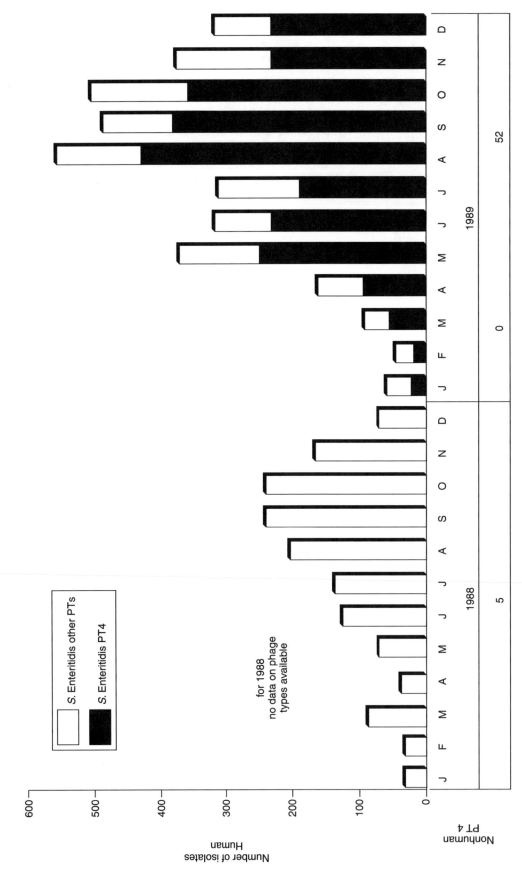

FIGURE 10.6 *Salmonella* Enteritidis PT4 and other phage types from human and nonhuman sources in Austria (general outbreaks excluded), 1988–89.

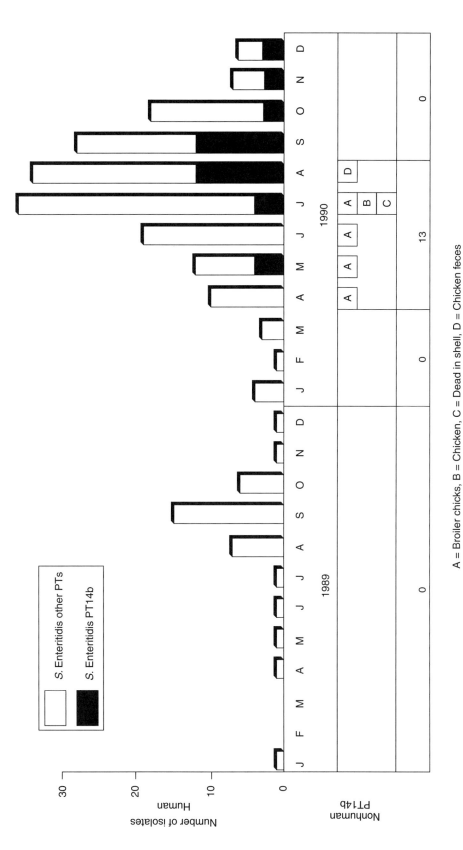

FIGURE 10.7 *Salmonella* Enteritidis PT14b and other phage types from humans and other sources in the district of Deutschlandsberg; population, 60,581 (general outbreaks excluded), 1989–90.

A = Broiler chicks, B = Chicken, C = Dead in shell, D = Chicken feces

99

This review demonstrates the impact of *S. Enteritidis* infections on the population at large, based on a simple but powerful tool of descriptive epidemiology: namely, to monitor and possibly fit together *S. Enteritidis* isolates from human and nonhuman origin over time and space, not at serovar level, as done by others (Bögel et al., 1995), but at phage-type level (Thiel, 1992).

SALMONELLA ENTERITIDIS PHAGE TYPES IN AUSTRIA

The epidemiological applications of phage typing are well documented (Threlfall and Frost, 1989). Faced with the sharp increase of *S. Enteritidis* in Austria by 1988, the NSC was keen to obtain Colindale typing phages (Ward et al., 1987), and in mid-1989 the method was incorporated into the routine identification procedure for all *S. Enteritidis* strains.

To get an idea of the phage-type situation in the preceding years, the existing strain collection was partly typed back to 1984. This analysis pointed out that, before 1988, phage type 8 (PT8) was dominant in humans and poultry, yet in low numbers (data not shown).

Having phage typed all human and nonhuman *S. Enteritidis* isolates during 1989, it became clear that PT4 had arrived on a large scale and was responsible for the observed dramatic increase of *S. Enteritidis* in humans, food, animals, and the environment (Thiel, 1991; Thiel et al., 1993).

In 1989, the seasonal curve for *S. Enteritidis* isolates showed a high rate of PT4 in humans (69% of all *S. Enteritidis*), with an incidence of 32 cases per 100,000 Austrian inhabitants (total population, 7,795,786) (Figs. 10.1, 10.6). From January to April 1989, no isolates of *S. Enteritidis* PT4 from domestic poultry were referred to the NSC, but by May all major domestic poultry-producing areas simultaneously referred a total of 52 *S. Enteritidis* PT4 strains from all production levels (for example, from chicks dead in shells, to parent chickens, to broiler chickens for retail sale) (Fig. 10.6). Since then, Austria has remained a *PT4 country,* and therefore the value of PT4 data for epidemiological purposes became rather limited. Even molecular fingerprinting could indicate only that PT4 comprised a genomic stable clone over years (Buchrieser et al., 1997). But what beyond the shadow of PT4, hidden under *serovar canvas,* might happen that could cause a call for action?

The following selected phage-type episodes (Figs. 10.2–10.5) represent regional epidemiological key phases:

PT14b. In 1989, only 29 infections with this phage type were registered in Austria, compared with 185 in 1990. The geographical distribution shows a very high incidence in the district of Deutschlandsberg, in which *S. Enteritidis* PT14b accounted for 23% of the total *S. Enteritidis* phage types (178). This phage type accounted for 1.9% of 7712 *S. Enteritidis* isolates from the other districts of Austria. On the nonhuman side, from April until July, 10 regional broiler farms were PT14b positive, with eight of them located in the same district (Fig. 10.7). In July, one PT14b

strain from a dead chick in a shell egg from a regional hatchery was referred to the NSC (Fig. 10.7). The NSC initiated a meeting with local general practitioners and public health officials to raise awareness and encouraged a private veterinarian voluntarily to destroy a PT14b-positive parent flock with 1400 birds at the age of 40 weeks.

PT5a. In 1990, there was only a small amount of this phage type in Austria (Fig. 10.3). Starting in the spring of 1991, increasing numbers of human PT5a infections in Oberösterreich and adjacent parts of Niederösterreich were registered: PT5a accounted for 9.2% of 1456 *S. Enteritidis* isolates from the region of Oberösterreich (infection incidence, 10 cases per 100,000 inhabitants) and accounted for 8% of 1325 *S. Enteritidis* isolates from the region of Niederösterreich (infection incidence, 7.1 cases per 100,000 inhabitants), whereas PT5a accounted for 1.2% of the 6208 *S. Enteritidis* isolates from the rest of Austria (infection incidence, 1.3 cases per 100,0000 inhabitants). During the same period and from the same region, 13 PT5a isolates from broiler chickens, chicks dead in shell eggs, feces from laying chickens, and chickens for retail sale were referred to the NSC. By tracing these strains, the NSC learned that most of the investigations were initiated through private interest. All information on import, holding conditions, and local chicken and egg retail sales was confidential and could therefore unfortunately not be reported to public health officials for intervention. High losses were reported; one veterinarian believed the problem was a temperature regulation failure in the breeder rather than an underlying infection, and nearly 400 chicks died.

PT21. This phage type was rare in Austria until the early 1990s (Fig. 10.4). From December 1994 onward, the NSC registered an increasing number of human infections with PT21 in Tirol. In early February, the LHAs were informed about the emerging cluster of this phage type. Later in February, the NSC initiated a Salm-Net inquiry: no similar observations were reported from the five countries that responded. In April 1995, a strain of *S. Enteritidis* PT21, isolated from a cloacal swab of a flock at the end of lay was sent to the NSC (this is the only compulsory investigation in the laying branch; all other salmonella screening is only a recommendation). The farm from where the isolate originated turned out to be the major egg producer in the region. The trade area correlated well with home addresses of patients, as did individual egg retail and food histories. Based on these circumstances, the LHA initiated bacteriological examination of eggs. Of 1200 eggs investigated, 13 pools of five eggs were positive for *S. Enteritidis* PT21 (Fig. 10.10). In mid-May, the farm was legally forbidden to sell fresh eggs. A dramatic decline in *S. Enteritidis* PT21 infections was observed in the region as a result of this intervention (Figs. 10.11, 10.12) (WHO, 1995a). This particular phage type had an incidence of 47 cases per 100,000 inhabitants for 1995 in the district of Tirol, accounting for 30.3% of the total *S. Enteritidis* isolates (981) in this area, compared with 1.8 cases per 100,000 inhabitants in the rest of Austria. In July 1996, *S. Enteritidis* PT21 strains were isolated from noodle preparations with an expiration date of January 1996.

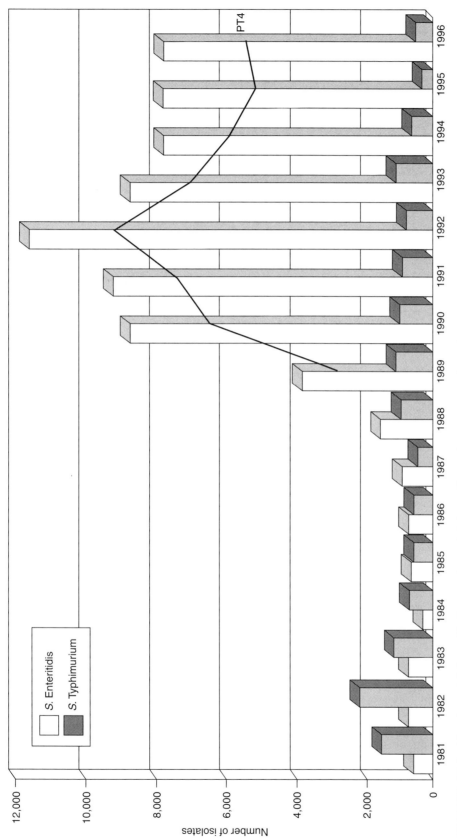

FIGURE 10.8 Number of *Salmonella* Enteritidis and *Salmonella* Typhimurium isolates from human sources in Austria, 1981–96.

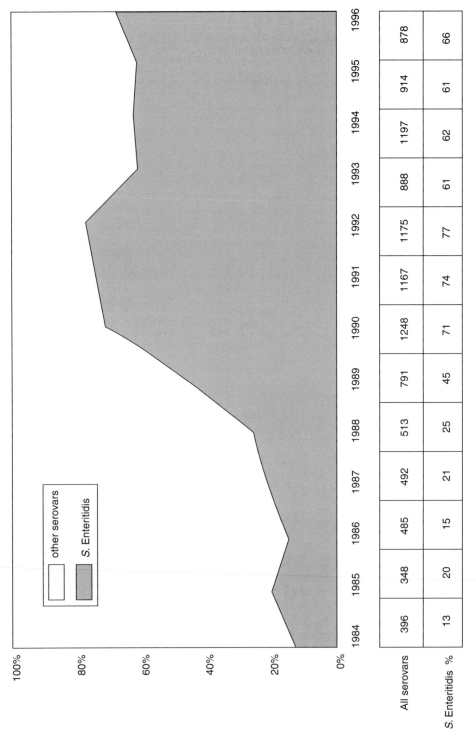

	1984	1985	1986	1987	1988	1989	1990	1991	1992	1993	1994	1995	1996
All serovars	396	348	485	492	513	791	1248	1167	1175	888	1197	914	878
S. Enteritidis %	13	20	15	21	25	45	71	74	77	61	62	61	66

FIGURE 10.9 *Salmonella* Enteritidis and other serovar isolates from food handlers in Austria, 1984–96.

These noodles were prepared with eggs from the same farm, which could indicate that the farm was already positive for *S.* Enteritidis PT21 in January 1995, simultaneously with the regional emergence of PT21 in humans.

PT6. Until 1993, this phage type was quite uncommon throughout Austria (Fig. 10.5). It increased in 1994, followed by an even greater increase in 1995, with an outstanding high incidence in Vorarlberg. This situation remained fairly unchanged during 1996 (Fig. 10.13). In November 1996, the regional food laboratory received an official routine sample of bulk curd with raw egg. This product sample yielded *S.* Enteritidis PT6. The NSC brought this to the attention of the local public health agencies, who in turn traced the eggs back to a large egg producer in the area. Bacteriological examination of the first four laying hens recovered *S.* Enteritidis PT6 from two of the birds.

The aforementioned *S.* Enteritidis events have features in common that allow a few general remarks:

- Based on phage typing, seemingly unrelated sporadic cases, excreters, and family outbreaks of serovar Enteritidis turn out to be phage-type clusters. When these clusters then correspond with a regionally distributed food vehicle of the same phage type, the clusters fulfill the criteria of an otherwise unrecognized community outbreak.
- These outbreaks are different: they tend to cover a larger geographical area, they are more diffuse, and they follow more or less the total seasonal epidemic curve over a longer period of time toward endemicity.
- With these facts in hand, why hesitate to claim similar modes of transmission and correlation for other phage types around?
- The Poultry Zoonosis Order—a law since 1992 (WHO, 1994)—without offering financial reimbursement for the destruction of *S.* Enteritidis–positive flocks, has had little impact on epidemiology of the disease.
- However, the isolates gained through compulsory investigations are valuable to epidemiologists. A rough comparison of the five most common phage types in humans and the respective rates in the domestic poultry and egg production shows an interesting relationship (Table 10.2).
- There are expectations based on serum antibody studies (Liesegang et al., 1997) that there is growing protective immunity against *S.* Enteritidis in the population. On the one hand, the episodes just described fit well into the ups and downs listed in Table 10.2 (except PT7, which is considered to be the result of a gut phenomenon of *S.* Enteritidis rather than a marker). On the other hand, if one looks at the overall epidemic curves, including food handlers, it is difficult to believe that *S.* Enteritidis has had its day as long as its cozy poultry niche keeps getting filled.
- This new understanding about the merely suspected epidemiological link between sporadic and single family-related infections as local or regional clusters

not only diminishes the bulk of sporadic infections but underlines the infective potential of single eggs and chickens.

- Rural markets, local bakeries, and other distributors at the community level may serve as amplifiers. This overall pattern also supports the hypotheses of a transient provision with a consignment of *S.* Enteritidis–infected shell eggs or chicken meat (Bögel et al., 1995).
- The relevant *S.* Enteritidis strains of nonhuman origin, either actively induced or as a lucky strike, served as *missing links,* favoring phage-type monitoring of *S.* Enteritidis strains from all sources (Schroeter et al., 1995).

At this point, it is important to realize that Austria is totally dependent on parent chickens imported mainly from Western Europe. Bearing that in mind and also knowing that poultry/egg production technology in Austria remained fairly unchanged in the critical late 1980s, the data presented should be seen against the background of the world map of *S.* Enteritidis phage types (Kühn, 1995), and the following comments apply:

- Under the given circumstances, the overflow with PT4 into Austria in 1988–89 was inevitable.
- The emergence of an endemic clone of PT4 with enhanced virulence, as argued by Pignato et al. (1996), is unlikely.
- Under different international dependencies on domestic poultry production, probably other phage types would have become dominant in Austria, as seen in other countries (Khakhria et al., 1991; László et al., 1993; Boyce et al., 1996; Cowden, 1996).

In other words, the ongoing infective pressure of *S.* Enteritidis on the community seems largely determined by the actual import practice and local conditions of the domestic poultry/egg industry, irrespective of the phage type involved.

SUMMARY

In conclusion, phage-type monitoring of isolates from human and nonhuman sources in time and space did bring an element of understanding into the epidemiological mosaic of *S.* Enteritidis in Europe, which would not have been achieved by serotyping alone. Furthermore, this monitoring opened an additional path for control measures.

Despite the limitations of phage typing (Rankin and Platt, 1995; Baggesen et al., 1997) and the undisputed need for other phenotypic or even genotypic markers, this method combined with antibiotic resistance typing is a basic tool for sero-subtyping of the serovar Enteritidis (Threlfall and Chart, 1993).

Salmonella reference laboratories in general are encouraged to act as catalysts among all of the sectoral responsibilities and traditional salmonella defense lines (Bögel et al., 1995) to create powerful and hopefully successful intervention teams. *Phage-type hunting* can support this goal.

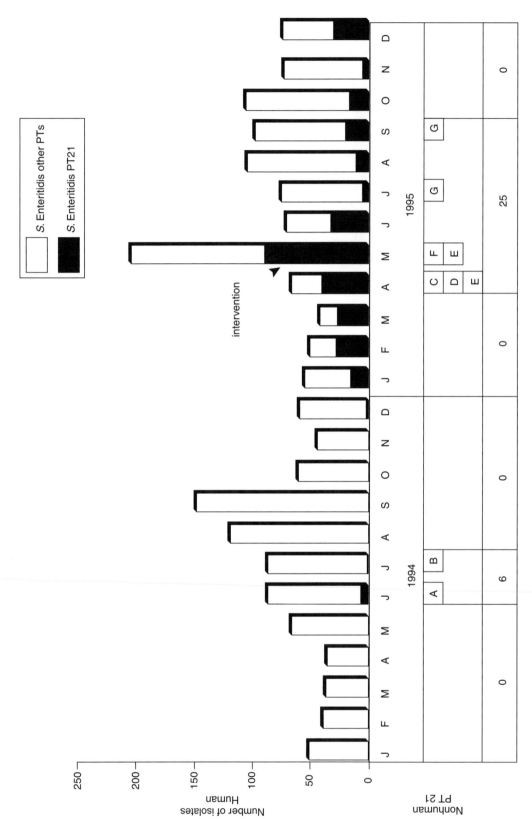

FIGURE 10.10 *Salmonella* Enteritidis PT21 and other phage types from human and nonhuman sources in Tirol; population, 631,410 (general outbreaks excluded), 1994–95.

A = Poultry, B = Poultry feces, C = Laying chicken cloacal swab, D = Laying chicken, E = Shell eggs, F = Liquid egg pasteurized, G = Noodles

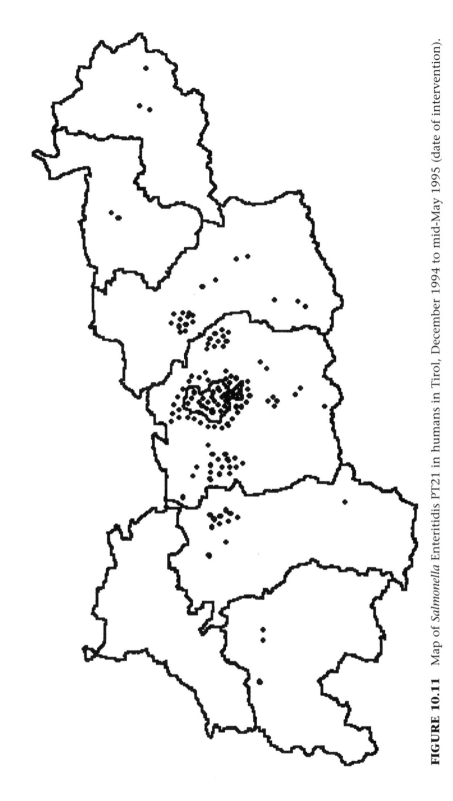

FIGURE 10.11 Map of *Salmonella* Enteritidis PT21 in humans in Tirol, December 1994 to mid-May 1995 (date of intervention).

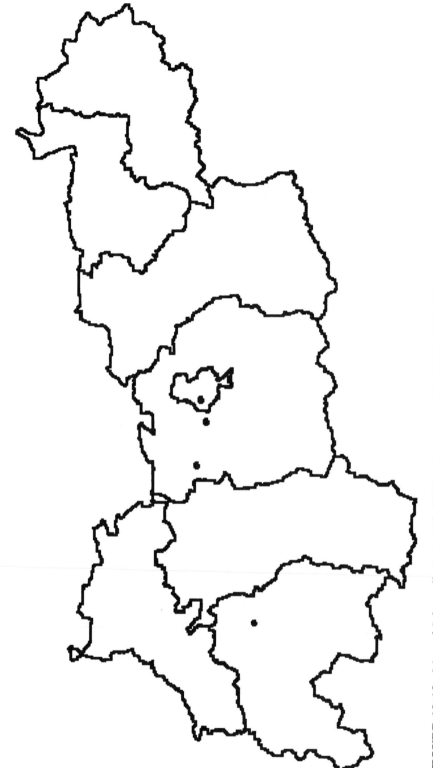

FIGURE 10.12 Map of *Salmonella* Enteritidis PT21 in humans in Tirol, July 1995 (after intervention).

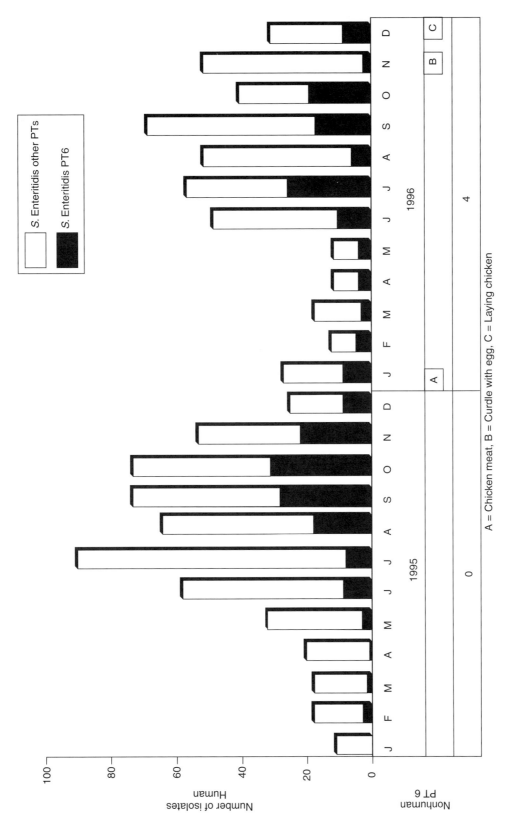

FIGURE 10.13 *Salmonella* Enteritidis PT6 and other phage types from human and nonhuman sources in Voralberg; population, 331,472 (general outbreaks excluded), 1995–96.

107

TABLE 10.2   Common *Salmonella* Enteritidis phage types (PTs) from human and nonhuman sources in Austria, 1993–96

S. Enteritidis	Year	Five most common PTs (1996) (%)					Five PTs	PT7
		PT4	PT8	PT21	PT6	PT1		
Total human								
8726	1993	79.5	9.4	0.7	0.5	4.0	94.1	0.3
7753	1994	74.9	10.2	1.5	1.9	5.5	94.0	0.4
7763	1995	65.9	10.5	5.5	8.4	3.9	94.2	0.3
7800	1996	69.8	14.9	3.8	3.7	1.9	94.1	0.4
Nonhuman[a]								
344	1993	47.7	9.3	0.9	2.0	6.7	66.6	21.2
331	1994	49.0	3.0	3.0	0.6	8.5	64.1	23.0
201	1995	46.0	3.9	3.4	17.0	2.9	71.8	20.0
310	1996	48.1	2.3	8.7	4.5	0.6	64.2	21.3

[a] Poultry, zoonosis order.

REFERENCES

Baggesen, D.L., Wegener, H.C., and Madsen, M. 1997. Correlation of conversion of *Salmonella enterica* serovar Enteritidis phage type 1, 4, or 6 to phage type 7 with loss of lipopolysaccharide. J. Clin. Microbiol. 35:330–333.

Bögel, K., Käsbohrer, A., Stöhr, K., Lehmacher, W., and Talaska, T. 1995. Pattern analysis of human *Salmonella enteritidis* infection. Zentralbl. Bakteriol. 282:474–497.

Boyce, T.G., Koo, D., Swerdlow, D.L., Gomez, T.M., Serrano, B., Nickey, N., Hickman-Brenner, F.W., Galcolm, G.B., and Griffin, P.M. 1996. Recurrent outbreaks of *Salmonella* Enteritidis infections in a Texas restaurant: phage type 4 arrives in the United States. Epidemiol. Infect. 117:29–34.

Buchrieser, C., Brosch, R., Buchrieser, O., Kristl, A., Luchansky, J.B., and Kaspar, C.W. 1997. Genomic analyses of *Salmonella enteritidis* phage type 4 strains from Austria and phage type 8 strains from the United States. Zentralbl. Bakteriol. 285:379–388.

Cowden, J.M. 1996. Outbreaks of salmonellosis: case control studies have their place, but their power should not be overestimated. BMJ 313:1094–1095.

Cowden, J.M., Lynch, D., Joseph, C.A., O'Mahoney, M., Mawer, S.L., Rowe, B., et al. 1989. Case control study of infections with *Salmonella enteritidis* phage type 4 in England. BMJ 299:771–773.

Khakhria, R., Duck, D., and Lior, H. 1991. Distribution of *Salmonella enteritidis* phage types in Canada. Epidemiol. Infect. 106:25–32.

Kist, M. 1995. Fall-Kontroll Studien zur Epidemiologie sporadischer Enteritidis-Salmonellosen. In: Küheng, H., and Tschäpe, H., eds. Salmonellosen des Menschen. Munich: RKI Referat Presse Schriften 3/95, pp. 41–60.

Kühn, H. 1995. Epidemiology of salmonellosis in Germany. Biotest Bull. 5:157–170.

László Vera, G., Csórián Erzsébet, Sz., and Milch, H. 1993. Comparison of two *Salmonella* Enteritidis phage typing methods. Acta Microbiol. Hung. 40:255–263.

Liesegang, A., Prager, R., Streckel, W., Rabsch, W., Gericke, B., Seltmann, G., Helmuth, R., and Tschäpe, H. 1997. Wird der Salmonella-enterica-Stamm DT104 des Serovars Typhimurium der neue führende Epidemietyp in Deutschland? Infektionsepidemiol. Forsch. (RKI Schriften InfFoI/97:6–10).

Pignato, S., Nastasi, A., Mammina, C., Fantasia, M., and Giammanco, G. 1996. Phage types and ribotypes of *Salmonella* Enteritidis in Southern Italy. Zentralbl. Bakteriol. 283:399–405.

Rankin, S., and Platt, D.J. 1995. Phage conversion in *Salmonella enterica* serotype Enteritidis: implications for epidemiology. Epidemiol. Infect. 114:227–236.

Schroeter, A., Bockhorst, W., Hartung, M., Protz, D., and Helmuth, R. 1995. Vorkommen des Salmonella-enteritidis-Phagentyps 6a in Deutschland. Bundesgesundheitsblatt 1:10–12.

Thiel, W. 1991. Zum Salmonellen-Geschehen in Österreich. Oesterr. Gefluegel Wirtsch. 5:147–151.

Thiel, W. 1992. Verbreitung bestimmter Phagentypen von S. Enteritidis in Österreich Schweizerische Gesellschaft für Mikrobiologie. 51. Jahresversammlung (Abstracts), 45.

Thiel, W., Bogiatzis, A., Feierl, G., and Sixl, W. 1993. Epidemiology of S. Enteritidis in Austria. WHO/CDS/VPH/93.123:17.

Threlfall, E.J., and Chart, H. 1993. Interrelationships between strains of *Salmonella enteritidis*. Epidemiol. Infect. 11:1–8.

Threlfall, J.A., and Frost, J.A. 1990. The identification, typing and fingerprinting of *Salmonella*: laboratory aspects and epidemiological applications. J. Appl. Bacteriol. 68:5–16.

Ward, L.R., de Sa, J.D.H., and Rowe, B. 1987. A phagetyping scheme for *Salmonella enteritidis*. Epidemiol. Infect. 99:291–294.

World Health Organization (WHO). 1993. WHO workshop on transmission characteristics of zoonotic salmonellosis with special reference to S. enteritidis, Hannover, March 1993. Document WHO/CDS/VPH/93. 123(Annex 3):17–18.

World Health Organization. 1994. Guidelines on detection and monitoring of *Salmonella* infected poultry flocks with particular reference to *Salmonella* Enteritidis, Zoon/94 173. Graz, Austria, pp. 18–25.

World Health Organization. 1995a. Austria: outbreak of infection with *Salmonella enteritidis* phage type 21 associated with shell eggs. Weekly Epidemiol. Rec. 34:244–245.

World Health Organization. 1995b. Surveillance programme for control of foodborne infections and intoxications in Europe. Sixth report, 1990–1992, Austria. Berlin: FAO/WHO, pp. 19–26.

11

Epidemiology of *Salmonella enterica* Serovar Enteritidis Infections in Italy

G. Scuderi

INTRODUCTION

In the broad spectrum of enteric infections, nontyphoidal salmonellosis, particularly *Salmonella enterica* serovar Enteritidis (*S.* Enteritidis) infections have become increasingly important in recent years in many parts of the world, including most European countries (Rodrigue et al., 1990). In Italy, data on human salmonella infections are collected through two main systems:

- The National Laboratory-based Surveillance System of Enteropathogenic Bacteria. This system was set up in 1971 and includes enteropathogenic bacteria isolated from humans, animals, and foods (Italy, Ministero della Sanità, 1967).
- The National Infectious Disease Reporting (NIDR) System (Sistema di Notifica delle Malattie Infettive), which was reviewed in 1990 (Italy, Ministero della Sanità, 1991). This system is based on clinical and laboratory data on sporadic cases and outbreak cases of foodborne salmonella infections.

Both systems have been recently computerized. The first system became part of the European *Salmonella* Laboratory Surveillance System—Salm-Net (*Salmonella* Network)—which was set up in Italy in 1992. The second (the NIDR) was started in 1994. This chapter focuses on human *S.* Enteritidis gastrointestinal infections in Italy, including the epidemiology, food sources, and public health and legislative measures introduced for controlling these infections.

THE ROLE OF FOOD SOURCES IN THE EPIDEMIOLOGY OF *SALMONELLA* ENTERITIDIS

In the NIDR system, cases caused by *S.* Enteritidis are reported as cases of nontyphoidal salmonellosis (ICD-9003) on the basis of both clinical and bacteriological findings. However, information on the specific agent is not collected, making it impossible to know how many cases are caused by this etiological agent. The total number of cases of salmonellosis were constant at about 10,000 per year through 1989, increased to about 20,000 per year from 1990 to 1994, and then decreased to about 15,000 in 1995 (Italy, Ministero della Sanità, 1996) (Fig. 11.1).

More specific information is available from the National Human Laboratory Surveillance system. The absolute numbers of isolates of *S.* Enteritidis from human samples have been previously described (Binkin et al., 1993): about 400 isolates per year in the early 1980s, increasing to 1100 in 1988; there were 6500 isolates in 1993 (M. Fantasia, unpublished data; see Table 11.1), decreasing to 5400 in 1994 and then to 4500 in 1995 (Fantasia et al., 1997). Data on the total number of *S.* Enteritidis and total salmonella isolates are also presented in Figure 11.1. Table 11.1 shows the total number of *S.* Enteritidis isolates for 1988–95 and their percentage of total salmonella isolates. With regard to the comparison of this serovar with others, *S.* Enteritidis increased from 7.4% in 1988 to 33.4% in 1990, reaching 57.4% in 1992 and decreasing to 37.2% in 1995. These data indicate that

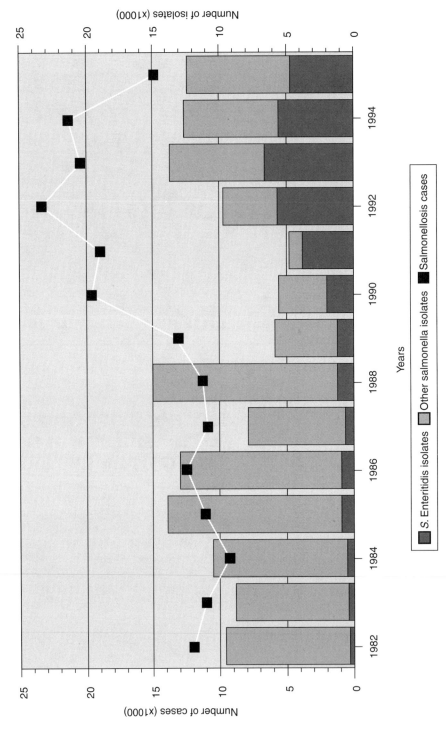

FIGURE 11.1   Salmonellosis in humans and a number of isolates of *Salmonella* Enteritidis and the total of salmonellae from humans in Italy, 1982–95. Note: Data for the isolates for 1987, 1990, and 1991 are incomplete.

TABLE 11.1 *Salmonella* **Enteritidis (number and percentages of the total salmonella isolates from humans)**

Year	No.	%
1988	1112	7.4
1989	1084	18.8
1990	1830	33.4
1991	3703	41.4
1992	5517	57.4
1993	6567	48.3
1994	5435	43.4
1995	4575	37.2

Source: M. Fantasia, unpublished data.

S. Enteritidis has been one of the five most commonly isolated salmonella serovars between 1973 and 1986 (Fantasia and Filetici, 1989). Furthermore, *S.* Enteritidis was the most frequently isolated salmonella serovar during 1989, 1992, and 1993, surpassing *S.* Typhimurium, which in previous years ranked first (Fantasia et al., 1991). Additionally, data from the Salm-Net system show that *S.* Enteritidis was the most commonly isolated salmonella serovar in 1994–95 (Fantasia et al., 1997).

Until 1993, data from laboratory surveillance were obtained by three sovra-regional centers, which surveyed the following regions particularly: Lombardy, Venetia, Toscany, and Sicily. All regions contributed to the Salm-Net surveillance system, but especially Venetia and Lombardy, where computerized archives were established in 1989 and 1993, respectively.

In Italy, the national surveillance of foodborne outbreaks started in 1991 (Italy, Ministero della Sanità, 1991). Based on data collected from the national foodborne-outbreak registration system, among 1379 salmonella outbreaks registered in Italy from 1991 to 1994, group-D salmonellae accounted for 68% of all salmonella isolates (Scuderi et al., 1993, 1996). The number of group-D salmonella outbreaks increased in 1991, peaked in 1992, and decreased between 1993 and 1994; the isolation rate was quite constant also for 1995 (Prete et al., 1996). Among the 946 group-D salmonella outbreaks registered, 473 (50%) were due to *S.* Enteritidis, which accounted for 34% of the total salmonella outbreaks (Scuderi et al., 1993, 1996). Data on the registered foodborne outbreaks caused by salmonella were obtained from the majority of the Italian regions, especially from regions with established surveillance systems, such as Emilia-Romagna, where surveillance has been in effect since 1983 (Casadio et al., 1992; Scuderi et al., 1992), Lombardy (Sodano, 1994), Molise (Manuppella et al., 1994), and Toscany (Levr et al., 1992).

In 31.4% of the total outbreaks caused by *S.* Enteritidis reported during 1991–94 (Scuderi et al., 1993) the vehicle was not ascertained, whereas in 58.1% of the outbreaks the vehicles were eggs and egg-containing foods, as in other countries (St. Louis et al., 1988). In 19.6% of these egg-associated outbreaks, *tiramisu* (a dessert made with raw eggs) was specifically implicated. In 12%, the vehicle implicated was reported generically as "eggs" in nonspecified form, including shell eggs or other egg food preparations: egg pasta was implicated in 7.8%, ice cream in 7.6%, foods with egg sauces in 5.1%, cakes or pastries filled with custard in 3.3%, and other egg foods in 2.7% of these foodborne outbreaks. In the rest of the outbreaks, other vehicles included poultry (2%) and other kinds of meat (such as beef, lamb, and pork) (2.5%); cakes (1.9%); shellfish (1.6%); tuna meat (veal with tuna sauce), which may or may not contain eggs (1%); milk or cheese (0.6%); pasta without eggs (0.4%); and salami (0.4%). In the majority (78%) of the outbreaks caused by *S.* Enteritidis, the food was ascertained on the basis of the epidemiological investigation. Only in the 22% of the outbreaks was the food confirmed by bacteriological analysis.

The distribution of the outbreaks caused by *S.* Enteritidis transmitted by an exposed person that were registered during 1991–94 revealed that low numbers of individuals were involved: four individuals were involved in 17.3% of outbreaks, three in 12.3%, five in 11.7%, and two in 8.6%. Large-scale community outbreaks, such as the outbreak that occurred in 1991, accounted for 2% of the total outbreaks (Scuderi et al., 1992).

As in other countries (Anon., 1988), a study of the *S.* Enteritidis isolates from 50 foodborne outbreaks in Italy revealed that phage type 4 (PT4) is the predominant phage type and that the majority of PT4 isolates carried the 38-MDa plasmid associated with virulence (Fantasia and Filetici, 1994). These strains were isolated from the following foods implicated in 50 outbreaks: eggs (8 of 50) or egg-containing foods, such as cakes and cream (13 of 50) and *tiramis* (6 of 50), ice cream (5 of 50), and mayonnaise or tuna sauce (2 of 50); in rare cases, the strains studied were isolated from vegetables, lamb cutlet, salmon, cheese, ground beef, or processed meat.

PUBLIC HEALTH AND LEGISLATIVE MEASURES

From the data presented in this report, it is clear that *S.* Enteritidis surveillance in Italy has been a prominent health issue in the field of gastrointestinal infections. Italian data on isolation rates from humans with respect to the total number of salmonella isolates in 1995 are comparable to those of other European countries (Fisher et al., 1997). The absolute numbers of *S.* Enteritidis isolates from the 1980s up to 1992 indicate that the trend was increasing, but the 1993–95 data indicate that some control was achieved, based on the lower isolation rate of this serovar. Of course, as with any surveillance system, our system suffers from underreporting. Moreover, many changes were made to the surveillance systems. The new version of the National Infectious Disease Reporting System came into effect in April 1991, and the numbers of registrations from each region are very different. The same situation exists for the National Laboratory Human Surveillance System: the figures refer to strains isolated and/or typed at the reference regional laboratories, and laboratory investigations often are not carried to the serovar level.

On the other hand, the evolving methodology of the surveillance systems and particularly their results might lead to a major emphasis on salmonella surveillance in general and especially on detecting the *S.* Enteritidis serovar.

In Italy, the control of *S.* Enteritidis human infection has been included in the control of human enteric pathogens, food-transmitted diseases, zoonoses, periodic examinations of the carrier status of food handlers, hygiene in food preparation, and animal infections. At the level of food hygiene production, many food industries have adopted the Hazard Analysis Critical Control Point methodology. Moreover, Italy follows the European Union recommendations. Special measures were adopted in 1992 after results of the second year of national surveillance became available and especially after some large outbreaks due to the consumption of egg-containing foods. The Ministry of Health, the National Institute of Health, and the National Health Council launched a concerted action to improve the surveillance of salmonellosis in humans, animals, and food. As in other countries, special attention was given to the transmission of *S.* Enteritidis through egg-containing foods (Scuderi et al., 1996).

The Department of Health of each region was warned of the high incidence of *S.* Enteritidis foodborne outbreaks and particularly those due to the consumption of egg-containing foods. The following recommendations were made:

1. Surveillance of human salmonellosis should include sporadic cases as well as outbreak cases. To enhance surveillance, guidelines for epidemiological and bacteriological analysis (Greco et al., 1993) during salmonella foodborne outbreaks were developed and distributed to all local health units.
2. The public should be educated regarding the preparation of egg-containing foods; a special warning was released about the hazards of consuming foods that contain raw eggs, especially those prepared in large quantities that use a large number of eggs and that might not be consumed for a long period of time, such as *tiramis* or other recipes in which cooking time and/or temperature are insufficient to kill the microorganism. For this reason, during epidemic periods, some regions prohibited the preparation and consumption of foods that contained fresh raw eggs. It was recommended that pasteurized eggs be used for commercial catering, for example, to schools, the military, hospitals, and homes for the elderly.
3. Special attention should be devoted to the surveillance and control of all animal farms, particularly poultry and hen farms, to avoid infections of eggs. Guidelines have been prepared for sampling and analysis for the bacteriological control of feeds, with particular reference to research and to isolation of salmonellae (Piccininno et al., 1992).

CONCLUSION

Data gathered during the last 4 years of laboratory-based and clinically based surveillance suggest that the legislative measures adopted have achieved some control of *S.* Enteritidis outbreaks and of bacteriological laboratory isolations. This has been associated with a concomitant reduction in cases among humans. This might be the result of all of the health measures that have been adopted, but it cannot be excluded that this is a "natural" decreasing trend, as often occurs with infections caused by other salmonella serovars. Many more years of surveillance will be necessary to confirm the essence of this decreasing trend.

ACKNOWLEDGMENTS

The author especially thanks Dr. S. Salmaso, who introduced her to the field of epidemiology and revised the manuscript; many thanks also to Mrs. P. Carbonari, Mrs. G. Canganella, Mrs. S. Lana, and Mr. M. Kanieff for secretarial assistance.

REFERENCES

Anonymous. 1988. *Salmonella enteritidis* phage type 4: chicken and egg. Lancet 1:720–722.

Binkin, N., Scuderi, G., Novaco, F., Giovanardi, G.L., Paganelli, G., Ferrari, G., Cappelli, O., Ravaglia, L., Zilioli, F., Amadei, V., Magliani, W., Viani, I., Ricci, D., Borrini, B., Magri, M., Alessandrini, A., Bursi, G., Barigazzi, G., Fantasia, M., Filetici, E., and Salmaso, S. 1993. Egg-related *Salmonella enteritidis*, Italy, 1991. Epidemiol. Infect. 110:227–237.

Casadio, P., Lanciotti, G., and Novaco, F. 1992. A pranzo con il killer. Come 1/2.

Fantasia, M., and Filetici, E. 1989. Italian experience in *Salmonella* spp. isolations from 1973 to 1986. Microbiologica 12:85–89.

Fantasia, M., and Filetici E. 1994. *Salmonella enteritidis* in Italy. Int. J. Food Microbiol. 21:7–13.

Fantasia, M., Filetici, E., Anastasio, M.P., Marcozzi, M.D., Gramenzi, M.P., and Aureli, P. 1991. Italian experience in *Salmonella enteritidis* 1978–1988: characterization of isolates from food and man. Int. J. Food Microbiol. 12:353–362.

Fantasia, M., Niglio, T., and Scuderi, G. 1997. Laboratory-based surveillance of *Salmonella* infections in human: Italy, 1994–1995 [Oral presentation]. In: Polydorou K., et al., eds. Proceedings of the W.A.V.M.I. 15th international symposium of salmonellosis/brucellosis, Cyprus, 16–21 February 1997.

Fisher, I., et al. 1997. *Salmonella* Enteritidis and *S.* Typhimurium in Western Europe for 1993–1995: a surveillance report from Salm-Net. Eurosurveillance 2:4–6.

Greco, D., Scuderi, G., Fantasia, M., Toti, L., Orefice, L., Aureli, P., Piccininno, G., Macrí, A., Squarcione, S., Maffei, C., Filippetti, F., Pandolfi, P., and Binkin, N. 1993. Linee guida per le indagini su epidemie di salmonellosi di origine alimentare. Rapporti ISTISAN 93/30. Istituto Superiore di Sanità.

Italy, Ministero della Sanità. Circolare 163 del 17.10.1967 Istituzione del Sistema Nazionale di Sorveglianza delle Salmonelle e degli Enterobatteri Patogeni.

Italy, Ministero della Sanità. D.M. 15 Dec. 1990. Sistema Informativo delle Malattie Infettive e Diffusive. Gazz Uff 8 Jan. 1991. Serie Gen 6.

Italy, Ministero della Sanità. Direzione Generale Servizi Igiene Pubblica Divisione Profilassi Malattie Infettive. Boll. Min. Sanità 1996.

Levr, E., Valentini, P., Pellegrini, G., and Caroli, G. 1992. At home as well as abroad: the epidemiological success of *Salmonella enteritidis*. J. Prev. Med. Hyg. 33:37–40.

Manuppella, A., Ricci, N., and Pede, V. 1994. Il sistema di Sorveglianza delle Salmonellosi nel Molise. Microbiol. Med. 9:32–33.

Piccininno, G., Achene, L., Adone, R., Pistoia, C., and Ciuchini, F. 1992. Metodi di campionamento e di analisi per il controllo microbiologico dei mangimi, con particolare riferimento alla ricerca ed isolamento delle salmonelle. Rapporti ISTISAN 92/18. Istituto Superiore di Sanità.

Prete, A.M., Vellucci, L., and Squarcione, S. 1996. Foodborne disease outbreaks: data from the national reporting system of infectious diseases. In: Cost action 97 workshop: prevention of contamination of poultry meat, eggs and egg products, Rome, 23–25 October.

Rodrigue, D.C., Tauxe, R.V., and Rowe, B. 1990. International increase in *Salmonella enteritidis*: a new pandemic? Epidemiol. Infect. 105:21–27.

Scuderi, G., Binkin, N., Novaco, F., Fantasia, M., Filetici, E., et al. 1992. *Salmonella enteritidis* in provincia di Parma. Ig. Mod. 98:867–887.

Scuderi, G., Squarcione, S., Giannico, F., Panatta, M., and Greco, D. 1993. Tossinfezioni da *Salmonella* in Italia: il sistema di notifica dei focolai epidemici. Ig. Mod. 100:218–239.

Scuderi, G., Fantasia, M., Filetici, E., and Anastasio, M.P. 1996. Foodborne outbreaks caused by *Salmonella* in Italy, 1991–4. Epidemiol. Infect. 116:257–265.

Sodano, L. Rapporto sui focolai epidemici di origine alimentare in Lombardia. Luglio, 1994.

St. Louis, M.E., Morse, D.L., Potter, M.E., De Melfi, T.M., Guzewich, J.J., Tauxe, R.V., Blake, P.A., and the *Salmonella enteritidis* Working Group. 1988. The emergence of grade A eggs as a major source of *Salmonella enteritidis* infection: new implications for the control of salmonellosis. JAMA 259:2103–2107.

12

Prevalence of *Salmonella enterica* Serovar Enteritidis and Other Salmonella Serovars Among Immunocompromised and Immunocompetent Persons in New York City, 1993–95

R. Gruenewald, R.J. Carter, T.P. Singh, S. Terry, G. Williams, and A. Ramon

INTRODUCTION

Salmonella infections are transmitted to humans primarily by ingestion of contaminated raw or undercooked eggs, poultry, meat, and dairy products, or foods that are cross-contaminated with these products (Angulo and Swerdlow, 1995). Compared with middle-aged individuals, the susceptibility and vulnerability of infants to salmonellosis is extremely high and that of the very old is above average (Blaser and Feldman, 1981; Blaser and Newman, 1982; Hargrett-Bean et al., 1988; Tauxe, 1996). Immunodeficient individuals, including those with acquired immunodeficiency syndrome (AIDS), are often much more vulnerable than are immunocompetent individuals to infections caused by a variety of microorganisms, including salmonellae (Wolfe et al., 1971; Mildvan et al., 1982; Kovacs and Masur, 1985; Centers for Disease Control, 1992; Gruenewald et al., 1994; Angulo and Swerdlow, 1995).

Between 1968 and 1987, *Salmonella* Typhimurium was the most frequently isolated serovar from humans in the United States (Blaser and Feldman, 1981; Levine et al., 1991). Between 1976 and 1985, the sixfold increase in the reported incidence of *Salmonella enterica* serovar Enteritidis (*S.* Enteritidis) infections in the northeastern United States was traced to its colonization of grade-A shell eggs, most likely via transovarian transmission (St. Louis et al., 1988; Gast and Beard, 1990; Altekruse and Swerdlow, 1996). Thereafter, the widespread presence of salmonellae in chicken eggs became established in many egg-product plants throughout the continental United States (Ebel et al., 1993; Vugia et al., 1993). It is, therefore, not surprising that, as of 1990, *S.* Enteritidis became the most frequently isolated serovar in the United States (Mishu et al., 1994; Altekruse and Swerdlow, 1996; Boyce et al., 1996). A sharp increase in the incidence of *S.* Enteritidis infections between 1979 and 1987 was also noted in Europe and South America (Rodrigue et al., 1990).

Although a number of salmonella serovars have been shown to possess enhanced invasiveness in persons with AIDS (Celum et al., 1987), *S.* Enteritidis may be particularly virulent in this group (Levine et al., 1991). A study of salmonella infections diagnosed between January 1985 and August 1988 in 20- to 59-year-old New York City (NYC) residents found that, among persons listed in the NYC AIDS Registry, salmonella septicemia and gastroenteritis were seen 197 and 51 times, respectively, more frequently than among persons not listed in this registry (Gruenewald et al., 1994). In this same study, *S.* Enteritidis was the most common serovar isolated, accounting for 76% of all septicemia cases and 39% of all cases of gastroenteritis.

Here we report the results of a study of NYC residents of all ages, without AIDS, and 20- to 59-year-old persons with AIDS, all of whom were infected with salmonellae between 1993 and 1995. This study compared persons of different ages, sex, and AIDS status, with respect to the frequency and sites of infection and infecting salmonella serovar. We then compared these findings with those of an earlier study of NYC residents infected with salmonellae between 1985 and 1988 (Gruenewald et al., 1994).

MATERIALS AND METHODS

Salmonellosis is a reportable condition as per the NYC Health Code. Each year the NYC Department of Health (NYCDOH) receives reports of salmonella infection in approximately 2000 NYC residents. Demographic information for each patient is collected by the Bureau of Communicable Disease. The Enteric Bacteriology Laboratory of the NYC Bureau of Laboratories routinely receives salmonella isolates from hospitals in all five boroughs of NYC and performs serological typing of subcultures according to the methods of Gruenewald et al. (1990).

Between 1 January 1993 and 31 December 1995, the NYCDOH received reports of more than 6000 NYC residents diagnosed with salmonella infection. Records missing information on sex, age, salmonella serovar, or site of infection were excluded from this analysis. Specimens identified as *Salmonella* Typhi were also excluded because 69% of these infections originated in foreign countries (NYCDOH Bureau of Communicable Disease, 1997). The name, sex, date of birth, and zip code for each case/patient was matched against the NYC AIDS Registry to identify persons with AIDS.

Persons were then divided into subgroups on the following basis: presence in the AIDS Registry, infecting salmonella serovar, body site infected, sex, and six age categories (0–1, 2–4, 5–19, 20–59, 60–79, and 80–98 years of age). Age categories were based on feeding patterns, immunological function and lifestyle. Because fewer than 4% of persons with salmonella infection and AIDS were younger than age 20 or older than age 59, we report results for only 20- to 59-year-old persons with AIDS. Comparisons between persons with and without AIDS were restricted to 20- to 59-year-olds.

All subgroups were compared with each other on the basis of total number of salmonella isolates and the number and proportion of each serovar. We report results for *Salmonella* serovars Enteritidis, Typhimurium, and Heidelberg separately. An additional 160 serovars were isolated from specimens; but because no other single serovar accounted for more than 4% of the total salmonella-infected population, we combined the results for these 160 serovars into an "other serovar" category. Statistical analysis was performed using Epi-Info 6.04 software (Dean et al., 1990). Categorical data were analyzed using the Mantel-Haenszel chi-squared test.

RESULTS

Between 1 January 1993 and 31 December 1995, the Bureau of Communicable Disease received 6213 reports of salmonella infection in NYC residents. Of these, 3231 (52%) were males, and 2982 (48%) were females; 475 (8%) were persons with AIDS and 840 (26%) were children less than 2 years of age. We report results for 3881 (62%) of these persons for whom information on age, sex, salmonella serovar, and site of infection was available. Of the 3881 cases, 3526 (1767 males and 1759 females) were persons without AIDS and 355 (274 males and 81 females) were persons with AIDS. Overall, *S.* Enteritidis accounted for 1514 (39%), *S.* Typhimurium for 875 (23%), *S.* Heidelberg for 319 (8%), and other serovars for 1173 (30%) of the 3881 infections.

Gastrointestinal Infections in Persons without AIDS

Of the 3526 persons without AIDS who were infected with salmonellae, 3050 (87%) had gastroenteritis, of whom 1014 (33%) were children less than 2 years of age. Thereafter, the incidence of gastroenteritis continuously decreased with advancing age but increased again slightly after age 60 (Table 12.1).

With respect to serovar distribution, in children less than 2 years of age with gastroenteritis, the number with *S.* Enteritidis (n = 239) was similar to that of *S.* Typhimurium (n = 254), and together accounted for 49% of the 1014 cases (Table 12.2). In this same age category, *S.* Heidelberg caused 94 (9%) of the gastrointestinal infections and other serovars accounted for 427 (42%) of the infections. In 5- to 79-year-old persons without AIDS, *S.* Enteritidis caused 40%–50% of all salmonella gastrointestinal infections and was 2–3 times more frequently isolated from stool than was *S.* Typhimurium. The only time after the age of 5 during which *S.* Enteritidis lost its dominant role as the cause of salmonella gastroenteritis was in 80- to 98-year-old persons, from whom *S.* Heidelberg was isolated more frequently.

Septicemia in Persons without AIDS

Of the 3526 persons without AIDS, 414 (12%) had septicemia, of whom 123 (30%) were under 2 years of age

TABLE 12.1   Case rates of salmonellosis by age group and site of infection among persons without AIDS

Age (years)	NYC population (1990)	Stool		Blood	
		Case total	Case rate[a]	Case total	Case rate[a]
0–1	229,731	1014	441	123	54
2–4	301,699	531	176	37	12
5–19	1,381,337	479	35	24	2
20–59	4,149,068	803	19	140	3
60–79	1,037,642	157	15	66	6
80–98	223,087	66	30	24	11

[a]Per 100,000 population.
NYC, New York City.

TABLE 12.2   Salmonella serovars isolated from the stool of persons without AIDS

Age (years)	Sex	No. serovars isolated (%)				
		Enteritidis	Typhimurium	Heidelberg	Other	Total
0–1	M	132 (26)	124 (24)	45 (9)	216 (42)	517 (100)
0–1	F	107 (22)	130 (26)	49 (10)	211 (42)	497 (100)
2–4	M	116 (38)	82 (27)	20 (7)	85 (28)	303 (100)
2–4	F	80 (35)	67 (29)	22 (10)	59 (26)	228 (100)
5–19	M	115 (49)	44 (19)	20 (9)	55 (24)	234 (100)
5–19	F	105 (43)	68 (28)	17 (7)	55 (22)	245 (100)
20–59	M	170 (46)	81 (22)	13 (3)	108 (29)	372 (100)
20–59	F	214 (50)	60 (14)	19 (4)	138 (32)	431 (100)
60–79	M	27 (42)	11 (17)	4 (6)	23 (35)	65 (100)
60–79	F	37 (40)	12 (13)	11 (12)	32 (35)	92 (100)
80–98	M	6 (30)	1 (5)	4 (20)	9 (45)	20 (100)
80–98	F	11 (24)	6 (13)	20 (43)	9 (20)	46 (100)
Total		1120 (37)	686 (22)	244 (8)	1000 (33)	3050 (100)

(Table 12.1). The case rate for septicemia decreased from age 2 through the 20- to 59-year-old age group and thereafter increased moderately through the 80- to 98-year-old age group.

Of the salmonellae isolated from the blood of 123 children younger than 2 years of age, 46 (37%) were *S.* Heidelberg and 29 (24%) were *S.* Enteritidis. After the age of 5 years, *S.* Enteritidis became the most frequent cause of septicemia, responsible for 126 (50%) of 254 septicemia cases in 5- to 98-year-old persons, whereas *S.* Typhimurium was responsible for 56 (22%) and *S.* Heidelberg for 14 (6%) (Table 12.3).

Among 20- to 59-year-old persons, men were almost twice as likely as women to have septicemia: 90 (64%) of the 140 persons with septicemia were men and 50 (36%) were women.

Salmonella Gastroenteritis and Septicemia in Persons with AIDS

Of the 355 persons with salmonellosis and AIDS, 90 (71 males and 19 females) had gastroenteritis and 234 (180 males and 54 females) had septicemia (Table 12.4). The higher proportion of males among persons with AIDS and salmonella infection parallels the 1993–95 NYCDOH AIDS

Registry information, which included three times more males than females. According to the AIDS Registry, there were an estimated 23,000 NYC residents between the ages of 20 and 59 living with AIDS between 1993–95. Using this figure as the population denominator, the case rates for gastroenteritis and septicemia were, respectively, 391 and 1017 cases per 100,000 persons living with AIDS. Of the 90 persons with gastroenteritis, 36 (40%) were caused by *S.* Enteritidis, 20 (22%) by *S.* Typhimurium, four (4%) by *S.* Heidelberg, and 30 (33%) by other serovars (Table 12.4). There were significant sex differences in the distribution of serovars ($\chi^2 = 10.2$; p = 0.02), with males more likely to have *S.* Typhimurium compared with females. Of the 234 persons with septicemia, 156 (67%) of the cases were caused by *S.* Enteritidis, 70 (30%) by *S.* Typhimurium, eight (3%) by other serovars, and none by *S.* Heidelberg.

Urinary-Tract and Other Body-Site Infections Occurring Among 20- to 59-Year-Olds

Among persons without AIDS who were between the ages of 20 and 59, a total of 31 had a urinary-tract infection.

TABLE 12.3 Salmonella serovars isolated from blood of persons without AIDS

Age (years)	Sex	No. serovars isolated (%)				
		Enteritidis	Typhimurium	Heidelberg	Other	Total
0–1	M	19 (28)	6 (9)	23 (34)	19 (28)	67 (100)
0–1	F	10 (18)	7 (12)	23 (41)	16 (29)	56 (100)
2–4	M	4 (22)	3 (17)	2 (11)	9 (50)	18 (100)
2–4	F	2 (11)	1 (5)	5 (26)	11 (58)	19 (100)
5–19	M	4 (36)	0 (0)	1 (9)	6 (55)	11 (100)
5–19	F	3 (23)	2 (15)	1 (8)	7 (54)	13 (100)
20–59	M	45 (50)	25 (28)	3 (3)	17 (19)	90 (100)
20–59	F	30 (60)	10 (20)	3 (6)	7 (14)	50 (100)
60–79	M	16 (50)	4 (13)	3 (9)	9 (28)	32 (100)
60–79	F	16 (47)	10 (29)	1 (3)	7 (21)	34 (100)
80–98	M	7 (78)	1 (11)	0 (0)	1 (11)	9 (100)
80–98	F	5 (33)	4 (27)	2 (13)	4 (27)	15 (100)
Total		161 (39)	73 (18)	67 (16)	113 (27)	414 (100)

TABLE 12.4 Salmonella serovars isolated from the stool or blood of persons with AIDS (aged 20–59 years)

Site of isolation	Sex	No. serovars isolated (%)				
		Enteritidis	Typhimurium	Heidelberg	Other	Total
Stool	M	28 (39)	19 (27)	1 (1)	23 (32)	71 (100)
Stool	F	8 (42)	1 (5)	3 (16)	7 (37)	19 (100)
Blood	M	124 (69)	50 (28)	0 (0)	6 (3)	180 (100)
Blood	F	32 (59)	20 (37)	0 (0)	2 (4)	54 (100)
Total		192 (59)	90 (28)	4 (1)	38 (12)	324 (100)

Salmonella Enteritidis was isolated from the urine of 14 of these persons, *S.* Typhimurium from three, *S.* Heidelberg from four, and other serovars from 10 (Table 12.5). Of 22 urine specimens obtained from persons with AIDS, nine *S.* Enteritidis, 10 *S.* Typhimurium, and three other salmonella serovars were isolated. The rate of salmonella urinary-tract infection for persons with AIDS (96 cases per 100,000 population) was much higher than for persons without AIDS (0.75 cases per 100,000 population).

Specimens obtained from other body sites included abscesses, lymph nodes, synovial fluid, and bone aspirates. The 31 persons without AIDS yielded 14 *S.* Enteritidis, eight *S.* Typhimurium, and nine isolates of other serovars (Table 12.6); these persons had an infection rate of 0.75 cases per 100,000 population. *Salmonella* Typhimurium was isolated from five persons with AIDS who were infected at other body sites, and *S.* Enteritidis was isolated from four such persons. This is equivalent to an infection rate of 39 cases per 100,000 population.

DISCUSSION

Consistent with previous studies, our results indicate that children younger than age 2, the very old, and persons with AIDS are more susceptible to salmonellosis than are most other individuals (Blaser and Feldman, 1981; Blaser and Newman, 1982; Celum et al., 1987; Hargrett-Bean et al., 1988; Levine et al., 1991; Gruenewald et al., 1994; Tauxe, 1996). Based on infection rates per 100,000 population, the rates of septicemia, gastroenteritis, urinary-tract infections, and infections at other body sites among persons with AIDS were, respectively, 339, 21, 128, and 52 times higher than among similarly aged persons without AIDS. The increased vulnerability of persons with AIDS to salmonella infection is consistent with the findings of our previous study of salmonella cases diagnosed between 1985 and 1988 (Gruenewald et al., 1994). The fact that, among 20- to 59-year-old persons without AIDS, men were almost twice as likely to have septicemia than women was also consistent with previous studies (Levine et al., 1991; Gruenewald et al., 1994) and may reflect men with HIV infection who did not yet have an AIDS-defining condition.

In the present study, *S.* Enteritidis was the most frequently isolated serovar (followed by *S.* Typhimurium) in both persons with AIDS and persons of all ages without AIDS and the most invasive serovar in persons with AIDS. Salmonellae infecting blood and various other extraintestinal body sites reach these destinations via the gastrointestinal tract (Snydman and Gorbach, 1982). In this study, the vulnerability to the dissemination of salmonellae from the gastrointestinal tract to various other body sites, and

TABLE 12.5   Salmonella serovars isolated from the urine of persons with and without AIDS (aged 20–59 years)

Listed in AIDS registry	Sex	No. serovars isolated (%)				
		Enteritidis	Typhimurium	Heidelberg	Other	Total
No	M	5	0	1	4	10
No	F	9	3	3	6	21
Yes	M	5	9	0	1	15
Yes	F	4	1	0	2	7
Total		23	13	4	13	53

TABLE 12.6   Salmonella serovars isolated from other sites of persons with and without AIDS (aged 20–59 years)

Listed in AIDS registry	Sex	No. serovars isolated (%)				
		Enteritidis	Typhimurium	Heidelberg	Other	Total
No	M	6	5	0	8	19
No	F	8	3	0	1	12
Yes	M	3	5	0	0	8
Yes	F	1	0	0	0	1
Total		18	13	0	9	40

the serovars causing such infections, were shown to differ in persons with AIDS and those without AIDS. Infections in persons with AIDS were predominantly extraintestinal (septicemia, urinary-tract infections, and infections at other body sites) rather than gastrointestinal, whereas the reverse was true among persons without AIDS. Among persons with AIDS, the invasive serovars responsible for these predominating extraintestinal infections consisted mainly of *S.* Enteritidis or *S.* Typhimurium, whereas *S.* Heidelberg was never isolated. In contrast, the relatively few extraintestinal infections occurring in persons without AIDS were often caused by salmonella serovars other than *S.* Enteritidis or *S.* Typhimurium. Persons with gastroenteritis were infected with *S.* Enteritidis, *S.* Typhimurium, or a variety of other salmonella serovars; however, serovar distribution was not associated with AIDS status.

In persons with AIDS, the predominance of extraintestinal infections and the serovars that caused them is reflected by ratios of cases of septicemia to cases of gastroenteritis. Thus, the ratio of cases of *S.* Enteritidis septicemia to *S.* Enteritidis gastroenteritis was 4.3:1 (156 septicemia cases and 36 gastroenteritis cases). The ratio of *S.* Typhimurium septicemia to gastroenteritis cases was 3.5:1 (70 cases of septicemia and 20 cases of gastroenteritis). In contrast, the ratio of septicemia to gastroenteritis cases caused by other salmonella serovars was only 1:3.7 (8 cases of septicemia and 30 cases of gastroenteritis). In an earlier study of salmonella-infected NYC residents, the ratio of septicemia to gastroenteritis cases in 20- to 59-year-old persons with AIDS was 3.0:1 for *S.* Enteritidis, 1:1.3 for *S.* Typhimurium, and 1:7.5 for other serovars (Gruenewald et al., 1994). When compared with the results of the previous study (Gruenewald et al., 1994), *S.* Typhimurium demonstrated in the present

study a substantial increase in invasiveness, reflected by the increased ratio of septicemia to gastroenteritis cases; the increase in the invasiveness of *S.* Enteritidis and other salmonellae was more moderate.

That *S.* Enteritidis and *S.* Typhimurium, the two most frequently isolated serovars, were found to be especially invasive in persons with AIDS can be considered to be the worst possible scenario: had these two serovars been no more invasive than most other serovars, one would have expected the incidence of extraintestinal infections in persons with AIDS to be substantially reduced. In fact, not all *S.* Enteritidis subpopulations were found to be invasive in persons with AIDS. In San Francisco, Celum et al. (1987) found that *S.* Enteritidis did not cause septicemia or even gastroenteritis in patients with AIDS but caused both types of infections in patients without AIDS. The *S.* Enteritidis subpopulation studied by Celum et al. between 1982 and 1986, as well as *S.* Heidelberg and other serovars isolated from NYC residents, may have lacked the virulence factors that enabled their frequent dissemination to extraintestinal sites even in immunodeficient persons with AIDS. Alternatively, these organisms may have been more vulnerable to host defense mechanisms that still function in persons with AIDS than were the *S.* Enteritidis and *S.* Typhimurium subpopulations isolated in NYC.

The ability of *S.* Enteritidis to colonize grade-A shell eggs produced in egg-product plants throughout the United States has been largely responsible for its prominence as the most frequently isolated serovar in this country (Ebel et al., 1993; Vugia et al., 1993; Mishu et al., 1994; Boyce et al., 1996). Children younger than age 2 and, to a lesser extent, the very old were found to be more susceptible to salmonellosis than were other age groups.

The very young and the very old were different from the AIDS cohort with regard to serovar distribution and site of infection. Infants have yet to achieve a fully functioning immune system and older persons, as well as persons with AIDS, have declining immune function. Each cohort, though, is greatly affected by exposure to salmonellae. Given the virulence of the two major serovars in persons with AIDS and the virulence of other serovars in persons without AIDS (that is, *Salmonella* Heidelberg in infants and the very old), it seems prudent to educate vulnerable individuals and their caretakers on ways to reduce their risk of salmonella infection, including thoroughly cooking eggs, poultry, and meat, and carefully washing hands after toileting and before eating.

ACKNOWLEDGMENTS

The authors acknowledge the assistance of Esbeth Bradly, Maggie Spencer, and the staff of the Bureau of Communicable Disease, and Dr. Susan Forlenza, Director, and the staff of the Office of AIDS Surveillance of the New York City Department of Health.

REFERENCES

Altekruse, S.F., and Swerdlow, D.L. 1996. The changing epidemiology of foodborne diseases. Am. J. Med. Sci. 311:23–29.

Angulo, F.J., and Swerdlow, D.L. 1995. Bacterial enteric infections in persons infected with human immunodeficiency virus. Clin. Infect. Dis. 21(Suppl. 1):S84–S93.

Blaser, M.J., and Feldman, R.A. 1981. *Salmonella* bacteremia: reports to the Centers for Disease Control, 1968–1979. J. Infect. Dis. 143:743–746.

Blaser, M.J., and Newman, L.S. 1982. A review of human salmonellosis. I. Infective dose. Rev. Infect. Dis. 4:1096–1106.

Boyce, T.G., Koo, D., Swerdlow, D.L., Gomez, T.M., Serrano, B., Nickey, L.N., Hickman-Brenner, F.W., Malcolm, G.B., and Griffin, P.M. 1996. Recurrent outbreaks of *Salmonella enteritidis* infections in a Texas restaurant: phage type 4 arrives in the United States. Epidemiol. Infect. 117:29–34.

Celum, C.L., Chaisson, R.E., Rutherford, G.W., Barnhart, J.L., and Echenberg, D.F. 1987. Incidence of salmonellosis in patients with AIDS. J. Infect. Dis. 156:998–1002.

Centers for Disease Control. 1992. 1993 Revised classification system for HIV infection and expanded surveillance case definition for AIDS among adolescents and adults. MMWR 41(RR-17).

Dean, A.G., Dean, J.A., Burton, A.H., and Dicker, R.C. 1990. Epi-Info, version 6.04: a word processing database and statistical program for epidemiology on microcomputers. Atlanta: Centers for Disease Control.

Ebel, E.D., Mason, J., Thomas, L.A., Ferris, K.E., Beckman, M.G., Cummins, D.R., Schroeder-Tucker, L., Sutherlin, W.D., Glasshoff, R.L., and Smithhisler, N.M. 1993. Occurrence of *Salmonella enteritidis* in unpasteurized liquid egg in the United States. Avian Dis. 37:135–142.

Gast, R.K., and Beard, C.W. 1990. Production of SE-contaminated eggs by experimentally infected hens. Avian Dis. 34:438–446.

Gruenewald, R., Dixon, D.P., Brun, M., Yappow, S., Henderson, R., Douglas, J.E., and Backer, M.H. 1990. Identification of *Salmonella* somatic and flagellar antigens by modified serological methods. Appl. Environ. Microbiol. 56:24–30.

Gruenewald, R., Blum, S., and Chan, J. 1994. Relationship between human immunodeficiency virus infection and salmonellosis in 20- to 59-year-old residents of New York City. Clin. Infect. Dis. 18:358–363.

Hargrett-Bean, N.T., Pavia, A.T., and Tauxe, R.V. 1988. *Salmonella* isolates from humans in the United States, 1984–1986. MMWR 37(SS-2:25–31).

Kovacs, J.A., and Masur, H. 1985. Opportunistic infections. In: Gallin, J.I., and Fauci, A.S., eds. Advances in host defense mechanisms, vol. 5. New York: Raven, pp. 35–58.

Levine, W.C., Buehler, J.W., Bean, N.H., and Tauxe, R.V. 1991. Epidemiology of nontyphoidal *Salmonella* bacteremia during the human immunodeficiency virus epidemic. J. Infect. Dis. 164:81–87.

Mildvan, D., Mathur, U., Enlow, R.W., Romain, P.L., Winchester, R.J., Colp, C., Singman, H., Adelsberg, B.R., and Spigland, I. 1982. Opportunistic infections and immune deficiency in homosexual men. Ann. Intern. Med. 96(Part 1):700–704.

Mishu, B., Koehler, J., Lee, L., Rodrigue, D., Hickman-Brenner, F., Blake, P., and Tauxe, R.V. 1994. Outbreaks of *Salmonella enteritidis* infections in the United States, 1985–1991. J. Infect. Dis. 169:547–552.

Rodrigue, D.C., Tauxe, R.V., and Rowe, B. 1990. International increase in *Salmonella enteritidis*: a new pandemic? Epidemiol. Infect. 105:21–27.

Snydman, D.R., and Gorbach, S.L. 1982. Salmonellosis: nontyphoidal. In: Evans, A.S., and Feldman, H.A., eds. Bacterial infections of humans: epidemiology and control. New York: Plenum Medical, pp. 463–485.

St. Louis, M.E., Morse, D.L., Potter, M.E., DeMelfi, T.M., Guzewich, J.J., Tauxe, R.V., and Blake, P.A. 1988. The emergence of grade A eggs as a major source of *Salmonella enteritidis* infections: new implications for the control of salmonellosis. JAMA 259:2103–2107.

Tauxe, R.V. 1996. An update on *Salmonella*. Health Environ. 10:1–4.

Vugia, D.J., Mishu, B., Smith, M., Tavris, D.R., Hickman-Brenner, F.W., and Tauxe, R.V. 1993. *Salmonella enteritidis* outbreak in a restaurant chain: the continuing challenge of prevention. Epidemiol. Infect. 110:49–61.

Wolfe, M.S., Armstrong, D., Louria, D.B., and Blevins, A. 1971. Salmonellosis in patients with neoplastic disease: a review of 100 episodes at Memorial Cancer Center over a 13-year period. Arch. Intern. Med. 128:546–554.

Part II
Molecular Epidemiology

13

Molecular Epidemiological Methods for Differentiation of *Salmonella enterica* Serovar Enteritidis Strains

M.C. Mendoza and E. Landeras

INTRODUCTION

Molecular epidemiology is based on the use of a series of techniques of molecular biology to analyze microbiological traits that enable the differentiation of strains and are useful as epidemiological markers. These techniques, called *molecular typing methods,* may be categorized into two broad groups on the basis of the type of traits or macromolecules targeted for typing: phenotypic methods (those that detect characteristics expressed by the organism) and genotypic methods (those that involve direct DNA analysis of chromosomal or extrachromosomal genetic elements) (Maslow et al., 1993; Swaminathan and Matar, 1993; Helmuth and Schroeter, 1994; Arbeit, 1995). The usefulness of a trait for typing is related to its stability in a given strain and its diversity among the strains forming one species. A bacterial clone can be defined as a population of cells showing so many identical traits that the most likely explanation for this identity is that all derive from one common ancestor. The typing methods are based on the premise that clonally related organisms share traits that can differentiate them from unrelated organisms.

In the 1990s, molecular typing methods based on the analysis of chromosomal DNA (DNA fingerprinting) have been shown to have broad applications in public health bacteriology and are being used—alone or in combination with standard, well-established methods (such as serotyping and phage typing)—for epidemiological purposes. They have become useful tools for the differentiation of pathogen from nonpathogen clones and for ascertaining whether the most frequent contemporary virulent isolates belong to one, a few, or many lineages. In addition, molecular methods are essential in different epidemiological settings, such as

- The differentiation of the number and types of bacterial clones present in a panel of strains representing the bacterial populations of a hospital, farm, country, or continent or worldwide; and the definition of pandemic, endemic, and sporadic pathogen clones.
- The study of the maintenance, dispersion, and evolution of clones.
- The determination of the natural reservoirs of pathogen clones and identification of the source of infection both in outbreaks and in sporadic diseases.
- The recognition of outbreaks in order to ascertain the number and type of strains implicated in each outbreak and their origin.
- The assurance that immunization programs lead to the eradication of the target pathogen instead of replacement with a variant subtype.

125

CRITERIA FOR EVALUATING MOLECULAR TYPING METHODS

A new typing method must be proposed after obtaining adequate knowledge of its effectiveness for a broad sample of strains, including well-characterized reference strains and epidemic and sporadic isolates, and after the comparison of the results with those of previously well-established approaches. Considered in evaluating the method are several criteria, which can be categorized as principal and secondary (Maslow et al., 1993; Arbeit, 1995).

The principal criteria are typeability, reproducibility, and sensitivity. *Typeability* refers to the proportion of strains that can be typed by the method. Essentially all strains are typeable by molecular methods, except for some hybridization techniques using probes for DNA sequences (loci) not present in all strains of a species. *Reproducibility* refers to the ability of a method to yield the same result when the same strain is tested repeatedly. The molecular methods should be well standardized to minimize false results; for example, incomplete digestion of DNA by a restriction enzyme (RE) may cause artifact bands to appear, falsely showing differences between strains. With some probes, it can be difficult to evaluate the faint bands that appear in a pattern after Southern hybridization; and in some procedures based on the *polymerase chain reaction* (PCR), if the amplification conditions are not well standardized, artifact bands can also appear. *Sensitivity* or *discriminatory power* refers to the ability to differentiate among unrelated strains. In determining discriminatory power, it is particularly informative to test epidemiologically unrelated strains that have proved to be indistinguishable by other methods. For determining the discriminating ability of a new method, Hunter and Gaston (1988) recommended the use of Simpson's index of diversity (DI), and a method is considered statistically useful if the DI > 0.95.

The following secondary criteria have to be considered. The method should be of *easy interpretation*. This will be more reliable if based on logical, objective, and readily applied criteria. In some genetic methods, the electrophoretic banding profiles can be complex and barely accurate. In an effort to make electrophoretic banding profiles more easily understandable and accessible for typing, a variety of equipment has been developed in order to digitalize patterns, and statistical programs for processing the results have been introduced. In addition, the ideal typing system should be *technically simple, rapid, inexpensive, and not require complex equipment,* in order to be applied to a wide variety of species, as well as to a large number of isolates simultaneously. These features do not normally apply to molecular procedures, some of which require multiple steps and/or specific and complex equipment. With these methods, the cost in terms of work, time, and money is relatively high in comparison to standard phenotypic methods, such as serotyping or phage typing.

On the contrary, most of the molecular methods show some advantages: they do not require the use of organism-specific reagents, are applicable for typing all strains, enable the objective evaluation of results and the statistical analysis of the data, and are amenable to automation. In addition, most methods based on genotype characterization appear to be suitable for studying both population genetic structure and evolutionary relationships within species and serovars.

EPIDEMIOLOGICAL SURVEILLANCE OF *SALMONELLA* ENTERITIDIS

Nontyphoidal salmonella serovars, which include *S. enterica* serovar Enteritidis (*S.* Enteritidis), are categorized as foodborne classic pathogens, which have a wide range of animal reservoirs and high spread potential and ability to survive in the environmental water. Improvement of epidemiological surveillance for these pathogens is currently necessary because of the continuing presence of disease in endemic areas. In addition, rapidly growing international food trade between countries that maintain widely different levels of hygiene conditions in the production and manufacture of foods and animal feeds has greatly facilitated the introduction of new salmonella lineages within the geographical boundaries of the importing countries. Salmonellae can be transferred not only by animal products, but also by fresh vegetables, spices, cheese, and aquacultural products, causing serious economic losses to the food industry [for a review, see D'Aoust (1994)]. The incidence of *S.* Enteritidis began to increase in European countries sometime in the mid-1980s and in the United States in 1979. It is currently the most frequent serovar causing human salmonellosis in most developed countries (Chalker and Blaser, 1988; Rodrigue et al., 1990; Stanley et al., 1992a,b; Usera et al., 1994; González-Hevia and Mendoza, 1995b; Suzuki et al., 1995). The wide spread of *S.* Enteritidis may be attributed to intensive practices of animal production, including poultry and hen eggs, together with the ability of this bacteria to be transmitted vertically (Thiagarajan et al., 1994; Braun and Fehlhaber, 1995). It is now well established that poultry and eggs are among the major sources of human infection with *S.* Enteritidis (Perales and Audicana, 1989; Rampling, 1993).

Accurate characterization of the prevalent *S.* Enteritidis pathogen clones that are associated with human and animal salmonellosis is needed to differentiate them from less-pathogenic clones and to study their origin, evolution, and major infection routes. This will improve both the epidemiological surveillance and the preventive and control measures. In recent years, phage typing has been used widely in epidemiological studies of *S.* Enteritidis. The scheme of Ward et al. (1987) has been most frequently used. In the present review, the phage types discussed always follow this scheme. Based on recent epidemiological studies, there is no doubt now that phage type 4 (PT4) in Europe and PT8 and PT13a in the United States are the *S.* Enteritidis phage types most frequently associated with food poisoning and with the concurrent widespread infection of commercial poultry and eggs (Stanley et al., 1992a; Helmuth and Schroeter, 1994; Usera et al., 1994; Fadl et al., 1995). It is important to emphasize that changes in phage type have been observed in isolates from the same clone, and that these changes may be related, at least, to plasmid acquisition, loss of the ability to express long-chain lipopolysaccharide (LPS), and spontaneous mutations affecting phage receptor sites (Chart et al., 1989; Frost et al., 1989; Threlfall and Chart, 1993; Powell et al., 1995).

Since the beginning of the 1990s, efforts to type *S.* Enteritidis at the molecular level have been undertaken and several molecular techniques have been applied. The results of molecular methods have been frequently correlated with phage typing in order to use them as complementary or alternative tools. Analysis by molecular methods of the non-phage-typeable strains may reveal the genotypic relationship among these strains and strains of known phage types. This review concentrates on the data obtained by using different molecular methods, mainly DNA fingerprinting, to discriminate among different strains and to define clonal groups of *S.* Enteritidis from different sources and geographical regions. Furthermore, this review describes the basic principles of each of the molecular techniques, as well as their strengths and weaknesses [for a more detailed review on the principles and applications of molecular typing methods, see Swaminathan and Matar (1993)].

MOLECULAR PHENOTYPIC METHODS FOR TYPING *SALMONELLA* ENTERITIDIS

The macromolecules targeted by the molecular phenotypic methods used for the typing of *S.* Enteritidis include LPS, outer-membrane proteins, and soluble metabolic enzymes. Results from these procedures have been revised and correlated with one another, and with respect to genetic methods, by Helmuth and Schroeter (1994) and used to define the epidemic PT4 clone present in Europe today.

In salmonellae, LPS is a major virulence factor and its analysis is a part of the serotyping scheme of Kauffman-White. Using this scheme, more than 2300 serovars have been described on the basis of the antigen structure of LPS (O antigen) and flagellar proteins (H antigen). The ability of salmonella isolates to transfer, acquire, and recombine the genes for O antigen (*rfb* cluster) and the genes for phase-I flagellin (*fliC*) explains the existence of such a large number of serovars, but it also represents a major limitation for the serological scheme. In fact, serotyping is a convenient and epidemiologically useful method of categorizing isolates, but it does not provide a basis for estimating evolutionary genetic relatedness among strains (Boyd et al., 1993). Some phylogenetic studies based on multilocus enzyme analysis (Beltran et al., 1988; Boyd et al., 1993), polymorphism of the rDNA region (Mendoza et al., 1996), and polymorphism of 16S–23S intergenic spacer region (Lagatolla et al., 1996) have shown that strains of the same

serovar may be distantly related, and/or that strains from different serovars appear to be closely related.

Sodium dodecyl sulfate–polyacrylamide gel electrophoresis (SDS-PAGE) of LPS has been evaluated in the study of salmonella mutants with different LPS chemotypes by Hitchcock and Brown (1983) and, within *S.* Enteritidis, it has also been correlated with phage typing by Chart et al. (1989) and by Threlfall and Chart (1993). Results from these studies showed that strains belonging to the majority of phage types, including the prevalent PT4, PT6, PT8, and PT13, expressed long-chain LPS, whereas PT30 strains showed a variable expression, and PT7 and PT23 did not synthesize typical LPS. Strains that did not synthesize the long chain of LPS were rough variants, a phenotype correlated with avirulence for mice; and strains PT23 and PT30 were thought to originate from smooth strains associated with poultry. All 16 PT4 strains analyzed, collected before and during the present epidemic, showed long-chain LPS [cited by Helmuth and Schroeter (1994)].

Whole cell and outer-membrane protein (OMP) profiles determined by SDS-PAGE are also used for typing *S.* Enteritidis. Helmuth and Schroeter (1994) reported that an initial investigation of OMPs of salmonellae suggested the existence of different patterns within seven common serovars. Later, these authors found a complete homogeneity of OMPs among ancestral and more than 400 contemporary *S.* Enteritidis PT4 strains isolated from poultry in Germany. A similarly high degree of OMP homogeneity had been previously described in poultry isolates from Maine in the United States by Singer et al. (1992). Soluble, cytoplasmic enzymes may show a high degree of polymorphism, which can be analyzed by starch-gel electrophoresis and the use of specific substrates. Variations in electrophoretic mobility of a constitutive enzyme within different strains of the same species can be attributed to isoenzymes (functionally similar forms of an enzyme, including polymers of subunits produced by different gene loci or by different alleles at the same locus) or to allozymes (variants of polypeptides representing different allelic alternatives at the same locus). The basic assumption in multilocus enzyme electrophoresis (MLEE) is that changes in the mobility of enzymes are a result of charge differences due to amino acid substitutions in the polypeptide sequence and that these charge differences reflect changes in the DNA encoding the polypeptide. Groups of strains carrying identical alleles form an electrotype and the genetic distances of different electrotypes can be calculated on the basis of dissimilar alleles. Once calculated, genetic distances can be represented in a dendrogram.

By using MLEE, Beltran et al. (1988) defined the population genetics of *S.* Enteritidis and seven other important salmonella serovars. Out of 257 strains of *S.* Enteritidis, 14 different electrotypes were defined. The most frequent of them (named En1) included 93% of the strains. These authors designed an MLEE-derived evolutionary dendrogram in which En1 and nine other *S.* Enteritidis electrotypes fell into a major cluster and could be considered as members of the same lineage. The other four electrotypes fell into three unusual lineages. These data support the fact that *S.* Enteritidis is a polyphyletic serovar. Helmuth and Schroeter (1994) reported that when their laboratory used MLEE to analyze 61 isolates belonging to PT4 from poultry, all of the isolates ascribed to the predominating electrotype, En1. These authors emphasized that these results, like the LPS and OMP homogeneity, supported the highly clonal nature of PT4 strains.

The appearance of LPS and the OMP profiles, both determined by SDS-PAGE, as well as the analysis of metabolic enzymes by MLEE, are relatively simple methods to establish an interrelationship among strains and to evaluate heterogeneity. As typing methods for *S.* Enteritidis, however, they have weak discriminatory power.

GENETIC METHODS FOR TYPING *SALMONELLA* ENTERITIDIS

Genetic typing methods used for *S.* Enteritidis include the analysis of plasmids and two groups of chromosomal DNA fingerprinting, each including several variants. The first group is based on the analysis of the restriction fragment length polymorphism, and the second is based on genetic amplification by the PCR.

Plasmid Analysis

The first DNA-based technique applied to epidemiological studies involved the analysis of plasmids. In the most basic procedure, plasmid DNA is obtained from each isolate and separated electrophoretically in an agarose gel to determine the number and size of the plasmids, which is called the *plasmid profile* (Fig. 13.1A). Additional information can be obtained by digesting the plasmid DNA with a restrictive enzyme (RE) and then comparing the number and size of the resulting fragments. Each RE cuts the DNA at a constant position within a specific recognition sequence, usually composed of 4–6 base pairs (bp). Complete digestion of a given DNA with an RE provides a reproducible array of fragments that can be separated by agarose-gel electrophoresis and visualized by staining with ethidium bromide. Examples of *plasmid restriction profiles* are shown in Figure 13.1B.

Considerable work on epidemiological subtyping of *S.* Enteritidis by plasmid profile analysis has been reported. Some plasmids in salmonellae have been considered as serovar-specific virulence plasmids because they exhibit a strong effect on bacterial virulence, and five virulence genes (named *spvRABCD*) have been identified [for a review, see Gulig et al. (1993)]. The typical virulence plasmid of *S.* Enteritidis is approximately 36–38 MDa in size, although plasmids of different molecular sizes, related to that of 36–38 MDa, have been reported. Virulence plasmids of 36–38, 59, and 45 MDa have been described in which the *spvC* gene is located on a conserved 3.5-kbp *Hin*dIII fragment, and this can be revealed by hybridization with an *spvC*-specific probe (Brown et al., 1993).

Threlfall et al. (1989) reported that the phage-type strains (representative of the first established phage types)

showed 11 plasmid profiles. In a further study, 25 plasmid profile types were revealed in a series of 1022 PT4 strains isolated from humans, chickens, and eggs in England and Wales in 1988–92 (Threlfall et al., 1994). The predominant profile carried the 38-MDa plasmid and comprised more than 90% of human and 70% of poultry isolates. Helmuth and Schroeter (1994) cited that about 80% of the strains, belonging to epidemiologically important phage types that had been isolated before 1985, carried only a 37-MDa virulence plasmid. They also cited that, in Germany, all *S.* Enteritidis isolates have been subject to plasmid profiling since 1990. The heterogeneity of the plasmid profiles found in strains isolated from different sources in other countries has also been reported (Rivera et al., 1991; Morris et al., 1992; Gruner et al., 1994; Vatopoulos et al., 1994; González-Hevia and Mendoza, 1995b; Millemann et al., 1995; Suzuki et al., 1995).

The following contributions of plasmid analysis to *S.* Enteritidis epidemiology can be used as examples:

- In the study of the changing clonal patterns in Maryland (United States) between 1985 and 1990, a strong increase was found (from 43% in 1985 to 88% in 1988–89) in the number of strains showing a profile consisting of the single 36-MDa plasmid (Morris et al., 1992).
- In outbreak diagnosis, the plasmid profile was useful in defining the type and number of strains implicated (González-Hevia et al., 1994; González-Hevia and Mendoza, 1995a,b).
- In the correlation of drug resistance with plasmids of different size, some of them have been transferable by conjugation. Among strains collected in a Spanish hospital, Rivera et al. (1991) found six conjugative resistance plasmids (between 32 and 114 kb) mediating resistance to ampicillin and other semisynthetic penicillins, streptomycin, kanamycin, chloramphenicol, and/or tetracycline. Frost et al. (1989) demonstrated that the acquisition of a 34-MDa plasmid, which encodes for ampicillin, streptomycin, and tetracycline resistance, converted *S.* Enteritidis PT4 to PT24. Vatopoulos et al. (1994) revealed that ampicillin resistance of *S.* Enteritidis strains from Greece was due to related 34-MDa plasmids encoding TEM-type β-lactamases.
- The usefulness of plasmid profile as a secondary marker to differentiate human pathogen strains from a specific health area was reported by González-Hevia and Mendoza (1995a). In that study, 12 types of plasmids (between 1.1 and 57 MDa) were found, forming 12 profiles, 10 of which included a 36-MDa virulence plasmid. Some profiles were encountered in both epidemic and sporadic strains collected over different years, and 8% were plasmid-free strains.

Technically, plasmid analysis is one of the simplest DNA-based methods, and it can be efficiently performed with basic electrophoretic equipment and commercially available reagents. It is a useful tool for identifying outbreak strains but not for large-scale strain comparisons in

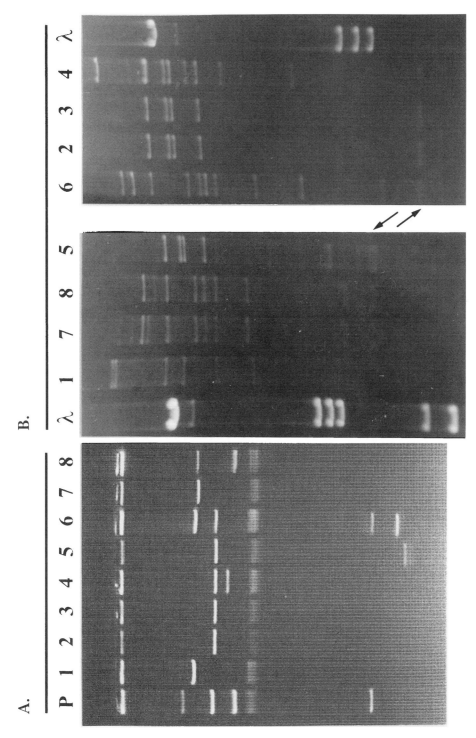

FIGURE 13.1   Analysis of plasmids from salmonella strains. **A.** Plasmid profiles. **B.** Plasmid restriction profiles generated by *HindIII*. Lane 1 shows the 60-MDa virulence plasmid from *Salmonella* Typhimurium ATCC 14028. Lane 2 shows the 38-MDa virulence plasmid from S. Enteritidis ATCC 13076. Lanes 3–8 show plasmids from Spanish clinical isolates: lane 3, 119/92; lane 4, 1961/94; lane 5, 1570/93; lane 6, 216/92; lane 7, 51/84; and lane 8, 138/87. Lane P, plasmid standard size; sizes of plasmids from top to bottom are 98, 42, 23.9, and 4.6 MDa. Lane l, bacteriophage lambda DNA cleaved with *PstI*; the sizes of the fragments from top to bottom are 14.16, 11.5, 5.08, 4.65, 4.50, 2.84, and 2.57 kb. The *arrows* show the 3.5-kb fragments carrying *Spv* genes.

retrospective or prospective epidemiological studies or for clonal analysis. The limitations and potential problems of plasmid analysis result from plasmids being extrachromosomal elements, which are not essential for normal bacterial growth and can be lost spontaneously or acquired readily by a host strain. The loss of the plasmid can occur either in the reservoir or in the natural environment or during subcultures and conservation of the host strain in the laboratory.

Chromosomal Restriction Analysis

Just as described for plasmid analysis, restriction site analysis of chromosomal DNA provides a cost-effective means of determining DNA sequence variations. Changes in the array of fragments generated by a specific RE are called restriction fragment length polymorphisms (RFLPs). RFLPs can result from sequence rearrangements, insertion or deletion of DNA, or base substitution within the RE cleavage site. Three RFLP variants are useful as epidemiological tools:

1. Restriction analysis using REs with relatively frequent restriction sites, and fragment separation by size using constant-field agarose electrophoresis, this being the oldest variant and thus usually called *restriction endonuclease analysis* (REA).
2. Restriction analysis using REs that have few restriction sites and fragment separation by size using *pulsed-field gel electrophoresis* (PFGE).
3. Restriction-hybridization analysis in which restriction fragments obtained in REA are transferred onto a nitrocellulose or nylon membrane and hybridized with a DNA probe: *restriction-hybridization techniques.*

RESTRICTION ENDONUCLEASE ANALYSIS (REA TYPING)

In the REA technique, the choice of the RE is very important in the restriction analysis (using REs with relatively frequent restriction sites and fragment separation by size with use of constant-field agarose electrophoresis) and should be based on two different criteria: (a) the size and frequency of the restriction fragments should be suitable for analysis (the best

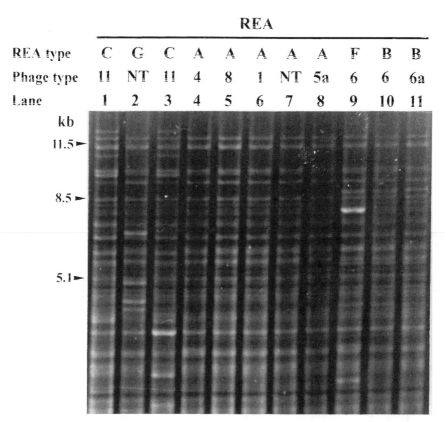

FIGURE 13.2   Restriction enzyme analysis of genomic DNA cleaved with *Hinc*II of *Salmonella* Enteritidis strains. The REA types shown correspond to Spanish clinical strains. The phage type of the strains is also indicated: lane 1, 51/84; lane 2, 98/87; lane 3, 138/87; lane 4, 801/91; lane 5, 5728/94; lane 6, 185/85; lane 7, 175/92; lane 8, 195/93; lane 9, 197/93; lane 10, 211/93; and lane 11, 217/93.

results are obtained with fragments ranging from 1000 to 15,000 bp), and (b) to avoid overlapping bands that may obscure differences, the fragments in this size range should not be too numerous. Appropriate REs can be selected empirically or more objectively following the method of Forbes et al., which is described by Swaminathan and Matar (1993).

REA has not been described as useful for typing *S.* Enteritidis probably because of the very complex fragment patterns originating with most REs. Nevertheless, Helmuth and Schroeter (1994) have cited that in an analysis of 14 PT4 strains, categorized as old and new, an identical pattern was found, data that were interpreted as the strains belonging to one clone. On the contrary, by using *Hinc*II, an RE with an ambiguous recognition sequence [CT(T/C) ↓ (A/G)AC], we were able to detect different profiles (Fig. 13.2). The two most frequent profiles were the named REA-A and REA-B, which corresponded to 66% and 24% of the strains tested, respectively. Both profiles were represented by strains from different sources (clinical, eggs, meat, and environmental water) collected in Spain in 1984–95 and ascribed to different phage types. REA-A was most frequent among strains ascribed to PT1 and PT4, whereas REA-B was ascribed to PT6 and PT6a (Mendoza et al., 1996; unpublished data).

This typing method is sensitive (because the entire genome is evaluated by RFLP), useful for comparing a few strains (preferably run in the same gel), and relatively easy to perform. It is not useful, though, for large-scale comparisons. Its disadvantage is that the genomic restriction fragments are too numerous and too closely spaced for both visual differentiation and scanning by densitometers or image-acquisition devices. To decrease the complexity of the restriction profiles, several alternative strategies have been proposed for RFLP analysis, and these are described next.

PULSED-FIELD GEL ELECTROPHORESIS (PFGE TYPING)

In the PFGE method, REs that cut DNA infrequently are used to generate large fragments of chromosomal DNA, which are separated by special electrophoretic procedures. DNA isolation involves the entrapment of bacteria in agarose plugs, where they are lysed with detergent, treated with proteinase K, and the contaminants removed by washing or dialysis. In a second step, the DNA is cleaved with an RE and the resulting large DNA fragments (between 10 and 800 kb) remain entrapped in the agarose-gel matrix. The entrapped DNA fragments can be resolved by cyclically altering the orientation of the electric field during electrophoresis. Various pulsed-field electrophoretic techniques used to separate restricted DNA fragments are listed by Swaminathan and Matar (1993). In Figure 13.3, examples of PFGE profiles generated by *Xba*I in *S.* Enteritidis strains are shown in comparison with *S.* Typhimurium profiles.

Using PFGE, a relatively wide diversity of *S.* Enteritidis types have been reported, some of which could be representative examples. Olsen et al. (1994) defined 10 *Not*I profiles (when bands >125 kb were used as the criterion for separation) within 62 *S.* Enteritidis of 33 phage types.

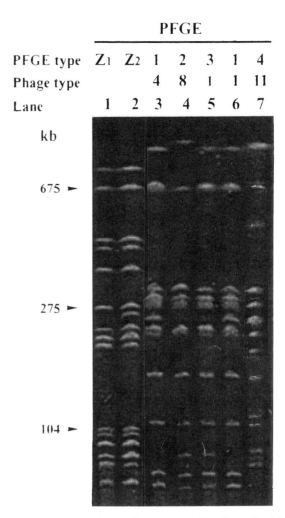

	PFGE						
PFGE type	Z₁	Z₂	1	2	3	1	4
Phage type			4	8	1	1	11
Lane	1	2	3	4	5	6	7

FIGURE 13.3   Analysis of genomic DNA cleaved with *Xba*I of salmonella strains by pulsed-field gel electrophoresis. The PFGE types shown in lanes 1 and 2 represent *S.* Typhimurium Spanish clinical strains: lane 1, 14/82; and lane 2, 247/94. Lanes 3–7 correspond to *Salmonella* Enteritidis strains: lane 3, strain of PT4; lane 4, strain of PT8; lane 5, ATCC 13073; lane 6, 20/84; and lane 7, 51/84 (these last two are Spanish clinical isolates).

In that study, strains belonging to 21 of 33 phage types formed one large cluster (which included strains from the most frequent phage types: PT4, PT6, PT8, and PT13). Also among strains belonging to the PT1, PT6, PT7, and PT14b, more than one PFGE profile was observed. Similar findings were reported by Liebisch and Schwarz (1996). These authors, using *Xba*I, *Spe*I, and *Not*I, identified four, five, and six PFGE profiles, respectively, among 31 strains isolated from animals and humans from Germany. The combination of results obtained with the three enzymes subdivided the series into nine genomic groups and increased the DI to 0.815. However, the genomic groups corresponded closely to the assignment of the isolates to different phage types, and it is noteworthy that isolates of phage types other than PT1 could not be differentiated further by PFGE typing. On the contrary, in a previous study, Powell et al. (1994) identified nine *Xba*I profiles among PT4 strains collected from different human and animal sources in 1967–92 from England and Wales. A profile was clearly predominant, being found in 30 of the 39 strains tested. Using the data from that report, we calculated the discriminatory index, as recommended by Hunter and Gaston (1988), and the DI obtained was 0.41. *Salmonella* Enteritidis strains collected in other countries have also been differentiated by PFGE performed with different REs. Thong et al. (1995), using *Xba*I, *Spe*I, and *Avr*II, identified four, two, and three PFGE profiles, respectively, in strains collected from humans and poultry from Switzerland, and only one or two PFGE profiles in human strains from Malaysia, and Suzuki et al. (1995), using *Xba*I and *Not*I, identified ten and four profiles, respectively, among 68 epidemic and sporadic human isolates collected in Japan.

Comparison of the banding patterns reported in some of the aforementioned studies is difficult, especially *Not*I patterns because this RE generates many DNA fragments. Fragments smaller than 100 kb from *Not*I, and smaller than 40 kb from other REs, can be sometimes detected between PFGE profiles, but they are frequently not well resolved and are too closely spaced for both visual differentiation and scanning by densitometers or image-acquisition devices.

The strength of PFGE as a molecular typing method is that it provides a highly reproducible restriction profile that typically shows distinct, well-resolved fragments, representing the entire bacterial chromosome in a single gel. This procedure is technically more demanding than conventional agarose-gel electrophoresis and requires more expensive, specialized equipment than do other molecular methods.

RESTRICTION-HYBRIDIZATION TECHNIQUES
In the restriction-hybridization techniques, the restriction fragments separated by agarose-gel electrophoresis for REA (as described in the preceding section on REA typing) are transferred to nitrocellulose or nylon membranes by Southern blotting and hybridized with one or more probes. A probe is a discrete DNA fragment labeled with high-energy radioisotopes (for example, ^{32}P) or chemically (for example, with biotin or digoxigenin). Only the genomic DNA fragments that contain loci homologous to the probe hybridize and can be detected. Variations in the number and size of the hybridized fragments reflect variations in both the number of loci that are homologous to the probe and the location of restriction sites within or flanking those loci. All strains carrying loci homologous to the probe are typeable, and the results are highly reproducible. Probes for typing include both specific or randomly cloned genomic DNA fragments, insertion sequences, bacteriophage DNA, and rRNA itself or the cloned ribosomal operon (ribotyping or riboprobing). For *S.* Enteritidis, several probes have been used, of which IS*200* and derived ribosomal RNA genes produced the most useful results.

IS*200* is an insertion sequence that has been found in almost all salmonella serovars and many *Shigella sonnei* and *Shigella flexneri* strains, but that is absent from other enterobacterias (Gilbert et al., 1990). It is one of the smallest insertion elements so far described (708 bp) and, because of its capability of transposing from one site to another, can be located on different DNA sites, which can be revealed after the digestion of chromosomal DNA with REs and subsequent Southern blotting and hybridization with a specific probe. Two internal IS*200* probes have been developed by Gilbert et al. (1990) and used to survey the presence of IS*200* in genomic DNA digested with REs that do not cut into IS*200*, such as *Pvu*II, *Ava*I, or *Pst*I. When genomic DNA of 18 *S.* Enteritidis strains, digested with any of the cited REs, was hybridized with one of the probes, it was found that all of these contained between 1 and 4 copies of IS*200*.

Researchers at the Central Public Health Laboratory of London have performed interesting work on the phylogenetics of *S.* Enteritidis, and IS*200* was among the markers used (Stanley and Baquar, 1994). Based on the copy number of IS*200* and the fragments into which it had been inserted, *S.* Enteritidis strains of different phage types were grouped into evolutionary lines. Among the phage-type strains, 26 fall into one of three main IS*200* band profiles, which showed only two IS*200* insertion sites per genome. These profiles were related by a conserved *Pst*I band of 4.5 kbp and differentiated by variable *Pst*I bands of 5.2 kbp (clonal line I, including PT1, PT4, PT6, and nine other infrequent phage types), 7 kbp (clonal line II, including PT6a, PT8, PT13, and five other infrequent phage types), or 3.9 kbp (clonal line III, which included PT11 and four other infrequent phage types). The strain of PT16 exhibited a unique IS*200* profile, with at least 12 insertion sites (Stanley et al., 1991). In addition, all epidemic PT4 strains from the United Kingdom that were studied showed the same IS*200* pattern (Stanley et al., 1992b).

Olsen et al. (1994) analyzed a series of 62 strains, including 33 phage-type strains of human and poultry origin from Denmark. Total DNA preparations were digested with *Pvu*II and *Pst*I, and probed with IS*200*. Eight and six different restriction patterns were respectively revealed for each RE. When results from both REs were used for grouping, a total of 11 groups were found, and the most frequent group included strains from 17 phage types. Four *Pst*I-IS*200* types included only two copies of IS*200* (three of these types—I, II, and IV—corresponded to the aforementioned clonal lines I, II, and III), whereas types V and VI included 15 and eight copies, respectively. In the same vein are the results from the German series analyzed by Liebisch and Schwarz (1996), which was differentiated into two *Pst*I-IS*200* types. These two types corresponded to clonal line I [strains ascribed to PT1, PT4, PT6, and strains with a lytic pattern that did not correspond to any recognized phage types or reacts but does not conform (RDNC)] and clonal line II (strains ascribed to PT8, PT13, and RDNC). In another study, Millemann et al. (1995) analyzed by *Pst*I-IS*200* profile 14 *S.* Enteritidis strains, which had not been phage typed, that had been isolated from poultry farms in France. The 14 strains fell into a single, new IS*200* type, which was characterized by the presence of three IS*200* copies located in fragments of 5.2, 4.5, and 1 kbp in size. These data suggest that natural *S.* Enteritidis populations, in different geographical areas, are undergoing different evolutionary changes.

Stanley et al. (1992b) analyzed sequence divergence at three loci of the chromosome in a series of salmonellae, including 12 pandemic strains and 12 PT4 U.K. isolates of *S.* Enteritidis, and seven subspecies-type strains. The genes screened were *fimA*, *rfaGBIJ*, and *umuDC*, which encode the type-1 fimbrial subunit, glycosyltransferases responsible for synthesis of the LPS core region, and mutagenic DNA repair, respectively. Chromosomal genetic loci exhibited characteristic DNA sequence divergence between subspecies of salmonellae, but no divergence was observed within *S.* Enteritidis, in which the locus *umuDC* was not found either. Related work (Olsen et al., 1994) evaluated as probes five randomly cloned fragments of the *S.* Enteritidis chromosome in a series represented by strains of 31 phage types. Four different restriction patterns were observed when the five chromosomal fragments were hybridized to *Pst*I-digested DNAs. Strains from 27 of these 31 phage types, including the phage types of major epidemiological importance, showed the same pattern, called RFLPI; PT3 and PT19 strains showed RFLPII; and PT14 and PT16 strains showed RFLPII and RFLPIV, respectively.

The data from RFLP analysis with the aforementioned probes revealed that these procedures are useful tools in establishing an interrelationship and in evaluating the heterogeneity of strains, but they had weak discriminatory power within *S.* Enteritidis.

Currently, an important part of our knowledge about genetic typing of *S.* Enteritidis strains stems from *ribotyping*. This method reveals the sequence divergence around and within rRNA gene loci, which are organized as polycistronic transcriptional units with the following organization (5'-promoter–16S–spacer region–23S–5S–3'), called *rrn* ribosomal operons (Brosius et al., 1981; Grimont and Grimont, 1986; Jensen et al., 1993). Ribotyping has two major advantages over other restriction-hybridization procedures: (a) the genes coding rRNA are highly conserved and therefore a single probe can be used for all eubacteria; and (b) since most bacteria contain multiple ribosomal operons, a reasonable number of fragments are obtained after probing, which enables interspecies and intraspecies discrimination. Salmonellae contain seven *rrn* loci distributed throughout the chromosome. If genomic DNA is digested with an RE that does not cut into the operons, seven or fewer DNA hybridizing fragments will be observed (an example is presented in Fig. 13.4, in which results from *Pst*I digestion are shown). However, if the RE cuts one or more times into some of the *rrn* loci, the number of fragments will be more than seven (see Fig. 13.4, which shows the results obtained after digestion with *Sph*I). The appropriate RE must be determined for each bacterial species and serovar, and the use of two or more

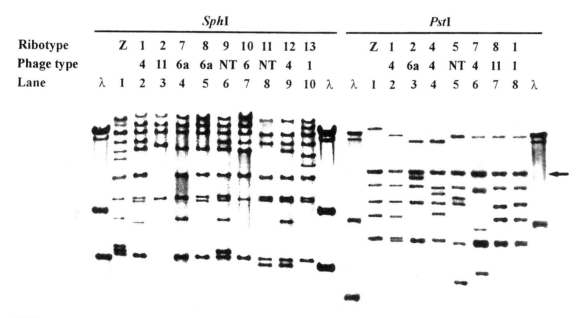

Ribotype			*Sph*I												*Pst*I						
	Z	1	2	7	8	9	10	11	12	13		Z	1	2	4	5	7	8	1	
Phage type		4	11	6a	6a	NT	6	NT	4	1			4	6a	4	NT	4	11	1	
Lane	λ	1	2	3	4	5	6	7	8	9	10	λ	λ	1	2	3	4	5	6	7	8	λ

FIGURE 13.4   Ribotyping performed independently with *Sph*I and *Pst*I of salmonella strains: lane 1, *Salmonella* Typhimurium ATCC 14028; lanes 2–10, Spanish clinical strains of *S.* Enteritidis (the phage type of these strains is also indicated). **_Sph_I ribotyping:** lane 2, 177/92; lane 3, 51/84; lane 4, 217/93; lane 5, 124/85; lane 6, 98/87; lane 7, 254/92; lane 8, 437/93; lane 9, 276/93; and lane 10, 11/94. **_Pst_I ribotyping:** lane 2, 177/92; lane 3, 124/85; lane 4, 175/94; lane 5, 475/93; lane 6, 80/87; lane 7, 51/84; and lane 8, 11/94. Lane l, bacteriophage lambda DNA cleaved with *Hin*dIII; the sizes of fragments from top to bottom are 27.5, 23.1, 9.4, and 6.6 kb.

REs can increase the discriminating power of the method but also increases the workload. The *rrnB* operon of *Escherichia coli* that has been cloned into pBR322 can be used as a probe (Brosius et al., 1981). Alternatively, cDNA synthesized from an rDNA 16S and 23S (or only 16S) template by reverse transcriptase is also employed. On the basis of the probe used, the complete rDNA regions, which include the *rrn* operons and adjacent sequences, or only the 16 rRNA genes and adjacent sequences, are analyzed. The banding patterns are called *ribotypes* in the first case and *16S ribotypes* in the second.

Researchers have evaluated different REs for ribotyping of *S.* Enteritidis, and those described as the most useful are *Sma*I (Gruner et al., 1994; Olsen et al., 1994; Usera et al., 1994), *Acc*I (Usera et al., 1994; Landeras et al., 1996; Lin et al., 1996), *Eco*RI, *Bgl*I, *Sal*I, *Hinc*II, and *Pst*I (Landeras et al., 1996). However, the strongest discriminatory power has been reported for *Sph*I, which differentiated between seven and 13 types in the different series analyzed (Gruner et al., 1994; Thong et al., 1995; Landeras et al., 1996; Lin et al., 1996). *Sph*I ribotyping was useful for discriminating strains belonging to the prevalent phage types, that is, PT4, PT8, and PT13 (Gruner et al., 1994; Lin et al., 1996), and we have also found differentiation within PT1, PT6, PT6a, RDNC, and non-phage-typeable (NPT) strains. However, it has also been found that strains ascribed to different PTs showed identical *Sph*I ribotypes. Some examples are shown in Figure 13.4: among PT1 strains, *Pst*I ribotypes labeled 1, 8, 9, and 13 were revealed; among PT4 strains, the labels 1, 4, 7, 9, 11, and 12; among PT6a, the labels 1, 6, and 8; and among NPT, the labels 1, 7, 9, 10, and 11. On the other hand, when we compared the nine *Sph*I ribotypes from poultry and/or human strains reported by Gruner et al. (1994) with the *Sph*I ribotypes found in our laboratory, we observed a different degree of likeness among them. Some of them seem to be identical or very similar. Thus, the ribotypes labeled B, F, and J by Gruner et al. (1994) and S7, S16, and S2 by Landeras et al. (1996) seem to be identical (S1, S2, and S7 ribotypes are labeled as 1, 2, and 7 in Fig. 13.4). The most frequent ribotypes in both series, labeled A and S1, respectively, differ only in that A shows a single fragment, whereas S1 shows a double band at a position corresponding to 9.6 kb. This difference could be real or due to a larger electrophoretic separation in the latter case. A similar comparison could not be made with other series, because in the reports by Thong et al. (1995) and Lin et al. (1996), the banding profiles corresponding to the reported ribotypes were not shown.

A two-way ribotyping procedure, which combines results from *Sph*I with results from *Pst*I, enabled us to differentiate 113 isolates (grouped into 58 strains) into 18 combined ribotypes. This procedure yielded a DI of 0.77, which was the highest DI found within pathogenic *S.* Enteritidis for both phenotypic and genotypic methods (Landeras et al., 1996). The data from banding profiles were used to construct a dendrogram of similarity that showed *S.* Enteritidis as a polyphyletic serovar, with a major lineage, including seven combined ribotypes and 77% of the strains tested. This definition as a polyphyletic

serovar had been previously described by using data from MLEE analysis (Beltran et al., 1988; Boyd et al., 1993).

Two-way ribotyping was used as an approach to trace the molecular epidemiology of *S.* Enteritidis isolates in Asturias (Spain), and certain points of interest were clarified. It enabled us to detect genotypic differences that grouped organisms causing 34 sporadic and unrelated episodes of human salmonellosis and others implicated in 20 outbreaks into 17 combined ribotypes or groups. Three of the groups included organisms collected over several years, and two of these groups included strains causing intestinal and extraintestinal infections, as well as strains collected from foods such as egg dishes and/or minced meat, that were identified as transmission vehicles. The three groups differed only in their *Sph*I ribotypes and could be considered as members of the same lineage, which may also include other organisms placed close together in the dendrogram. Organisms from other lineages are infrequently collected and are therefore playing a less important role in human illness in Asturias, Spain.

A variant of ribotyping (which we designated as *one-way ribotyping*), in which the DNA is digested with a mixture of *Pst*I and *Sph*I, is being evaluated in our laboratory with excellent results. It is yielding a somewhat higher discriminatory power than two-way ribotyping (because it differentiates some strains of the prevalent *Sph*I-*Pst*I ribotype) and has showed two other additional advantages. First, the banding patterns (PS ribotypes) consisted of 7–14 fragments, with sizes from 2.8 up to 27.5 kb, which are visually well interpretable. The differentiation of uncommon fragments was more accurate than in some of the *Pst*I or *Sph*I ribotypes. In fact, the differences between pairs of ribotypes usually affected more than one fragment (some examples are shown in Fig. 13.5). Second, it is a one-way procedure, which should be less costly in terms of work, time, and reagents. At the moment, we have differentiated 33 PS ribotypes (14 within PT4, of which four are shown in Fig. 13.5; six within PT1 and PT6a; three within PT6 and PT8; eight within NPT; and two within RDNC) in *S.* Enteritidis strains from different sources (clinical samples, eggs, chicken, meat, and water) in different geographical areas in the Iberian Peninsula and Canary Islands and collected during 1984–96. ATCC 13076, which is ascribed to PT1, and strains of PT4, PT6, PT6a, PT8, PT9, and PT13a of Ward et al. (1987) were also tested. While strains PT4 and PT6 showed identical PS ribotypes, each one of the others showed a different PS ribotype (Fig. 13.5). Conversely, some strains ascribed to PT1, PT4, PT6, PT6a, PT34, NPT, and RDNC showed a PS1 ribotype, just as some strains of PT1, PT4, PT7, and RDNC showed a PS3 ribotype.

The heterogeneity of types that can be differentiated with this one-way ribotyping procedure is greater than that usually described within *S.* Enteritidis of prevalent phage types, using data from molecular phenotypic and genetic methods. The major disadvantage of ribotyping, as well as the other restriction-hybridization procedures, is that multiple steps are required (DNA isolation, restriction, electrophoresis, Southern blotting, probe preparation, and hybridization), which are time-consuming and labor-intensive. Despite this disadvantage, we propose PS ribotyping as the most useful

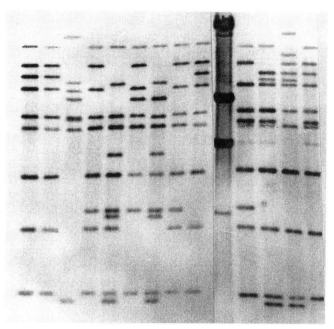

	*Sph*I-*Pst*I												
Ribotype	1	1	31	3	32	33	34	3	1		3	5	10	1
Phage type	4	6	6a	7	8	13a	9	1	34		4	4	4	4
Lane	1	2	3	4	5	6	7	8	9	λ	10	11	12	13

FIGURE 13.5 Ribotyping performed with a mixture of *Pst*I and *Sph*I of *Salmonella* Enteritidis strains. Lanes 1–3, 5, 6, and 7 show PS ribotypes of strains of PT4, PT6, PT6a, PT8, Pt13a, and PT9, respectively, from the Central Public Health Laboratory of London. Lanes 4, 8, and 9 show strains representing PT7, PT1, and PT34 from the Spanish *Salmonella* Reference Laboratory. Lanes 10–13 show Spanish clinical isolates ascribed to PT4: lane 10, 424/93; lane 11, 418/93; lane 12, 408/93; and lane 13, 398/93. Lane l, DNA from lambda phage digested with *Hin*dIII; the sizes of fragments from top to bottom are 27.5, 23.1, 9.4, 6.6, and 4.3 kb.

tool, for the moment, for differentiating *S.* Enteritidis strains, a proposal that is supported by two important observations: (a) its high sensitivity for differentiating strains ascribed to prevalent phage types, and (b) both the high reproducibility and ease of interpretation of the ribotypes that include distinct and well-resolved fragments, which will guarantee the comparison of results obtained from different series in different laboratories.

Typing Methods Based on the Polymerase Chain Reaction

The most recently introduced assays for typing bacterial DNA are the methods applying PCR, which have been reviewed by Arbeit (1995). The essential feature of PCR is the ability to replicate (amplify) a particular DNA sequence rapidly and exponentially. This sequence should represent a relatively small fragment of DNA, typically 0.5–2.0 kb, because larger sequences are difficult to amplify efficiently. The PCR-based typing methods may be categorized into two major types. The first type, *PCR-RFLP*, involves amplification of a known sequence, cutting with REs, and comparison of restriction fragments corresponding to an amplified DNA sequence from different strains. Virulence genes, repetitive chromosomal sequences, insertion sequences, and ribosomal operons are among the candidate traits for PCR-RFLP subtyping in *S.* Enteritidis. The second type involves random amplification of segments of the target DNA by using a single primer and is called *random amplification of polymorphic DNA* (RAPD) or arbitrarily primed PCR. The *RAPD method* does not require restriction of the amplicon, because several fragments of various sizes are generated during the PCR. The amplified DNA fragments are separated by electrophoresis on agarose gels and visualized by staining with ethidium bromide. The selection of appropriate primers and optimization of PCR conditions are of great importance in order to avoid the generation of artifacts or nonspecific DNA fragments in a profile and to maximize the discriminatory power of the method.

PCR RIBOTYPING

Two regions can be distinguished in the 16S–23S transcriptional units: the highly conserved genes for rRNA (which are so conserved that the same primers can recognize sequences in most bacteria) and the intergenic spacer region, which shows a significant degree of variation in length and sequence among species and a lower degree within species (Brosius et al., 1981; Jensen et al., 1993). The intergenic spacer region is being analyzed by a simple procedure, called *PCR ribotyping* (which can be complemented by cutting the amplified DNA with REs), which uses oligonucleotide primers complementary to conserved regions of the 16S and 23S rRNA genes. In a study by Jensen et al. (1993) on the identification of bacteria by PCR-amplified ribosomal DNA spacer polymorphisms, primers of only 15 nucleotides were used for both the 16S and the 23S regions. The size chosen was limited because of the variations in sequence beyond these highly conserved regions. With this procedure, bacteria belonging to eight genera and 28 species or serovars were tested, including six salmonella serovars. The only two *S.* Enteritidis strains analyzed showed a single profile that included three DNA-amplified fragments of 665, 610, and 480 bp. Recently, Lagatolla et al. (1996) analyzed a panel of 218 salmonella strains (belonging to 10 serovars and isolated from patients with diarrhea, and food of poultry origin, in Italian laboratories in 1977–94) by using two other primers of 19 and 22 nucleotides, complementary to conserved regions of the 16S and 23S rRNA genes, respectively. These primers had been previously described by Kostman et al. (1992). This typing method enabled the identification of seven different and specific electrophoretic profiles for seven serovars, which included *S.* Enteritidis. While in *S.* Typhimurium, *S.* Infantis, and *S.* Derby, eight, six, and four different profiles were identified, respectively. The 41 *S.* Enteritidis isolates analyzed showed an identical banding profile, which included four DNA-amplified fragments along the region between 1100 and 700 bp. This profile was different from profiles of other serovars.

Using the primers described by Kostman et al. (1992), we have also tested a series of salmonellae, which included *S.* Enteritidis strains representing 10 phage types and 18 PS ribotypes, and it was found that all *S.* Enteritidis strains showed an identical PCR ribotype, which is shown in Figure 13.6. This PCR ribotype was similar to the PCR ribotype of *S.* Typhimurium ATCC 14028 (differing only in the intensity of one of the three amplified DNA fragments) but different from PCR ribotypes of clinical strains of some other serovars (a clinical isolate classified as *S.* Ohio is included in Fig. 13.6) and different from the PCR ribotype of *S.* Enteritidis revealed in the series analyzed by Lagatolla et al. (1996). Since salmonellae have seven rRNA operons per genome, but only three or four rDNA-amplified fragments

were detected in the *S.* Enteritidis strains analyzed, it can be deduced that the intergenic spacer region of some of the seven operons has an identical or very similar size. PCR ribotyping is one of the most rapid and easily performed methods for molecular typing, but the results commented on before strongly suggest that it can be a useful tool for phylogenetic purposes between salmonella serovars but not within *S.* Enteritidis.

RANDOM AMPLIFICATION OF POLYMORPHIC DNA (RAPD TYPING)

The application of *RAPD fingerprinting* as a molecular tool requires the identification of oligonucleotide primers that are capable of recognizing DNA polymorphisms among isolates. Unfortunately, there is no way of predicting which oligonucleotide sequences will be useful. The first RAPD analysis applied to *S.* Enteritidis was developed by Fadl et al. (1995) by using a primer of 15 nucleotides selected in their laboratory. The method was used to analyze *S.* Enteritidis from 12 human outbreaks (belonging to PT8, PT13a, and NPT) and from 20 avian sources (belonging to PT8, PT13a, and PT14b). Nine distinct, randomly amplified DNA patterns were found (six in PT13a, and three in PT8 and PT14b), which showed two common and several uncommon fragments. Four patterns were found in strains from both human and avian sources. The results showed that this procedure may be useful to determine differences among isolates within the same phage types, and for tracing back the source of *S.* Enteritidis outbreaks in humans more precisely. In addition, the differences observed in the DNA patterns among PT8, PT13a, and PT14b isolates, as well as the identical banding patterns found among isolates belonging to different phage types, support previous findings suggesting that one phage type may be the progenitor of another phage type (Chart et al., 1989; Threlfall and Chart, 1993; Powell et al., 1994). In another recent study, Lin et al. (1996) screened 65 arbitrary primers with *S.* Enteritidis isolates. A panel of six primers was selected and used to test 28 *S.* Enteritidis isolates, collected in different U.S. states and one in Germany, which had been previously characterized by other typing methods (phage typing, ribotyping performed with *Acc*I and *Sph*I, and PFGE performed with *Xba*, *Avr*II, and *Apa*I). The genomic DNA was obtained by boiling the bacterial sample, to simplify the procedure, and determination of the appropriate concentrations of primer, DNA template, and Mg^{2+} was necessary for optimal reproducibility and discriminatory power. Different primers produced different numbers of patterns (which ranged between three and five), and, by combining the results from the six primers, a total of 14 RAPD subtypes were revealed. The RAPDs provided a greater number of types or groups than any of the other typing methods when applied individually.

We are also evaluating different primers for RAPD, in the same panel of *S.* Enteritidis strains that had been previously evaluated by ribotyping and PCR ribotyping. Many of the primers tested generated nonreproducible profiles, and/or fragments that are not well resolved. With none of the primers was the reproducibility 100%, and with each of

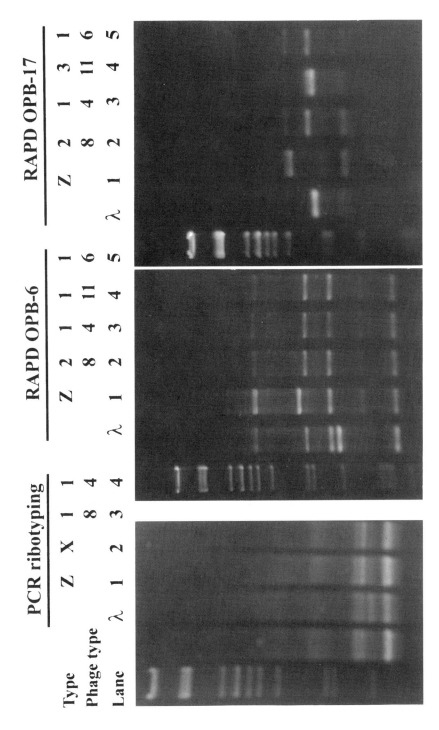

FIGURE 13.6 Analysis of genomic DNA of salmonella strains by PCR-based methods. In **PCR ribotyping**, the patterns shown correspond to: lane 1, *Salmonella* Typhimurium ATCC 14028; lane 2, 50/94, which is a clinical isolate ascribed to *S.* Ohio; and lanes 3 and 4, strains of PT8 and PT4, respectively, of *S.* Enteritidis. In both **RAPDs**, the patterns shown correspond to: Lane 1, *S.* typhimurium ATCC 14028. Lanes 2–5, *S.* Enteritidis strains: lane 2, strain of PT8; and lane 3, strain of PT4. Lane 4, the Spanish clinical isolate 51/84; and lane 5, strain of PT6. Lane l, DNA from lambda phage digested with *Pst*I; the size of fragments from top to bottom are 14.16, 5.08, 4.5, 2.8, 2.5, 2.1, 2.0, 1.7, 1.2, 1.1, 0.8, 0.5, and 0.4 kb.

them the differentiation was much lower than with PCR ribotyping. Obviously, badly defined profiles cannot be used to compare results from different series or laboratories. An example of RAPD profiles that we found is that obtained with two of the primers, called OPB-6 and OPB-17, described by Lin et al. (1996), and shown in Figure 13.6. With both primers, a similar but not identical, differentiation of strains was found, given that all *S.* Enteritidis strains tested (which included strains representing 10 phage types and 18 PS ribotypes) showed identical RAPD profiles, called OPB-6/1 and OPB-17/1, with three exceptions: ATCC 13076 and the strain of PT8 showed different profiles with both primers, which were called OPB-6/2 and OPB-17/2; the strain of PT13a yielded OPB-17/2; and the only two PT11 strains tested yielded OPB-17/3. The profiles labeled OPB-6/2 and OPB-17/2 seem to be identical to profiles OPB-6/A and OPB-17/C, respectively, described by Lin et al. (1996).

The great advantage of PCR-based methods is that they are faster, relatively simple, and more economical than other genomic typing methods. For this, RAPD procedures that analyze the entire bacterial chromosome emerge as a particularly attractive method for typing of *S.* Enteritidis. However, we think that more work is still necessary to propose a well-standardized RAPD procedure, using a low number of selected primers that give specific and well-defined DNA-amplified profiles enabling the comparison of results from different series and laboratories. Only then could RAPD typing be an alternative to PCR ribotyping.

CORRELATION AMONG MOLECULAR TYPING METHODS AND APPLICATION TO CLONAL ANALYSIS OF *SALMONELLA* ENTERITIDIS

In previous sections, it has been shown that none of the molecular techniques proposed for the typing of *S.* Enteritidis meets all of the principal and secondary criteria that a typing method should fulfill for epidemiological and phylogenetic purposes. In fact, there is no preferred method for all clinical or epidemiological settings, and in critical situations such as the characterization and surveillance of highly virulent strains causing severe diseases, outbreaks, or epidemics, it will be necessary to apply several subtyping methods. For example, Powell et al. (1995), using PFGE and 16S *rrn* analysis, have demonstrated the in vivo derivation of PT9a and PT7 strains from a PT4 strain that was isolated from a single patient over a 6-week period. PT9a and PT7 could have been independently derived from PT4 during the disease, either as the result of a spontaneous mutation probably affecting phage receptor sites (PT9a) or due to the ability to express LPS (PT7).

As just described, studies of *S.* Enteritidis have shown that the use of several REs in RFLP analysis (Olsen et al., 1994; Suzuki et al., 1995; Thong et al., 1995; Landeras et al., 1996; Liebisch and Schwarz, 1996) or several primers

in RAPD (Lin et al., 1996) can efficiently increase discriminatory values (with respect to the use of a single RE or primer), just as with different genetic methods (Olsen et al., 1994; Suzuki et al., 1995; Thong et al., 1995; Liebisch and Schwarz, 1996). These combinations are useful tools for defining the number of clones in a panel of strains, for defining the number of strains associated with an outbreak, and for tracing back more precisely the source of *S.* Enteritidis outbreaks among humans.

The combination of results from different molecular methods might also be needed to differentiate strains, define clones and clonal lineages, and trace their phylogenetic relationship. The use of several typing procedures can also reveal the degree of evolutionary divergence among isolates ascribed to a single clonal lineage. In this sense, we should stress the homogeneity of results obtained from different series of PT4 strains when they were analyzed by different molecular typing methods (including OMPs, LPS, MLEE, IS*200*, and ribotyping performed with REs other than *Pst*I and *Sph*I). These results revealed a prevalent clonal structure among contemporary PT4 isolates and showed that the prevalent clonal lineage observed today emerged from a heterogeneous population before the onset of the current epidemic (Stanley et al., 1992b; Helmuth and Schroeter, 1994). However, it has also been observed that PT4 strains can be discriminated by PFGE (Powell et al., 1994) and by ribotyping (Figs. 13.4, 13.5) (Gruner et al., 1994). In each series analyzed with each of these methods, a profile was clearly more frequent, and strains belonging to each prevalent profile can be regarded as clonal. The polymorphisms identified in other isolates may represent evolutionary divergence, reflecting several classes of genetic rearrangements within *S.* Enteritidis PT4 genome.

For clonal analysis, several typing procedures can be used both to form clusters and to reveal the degree of convergence among clusters. An example is the work of Olsen et al. (1994), in which a series of 62 selected strains, of 33 phage types and one strain RDNC, were characterized by four genetic methods. By three of the methods (PFGE with *Not*I, ribotyping with *Sma*I, and probing with five randomly cloned fragments of the *S.* Enteritidis chromosome), one major group containing strains of the most commonly encountered phage types, and eight, six, and six minor groups, respectively, were found. The fourth method, based on IS*200* hybridization patterns resulting from the combination of results from *Pvu*II and *Pst*I revealed two major and seven minor groups. With the combined use of the four methods, two groups of strains, representing eight (PT4, PT4a, PT6, PT6a, PT7, PT21, PT25, and PT31) and seven (PT2, PT8, PT13, PT13a, PT22, PT23, and PT24) phage types, were formed and considered as the main evolutionary lines of *S.* Enteritidis; strains of the remaining phage types belonged to other groups and are currently playing a lesser role in salmonellosis.

In conclusion, monitoring *S.* Enteritidis by molecular techniques provides sufficient specificity to identify clones of organisms that can be traced temporally and geographically. The use of multiple typing methods can give an indication of the continuously occurring evolution of strains in nature, reflecting changes in biochemistry, lysogeny, extra-chromosomal DNA content, and nucleotide sequence of chromosomal DNA, which can be exploited for both epidemiological and phylogenetic purposes.

REFERENCES

Arbeit, R.D. 1995. Laboratory procedures for epidemiologic analysis of microorganisms. In: Murray, P.R., Baron, E.J., Pfaller, M.A., Tenover F.C., and Yolken, R.H., eds. Manual of clinical microbiology. Washington, DC: American Society for Microbiology, pp. 190–208.

Beltran, P., Musser, J.M., Helmuth, R., Farmer III, J.J., Frerichs, W.M., Wachsmuth, I.K., Ferris, K., McWhorter, A.C., Wells, J.G., Cravioto, A., and Selander, R.K. 1988. Toward a population genetic analysis of *Salmonella*: genetic diversity and relationships among strains of serotypes *S. choleraesuis, S. derby, S. dublin, S. enteritidis, S. heidelberg, S. infantis, S. newport,* and *S. typhimurium.* Proc. Natl. Acad. Sci. U.S.A. 85:7753–7757.

Boyd, E.F., Wang, F.U., Beltran, P., Plock, S.A., Nelson, K., and Selander, R. 1993. *Salmonella* reference collection B (SARB): strains of 37 serovars of subspecies. Int. J. Gen. Microbiol. 139:1125–1132.

Braun, P., and Fehlhaber, K. 1995. Migration of *Salmonella enteritidis* from the albumen into the egg yolk. Int. J. Food Microbiol. 25:95–99.

Brosius, J., Ullrich, A., Raker, M.A., Gray, A., Dull, T.J., Gutell, R.R., and Noller, H.F. 1981. Construction and fine mapping of recombinant plasmid containing the *rrnB* ribosomal RNA operon of *E. coli.* Plasmid 6:112–118.

Brown, D.J., Threlfall, E.J., Hampton, M.D., and Rowe, B. 1993. Molecular characterization of plasmids in *Salmonella enteritidis* phage types. Epidemiol. Infect. 110:209–216.

Chalker, R.B., and Blaser, M.J. 1988. A review of human salmonellosis. III. Magnitude of salmonellosis infection in the United States. Rev. Infect. Dis. 10:111–124.

Chart, H., Rowe, B., Threlfall, E.J., and Ward, L.R. 1989. Conversion of *Salmonella enteritidis* phage type 4 to phage type 7 involves loss of lipopolysaccharide with a concomitant loss of virulence. FEMS Microbiol. Lett. 60:37–40.

Chart, H., Threlfall, E.J., Ward, L.R., and Rowe, B. 1993. Unusual expression of lipopolysaccharide by strains of *Salmonella enteritidis* phage type 30. Lett. Appl. Microbiol. 16:87–90.

D'Aoust, J.Y. 1994. *Salmonella* and the international food trade. Int. J. Food Microbiol. 24:11–31.

Fadl, A.A., Nguyen, A.V., and Khan, M.I. 1995. Analysis of *Salmonella enteritidis* isolates by arbitrarily primed PCR. J. Clin. Microbiol. 33:987–989.

Frost, J.A., Ward, L.R., and Rowe, B. 1989. Acquisition of a drug resistance plasmid converts *Salmonella enteritidis* phage type 4 to phage type 24. Epidemiol. Infect. 103:243–248.

Gilbert, I., Barbé, J., and Casadesús, J. 1990. Distribution of insertion sequence IS*200* in *Salmonella* and *Shigella.* J. Gen. Microbiol. 136:2555–2560.

González-Hevia, M.A., Llaneza, J., and Mendoza, M.C. 1994. Differentiation of strains from a food-borne outbreak of

Salmonella enterica by phenotypic and genetic typing methods. Int. J. Food Microbiol. 22:97–103.

González-Hevia, M.A., and Mendoza, M.C. 1995a. Differentiation of strains from a food-borne outbreak of *Salmonella enterica* by phenotypic and genetic typing methods. Eur. J. Epidemiol. 11:479–482.

González-Hevia, M.A., and Mendoza, M.C. 1995b. Polymorphism of rRNA genes and plasmid analysis in the typing of *Salmonella enterica* serovar Enteritidis from a Spanish health area. Microbiologica 18:377–384.

Grimont, F., and Grimont, P.A.D. 1986. Ribosomal ribonucleic acid gene restriction patterns as potential taxonomic tools. Ann. Inst. Pasteur Microbiol. 137B:165–175.

Gruner, E., Martinetti Lucchini, G., Hoop, R.K., and Altwegg, M. 1994. Molecular epidemiology of *Salmonella enteritidis.* Eur. J. Epidemiol. 10:85–89.

Gulig, P.A., Danbara, H., Guiney, D.G., Lax, A.J., Norel, F., and Rhen, M. 1993. Molecular analysis of *spv* virulence genes of the salmonella virulence plasmids. Mol. Microbiol. 7:825–830.

Helmuth, R., and Schroeter, A. 1994. Molecular typing methods for *S. enteritidis.* Int. J. Food Microbiol. 21:69–77.

Hitchcock, P.J., and Brown, T.M. 1983. Morphological heterogeneity among *Salmonella* lipopolysaccharide chemotypes in silver-stained polyacrylamide gels. J. Bacteriol. 154:269–277.

Hunter, P.R., and Gaston, M.A. 1988. Numerical index of the discriminatory ability of typing systems: an application of Simpson's index of diversity. J. Clin. Microbiol. 26:2465–2466.

Jensen, M.A., Webster, J.A., and Strauss, N.R. 1993. Rapid identification of bacteria on the basis of polymerase chain reaction–amplified ribosomal DNA spacer polymorphisms. Appl. Environ. Microbiol. 59:945–952.

Kostman, J.R., Edlind, T.D., LiPuma, J.J., and Stull, T.L. 1992. Molecular epidemiology of *Pseudomonas cepacia* determined by polymerase chain reaction ribotyping. J. Clin. Microbiol. 30:2084–2087.

Lagatolla, C., Dolzani, L., Tonin, E., Lavenia, A., Di Micheli, M., Tommasini, T., and Monti-Bragadin, C. 1996. PCR ribotyping for characterizing *Salmonella* isolates of different serotypes. J. Clin. Microbiol. 34:2440–2443.

Landeras, E., Alzugaray, R., Gonzalez-Hevia, M.A., and Mendoza, M.C. 1996. Epidemiological differentiation of pathogenic strains of *Salmonella enteritidis* by ribotyping. J. Clin. Microbiol. 34:2294–2296.

Li, J., Nelson, K., McWhorter, A.C., Whittam, T.S., and Selander, R.K. 1994. Recombinational basis of serovar diversity in *Salmonella enterica.* Proc. Natl. Acad. Sci. U.S.A. 91:2552–2556.

Liebisch, B., and Schwarz, S. 1996. Molecular typing of *Salmonella enterica* subsp. *enterica* serovar Enteritidis isolates. J. Med. Microbiol. 44:52–59.

Lin, A.W., Usera, M.A., Barret, T.J., and Goldsby, R.A. 1996. Application of random amplified polymorphic DNA analysis to differentiate strains of *Salmonella enteritidis.* J. Clin. Microbiol. 34:870–876.

Maslow, J.N., Mulligan, M.E., and Arbeit, R.D. 1993. Molecular epidemiology: application of contemporary techniques to the typing of microorganisms. Clin. Infect. Dis. 17:153–164.

Mendoza, M.C., Guerra, B., Landeras, E., Lobato, M.J., Alvarez-Granda, Y., and Gonzalez-Hevia, M.A. 1996. *Salmonella enterica* en aguas: relación filogenética mediante analisis de restricción y ribotipificación con *Hinc*II. In: Microbiología de las aguas de abastecimiento. Madrid: Ministerio de Sanidad y Consumo and Asociación Española de Abastecimientos de Agua y Saneamiento, pp. 57–75.

Millemann, Y., Lesage, M.-C., Chaslus-Dancla, E., and Lafont, J.P. 1995. Value of plasmid profiling, ribotyping, and detection of IS200 for tracing avian isolates of *Salmonella typhimurium* and *S. enteritidis*. J. Clin. Microbiol. 33:173–179.

Morris, J.G., Dwyer, D.M., Hoge, C.W., Stubbs, A.D., Tilghman, D., Groves, C., Israel, E., and Libonatt, J. 1992. Changing clonal patterns of *Salmonella enteritidis* in Maryland: evaluation of strains isolated between 1985 and 1990. J. Clin. Microbiol. 30:1301–1303.

Olsen, J.E., Skov, M.N., Threlfall, E.J., and Brown, D.J. 1994. Clonal lines of *Salmonella enterica* serotype Enteritidis documented by IS200, ribotyping, pulsed-field gel electrophoresis and RFLP typing. J. Med. Microbiol. 40:15–22.

Perales, I., and Audicana, A. 1989. The role of hens' eggs in outbreaks of salmonellosis in north Spain. Int. J. Food Microbiol. 8:175–180.

Powell, N.G., Threlfall, E.J., Chart, H., and Rowe, B. 1994. Subdivision of *Salmonella enteritidis* PT4 by pulsed-field electrophoresis: potential for epidemiological surveillance. FEMS Microbiol. Lett. 119:193–198.

Powell, N.G., Threlfall, E.J., Chart, H., Schofield, S.L., and Rowe, B. 1995. Correlation of change in phage type with pulsed field profile and 16S *rnn* profile in *Salmonella enteritidis* phage types 4, 7 and 9a. Epidemiol. Infect. 114:403–411.

Rampling, A. 1993. *Salmonella enteritidis* five years on. Lancet 342:317–318.

Rivera, M.J., Rivera, N., Castillo, J., Rubio, M.C., and Gomez-Lus, R. 1991. Molecular and epidemiological study of *Salmonella* clinical isolates. J. Clin. Microbiol. 29:927–932.

Rodrigue, D.C., Tauxe, R.V., and Rowe, B. 1990. International increase in *Salmonella enteritidis*: a new pandemic? Epidemiol. Infect. 105:21–27.

Singer, T.J., Opitz, H.M., Gershman, M., Hall, M., Muñiz, I., and Shobba, V.R. 1992. Molecular characterization of *Salmonella enteritidis* isolates from Maine poultry and poultry farm environments. Avian Dis. 36:324–333.

Stanley, J., and Baquar, N. 1994. Phylogenetics of *Salmonella enteritidis*. Int. J. Food Microbiol. 21:79–87.

Stanley, J., Jones, C.S., and Threlfall, E.J. 1991. Evolutionary lines among *Salmonella enteritidis* phage types are identified by insertion sequence IS200 distribution. FEMS Microbiol. Lett. 82:83–90.

Stanley, J., Burnes, A.P., Threlfall, E.J., Chowdry, N., and Goldsworthy, M. 1992a. Genetic relationships among strains of *Salmonella enteritidis* in a national epidemic in Switzerland. Epidemiol. Infect. 108:213–220.

Stanley, J., Goldsworthy, M., and Threlfall, E.J. 1992b. Molecular phylogenetic typing of pandemic isolates of *Salmonella enteritidis*. FEMS Microbiol. Lett. 90:153–160.

Suzuki, Y., Ishihara, M., Matsumoto, M., Arakawa, S., Saito, M., Ishikawa, N., and Yokochi, T. 1995. Molecular epidemiology of *Salmonella enteritidis*: an outbreak and sporadic cases studied by means of pulsed-field gel electrophoresis. J. Infect. 31:211–217.

Swaminathan, B., and Matar, G.M. 1993. Molecular typing methods. In: Persing, D.H., Smith, T.F., Tenover, F.C., and White, T.J., eds. Diagnostic molecular microbiology: principles and applications. Washington, DC: American Society for Microbiology, pp. 26–45.

Thiagarajan, D., Saeed, A.M., and Asem, E.K. 1994. Mechanism of transovarian transmission of *Salmonella enteritidis* in laying hens. Poult. Sci. 73:89–98.

Thong, K.L., Ngeow, Y.F., Altwegg, M., Navaratnam, P., and Pang, T. 1995. Molecular analysis of *Salmonella enteritidis* by pulsed-field gel electrophoresis and ribotyping. J. Clin. Microbiol. 33:1070–1074.

Threlfall, E.J., and Chart, H. 1993. Interrelationships between strains of *Salmonella enteritidis*. Epidemiol. Infect. 111:1–8.

Threlfall, E.J., Rowe, B., and Ward, L. 1989. Subdivision of *Salmonella enteritidis* phage types by plasmid profile typing. Epidemiol. Infect. 102:459–465.

Threlfall, E.J., Hampton, M.D., Chart, H., and Rowe, B. 1994. Use of plasmid profile typing for surveillance of *Salmonella enteritidis* phage type 4 from humans, poultry and eggs. Epidemiol. Infect. 112:25–31.

Usera, M.A., Popovic, T., Bopp, C.A., and Strockbine, A.S. 1994. Molecular subtyping of *Salmonella enteritidis* phage type 8 strains from the United States. J. Clin. Microbiol. 32:194–198.

Vatopoulos, A.C., Mainas, E., Balis, E., Threlfall, E.J., Kanelopoulou, M., Kalapothaki, V., Malamou-Lada, H., and Legakis, N. 1994. Molecular epidemiology of ampicillin resistant clinical isolates of *Salmonella enteritidis*. J. Clin. Microbiol. 32:1322–1325.

Ward, L.R., De Sa, J., and Rowe, B.A. 1987. A phage typing scheme for *S. enteritidis*. Epidemiol. Infect. 99:291–294.

14

Rational Approach to the Choice of Molecular Markers Applicable to the Tracing of *Salmonella enterica* Serovar Enteritidis

E. Chaslus-Dancla and Y. Millemann

INTRODUCTION

The incidence of infections caused by *Salmonella enterica* serovar Enteritidis (*S.* Enteritidis) has increased throughout the world (Rodrigue et al., 1990; Canarelli et al., 1995). Currently, *S.* Enteritidis is the most common cause of human gastroenteritis and also the predominant serovar isolated from poultry products in many countries. Phenotypic and genotypic techniques have been carried out for subtyping *S.* Enteritidis isolates as a part of the epidemiological investigations that were conducted to investigate the origin of outbreaks. Phenotypic, including biochemical, characterization has been used for epidemiological studies of *S.* Enteritidis but has a limited discriminative power (Katouli et al., 1993; Poppe et al., 1993; Stubbs et al., 1994).

Phage typing is of interest because of its high correlation with pathogenicity. It has been used in studies on *S.* Enteritidis strains (Hickman-Brenner et al., 1991; Rodrigue et al., 1992; Brown et al., 1994), with discriminatory power and reproducibility. However, this method is time-consuming and restricted to reference laboratories. Moreover, instability can occur, because the phage type can be modified by the acquisition of a plasmid (Frost et al., 1989; Threlfall et al., 1993; Ridley et al., 1996) or a phage (Rankin and Platt, 1995) or by modifi-

cation of lipopolysaccharide (Chart et al., 1989; Baggesen et al., 1997). Increased frequency of *S.* Enteritidis involved in sporadic or epidemic cases and belonging to a restricted number of phage types has made this approach alone inadequate for epidemiological investigations (Nastasi and Mammina, 1996).

Epidemiological studies of *S.* Enteritidis infections thus require the use of additional efficient molecular markers to trace precisely the diffusion of clonal strains, and to demonstrate the persistence of particular clones in the environment. These markers must be discriminatory to distinguish epidemic and nonepidemic strains, applicable to a large number of isolates, reproducible and stable.

The analysis of phenotypic and genotypic characters enables the determination of the similarities between the isolates and the construction of dendrograms. The clonal lineages define groups of bacteria with extensive phenotypic and genotypic similarities, which enables one to hypothesize a common ancestor (Ørskov and Ørskov, 1983).

In this chapter, we review the different approaches for characterization with markers useful for epidemiological studies and develop a tentative hierarchy of their applicability to such studies. We focus mainly on phenotypic characters such as resistance to antibiotics and plasmids, and on genotypic characterization, with chromosomal fingerprints for rRNA (ribotyping) and for IS*200*, as well as amplification fingerprints of chromosomal DNA with two different approaches.

RESISTANCE TO ANTIBIOTICS

Salmonella Enteritidis strains isolated from humans are generally susceptible to antibiotics. In England and Wales until 1990, only 11% of the isolates from humans were resistant to antibiotics and 1% were multiresistant. Phage type 4 (PT4) was no exception in this respect, and, under such conditions, discrimination based on drug resistance was of limited interest. Nevertheless, some outbreaks were studied on the basis of the resistance phenotypes, such as the London outbreak of *S.* Enteritidis PT4 with the spread of *S.* Enteritidis PT24 derived from PT4 after the acquisition of a resistant plasmid (Threlfall and Chart, 1993).

A decrease in susceptibility to antibiotics was observed in strains from animals during the last few years, but most of the strains remained susceptible in England (Wray et al., 1993), Belgium (Pohl et al., 1991), Eastern Europe (Hasenson et al., 1992), or the United States (Singer et al., 1992). In France, more than 90% of *S.* Enteritidis strains from poultry are still susceptible to antibiotics (Brisabois et al., 1997).

Nevertheless, some authors reported resistance to a limited number of antibiotics. This resistance was generally observed against the β-lactams (Poppe et al., 1993; Vatopoulos et al., 1994) or β-lactams and tetracycline (Nair et al., 1995). In the latter study, there was a difference of resistance between strains of human or nonhuman origin. Resistance to penicillin alone was more frequently encountered in strains of human origin and resistance to different β-lactams and to tetracycline in strains with nonhuman sources. Whatever their origin, however, more than 40% of strains were resistant to tetracycline, but resistance to aminoglycosides, chloramphenicol, trimethoprim–sulfamethoxazole, and quinolones was uncommon. Some mechanisms of resistance were identified in clinical strains [for example, to the TEM1 β-lactamase (Rivera et al., 1991)], and recently an unusual resistance to β-lactams, including cephalosporins (DHA-1), was identified (Gaillot et al., 1997).

The relatively high frequency of resistance to β-lactams was also reported in a smaller collection of strains isolated from healthy chickens at slaughter. The *S.* Enteritidis strains were resistant only to β-lactams, in contrast with salmonella strains of other serovars, which were resistant to gentamicin, streptomycin, and tetracycline (Lee et al., 1993b). In some strains of *S.* Enteritidis isolated from pigs in England, resistance to tetracycline was recorded (Lee et al., 1993a).

Other recent studies showed an increase in resistance to the new fluoroquinolones in strains isolated from food animals and human food, and in clinical situations before and after treatment (Brown et al., 1996; Frost et al., 1996; Ouabdesselam et al., 1996).

From the literature, even if the situation has evolved somewhat in the last few years, it is still clear that resistance to antibiotics does not appear as a useful epidemiological

marker (Rodrigue et al., 1992), except in some limited cases of diffusion of particular clones. This situation is quite different from that observed with *S.* Typhimurium but is shared with *S.* Dublin (Martel et al., 1996).

In our experience, strains from poultry generally have been susceptible to antibiotics. Few have been resistant to nalidixic acid, to oxolinic acid, or to pefloxacin. They have been isolated in newborn ducks and not recovered later from adults. On one occasion, the acquisition of resistance to nalidixic acid was observed in strains isolated from rabbits during therapy.

Antibiograms were realized using solid medium according to the method of Bauer et al. (1966). Aminoglycosides, β-lactams, chloramphenicol and florfenicol, tetracycline, trimethoprim, and quinolones including the recent veterinary fluoroquinolones, enrofloxacin and danofloxacin, were considered as the most relevant antibiotics to be tested.

PLASMID PROFILES AND PLASMID FINGERPRINTS

Salmonella strains can harbor plasmids of different molecular sizes, ranging from about 1 to 200 kb. Strain characterization can be obtained from the plasmid profiles, which reveal information about the number and molecular sizes of the plasmids harbored. Further information can be drawn from the corresponding plasmid fingerprints obtained after digestion of the plasmids with restriction enzymes and separation of the generated fragments by electrophoresis.

Plasmid analysis has proved useful in several studies. In surveys of strains of *S.* Enteritidis from different sources (human or animal), distinct plasmid profiles were identified and used to distinguish isolates (Wachsmuth et al., 1991; Dorn et al., 1992). Strains of *S.* Enteritidis were subclassified according to their plasmid profiles in isolates from different outbreaks (Lujan et al., 1990). A good correlation between outbreaks and a single plasmid profile was observed in most cases and supported the conclusion of the usefulness of this approach. The usefulness of plasmid profiles was also shown in a study of more than 200 *S.* Enteritidis strains isolated from patients in a rural community (Rivera et al., 1991). Although only 10 were resistant to antibiotics and 15 different plasmid profiles were detected, including a predominant one characterized by a unique 54-kb plasmid, discrimination among strains was possible.

In several cases, however, a limited number of plasmids were present, with often a unique plasmid of about 55 kb (38 MDa), and, in such conditions, plasmid profiling appeared to be less sensitive than phage typing (Threlfall et al., 1989; Poppe et al., 1993). This low diversity of plasmid profiles limited the tracing of *S.* Enteritidis from poultry flocks to human infection, except when the presence of additional plasmids could be used to document this transmission (Dorn et al., 1993). In another study, the surveillance of susceptible strains of *S.* Enteritidis PT4 isolated from humans and poultry (chickens and eggs) was realized

(Threlfall et al., 1994). More than 1000 strains were studied and 25 plasmid profiles identified. The predominant plasmid profile was characterized by a single 38-MDa plasmid present in more than 90% of the strains from humans and 70% from poultry. A similar situation was encountered in a study of 203 *S*. Enteritidis strains isolated from sporadic cases or from outbreaks in Maryland between 1985 and 1990, where 10 plasmid profiles were identified (Morris et al., 1992). The emergence of a single profile, with only one plasmid of approximately 55 kb and associated with a particular phage type, restricted the interest in this approach.

A study of strains isolated from patients and belonging to different phage types, including the predominant PT4 but also different phage types of epidemiological importance, such as PT6a, PT1, and PT8, resulted in the hypothesis that a plasmid of the IncX group could be responsible for the conversion of PT4 or PT1 into PT6a (Ridley et al., 1996). Phage conversions were obtained by introducing unique plasmid strains of different phage types (Threlfall et al., 1993). Correlation of phage types and plasmid profiles was also observed in a survey of strains isolated from different sources (poultry and environment) (Singer et al., 1992). The strains were all susceptible to antibiotics, and different plasmid profiles were associated with PT13a and PT14.

From the literature, it appears that plasmid typing alone can be helpful on some occasions with *S*. Enteritidis strains, but for epidemiological studies, more information may be obtained with plasmid typing associated with other typing methods.

We studied strains from different animal origins. A plasmid of about 54 kb was present in every strain and sometimes with two additional plasmids of about 50 and 3.8 kb. Plasmid fingerprints of the 54-kb plasmids suggested they were closely related.

Different methods of plasmid DNA extraction (Birnboim and Doly, 1979; Kado and Liu, 1981) have been shown to be appropriate and were used in several epidemiological studies. We routinely used the method described by Takahashi and Nagano (1984), which, in our experience, has provided good results with plasmids from 1 to 120 kb.

CHROMOSOMAL FINGERPRINTS

Chromosomal fingerprinting appears to be better for the study of clonal diffusion.

Direct Electrophoresis

Chromosomal DNA can be digested with restriction enzymes. If these enzymes recognize frequent sites of restriction, more than 100 fragments can be generated and separated by electrophoresis. A direct comparison of such restriction profiles by *restriction endonuclease analysis* is difficult. The use of an enzyme that recognizes only rare restriction sites enables one to obtain a limited number of fragments (about 20–30). These high-molecular-weight fragments can be separated by *pulsed-field gel electrophoresis* (PFGE). Numerous techniques have been developed, of which *contour-clamped homogeneous electrophoretic field* is the most often used (Olsen et al., 1994; Powell et al., 1994; Thong et al., 1995; Liebisch and Schwarz, 1996; Lin et al., 1996).

Pulsed-field profiles (pulsotypes) were compared with ribotypes and seemed to be slightly less sensitive in their ability to discriminate between isolates, although a good concordance is generally observed between both methods (Thong et al., 1995). An equivalent discriminatory power has been observed in a work aimed at evaluating genetic relationships in apparently unrelated *S*. Enteritidis phage types isolated from a single patient during an infection (Powell et al., 1995). Recently, PFGE separation provided a higher level of discrimination than did ribotyping in a study of a collection of 31 epidemiologically unrelated strains (Liebisch and Schwarz, 1996). PFGE also provided a means of discrimination and appeared as suitable for epidemiological investigations of 39 *S*. Enteritidis PT4 strains, among which nine distinct pulsed-field profiles were identified (Powell et al., 1994).

The choice of enzymes appropriate for epidemiological studies is of particular importance. Some authors have preliminarily tested as many as 20 different restriction enzymes, and those most often retained have been *Xba*I, *Spe*I, and *Not*I. Several methods of DNA extraction have been developed in order to obtain intact chromosomal DNA. Generally, after an overnight broth culture, cells are embedded in a low-melting agarose and then lysed (with lysozyme or proteinase K); after numerous rinses (with water or triethanolamine), slices of agarose blocks containing DNA are then digested with restriction enzymes. Electrophoresis is generally conducted in 1% agarose gels.

Hybridization

Chromosomal restriction profiles can be more easily read after hybridization of DNA with a probe revealing a limited number of selected fragments in *restriction fragment length polymorphism*.

RIBOTYPES
Endonuclease-cleaved chromosomal DNA can be hybridized with the universal 16 + 23S rRNA probe corresponding to highly conserved sequences. Different probes can be used, 16 + 23S rRNA (Grimont and Grimont, 1986), cDNA obtained after reverse transcription (Picard-Pasquier et al., 1989), or fragments amplified within a conserved sequence of rRNA (Grimont and Grimont, 1996).

The excellent reproducibility of this method in standard conditions has led to its use in taxonomic and phylogenetic studies, for instance, for the characterization of strains of numerous serovars (Esteban et al., 1993). Ribotyping has also proved useful for the epidemiological surveys of *S*. Enteritidis isolates (Martinetti and Altwegg, 1990; Olsen et al., 1994; Thong et al., 1995). It can also help to identify clonal relations between strains of various phage types (Powell et al., 1995).

The essential choice of the most adequate enzymes can be made after preliminary studies (Martinetti and Altwegg, 1990; Landeras et al., 1990) to obtain clear and distinct banding patterns. The three restriction endonucleases SmaI, SphI, and AccI have thus been often retained for ribotyping of S. Enteritidis isolates (Martinetti and Altwegg, 1990; Olsen et al., 1994; Usera et al., 1994; González-Hevia and Mendoza, 1995; Landeras et al., 1996; Lin et al., 1996).

Most authors have used nonradioactive labeling with digoxigenin (Usera et al., 1994) or biotin (Martinetti and Altwegg, 1990; Pignato et al., 1990) as an alternative to radioactive labeling, but no difference in the results by using radioactive and nonradioactive labeling has been reported.

We have applied ribotyping to an epidemiological study on S. Enteritidis strains isolated from three avian species reared on four poultry farms and with probable clonal ties. A number of enzymes were tested in preliminary assays on S. Enteritidis isolates, and four of them (HindIII, BglII, PvuII, and SmaI) were chosen. We did not detect any difference among these particular S. Enteritidis isolates (Fig. 14.1A) (Millemann et al., 1995), but discrimination was observed between other S. Enteritidis strains of distant origins (unpublished data).

INSERTION SEQUENCE TYPES (ISOTYPES)

Insertion sequences are transposable elements present in several copies within the genome of prokaryotes. Their use has been suggested as epidemiological markers to discriminate related strains of various bacterial species, such as *Staphylococcus aureus* (IS256) (Monzon-Moreno et al., 1991), and *Mycobacterium tuberculosis* (IS986 or IS6110) (van Soolingen et al., 1991; Cave et al., 1994). Some other insertion sequences, IS1 and IS3, first described in *Escherichia coli* strains, and IS630 in *Shigella sonnei* isolates, have also been detected in salmonella serovars (Bisercic and Ochman, 1993; Matsutani and Ohtsubo, 1993) and might constitute additional markers of the strains.

IS200 has been identified in a strain of *Salmonella* Typhimurium (Lam and Roth, 1983). This short IS (700 bp long) appeared first to be specific to salmonella serovars, and copies were detected on the chromosomes of most of them, as well as copies on plasmids in S. Enteritidis isolates (Stanley et al., 1991). Exceptions are salmonella strains of serovars Agona, Typhisuis, and Arizona (Lam and Roth, 1983), where no IS200 copies were detected. IS200 copies were also detected in E. coli and Shigella serovars (Gibert et al., 1990; Bisercic and Ochman, 1993).

The number of IS200 copies on the chromosome greatly depends on the serovar. For S. Typhimurium strains, this number generally ranges from six to 10 (Lam and Roth, 1983; Gibert et al., 1990; Bisercic and Ochman, 1993), whereas it appears to be limited to two or three copies in S. Enteritidis isolates (Stanley et al., 1991, 1992; Millemann et al., 1995).

Studies have already been carried out on the copy number and location of IS200 for collections of S. Enteritidis PT4 or PT8 strains (Stanley et al., 1992; Usera et al., 1994). In general, isolates could be assigned to one of the three clonal lineages defined by Stanley et al. (1991).

The restriction enzymes selected to define restriction profiles for IS200 should not cut within the insertion sequence. The most often retained enzyme was PstI, which yields clear banding patterns. Nevertheless, BglII or PvuII can also be helpful. The probe can be obtained after amplification and digestion of plasmids pIZ45 or pIZ46 harboring an internal 300-bp HindIII-EcoRI fragment or a corresponding dimer, respectively (Gibert et al., 1990).

In our studies, we did not detect any differences by IS200 typing between related S. Enteritidis strains with either PstI, BglII, or PvuII. However, we did detect three bands in our S. Enteritidis isolates, leading to the proposal of the definition of S. Enteritidis clonal line (SECL) IV, differing from SECLI (grouping the great majority of the European PT4 pandemic isolates) by only one additional 1-kb band (Fig. 14.1B) (Millemann et al., 1995). By contrast, we could distinguish S. Enteritidis strains of distant origins when using PstI (unpublished data).

Radioactive labeling can be used, either with ^{32}P (Millemann et al., 1995) or ^{35}S (Stanley et al., 1992). The use of nonradioactive methods such as digoxigenin labeling (Olsen et al., 1994) or a chemiluminescent system (Liebisch and Schwarz, 1996) is increasing. In our experience, both approaches have been of equivalent quality (sensitivity and pattern clarity), but nonradioactive labeling was, of course, less exacting.

Despite good sensitivity and reproducibility, the current genotypic methods used for typing salmonella strains have some disadvantages. DNA hybridization allows a clear interpretation, but the method is cumbersome, time-consuming, and requires appreciable amounts of DNA. Therefore, rapid methods requiring only small amounts of template DNA and using the *polymerase chain reaction* (PCR) have been developed.

AMPLIFICATION PROFILES (PCR TYPES)

Various approaches have been considered with either defined primers or randomly chosen primers.

PCR Ribotypes

A method has been developed that consists of the amplification of the intergenic 16S–23S regions (Kostman et al., 1995; Gürtler and Stanisich, 1996). This technique of PCR ribotyping focuses on the polymorphism of the selected regions, either by a direct analysis of the amplification products or after their digestion by restriction enzymes.

Results were in close agreement with those of ribotyping when applied to S. Typhimurium strains (Nastasi and Mammina, 1995). In a recent study of S. Enteritidis isolates, PCR ribotyping enabled the subdivision of S. Enteritidis isolates of clinical interest. One of the PCR ribotypes was closely related to PT8, whereas 11 patterns were recognizable within PT4 and five within PT1. This work concluded in the epidemic circulation of multiple clones of S. Enteritidis PT4 (Nastasi and Mammina, 1996).

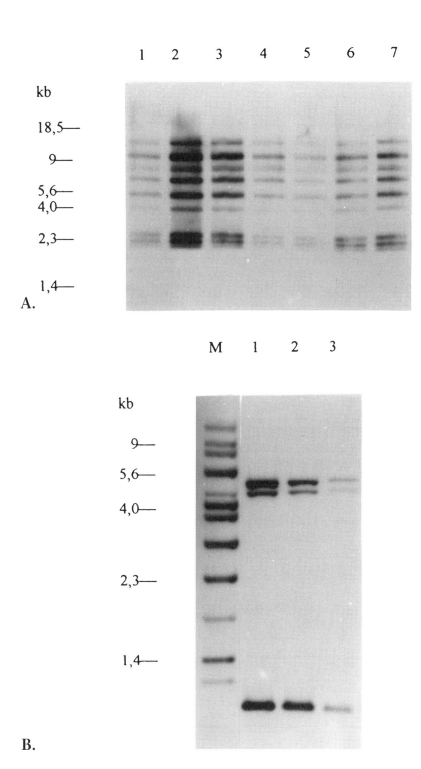

FIGURE 14.1   **A.** Ribotypes of *Salmonella* Enteritidis isolates, after cleavage by *Pvu*II. Lanes 1–7: different representative strains. **B.** IS*200* types of *S.* Enteritidis isolates, after cleavage by *Pst*I. Lanes 1–3: different representative strains.

Repetitive Extragenic Palindromic PCR

Repetitive and conserved sequences of the genome, such as the *repetitive extragenic palindromic* (REP) and *enterobacterial repetitive intergenic consensus* (ERIC) sequences have been described in Enterobacteriaceae.

Specific primers enabled DNA fragments located between these sequences to be amplified in REP PCR (Versalovic et al., 1991). Amplified fragments were separated by agarose-gel electrophoresis.

An ERIC sequence is a short, interspersed repetitive nucleic acid sequence originally found in *E. coli* and *S.* Typhimurium. The use of outward-facing primers complementary to each end of these repeats in PCR has been described and termed ERIC PCR (Versalovic et al., 1991). This technique has recently proved to be useful in epidemiological studies of *Enterobacter aerogenes* and *E. coli* isolates (Georghiou et al., 1991; Lipman et al., 1995). Applied to salmonellae of diverse serovars, it suggested the existence of "serovar-specific profiles" (van Lith and Aarts, 1994).

In our studies, both primers ERIC1R (5'-ATGTAAGCTC-CTGGGGATTCAC-3') and ERIC2 (5'-AAGTAAGTGACT-GGGGTGAGCG-3') were added to the reaction volume. The amplification conditions (deoxyribonucleoside triphosphate concentration, temperature and duration of extension, and DNA concentration) were tested to obtain a good reproducibility of banding patterns. ERIC PCR products were analyzed after electrophoresis in 1% agarose gel. Only one reproducible fingerprint was found among the *S.* Enteritidis strains, whereas two fingerprints were observed in the *S.* Typhimurium isolates. One of these fingerprints was shared by seven strains of *S.* Typhimurium and by all of the *S.* Enter-

itidis strains (Fig. 14.2) (Millemann et al., 1996). These results suggested this approach was not fully relevant for epidemiological studies of salmonellae.

RAPD and Arbitrarily Primed PCR

Random amplified polymorphic DNA (RAPD) analysis (Williams et al., 1990), or *arbitrarily primed PCR* (Welsh and McClelland, 1990), is a DNA-fingerprint technique using single, short primers of an arbitrarily selected sequence to amplify genomic DNA in a low-stringency PCR. The banding patterns obtained after electrophoresis of the PCR products have been used to fingerprint strains. RAPD does not require preliminary knowledge of nucleotidic sequences and is thus simple and rapid.

The main disadvantage of RAPD might be a lack of reproducibility. Numerous variation factors have been identified, such as the concentration and quality (the need for a unique batch) of the primer and *Taq* DNA polymerase, concentration of $MgCl_2$, concentration and quality of DNA, amplification conditions, and thermocycler. This implies preliminary studies to optimize conditions (Hilton et al., 1997; Tyler et al., 1997). Nevertheless, under uniform and optimized conditions, reproducible profiles are obtained by RAPD (Swaminathan and Barrett, 1995).

This method has been applied to the analysis of 33 unrelated avian and human *S.* Enteritidis isolates of different phage types and resulted in discrimination within a single phage type, suggesting its usefulness in tracing *S.* Enteritidis isolates from human outbreaks (Fadl et al., 1995). Recently, a panel of 29 *S.* Enteritidis strains already characterized by other methods was studied by RAPD analysis, which discriminated isolates within a single phage type and

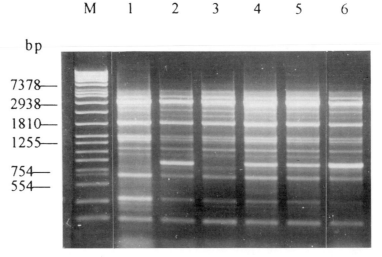

FIGURE 14.2   Enterobacterial repetitive intergenic ERIC PCR fingerprints of *Salmonella* Typhimurium isolates (lanes 1–3) and *Salmonella* Enteritidis isolates (lanes 4–6). Lanes 1 and 3: profile 1; and lanes 2 and 4–6: profile 2. M, molecular weight marker Raoul (Appligene).

enabled as many as 14 subtypes to be defined among the 29 isolates (Lin et al., 1996).

Nevertheless, the latter study underlined the crucial importance of the preliminary choice of the primers. Six were selected from 65. The criteria for such a choice were the obtaining of clear banding patterns, amplification, and discrimination among the test population. Therefore, although time-consuming, an accurate choice of primers in preliminary assays is a prerequisite for the sensible use of this method. When appropriately constituted primer sets are identified and employed, RAPD analysis provides a simple, rapid, and powerful method for subtyping *S.* Enteritidis.

Numerous batches of primers are available from different manufacturers. Rapid extraction of DNA by the boiling method may be considered, because it generally results in fingerprint patterns similar to those obtained from purified DNA.

In our laboratory, preliminary studies were realized with 40 primers (Operon Technologies, U.S.A.) on three strains of each serovar, *S.* Enteritidis and *S.* Typhimurium. From these results, two primers, OPG08 (5'-TCACGTCCAC-3'), and OPH13 (5'-GACGCCACAC-3'), were retained for subsequent studies (Fig. 14.3). The reproducibility of RAPD fingerprints was confirmed with both primers. RAPD analysis separated the *S.* Enteritidis strains into three groups, based on their origins and phenotypic characteristics. The presence of two different clonal strains in one flock could thus be hypothesized, whereas our former results with ribotyping did not enable discrimination of the

isolates. Confirmation was provided by phage typing. The presence of three strains with different RAPD types in another flock could suggest independent contaminations possibly due to a lack of sanitary protection. Very close patterns were observed among strains from related origins. In our work, RAPD analysis thus appeared as a method that improved the tracing of avian *S.* Enteritidis strains (Millemann et al., 1996).

METHODS OF ANALYSIS

Typeability, reproducibility, and discriminatory power must be evaluated to assess which method is the most efficient. The discriminatory power of a typing method is its ability to distinguish between unrelated strains and can be determined by the calculation of a discriminatory index. The construction of dendrograms showing the genetic relationships between clonal lineages can reinforce this analysis.

Calculation of the Index of Discrimination (Hunter and Gaston, 1988; Hunter, 1990)

Calculation of the index of discrimination is based on the probability of two unrelated strains being characterized as the same type. It must therefore be applied to a collection of unrelated isolates rather than to strains from related origins. Moreover, as typing schemes should not be validated

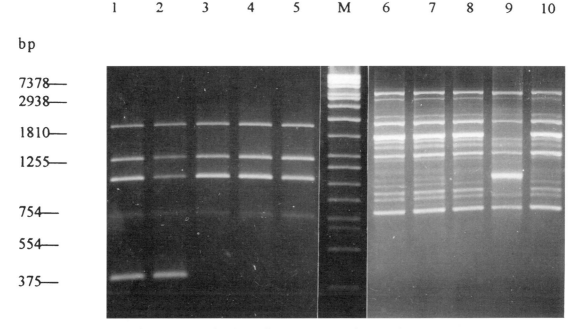

FIGURE 14.3   RAPD fingerprints of *Salmonella* Enteritidis isolates with primers OPG08 (lanes 1–5) and OPH13 (lanes 6–10). Lanes 1 and 2: profile I; lanes 3–5: profile II; lanes 6–8, 10: profile III; and lane 9: profile IV.

with small samples, no correcting factor for small populations has been made. The equation used for calculation is

$$D = 1 - \frac{1}{N(N-1)} \sum_{j=1}^{s} n_j(n_j - 1)$$

where N is the total number of strains tested, s is the number of different profiles (or types), and n_j is the number of strains within each type.

This index is therefore influenced by the number of the total isolates in the test population, the number of the different types detected, and the distribution of the strains within each type. A higher D (index of discrimination) will be obtained when strains are evenly distributed in the different types rather than in a predominant type. The discriminatory power of typing methods and of combined typing schemes can be compared with this analysis.

The acceptable level of discrimination will depend on a number of factors and should be as close to 1 as possible. The relative values obtained allow the classification of the different markers that are being compared and evaluated.

Construction of a Dendrogram

The dendrogram groups the strains according to the percentage of similarity between the profiles obtained with the different methods of typing. The most adapted grouping method is *single linkage,* whereas the *unweighted pair group method with arithmetic averages* (UPGMA) has a more taxonomic indication (Grimont and Grimont, 1996). Other methods (parsimony and correspondence analysis) can also be applied to confirm the results of single linkage or UPGMA. The numerical approach of the comparison of restriction and/or amplification profiles does not, of course, have a taxonomic or phylogenetic aim, but it helps considerably to interpret and to propose an epidemiological hypothesis.

Single linkage (or UPGMA) dendrograms have been successfully applied to epidemiological studies on salmonella isolates (Millemann et al., 1995; Landeras et al., 1996; Nastasi and Mammina, 1996).

CONCLUSION

Several phenotypic and genotypic markers are now available for epidemiological studies of salmonella isolates. In addition to their applicability, the essential properties of these markers must be reproducibility, stability, and discriminatory power. Reproducibility should be accurately studied through optimization of technical conditions particularly when amplification methods are used. Even if preliminary studies are time-consuming, the quality of the results depends greatly on them.

Stability of the markers should be demonstrated in both in vitro and in vivo conditions. Instability has been already reported for plasmid profiles and phage types, but stability should be studied for the amplification and restriction profiles. Some authors have tested the in vitro stability (van Soolingen et al., 1991; Murase et al., 1996), whereas others

have focused on in vivo stability (Millemann et al., 1995). In these experiments, axenic chickens reared in isolators under very controlled conditions were administered a unique salmonella strain. The stability of the different markers was confirmed on isolates recovered regularly from feces during the 15 weeks of rearing.

Discriminatory power must be considered after a collection of well-documented, related and unrelated isolates of known origins is established. Once this condition is fulfilled, markers can be compared and a hierarchy established between them with the help of the index of discrimination and of dendrograms.

Most authors have simultaneously compared several markers, such as phage types, plasmid profiles, isotypes, or ribotypes, and generally concluded that a combination of several markers is the best approach.

In our studies, several markers were tested, and their use in combination was proposed for epidemiological purposes. We underlined the interest in antibiotypes, although infrequently encountered, and of plasmid profiles, even in limited number. We stressed the interest in RAPD to trace precisely the diffusion of avian *S. Enteritidis* field isolates, in contrast with results obtained with *S. Typhimurium* strains.

ACKNOWLEDGMENTS

We thank Sabine Leroy-Sétrin and Jean-Pierre Lafont for critical reading of the manuscript and Stefan Schwarz for helpful discussion.

REFERENCES

Baggesen, D.L., Wegener, H.C., and Madsen, M. 1997. Correlation of conversion of *Salmonella enterica* serovar Enteritidis phage type 1, 4, or 6 to phage type 7 with loss of lipopolysaccharide. J. Clin. Microbiol. 35:330–333.

Bauer, A., Kirby, W.M.M., Cherris, J.C., and Turck, M. 1966. Antibiotic susceptibility testing by a standardized single disk method. Am. J. Clin. Pathol. 45:493–496.

Birnboim, H.C., and Doly, J. 1979. A rapid alkaline extraction procedure for screening recombinant plasmid DNA. Nucleic Acids Res. 7:1513–1522.

Bisercic, M., and Ochman, H. 1993. The ancestry of insertion sequences common to *Escherichia coli* and *Salmonella typhimurium*. J. Bacteriol. 175:7863–7868.

Brisabois, A., Fremy, S., Moury, F., Oudart, C., Piquet, C., and Pires Gomes, C. 1997. L'inventaire des Salmonellas 1994–1995. Maisons-Alfort, France: Centre National d'Etudes Veterinaires Alimentaires.

Brown, D.J., Baggesen, D.L., Hansen, H.B., and Bisgaard, M. 1994. The characterization of Danish isolates by *Salmonella enterica* serovar Enteritidis by phage typing and plasmid profiling 1980–1990. Acta Pathol. Microbiol. Scand. 102:208–214.

Brown, J.C., Thomson, C.J., and Amyes, S.G.B. 1996. Mutations of the *gyrA* gene of clinical isolates of *Salmonella typhimurium* and three other *Salmonella* species leading to decreased susceptibilities to 4-quinolone drugs. J. Antimicrob. Chemother. 37:351–356.

Canarelli, B., Laurans, G., Thomas, D., Zadwadzki, P., and Eb, F. 1995. Epidémiologie des *Salmonella* solées de 1978 à 1992 au CHU d'Amiens (908 souches). Med. Mal. Infect. 25:716–720.

Cave, M.D., Eisenach, K.D., Templeton, G., Salfinger, M., Mazurek, G., Bate, J.H., and Crawford, J.T. 1994. Stability of DNA fingerprint pattern produced with IS*6110* in strains of *Mycobacterium tuberculosis*. J. Clin. Microbiol. 32:262–266.

Chart, H., Rowe, B., Threlfall, E.J., and Ward, L.R. 1989. Conversion of *Salmonella enteritidis* phage type 4 to phage type 7 involves loss of lipopolysaccharide with concomitant loss of virulence. FEMS Microbiol. Lett. 60:37–40.

Dorn, C.R., Silapanuntakul, R., Angrick, E.J., and Shipman, L.D. 1992. Plasmid analysis and epidemiology of *Salmonella enteritidis* infection in three commercial layer flocks. Avian Dis. 36:844–851.

Dorn, C.R., Silapanuntakul, R., Angrick, E.J., and Shipman, L.D. 1993. Plasmid analysis of *Salmonella enteritidis* isolated from human gastroenteritis cases and from epidemiologically associated poultry flocks. Epidemiol. Infect. 111:239–243.

Esteban, E., Snipes, K., Hird, D., Kasten, R., and Kinde, H. 1993. Use of ribotyping for characterization of *Salmonella* serotypes. J. Clin. Microbiol. 31:233–237.

Fadl, A.A., Nguyen, A.V., and Khan, M.I. 1995. Analysis of *Salmonella enteritidis* isolates by arbitrarily primed PCR. J. Clin. Microbiol. 33:987–989.

Frost, J.A., Ward, L.R., and Rowe, B. 1989. Acquisition of a drug resistance plasmid converts *Salmonella enteritidis* phage type 4 to phage type 24. Epidemiol. Infect. 103:243–248.

Frost, J.A., Kelleher, A., and Rowe, B. 1996. Increasing ciprofloxacin resistance in salmonellas in England and Wales 1991–1994. J. Antimicrob. Chemother. 37:85–91.

Gaillot, O., Clément, C., Simonet, M., and Philippon, A. 1997. Novel β-lactam resistance with cephalosporinase characteristics in *Salmonella enteritidis*. J. Antimicrob. Chemother. 39:85–87.

Georghiou, P.R., Hamill, R.J., Wright, C.E., Versalovic, J., Koeuth, T., Watson, D.A., and Lupski, J.R. 1991. Molecular epidemiology of infections due to *Enterobacter aerogenes*: identification of hospital-associated strains by molecular techniques. Clin. Infect. Dis. 20:84–94.

Gibert, I., Barbé, J., and Casadesùs, J. 1990. Distribution of insertion sequence IS*200* in *Salmonella* and *Shigella*. J. Gen. Microbiol. 136:2555–2560.

González-Hevia, M.A., and Mendoza, M.C. 1995. Polymorphism of rRNA genes and plasmid analysis in the typing of *Salmonella enterica* serovar Enteritidis from a Spanish health area. New Microbiol. 18:377–384.

Grimont, F., and Grimont, P.A.D. 1986. Ribosomal ribonucleic acid gene restriction patterns as potential taxonomic tools. Ann. Inst. Pasteur Microbiol. 137B:165–175.

Grimont, P.A.D., and Grimont, F. 1996. Apport de la biologie moléculaire au typage: données méthodologiques. Med. Mal. Infect. 26:379–385.

Gürtler, V., and Stanisich, V.A. 1996. New approaches to typing and identification of bacteria using the 16S–23S rDNA spacer region. Microbiology 142:3–16.

Hasenson, L.B., Kaftyreva, L., Laszlo, V.G., Woitenkova, E., and Nesterova, M. 1992. Epidemiological and microbiological data on *Salmonella enteritidis*. Acta Microbiol. Hung. 39:31–39.

Hickman-Brenner, F.W., Stubbs, A.D., and Farmer III, J.J. 1991. Phage typing of *Salmonella enteritidis* in the United States. J. Clin. Microbiol. 29:2817–2823.

Hilton, A.C., Banks, J.G., and Penn, C.W. 1997. Optimization of RAPD for fingerprinting *Salmonella*. Lett. Appl. Microbiol. 24:243–248.

Hunter, P.R. 1990. Reproducibility and indices of discriminatory power of microbial typing methods. J. Clin. Microbiol. 28:1903–1905.

Hunter, P.R., and Gaston, M.A. 1988. Numerical index of discriminatory ability of typing systems: an application of Simpson's index of diversity. J. Clin. Microbiol. 26:2465–2466.

Kado, C.I., and Liu, S.-T. 1981. Procedure for the detection of large and small plasmids. J. Bacteriol. 145:1365–1373.

Katouli, M., Seuffer, R.H., Wollin, R., Kühn, I., and Möllby, R. 1993. Variations in biochemical phenotypes and phage types of *Salmonella enteritidis* in Germany 1980–92. Epidemiol. Infect. 111:199–207.

Kostman, J.R., Alden, M.B., Mair, M., Edlind, T.D., LiPuma, J.J., and Stull, T.L. 1995. A universal approach to bacterial molecular epidemiology by polymerase chain reaction ribotyping. J. Infect. Dis. 171:204–208.

Lam, S., and Roth, J.R. 1983. IS*200*: a *Salmonella*-specific insertion sequence. Cell 34:951–960.

Landeras, E., González-Hevia, M.A., Alzugaray, R., and Mendoza, M.C. 1996. Epidemiological differentiation of *Salmonella enteritidis* by ribotyping. J. Clin. Microbiol. 34:2294–2296.

Lee, C., Langlois, B.E., and Dawson, K.A. 1993a. Detection of tetracycline resistance determinants in pig isolates from three herds with different histories of antimicrobial agent exposure. Appl. Environ. Microbiol. 59:1467–1472.

Lee, L.A., Threatt, V.L., Puhr, N.D., Levine, P., Ferris, K., and Tauxe, R.V. 1993b. Antimicrobial-resistant *Salmonella* spp isolated from healthy broiler chickens after slaughter. J. Am. Vet. Med. Assoc. 202:752–755.

Liebisch, B., and Schwarz, S. 1996. Molecular typing of *Salmonella enterica* subsp. *enterica* serovar Enteritidis isolates. J. Med. Microbiol. 44:52–59.

Lin, A.W., Usera, M.A., Barrett, T.J., and Goldsby, R.A. 1996. Application of random amplified polymorphic DNA analysis to differentiate strains of *Salmonella enteritidis*. J. Clin. Microbiol. 34:870–876.

Lipman, L.J.A., de Nijs, A., Lam, T.J.G.M., and Gaastra, W. 1995. Identification of *Escherichia coli* strains from cows with clinical mastitis by serotyping and DNA polymorphism patterns with REP and ERIC primers. Vet. Microbiol. 43:13–19.

Lujan, R., Echeita, A., Usera, M.A., Martinez-Suarez, J.V., Alonso, R., and Saez-Nieto, J.A. 1990. Plasmid profiles as an epidemiological marker for *Salmonella enterica* serotype Enteritidis foodborne outbreaks. Microbiologia 6:45–50.

Martel, J.L., Chaslus-Dancla, E., Coudert, M., and Lafont, J.P. 1996. Evolution de la sensibilité aux antibiotiques des salmonelles d'origine bovine en France. Med. Mal. Infect. 26:415–419.

Martinetti, G., and Altwegg, M. 1990. rRNA gene restriction patterns and plasmid analysis as tool for typing *Salmonella enteritidis*. Res. Microbiol. 141:1151–1162.

Matsutani, S., and Ohtsubo, E. 1993. Distribution of the *Shigella sonnei* insertion elements in Enterobacteriaceae. Gene 127:111–115.

Millemann, Y., Lesage, M.-C., Chaslus-Dancla, E., and Lafont, J.-P. 1995. Value of plasmid profiling, ribotyping and detection of IS*200* for tracing avian isolates of *Salmonella typhimurium* and *enteritidis*. J. Clin. Microbiol. 33:173–179.

Millemann, Y., Lesage-Descauses, M.-C., Lafont, J.-P., and Chaslus-Dancla, E. 1996. Comparison of random amplified polymorphic DNA analysis and enterobacterial repetitive intergenic consensus-PCR for epidemiological studies of *Salmonella*. FEMS Immunol. Med. Microbiol. 14:129–134.

Monzon-Moreno, C., Aubert, S., Morvan, A., and El Solh, N. 1991. Usefulness of three probes in typing isolates of methicillin-resistant *Staphylococcus aureus* (MRSA). J. Med. Microbiol. 35:80–88.

Morris, J.G., Jr., Dwyer, D.M., Hoge, C.W., Stubbs, A.D., Tilghman, D., Groves, C., Israel, E., and Libonati, J.P. 1992. Changing clonal patterns of *Salmonella enteritidis* in Maryland: evaluation of strains isolated between 1985 and 1990. J. Clin. Microbiol. 30:1301–1303.

Murase, T., Nakamura, A., Matsushima, A., and Yamai, S. 1996. An epidemiological study of *Salmonella enteritidis* by pulsed-field electrophoresis (PFGE): several PFGE patterns observed in isolates from a food poisoning outbreak. Microbiol. Immunol. 40:873–875.

Nair, U.S., Saeed, A.M., Muriana, P.M., Kreisle, R.A., Barrett, B., Sinclair, C.L., and Fleissner, M.L. 1995. Plasmid profiles and resistance to antimicrobial agents among *Salmonella enteritidis* isolates from human beings and poultry in the midwestern United States. J. Am. Vet. Med. Assoc. 206:1339–1344.

Nastasi, A., and Mammina, C. 1995. Epidemiological evaluation by PCR ribotyping of sporadic and outbreak-associated strains of *Salmonella enterica* serotype Typhimurium. Res. Microbiol. 146:99–106.

Nastasi, A., and Mammina, C. 1996. Epidemiology of *Salmonella enterica* serotype Enteritidis infections in southern Italy during the years 1980–1994. Res. Microbiol. 147:393–403.

Olsen, J.E., Skov, M.N., Threlfall, E.J., and Brown, D.J. 1994. Clonal lines of *Salmonella enterica* serotype Enteritidis documented by IS*200*-, ribo-, pulsed-field gel electrophoresis and RFLP typing. J. Med. Microbiol. 40:15–22.

Ørskov, F., and Ørskov, I. 1983. Summary of a workshop on the clone concept in the epidemiology, taxonomy, and evolution of the Enterobacteriaceae and other bacteria. J. Infect. Dis. 148:346–357.

Ouabdesselam, S., Tankovic, J., and Soussy, C.J. 1996. Quinolone resistance mutations in the *gyrA* gene of clinical isolates of *Salmonella*. Microb. Drug Resist. 2:299–302.

Picard-Pasquier, N., Ouagued, M., Picard, B., Goullet, P., and Krishnamoorthy, R. 1989. A simple, sensitive method of analyzing bacterial ribosomal DNA polymorphism. Electrophoresis 10:186–189.

Pignato, S., Nastasi, A., Mammina, C., Fantasia, M., and Giammanco, G. 1996. Phage types and ribotypes of *Salmonella* Enteritidis in southern Italy. Zentralbl. Bakteriol. 283:399–405.

Pohl, P., Lintermans, P., Marin, M., and Couturier, M. 1991. Epidemiological study of *Salmonella enteritidis* strains of animal origin in Belgium. Epidemiol. Infect. 106:11–16.

Poppe, C., McFadden, K.A., Brower, A.M., and Demczuk, W. 1993. Characterization of *Salmonella enteritidis* strains. Can. J. Vet. Res. 67:176–184.

Powell, N.G., Threlfall, E.J., Chart, H., and Rowe, B. 1994. Subdivision of *Salmonella enteritidis* PT4 by pulsed-field gel electrophoresis: potential for epidemiological surveillance. FEMS Microbiol. Lett. 119:193–198.

Powell, N.G., Threlfall, E.J., Chart, H., Schofield, S.L., and Rowe, B. 1995. Correlation of change in phage type with pulsed field profile and 16S *rrn* profile in *Salmonella enteritidis* phage types 4, 7 and 9a. Epidemiol. Infect. 114:403–411.

Rankin, S., and Platt, D.J. 1995. Phage conversion in *Salmonella enterica* serotype Enteritidis: implications for epidemiology. Epidemiol. Infect. 114:227–236.

Ridley, A.M., Punia, P., Ward, L.R., Rowe, B., and Threlfall, E.J. 1996. Plasmid characterization and pulsed-field electrophoretic analysis demonstrate that ampicillin-resistant strains of *Salmonella enteritidis* phage type 6a are derived from *Salm. enteritidis* phage type 4. J. Appl. Bacteriol. 81:613–618.

Rivera, M.J., Rivera, N., Castillo, J., Rubio, M.C., and Gomez-Lus, R. 1991. Molecular and epidemiological study of *Salmonella* clinical isolates. J. Clin. Microbiol. 29:927–932.

Rodrigue, D.C., Tauxe, R.V., and Rowe, B. 1990. International increase in *Salmonella enteritidis*: a new pandemic? Epidemiol. Infect. 105:21–27.

Rodrigue, D.C., Cameron, D.N., Puhr, N.D., Brenner, F.W., St. Louis, M.E., Wachsmuth, I.K., and Tauxe, R.V. 1992. Comparison of plasmid profiles, phage types, and antimicrobial resistance patterns of *Salmonella enteritidis* isolates in the United States. J. Clin. Microbiol. 30:854–857.

Singer, J.T., Opitz, H.M., Gershman, M., Hall, M.M., Muniz, I.G., and Rao, S.V. 1992. Molecular characterization of *Salmonella enteritidis* isolates from Maine poultry and poultry farm environments. Avian Dis. 36:324–333.

Stanley, J., Jones, C.S., and Threlfall, E.J. 1991. Evolutionary lines among *Salmonella enteritidis* phage types are identified by insertion sequence IS*200* distribution. FEMS Microbiol. Lett. 82:83–90.

Stanley, J., Goldsworthy, M., and Threlfall, E.J. 1992. Molecular phylogenetic typing of pandemic isolates of *Salmonella enteritidis*. FEMS Microbiol. Lett. 90:153–160.

Stubbs, A.D., Hickman-Brenner, F.W., Cameron, D.N., and Farmer III, J.J. 1994. Differentiation of *Salmonella enteritidis* phage type 8 strains: evaluation of three additional phage typing systems, plasmid profiles, antibiotic susceptibility patterns, and biotyping. J. Clin. Microbiol. 32:199–201.

Swaminathan, B., and Barrett, T.J. 1995. Amplification methods for epidemiologic investigations of infectious disease. J. Microbiol. Methods 23:129–139.

Takahashi, S., and Nagano, Y. 1984. Rapid procedure for isolation of plasmid DNA and application to epidemiological analysis. J. Clin. Microbiol. 20:608–613.

Thong, K.L., Ngeow, Y.F., Altwegg, M., Navaratnam, P., and Pang, T. 1995. Molecular analysis of *Salmonella enteritidis* by pulsed-field gel electrophoresis and ribotyping. J. Clin. Microbiol. 33:1070–1074.

Threlfall, E.J., and Chart, H. 1993. Interrelationships between strains of *Salmonella enteritidis*. Epidemiol. Infect. 111:1–8.

Threlfall, E.J., Rowe, B., and Ward, L.R. 1989. Subdivision of *Salmonella enteritidis* phage types by plasmid profile typing. Epidemiol. Infect. 102:459–465.

Threlfall, E.J., Chart, H., Ward, L.R., de Sa, J.D., and Rowe, B. 1993. Interrelationships between strains of *Salmonella enteritidis* belonging to phage types 4, 7, 7a, 8, 13, 13a, 23, 24, and 30. J. Appl. Bacteriol. 75:43–48.

Threlfall, E.J., Hampton, M.D., Chart, H., and Rowe, B. 1994. Use of plasmid typing surveillance of *Salmonella enteritidis* phage type 4 from humans, poultry and eggs. Epidemiol. Infect. 112:25–31.

Tyler, K.D., Wang, G., Tyler, D., and Johnson, W.M. 1997. Factors affecting reliability and reproducibility of amplification-based DNA fingerprinting of representative bacterial pathogens. J. Clin. Microbiol. 35:339–346.

Usera, M.A., Popovic, T., Bopp, C.A., and Strockbine, N.A. 1994. Molecular subtyping of *Salmonella enteritidis* phage type 8 strains from the United States. J. Clin. Microbiol. 32:194–198.

Van Lith, L.A.J.T., and Aarts, H.J.M. 1994. Polymerase chain reaction identification of *Salmonella* serotypes. Lett. Appl. Microbiol. 19:273–276.

Van Soolingen, D., Hermans, P.W.M., de Haas, P.E.W., Soll, D.R., and van Embden, J.D.A. 1991. Occurrence and sta- bility of insertion sequences in *Mycobacterium tuberculosis* complex strains: evaluation of an insertion sequence–dependent DNA polymorphism as a tool in the epidemiology of tuberculosis. J. Clin. Microbiol. 29:2758–2786.

Vatopoulos, A.C., Mainas, E., Balis, E., Threlfall, E.J., Kanelopoulou, M., Kalapothaki, V., Malamou-Lada, H., and Legakis, N.J. 1994. Molecular epidemiology of ampicillin-resistant clinical isolates of *Salmonella enteritidis*. J. Clin. Microbiol. 32:1322–1325.

Versalovic, J., Koeuth, T., and Lupski, J.R. 1991. Distribution of repetitive DNA sequences in eubacteria and application to fingerprinting of bacterial genomes. Nucleic Acids Res. 19:6823–6831.

Wachsmuth, I.K., Kiehlbauch, J.A., Bopp, C.A., Cameron, D.N., Strockbine, N.A., Wells, J.G., and Blake, P.A. 1991. The use of plasmid profiles and nucleic acid probes in epidemiologic investigations of foodborne, diarrheal diseases. Int. J. Food Microbiol. 12:77–89.

Welsh, J., and McClelland, M. 1990. Fingerprinting genomes using PCR with arbitrary primers. Nucleic Acids Res. 18:7213–7218.

Williams, J.G.K., Kubelik, A.R., Livak, K.J., Rafalski, J.A., and Tingey, S.V. 1990. DNA polymorphisms amplified by arbitrary primers are useful as genetic markers. Nucleic Acids Res. 18:6531–6535.

Wray, C., McLaren, I.M., and Beedell, Y.E. 1993. Bacterial resistance monitoring of salmonellas isolated from animals: national experience of surveillance schemes in the United Kingdom. Vet. Microbiol. 35:313–319.

15

Phenotypic and Genotypic Characterization of *Salmonella enterica* Serovar Enteritidis

B.A.M. van der Zeijst and Y. Zhao

INTRODUCTION

The sudden emergence of *Salmonella enterica* serovar Enteritidis (*S.* Enteritidis) infections has required reliable and specific detection and identification methods for diagnosis and epidemiology. Understandably, advantage was taken from the enormous amount of serotyping done on salmonellae that was based on the Kauffmann-White typing scheme (Kauffmann, 1964). The scheme is based on somatic antigens [O antigens of lipopolysaccharides (LPS)], the flagellin (H antigen, phases 1 and 2), and occasionally capsular (Vi) antigen. Antigen profiles are derived from agglutination reactions with homologous antisera. Salmonellae containing related O antigens are clustered in serogroups. Within each serogroup, serovars are determined by means of the combination of O and H antigens. Using this scheme, more than 2200 serologically distinct types of salmonella serovars can be discriminated (LeMinor and Popoff, 1988). The original scheme is based on polyclonal antisera. To discriminate between *S.* Enteritidis and other salmonellae sharing the same antigenic specificities, highly discriminatory, preferably monoclonal, antibodies are required. Also, information on the exact structure of the epitopes recognized by such antibodies is desirable. *Salmonella* Enteritidis belongs to serogroup D1. It has the antigenic formula 1,9,12:g,m:- representing the O antigens and the phase-1 H antigens.

This chapter reviews the available information on the O antigens and flagellin of *S.* Enteritidis. Also, where available, information on the biological activity of these antigens is discussed. The second topic is the genetic characterization of *S.* Enteritidis, either by multilocus enzyme electrophoresis or by DNA-based methods.

Since 1978, *S.* Enteritidis has been increasingly responsible for outbreaks of salmonellosis in Spain (Perales and Audicana, 1988). In 1983, *S.* Enteritidis accounted for about 80% of such outbreaks [World Health Organization (WHO), 1990]. In 1988, St. Louis et al. reported an alarming rise in the number of outbreaks and cases of human salmonellosis caused by *S.* Enteritidis in the northeastern United States. Retrospective analysis of available data revealed that in that part of the United States, the number of *S.* Enteritidis isolates had increased steadily since 1976 (Mason, 1994). Over the past decades, a similar emergence of *S.* Enteritidis among humans was observed in Great Britain (Anon., 1988), as well as in many other countries (WHO, 1989; Rodrigue et al., 1990).

Such a sudden increase in the incidence of disease caused by a bacterium points to clonal expansion of this pathogen. Bacteria always evolve, which may result in bacterial clones that are so well adapted to their host that they have an advantage over other clones of the same bacterial species. This results in rapid epidemic expansion of the clone, followed by only a few additional mutations (Achtman, 1997). We review the available information in this light.

GENOTYPIC CHARACTERIZATION

Various methods have been used to characterize *S.* Enteritidis genomes in comparison with other salmonellae. Multilocus enzyme electrophoresis (MEE) has contributed most (Beltran et al., 1988). Restriction fragment length polymorphism in various forms has contributed also (Tompkins et al., 1986; Martinetti and Altwegg, 1990; Stanley et al., 1991, 1992; Thong et al., 1995). More recently, pulsed-field gel electrophoresis (Powell et al., 1995; Suzuki et al., 1995; Thong et al., 1995), and the polymerase chain reaction (PCR) (Fadl et al., 1995; Lampel et al., 1996) have been used. These methods were targeted to the genome, but other studies have also focused on plasmids (Threlfall et al., 1989; Brown et al., 1993; Mills et al., 1995).

An extensive study of the genetic structure of salmonellae by Selander and coworkers using MEE (Beltran et al., 1988) showed that the majority of the strains clustered together, supporting a clonal origin. Also DNA-based methods indicated that most *S*. Enteritidis strains belonged to two large clusters (Olsen et al., 1994).

The question about the origin of *S*. Enteritidis, possibly from (genetically) related salmonellae, is relevant. From MEE and comparison of *fliC* genes, encoding phase-1 flagellin, it became clear that *Salmonella* Dublin clones are closely related to a globally predominant *S*. Enteritidis clone (Selander et al., 1992). *Salmonella* Dublin is a 1,9,12:g,p:- serovar. Based on MEE, another close relationship exists with *Salmonella* Gallinarum and *Salmonella* Pullorum (Li et al., 1993). In fact, *S*. Pullorum becomes mobile under the appropriate culture conditions (Holt and Chaubal, 1997). These two strains are both economically important pathogens for poultry, where they cause fowl typhoid and pullorum disease, respectively. They share the O:1,9,12 antigens with *S*. Enteritidis and *S*. Dublin but are nonmotile because they do not possess flagella. This is not because they lack a flagellin gene. In fact, both *S*. Gallinarum and *S*. Pullorum contain an *fliC* gene that is (almost) identical to that of *S*. Enteritidis (Li et al., 1993). Li et al. speculate that *S*. Pullorum and *S*. Gallinarum are descendants of *S*. Enteritidis, but obviously the reverse order could also be true. The close relationship among *S*. Enteritidis, *S*. Gallinarum, *S*. Pullorum, and *S*. Dublin was also confirmed by IS*200* pattern typing (Olsen et al., 1996). Thus, these four salmonellae seem to have a common ancestry.

SEROTYPING

Lipopolysaccharides

LPS is a major component of Gram-negative bacteria. It is anchored in the bacterial outer membrane, where it constitutes about 73% of the surface (Nikaido, 1996). LPS consists of three parts. Lipid A is inserted into the membrane lipids. Directly attached to the lipid A is the inner core, followed by the outer core. In many bacteria, O antigen is bound to the core. O antigen consists of repeating oligosaccharide units protruding far from the outer membrane.

STRUCTURE

Detailed information is known about the structure of the O antigens of a number of salmonellae. The gene loci encoding the enzymes responsible for the synthesis of the O antigens have been cloned and characterized for a number of strains (Reeves, 1993). Also, the structure of the O antigen of *S*. Enteritidis is known. It very much resembles that of *S. typhi*, which is serovar 9,12,[Vi]:d,- (Hellerqvist et al., 1969) (Fig. 15.1). One monoclonal antibody against the O:9 specificity of *S*. Enteritidis is available (Hoorfar et al., 1994). The structure recognized by this monoclonal antibody has not been determined, but it is assumed that the tyvelosyl residue determines the O:9 specificity and the glucose the O:12 specificity. No information is available on the structures that determine the O:1 specificity.

The gene cluster encoding the *S. typhi* O antigen has been cloned and characterized (Verma et al., 1988). It is located on the bacterial chromosome. However, there are clear indications that the O antigens of *S*. Enteritidis are at least partially plasmid encoded.

ROLE IN PATHOGENESIS

O antigens have important biological properties. They increase the resistance of bacteria against complement and other components of serum and against phagocytosis (Pluschke and Achtman, 1984; Cross et al., 1986; Grossmann et al., 1987). Mutants in which O antigen synthesis is

$$\alpha\text{-Tyv} \qquad\qquad\qquad [\alpha\text{-D-Glc}]_n$$
$$1 \qquad\qquad\qquad\qquad 1$$
$$\downarrow \qquad\qquad\qquad\qquad \downarrow$$
$$3 \qquad\qquad\qquad\qquad 4$$
$$\rightarrow 2\text{-}\beta\text{-Man-1}\rightarrow 4\text{-}\alpha\text{-L-Rha-1}\rightarrow 3\text{-}\alpha\text{-D-Gal-1}\rightarrow$$

FIGURE 15.1 Structure of the O-antigen repeating oligosaccharide unit from *Salmonella* Enteritidis and *S. typhi* (Hellerqvist et al., 1969; Rahman et al., 1997). The level of glycosylation of Gal is variable. Gal, galactose; Glc, glucose; Man, mannose; Rha, rhamnose; and Tyv, tyvelose.

abolished become avirulent (Binns et al., 1985; Finlay et al., 1988; Chart et al., 1989; Miller et al., 1989; Mroczenski-Wildey et al., 1989; Nnalue and Lindberg, 1990). In *S.* Enteritidis, loss of long-chain LPS was accompanied with loss of virulence for Balb/c mice (Chart et al., 1989). Also, virulence and invasiveness of strains with high-molecular-weight O antigen have been reported to be higher than those of strains with low-molecular-weight O antigen (Guard-Petter et al., 1996). A virulent isolate of *S.* Enteritidis was found to have a glucose–galactose ratio of 1:2 (as *S. typhi* does) whereas, in an attenuated *S.* Enteritidis strain, this ratio was only 1:8 (Rahman et al., 1997). So glycosylation, a late step in the biosynthesis of the O antigen (Nikaido et al., 1971), may lead to increased virulence of *S.* Enteritidis.

ROLE IN PHAGE ATTACHMENT

A total of 27 *S.* Enteritidis phage types are distinguished by the internationally recognized British phage-typing system (Ward et al., 1987), and a further 17 have subsequently been identified (Threlfall et al., 1993). Phage type 4 (PT4) predominates in Europe (Ward et al., 1987), whereas PT8 is one of the most abundant types in North America (Hickman-Brenner et al., 1991; Khakhria et al., 1991; Rodrigue et al., 1992).

Changes in phage type occur frequently and have been shown to be related to both plasmid acquisition and loss of the ability to express long-chain LPS. For example, the acquisition of incompatibility group-N drug-resistance plasmids has been shown to result in the conversion of *S.* Enteritidis PT4 to *S.* Enteritidis PT24 (Frost et al., 1989). These studies were extended (Threlfall and Chart, 1993; Threlfall et al., 1993). Likewise, the loss of the ability to express long-chain LPS and O:9,12 antigen has been shown to result in the conversion of *S.* Enteritidis PT4 to *S.* Enteritidis PT7 (Chart et al., 1989).

Powell et al. (1995) have investigated strains with different serovars isolated from a single patient during a 6-week period. Both ribotyping and pulsed-field gel electrophoresis indicated that in this patient, PT4 had mutated independently to PT7 and PT9a. PT7 had a changed LPS. Infection with temperate phages can also lead to phage-type conversion (Rankin and Platt, 1995).

Flagella

STRUCTURE AND BIOSYNTHESIS

An important feature of *Salmonella* and many other bacterial genera are the flagella, which confer motility to the bacterium and in this way contribute to colonization (Wilson and Beveridge, 1993). The flagellar filament of salmonellae is a multimer of a single protein: the flagellin. Comparison of the amino acid sequences of salmonella flagellins has led to the definition of eight regions of different variability (Wei and Joys, 1985). The amino-terminal and carboxy-terminal sequences (regions I and II and VIII, respectively) are conserved. The middle part, however, especially regions IV, V, and VI, is (hyper)variable and determines the serovar-specific H antigen (Wei and Joys, 1985; Newton et al., 1991b). The properties of the regions become directly evident from three-dimensional models for the *Salmonella* Typhimurium

flagellin (Fig. 15.2) (Mimori et al., 1995; Morgan et al., 1995). The essence of this model is that each of the several thousands of individual flagellins is folded in a horseshoe-like structure. The termini of the flagellin are the legs of the horseshoe, each consisting of the domains D1 and D2, as defined by Mimori et al. (1995), are in the center of the flagellum near the central cavity. They are crucial in holding the flagellum together and, in contrast to the middle part of the flagellin, do not tolerate insertions and deletions (Newton et al., 1989, 1991a,b; Hyman and Trachtenberg, 1991; Kanto et al., 1991). The middle part of the flagellin (D3) is at the surface of the flagellar filament.

EPITOPE MAPPING

Most salmonella serovars are capable of flagellin phase variation. They contain two flagellar genes at different locations on the chromosome. There is a regulatory mechanism that ensures that only one gene is expressed at a given time (Wilcox et al., 1977). But only one flagellin gene is present in *S.* Enteritidis (Van Asten et al., 1995). Attempts have been made to map the serospecific epitopes of salmonella flagellins, based on sequence comparison, Pepscan (peptide-scanning procedure), and the generation of deletion mutants. This approach has been successful for the d serovar. This antigen appears to be determined mainly by region IV (Frankel et al., 1989; Newton et al., 1991b), although contributions from regions V and VI were also found (Joys and Schodel, 1991). Van Asten et al. (1995) succeeded in identifying the epitope responsible for the g,m antigen. They screened expression products representing parts of the flagellin of *S.* Enteritidis for their reactivity with polyclonal and monoclonal antisera. In this way, they were able to narrow the g,m epitope down to amino acids 258 and 348 of the flagellin (Fig. 15.3). This approach also showed that the region between amino acids 258 and 284 contributed to the epitope, although it was not responsible for the difference in serovar between *S.* Enteritidis, *S.* Dublin var. Thailand, *S.* Dublin, *S.* Rostock, *S.* Moscow, and *S.* Derby. For the first four strains, the difference in serovar is wholly determined by the sequence of region V, whereas the differences in region IV may also play a role in the case of the last two strains. Another indication for a contribution by the carboxy-terminal part of region IV to the g,m epitope came from a clone with a PCR (C1-3*) differing by just one nucleotide, at position 893 (T → C). The resulting change from Ser to Pro (amino acid 298) destroyed the reactivity of the protein with the monoclonal antibodies.

These results also showed that the g,m epitope as recognized by the monoclonal antibody is conformation independent.

ROLE IN PATHOGENESIS

Flagellins of a number of bacteria have been shown to be important for virulence and colonization [see O'Toole et al. (1996)]. Likewise, for salmonellae it has been shown that motility is essential for the invasion of HeLa cell layers by *S. typhi* (Liu et al., 1988) and of HeLa and Henle's cell layers by *S.* Typhimurium (Khoramian-Falsafi et al., 1990; Lockman and Curtiss, 1990). The presence of a paralyzed

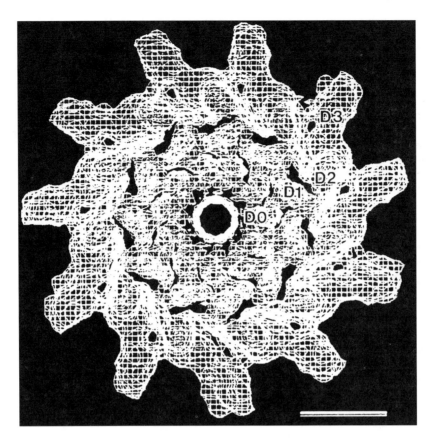

FIGURE 15.2   Cross section of the salmonella flagellum [modified from Mimori et al. (1995)]. There are 11 spokelike individual flagellins. In one of them, the D domains are indicated. The g,m-specific domain of *Salmonella* Enteritidis is located in D3. The scale bar represents 50 Å.

flagellum does not confer invasiveness. Inactivation of the *fliC* gene of two independent different *S.* Enteritidis strains leads to a 50-fold reduction in invasion of Caco-2 cells, whereas adhesion remains the same (A.J.A.M. van Asten, H.G.C.J.M. Hendriks, J.F.J.C. Koninkx, and B.A.M. Van der Zeijst, unpublished observations).

PRACTICAL ASPECTS OF *SALMONELLA* ENTERITIDIS CHARACTERIZATION: PROBLEMS WITH SPECIFICITY AND SENSITIVITY

From a practical point of view, serology is the preferred method for monitoring *S.* Enteritidis infections in poultry. Enzyme-linked immunosorbent assays (ELISAs) for the flagellin or the LPS have been the logical choices. An ELISA for fimbriae is another possibility. The methods in use have been compared (Barrow, 1996), but this comparison did not address such questions as the possibility of cross-reactions

of *S.* Enteritidis LPS with antibodies against salmonellae of serogroups B and D and the difference in kinetics in antibody responses to flagella and LPS.

The immune response to LPS is delayed compared with that against the g,m epitope on the flagellin (Van Zijderveld et al., 1992; Baay and Huis in 't Veld, 1993). Nevertheless, in practice, often the less-specific indirect LPS-based ELISA is used rather than the highly specific ELISA directed at the g,m epitope (Van Zijderveld et al., 1992). Monoclonal antibodies that may be used in a similar specific assay have also been developed (Keller et al., 1993).

CONCLUSIONS AND PROSPECTS

The sudden rise in the incidence of *S.* Enteritidis infections, together with the clustering in MEE of most clones, indicates that *S.* Enteritidis may have evolved from a closely related salmonella by acquiring new colonization and virulence factors. *Salmonella* Gallinarum and *S.* Pullorum are likely candidates because they colonize poultry very well.

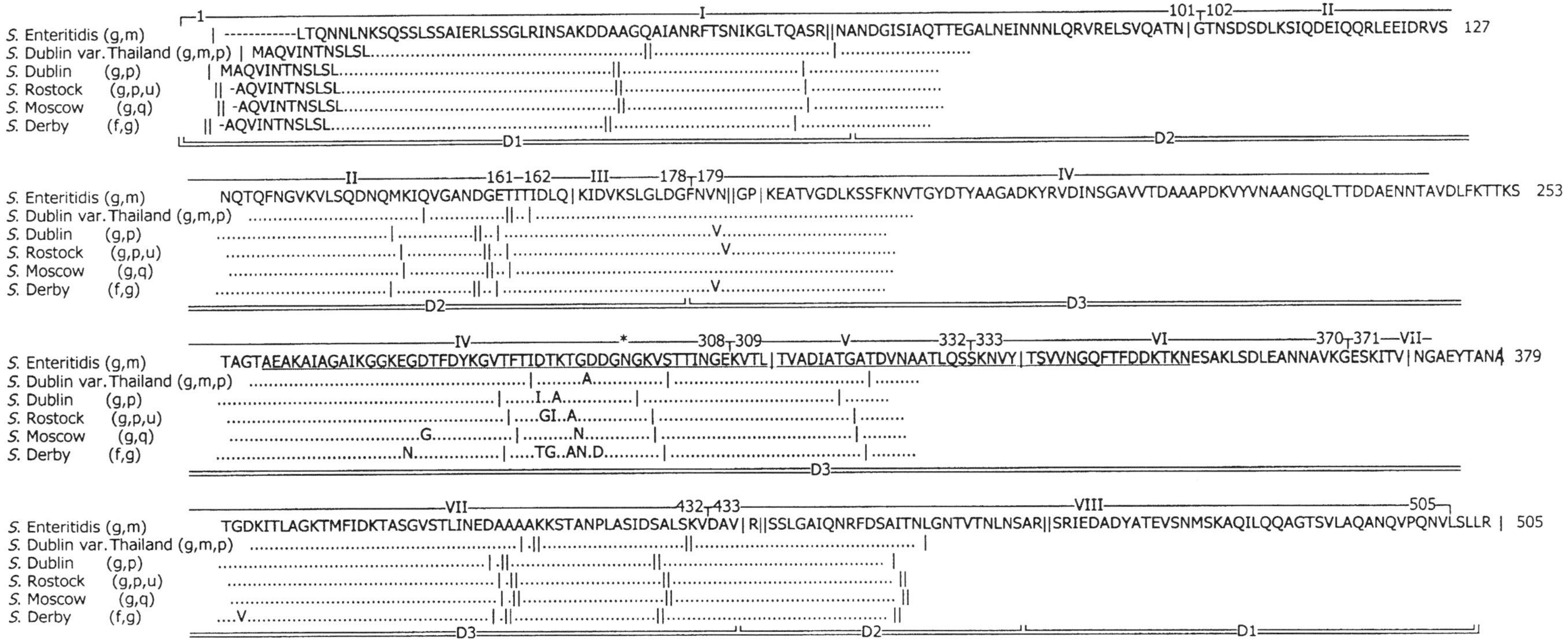

S. Enteritidis (g,m)
S. Dublin var. Thailand (g,m,p)
S. Dublin (g,p)
S. Rostock (g,p,u)
S. Moscow (g,q)
S. Derby (f,g)

```
                                                                                     101—102
      1                                                                        I                    II
            ------------LTQNNLNKSQSSLSSAIERLSSGLRINSAKDDAAGQAIANRFTSNIKGLTQASR||NANDGISIAQTTEGALNEINNNLQRVRELSVQATN||GTNSDSDLKSIQDEIQQRLEEIDRVS   127
                | MAQVINTNSLSL......
                | MAQVINTNSLSL......
               ||-AQVINTNSLSL......
               ||-AQVINTNSLSL......
               ||-AQVINTNSLSL......
                              II                              III                       178—179
                                          161—162                          IV
                                                                                                              D2
      NQTQFNGVKVLSQDNQMKIQVGANDGETTTIDLQ|KIDVKSLGLDGFNVN||GP|KEATVGDLKSSFKNVTGYDTYAAGADKYRVDINSGAVVTDAAAPDKVYYNAANGQLTTDDAENNTAVDLFKTTKS   253
                                  D1                                                    V.
                                                                                        V.
                                                                                        V.
                              IV                          *   308—309           V   332—333        370—371—ViI—
                                                                                                              VI
      TAGTAEEAKAIAGAIKGGKEGDTFDYKGVTFTIDTKTGDDGNGKVSTTINGEKVTL|TVADIATGATDVNAATLQSSKNVY|TSVVNGQFTFDDKTKNESAKLSDLEANNAVKGESKITV|NGAEYTANA   379
                              |.I.A.
                              |.GI.A.
                          .G.     |.N.
                          .N.     |.TG.AN.D.
                                                                                D3
                              VII                             432—433                  VIII              505
      TGDKITLAGKTMFIDKTASGVSTLINEDAAAAKKSTANPLASIDSALSKVDAV|R||SSLGAIQNRFDSAITNLGNTVTNLNSAR||SRIEDADYATEVSNMSKAQILQQAGTSVLAQANQVPQNVLSLLR |   505
                              .V.                                                       D2
                                                                                        D3
```

FIGURE 15.3 Alignment of the amino acid sequences of flagellins; *Salmonella* Enteritidis, U129630 (accession number). The sequences were translated from DNA sequences with the following accession numbers: S. Dublin var. Thailand, M84973; S. Dublin, 84972; S. Rostock, Z15071; S. Moscow, Z15086; and S. Derby, Z15066. The H type of each strain is indicated. Identical amino acids are indicated by a dot. The structural domains recognized in the electron-density map of the flagellum are represented by double lines. The eight regions described by Wei and Joys (1985) on the basis of amino acid homology are demarcated as single lines. Amino acid positions are indicated. The shaded part of S. Enteritidis represents the smallest part tested, which still reacts with the g,m-specific monoclonal antibody.

The resulting changes would have resulted in more virulence for humans and possibly an even better adaptation to avian hosts. *Salmonella* Enteritidis strains that do not belong to the main clonal population are likely the result of horizontal gene transfer. Phylogenetic trees constructed from MEE were compared with those from sequences of the variable region of the *fliC* gene (Li et al., 1994). Both trees had a different topology, indicating that DNA had recombined, presumably by horizontal gene transfer. Similar data have been found for the gene of the *rfb* cluster that mediates the synthesis of O antigen (Selander, 1997).

Are O antigens or H antigens important for virulence and colonization? LPS is clearly involved in the virulence of *S.* Enteritidis, but it seems unlikely that the O:1,9,12 antigens change salmonellae into *S.* Enteritidis. At least in some cases, clearly the change in phage type is accompanied by the loss of the O-antigen serovar (Chart et al., 1989; Threlfall et al., 1993). Nevertheless, it may be possible that the strains that seem to have lost their O antigens still contain a single repeat of the O antigen.

It is surprising that the locus (or loci) encoding the O antigen of *S.* Enteritidis has not yet been cloned and characterized. The situation may be more complicated than in other salmonellae, in view of the involvement of plasmid-encoded genes, but DNA clones from *S. typhi* and other salmonellae are available to be used as probes to find the locus.

There seems to be a stronger case for the involvement of the g,m epitope of the flagellin in colonization or virulence. This epitope is almost unique for *S.* Enteritidis and is most frequently associated with fowl. Another relevant observation is the close relationship with *S.* Dublin, a strain regarded to be strongly host adapted to cattle (Selander et al., 1992). The results presented in Figure 15.3 show that only two amino acid changes in the epitope have led to the change from the g,m serovar to the g,p specificity. Nevertheless, there are other differences between *S.* Enteritidis and *S.* Dublin, such as the virulence plasmid and a different auxotrophy (Selander et al., 1992). However, it is now technically possible to change the g,m epitope of *S.* Enteritidis into a g,p epitope and vice versa, and test the resulting isogenic mutants in animals.

REFERENCES

Achtman, M. 1997. Spread of serogroup A meningococci: a paradigm for bacterial microevolution. In: Van der Zeijst, B.A.M., Hoekstra, W.P.M., van Embden, J.D.A., and van Alphen, A.J.W., eds. Ecology of pathogenic bacteria: molecular and evolutionary aspects. Amsterdam: KNAW Verhandelingen, Afd. Natuurkunde, Tweede Reeks, deel 96, pp. 215–223.

Anonymous. 1988. *Salmonella enteritidis* phage type 4: chicken and eggs. Lancet 2:720–722.

Baay, M.F., and Huis in 't Veld, J.H. 1993. Alternative antigens reduce cross-reactions in an ELISA for the detection of *Salmonella enteritidis* in poultry. J. Appl. Bacteriol. 74:243–247.

Barrow, P.A., Desmidt, M., Ducatelle, R., Guittet, M., van der Heijden, H.M., Holt, P.S., Huis in 't Veld, J.H., McDonough, P., Nagaraja, K.V., Porter, R.E., Proux, K., Sisak, F., Staak, C., Steinbach, G., Thorns, C.J., Wray, C., and van Zijderveld, F. 1996. World Health Organisation–supervised interlaboratory comparison of ELISAs for the serological detection of *Salmonella enterica* serotype Enteritidis in chickens. Epidemiol. Infect. 117:69–77.

Beltran, P., Musser, J.M., Helmuth, R., Farmer III, J.J., Frerichs, W.M., Wachsmuth, I.K., Ferris, K., McWhorter, A.C., Wells, J.G., Cravioto, A., and Selander, R.K. 1988. Toward a population genetic analysis of *Salmonella*: genetic diversity and relationships among strains of serotypes *S. choleraesuis, S. derby, S. dublin, S.* Enteritidis, *S. heidelberg, S. infantis, S. newport,* and *S. typhimurium.* Proc. Natl. Acad. Sci. U.S.A. 85:7753–7757.

Binns, M.M., Vaughan, S., and Timmis, K.N. 1985. 'O'-antigens are essential virulence factors of *Shigella sonnei* and *Shigella dysenteriae* 1. Zentralbl. Bakteriol. Hyg. 181:197–205.

Brown, D.J., Threlfall, E.J., Hampton, M.D., and Rowe, B. 1993. Molecular characterization of plasmids in *Salmonella enteritidis* phage types. Epidemiol. Infect. 110:209–216.

Chart, H., Row, B., Threlfall, E.J., and Ward, L.R. 1989. Conversion of *Salmonella enteritidis* phage type 4 to phage type 7 involves loss of lipopolysaccharide with concomitant loss of virulence. FEMS Microbiol. Lett. 51:37–40.

Cross, A.S., Kim, K.S., Wright, D.C., Sadoff, J.C., and Gemski, P. 1986. Role of lipopolysaccharide and capsule in the serum resistance of bacteremic strains of *Escherichia coli.* J. Infect. Dis. 154:497–503.

Fadl, A., Nguyen, A.V., and Khan, M.I. 1995. Analysis of *Salmonella enteritidis* isolates by arbitrarily primed PCR. J. Clin. Microbiol. 33:987–989.

Finlay, B.B., Starnbach, M.N., Francis, C.L., Stocker, B.A.D., Chatfield, S., Dougan, G., and Falkow, S. 1988. Identification and characterization of TnphoA mutants of *Salmonella* that are unable to pass through a polarized MDCK epithelial cell monolayer. Mol. Microbiol. 2:757–766.

Frankel, G., Newton, S.M.C., Schoolnik, G.K., and Stocker, B.A.D. 1989. Intragenic recombination in a flagellin gene: characterization of the H1-j gene of *Salmonella typhi.* EMBO J. 8:3249–3252.

Frost, J.A., Ward, L.R., and Rowe, B. 1989. Acquisition of a drug resistance plasmid converts *Salmonella enteritidis* phage type 4 to phage type 24. Epidemiol. Infect. 103:243–248.

Grossmann, N., Schmetz, M.A., Foulds, J., Klima, E.N., Jiminez, V., Leive, L.L., and Joiner, K.A. 1987. Lipopolysaccharide size and distribution determine serum resistance in *Salmonella montevideo.* J. Bacteriol. 169:856–863.

Guard-Petter, J., Keller, L.H., Rahman, M.M., Carlson, R.W., and Silvers, S. 1996. A novel relationship between O-antigen variation, matrix formation, and invasiveness of *Salmonella enteritidis.* Epidemiol. Infect. 117:219–231.

Hellerqvist, C.G., Lindberg, B., Svenson, S., Holme, T., and Lindberg, A.A. 1969. Structural studies on the O-specific side chains of the wall lipopolysaccharides from *Salmonella typhi* and *S. enteritidis.* Acta Chem. Scand. 23:1588–1596.

Hickman-Brenner, F.W., Stubbs, A.D., and Farmer, J.J. 1991. Phage typing of *Salmonella enteritidis* in the United States. J. Clin. Microbiol. 29:2817–2823.

Holt, P.S., and Chaubal, L.H. 1997. Detection of motility and putative synthesis of flagellar proteins in *Salmonella pullorum* cultures. J. Clin. Microbiol. 35:1016–1020.

Hoorfar, J., Feld, N.C., Schirmer, A.L., Bitsch, V., and Lind, P. 1994. Serodiagnosis of *Salmonella dublin* infection in Danish dairy herds using O-antigen based enzyme-linked immunosorbent assay. Can. J. Vet. Res. 38:268–274.

Hyman, H.C., and Trachtenberg, S. 1991. Point mutations that lock *Salmonella typhimurium* flagellar filaments in the straight right-handed and left-handed forms and their relation to filament superhelicity. J. Mol. Biol. 220:79–88.

Joys, T.M., and Schodel, F. 1991. Epitope mapping of the d flagella antigen of *Salmonella muenchen*. Infect. Immun. 59:3330–3332.

Kanto, S., Okino, H., Aizawa, S.I., and Yamaguchi, S. 1991. Amino acids responsible for flagellar shape are distributed in terminal regions of flagellin. J. Mol. Biol. 219:471–480.

Kauffmann, F. 1964. Da Kauffmann-White-Scheme. In: Van Oye E., ed. The world problem of salmonellosis. The Hague: W. Junk, pp. 21–66.

Keller, L.H., Benson, C.E., Garcia, V., Nocks, E., Battenfelder, P., and Eckroade, R.J. 1993. Monoclonal antibody-based detection system for *Salmonella enteritidis*. Avian Dis. 37:501–507.

Khakhria, R., Duck, D., and Lior, H. 1991. Distribution of *Salmonella enteritidis* phage types in Canada. Epidemiol. Infect. 105:21–27.

Khoramian-Falsafi, T., Harayami, S., Kutsukake, K., and Pechere, J.C. 1990. Effect of motility and chemotaxis on the invasion of *Salmonella typhimurium* into HeLa cells. Microb. Pathog. 9:47–53.

Lampel, K.A., Keasler, S.P., and Hanes, D.E. 1996. Specific detection of *Salmonella enterica* serotype Enteritidis using the polymerase chain reaction. Epidemiol. Infect. 116:137–145.

LeMinor, L., and Popoff, M.Y. 1988. Antigenic formulas of the *Salmonella* serovars, 5th ed. Paris: World Health Organization Collaborating Centre for Reference and Research on *Salmonella*, Pasteur Institute, pp. 1–146.

Li, J., Smith, N.H., Nelson, K., Crichton, P.B., Old, D.C., Whittam, T.S., and Selander, R.K. 1993. Evolutionary origin and radiation of the avian-adapted non-motile salmonellae. J. Med. Microbiol. 38:129–139.

Liu, S.-L., Takayuki, E., Miura, H., Matsui, K., and Yabuuchi, E. 1988. Intact motility as a *Salmonella typhi* invasion-related factor. Infect. Immun. 56:1967–1973.

Lockman, H.A., and Curtiss, R. 1990. *Salmonella typhimurium* mutants lacking flagella or motility remain virulent in Balb/c mice. Infect. Immun. 58:137–143.

Martinetti, G., and Altwegg, M. 1990. rRNA gene restriction patterns and plasmid analysis as a tool for typing *Salmonella enteritidis*. Res. Microbiol. 141:1151–1162.

Mason, J. 1994. *Salmonella enteritidis* control programs in the United States. Int. J. Food Microbiol. 21:155–169.

Miller, I., Maskell, D., Hormaeche, C., Johnson, K., Pickard, D., and Dougan, G. 1989. Isolation of orally attenuated *Salmonella typhimurium* following TnphoA mutagenesis. Infect. Immun. 57:2758–2763.

Mills, L., Woolcock, J.B., and Cox, J.M. 1995. Plasmid analysis of Australian strains of *Salmonella enteritidis*. Lett. Appl. Microbiol. 20:85–88.

Mimori, Y., Yamashita, I., Murata, K., Fujiyoshi, Y., Yonekura, K., Toyoshima, C., and Namba, K. 1995. The structure of the R-type straight flagellar filament of *Salmonella* at 9 Å resolution by electron cryomicroscopy. J. Mol. Biol. 249:69–87.

Morgan, D.G., Owen, C., Melanson, L.A., and DeRosier, D.J. 1995. Structure of bacterial flagellar filaments at 11 Å resolution: packing of the α-helices. J. Mol. Biol. 249:88–110.

Mroczenski-Wildey, M.J., DiFabio, J.L., and Cabello, F.C. 1989. Invasion and lysis of HeLa cell monolayers by *Salmonella typhi*: the role of lipopolysaccharide. Microb. Pathog. 6:143–152.

Newton, S.M.C., Jacob, C.O., and Stocker, B.A.D. 1989. Immune response to cholera toxin epitope inserted in *Salmonella* flagellin. Science 244:70–72.

Newton, S.M.C., Kotb, M., Poirier, T.P., Stocker, B.A.D., and Beachey, E.H. 1991a. Expression and immunogenicity of a streptococcal M protein epitope inserted in *Salmonella* flagellin. Infect. Immun. 49:2158–2165.

Newton, S.M.C., Wasley, R.D., Wilson, A., Rosenberg, L.T., Miller, J.F., and Stocker, B.A.D. 1991b. Segment-IV of a *Salmonella*-flagellin gene specifies flagellar antigen epitopes. Mol. Microbiol. 5:419–425.

Nikaido, H. 1996. Outer membrane in *Escherichia coli* and *Salmonella*. In: Neidhardt, F.C., ed. *Escherichia coli* and *Salmonella*: cellular and molecular biology, 2nd ed. Washington, DC: American Society for Microbiology, pp. 29–47.

Nikaido, H., Nikaido, K., Nakae, T., and Makela, P.H. 1971. Glycosylation of lipopolysaccharide in *Salmonella*: biosynthesis of O-antigen factor 12_2. 1. Over-all reaction. J. Biol. Chem. 246:3902–3911.

Nnalue, N.A., and Lindberg, A.A. 1990. *Salmonella-choleraesuis* strains deficient in O-antigen remain fully virulent for mice by parenteral inoculation but are avirulent by oral administration. Infect. Immun. 58:2493–2501.

Olsen, J.E., Skov, M.N., Threlfall, E.J., and Brown, D.J. 1994. Clonal lines of *Salmonella enterica* serotype *Enteritidis* documented by IS*200*-, ribo-, pulsed-field gel electrophoresis and RFLP typing. J. Med. Microbiol. 40:15–22.

Olsen, J.E., Skov, M.N., Christensen, J.P., and Bisgaard, M. 1996. Genomic lineage of *Salmonella enterica* serotype Gallinarum. J. Med. Microbiol. 45:413–418.

O'Toole, R., Milton, D.L., and Wolf-Watz, H. 1996. Chemotactic motility is required for invasion of the host by the fish pathogen *Vibrio anguillarum*. Mol. Microbiol. 19:625–637.

Perales, I., and Audicana, A. 1988. *Salmonella enteritidis* and eggs. Lancet 1133.

Pluschke, G., and Achtman, M. 1984. Degree of antibody-independent activation of the classical complement pathway by K1 *Escherichia coli* differs with O-antigen type and correlates with virulence of meningitis in newborns. Infect. Immun. 43:684–692.

Powell, N.G., Threlfall, E.J., Chart, H., Schofield, S.L., and Rowe, B. 1995. Correlation of change in phage type with pulsed field profile and 16S rrn profile in *Salmonella enteritidis* phage types 4, 7 and 9a. Epidemiol. Infect. 114:403–411.

Rahman, M.M., Guard-Petter, J., and Carlson, R.W. 1997. A virulent isolate of *Salmonella enteritidis* produces a *Salmonella typhi*-like lipopolysaccharide. J. Bacteriol. 179:2126–2131.

Rankin, S., and Platt, D.J. 1995. Phage conversion in *Salmonella enterica* serotype Enteritidis: implications for epidemiology. Epidemiol. Infect. 114:227–236.

Reeves, P. 1993. Evolution of *Salmonella* O antigen variation by interspecific gene transfer on a large scale. Trends Genet. 9:17–22.

Rodrigue, D.C., Tauxe, R.V., and Rowe, B. 1990. International increase in *Salmonella enteritidis:* a new pandemic? Epidemiol. Infect. 105:21–27.

Rodrigue, D.C., Cameron, D.N., and Puhr, N.D. 1992. Comparison of plasmid profiles, phage types, and antimicrobial resistance patterns of *Salmonella enteritidis* isolates in the United States. J. Clin. Microbiol. 30:854–857.

Selander, R.K. 1997. DNA sequence analysis of the genetic structure and evolution of *Salmonella enterica*. In: Van der Zeijst, B.A.M., Hoekstra, W.P.M., van Embden, J.D.A., and van Alphen, A.J.W., eds. Ecology of pathogenic bacteria: molecular and evolutionary aspects. Amsterdam: KNAW Verhandelingen, Afd. Natuurkunde, Tweede Reeks, deel 96, pp. 191–213.

Selander, R.K., Smith, N.H., Li, J., Beltran, P., Ferris, K.E., Kopecko, D.J., and Rubin, F.A. 1992. Molecular evolutionary genetics of the cattle-adapted serovar *Salmonella dublin*. J. Bacteriol. 174:3587–3592.

St. Louis, M.E., Morse, D.L., Potter, M.E., DeMelfi, T.M., Guzewich, J.J., Tauxe, R.V., and Blake, P.A. 1988. The emergence of grade A eggs as a major source of *Salmonella enteritidis* infections: new implications for the control of salmonellosis. JAMA 259:2103–2107.

Stanley, J., Jones, C.S., and Threlfall, E.J. 1991. Evolutionary lines among *Salmonella enteritidis* phage types are identified by insertion sequence IS*200* distribution. FEMS Microbiol. Lett. 82:83–90.

Stanley, J., Goldsworthy, M., and Threlfall, E.J. 1992. Molecular phylogenetic typing of pandemic isolates of *Salmonella enteritidis*. FEMS Microbiol. Lett. 90:153–160.

Suzuki, Y., Ishihara, M., Matsumoto, M., Arakawa, S., Saitu, M., Ishikawa, N., and Yokochi, T. 1995. An outbreak and sporadic cases studied by means of pulsed-field gel electrophoresis. J. Infect. 31:211–217.

Thong, K.L., Ngeow, Y.F., Altwegg, M., Navaratnam, P., and Pang, T. 1995. Molecular analysis of *Salmonella enteritidis* by pulsed-field gel electrophoresis and ribotyping. J. Clin. Microbiol. 33:1070–1074.

Threlfall, E.J., and Chart, H. 1993. Interrelationships between strains of *Salmonella enteritidis*. Epidemiol. Infect. 111:1–8.

Threlfall, E.J., Rowe, B., and Ward, L.R. 1989. Subdivision of *Salmonella enteritidis* phage types by plasmid profile typing. Epidemiol. Infect. 102:459–465.

Threlfall, E.J., Chart, H., Ward, L.R., de Sa, J.D., and Rowe, B. 1993. Interrelationships between strains of *Salmonella enteritidis* belonging to phage types 4, 7, 7a, 8, 13, 13a, 23, 24 and 30. J. Appl. Bacteriol. 75:43–48.

Tompkins, L.S., Troup, N., Labaigne-Roussel, A., and Cohen, M. 1986. Cloned random chromosomal sequences as probes to identify *Salmonella* species. J. Infect. Dis. 154:156–162.

Van Asten, A.J., Zwaagstra, K.A., Baay, M.F., Kusters, J.G., Huis in 't Veld, J.H., and van der Zeijst, B.A. 1995. Identification of the domain which determines the g,m-serotype of the flagellin of *Salmonella enteritidis*. J. Bacteriol. 177:1610–1613.

Van Zijderveld, F.G., van Zijderveld-van Bemmel, A.M., and Anakotta, J. 1992. Comparison of four different enzyme-linked immunosorbent assays for serological diagnosis of *Salmonella enteritidis* infections in experimentally infected chickens. J. Clin. Microbiol. 30:2560–2566.

Verma, N.K., Quigley, N.B., and Reeves, P.R. 1988. O-antigen variation in *Salmonella* spp.: *rfb* gene clusters of three strains. J. Bacteriol. 170:103–107.

Ward, L.R., de Sa, J.D.H., and Rowe, B. 1987. A phage typing scheme for *Salmonella enteritidis*. Epidemiol. Infect. 99:291–294.

Wei, L.N., and Joys, T.M. 1985. Covalent structure of three phase-1 flagellar filament proteins of *Salmonella*. J. Mol. Biol. 186:791–803.

Wilcox, G., Abelson, J., and Fox, C.F. 1977. Molecular approaches to eukaryotic genetic systems. New York: Academic.

Wilson, D.R., and Beveridge, T.J. 1993. Bacterial flagellar filaments and their component flagellins. Can. J. Microbiol. 39:451–472.

World Health Organization (WHO). 1989. Report of WHO on epidemiological emergence in poultry and egg salmonellosis. WHO report on WHO/CDS/VPH/92.110. Geneva: WHO.

World Health Organization (WHO). 1990. WHO surveillance programme for control of foodborne infections and intoxications in Europe. Fourth report 1983/1984. Berlin: Robert von Ostertag Institute, p. 118.

16

Use of Molecular Biological Markers in the Epidemiological Study of *Salmonella enterica* Serovar Enteritidis Infections in Humans and Animals

A.M. Saeed and U.S. Nair

INTRODUCTION

Salmonella enterica serovar Enteritidis (*S.* Enteritidis) has become one of the main causes of foodborne illness worldwide [Baird-Parker, 1990; Rodrigue et al., 1990; Hedberg et al., 1993; Vatopoulos et al., 1994; Centers for Disease Control (CDC), 1996]. The number of infections attributable to *S.* Enteritidis increased from 1700 during 1976 to over 10,000 during 1995, representing a fivefold increase during that period, especially in the New England and Mid-Atlantic regions of the United States. By 1990, *S.* Enteritidis surpassed *S.* Typhimurium to become the most predominant salmonella serovar among human beings and animals (CDC, 1987, 1990).

In the United States, between 1985 and 1991, a total of 340 outbreaks of foodborne *S.* Enteritidis infections were reported. Food vehicles were identified only in 151 (44%) of the 340 outbreaks. Eggs were implicated in 125 (83%) of the 151 foodborne *S.* Enteritidis outbreaks (Mishu et al., 1994).

Identification of major sources for human infection with *S.* Enteritidis is the most important part of prevention and control efforts. Epidemiological association of certain foods with cases of *S.* Enteritidis food poisoning may not be adequate to establish a sufficient causal relationship between the food item and clinical cases in affected individuals.

Moreover, no single attribute characterizes *S.* Enteritidis isolates from different sources. Therefore, several tools are often needed to demonstrate relatedness among *S.* Enteritidis isolates from human and nonhuman sources.

In this report, *S.* Enteritidis isolates from sporadic infections of human beings during 1990–92 were compared with *S.* Enteritidis isolates collected from several nonhuman sources, particularly poultry, eggs, and the environment, during the same period. Prevalence of different phage types, antimicrobial resistance, and plasmid profile patterns of these isolates were compared to clarify the possible mode of transmission of *S.* Enteritidis organisms from foods of animal origin and from the environment to human beings (Holmberg et al., 1984c).

MATERIALS AND METHODS

Bacterial Isolates

A total of 588 *S.* Enteritidis isolates were collected from human beings and nonhuman sources in the nine states that constitute the North Central Region of the United States; 121 *S.* Enteritidis isolates were from sporadic human infections. Nonhuman *S.* Enteritidis sources included chickens, eggs, and the environment; all of the 92 S. Enteritidis isolates were from 5000 pools of cecal samples obtained from 25,000 hens (five pairs of ceca per pool) from the nine states. The isolates from tissues of chickens were mainly from liver, yolk sac, and spleen. Egg isolates were from egg surveys conducted by the U.S. Department of Agriculture and cultured in the authors' laboratory. Environmental isolates were from surveys of poultry houses conducted by the authors in the Midwestern states and included mice trapped in these houses, cages, and manure pits. Isolates were also obtained from miscellaneous sources (n = 39), including isolates from poultry, horses, cattle, dogs, and swine.

Phage Typing

Most of the S. Enteritidis isolates of animal, eggs, and environmental sources were phage typed at the National Veterinary Services Laboratories (Ames, IA, U.S.A.). Most human S. Enteritidis isolates were phage typed at the CDC (Atlanta, GA, U.S.A.). Phage typing was performed using the method of Ward et al. (1994).

Antimicrobial Resistance Profiles

Isolates were tested for antimicrobial susceptibility by the standard *minimal inhibitory concentration* (MIC) method (Sahm and Washington, 1991). All isolates were tested for their susceptibility to antimicrobials commonly used in human medicine. An isolate was determined to be resistant to an antimicrobial if it was resistant to the assigned concentration of antimicrobial at which it was tested, and multiresistant if it was resistant to more than one antimicrobial agent. The MICs of the various antimicrobials used were penicillin, 8 µg/ml; amoxicillin, 32 µg/ml; ampicillin, 32 µg/ml; piperacillin, 128 µg/ml; cefotaxime, 64 µg/ml; cephalothin, 32 µg/ml; amikacin, 64 µg/ml; gentamicin, 16 µg/ml; tetracycline, 16 µg/ml; chloramphenicol, 32 µg/ml; ciprofloxacin, 4 µg/ml; and trimethoprim–sulfamethoxazole, 160 µg/ml. Resistance of isolates to antimicrobial agents was determined to belong to one of five groups:

- Group 1: resistant to β-lactam antibiotics consisting of penicillin, amoxicillin, ampicillin, piperacillin, cefotaxime, and cephalothin
- Group 2: resistant to β-lactam antibiotics and tetracycline
- Group 3: resistant to β-lactam antibiotics, aminoglycosides, and tetracycline
- Group 4: resistant to β-lactam antibiotics and aminoglycosides
- Group 5: susceptible to all antimicrobials used, except penicillin

Plasmid Profile Analysis

A representative number of S. Enteritidis isolates (n = 362) from human and nonhuman sources were analyzed for their plasmid pattern. Plasmid DNA was extracted from S. Enteritidis isolates by the methods described in the *Molecular Cloning Laboratory Manual* (Sambrook et al., 1989).

Plasmids that ranged from 2 to 16 kb were grouped as low molecular weight (LMW), and plasmids that ranged from 40 to 75 kb were grouped as high molecular weight (HMW).

Statistical Analysis

Chi-squared test and Fisher's exact tests were performed using the Statistical Analysis System (SAS Institute, 1989). Significance was defined as $\alpha = 0.05$.

RESULTS

Distribution of *Salmonella* Enteritidis Phage Types Among Different Age Groups in Human Cases

Examination of the seasonal occurrence of sporadic cases of human S. Enteritidis infections revealed that most of the cases occurred during the summer (June, July, and August). These cases included age groups that ranged between 1-month-old infants to 81-year-old individuals (Fig. 16.1). The median age of infected individuals was 30 years, and the mean age was 32 years. Almost equal proportions of males (48%) and females (52%) were affected. On analyzing the geographical distribution of the strains, no particular trend was noticed, although about 20% of the isolates were from individuals in a single county and all of the other cases were rather randomly located. On further examination of the data and the sources/hospitals for fecal samples, no particular pattern was seen.

Salmonella Enteritidis phage types 8, 13a, and 28 were the common ones seen among human sporadic cases in this study. In 1990, 96% of the isolates were of phage type 8 (PT8), and 4% of the isolates were of PT28. Isolates of PT13a were not reported. In 1991, 45% of the isolates were of PT8, 16% were of PT13a, and 8% were of PT28, while an increase in the prevalence of PT13a to 44% was observed in 1992, followed by 28% for PT8 and 13% for PT28 (Fig. 16.2). The distribution of S. Enteritidis PT8, PT13a, and PT28 in different age groups of sporadic cases of human salmonellosis is shown in Figure 16.3.

Frequency of Various *Salmonella* Enteritidis Phage Types in Samples from Human and Nonhuman Sources

A total of 555 S. Enteritidis isolates from all sources were phage typed. Of these, 258 (46%) were of PT8, 108 (19%) were of PT13a, 99 (18%) were of PT28, 42 (7%) were of PT23, seven (1%) were of PT13, seven (1%) were of PT4, and 34 (6%) were untypeable (Table 16.1). Other phage types—PT24, PT4, PT6a, PT2, and PT1—not commonly isolated in the United States were also observed. This frequency distribution indicates that S. Enteritidis PT8, PT13a, and PT28 were the most common phage types. Twenty (48%) of S. Enteritidis isolates from eggs, five (3%) of the environmental S. Enteritidis isolates, and nine (22%) of the isolates from

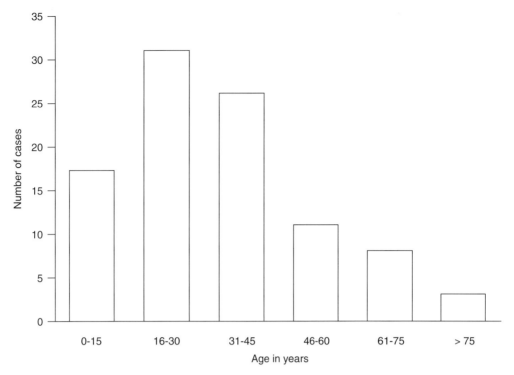

FIGURE 16.1   Age distribution of sporadic cases of human *Salmonella* Enteritidis infections during 1990–92. All cases for which age was known were included; age was not known for 25 cases.

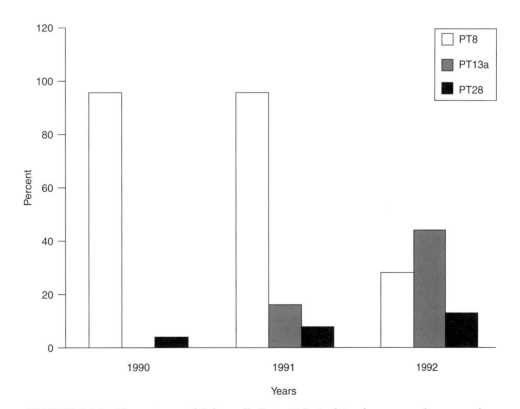

FIGURE 16.2   Phage types of *Salmonella* Enteritidis isolates from sporadic cases of human infections during 1990–92. Predominant *S.* Enteritidis phage types 8, 13a, and 28 are presented here.

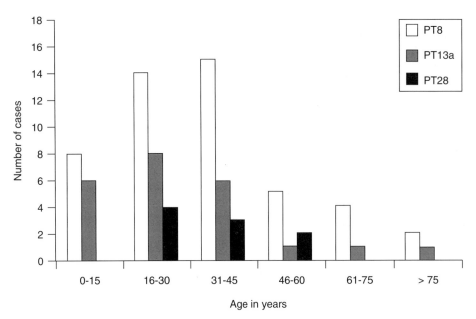

FIGURE 16.3 Distribution of *Salmonella* Enteritidis PT8, PT13a, and PT28 in different age groups of sporadic cases of human salmonellosis during 1990–92. Age was unknown for 25 cases.

TABLE 16.1   Phage types of *Salmonella* Enteritidis isolates from humans, environment, hen ceca, tissues, eggs, and other sources (n = 550)

Sources	No. of isolates	Phage types						
		8 No. (%)	13a No. (%)	28 No. (%)	23 No. (%)	13 No. (%)	4 No. (%)	Untypeable No. (%)
Humans[a]	98	59 (60)	24 (24)	10 (10)	1 (1)	0	4 (4)	0
Environment	182	78 (43)	18 (10)	43 (24)	37 (20)	1 (0)	0	5 (3)
Ceca	92	35 (38)	47 (51)	0	2 (2)	4 (4)	3 (3)	1 (1)
Tissue	109	50 (46)	12 (11)	44 (40)	1 (1)	1 (1)	0	1 (1)
Eggs	42	20 (48)	0	1 (2)	1 (2)	0	0	20 (48)
Others	32	16 (50)	7 (22)	1 (3)	0	1 (3)	0	7 (22)
Total	550	258 (45)	108 (19)	99 (17)	42 (7)	7 (1)	7 (1)	34 (6)

[a]The following phage types were also observed: PT34 (3), PT24 (6), PT14B (2), PT1 (2), PT2 (1), and PT6A (1).

other sources were untypeable. It is evident that the prevalence of *S.* Enteritidis PT8 in humans is not different from its prevalence among isolates from eggs, the environment, tissue, and other sources. However, *S.* Enteritidis PT8 strains were more likely to be isolated from humans than from chicken cecal samples ($\chi^2 = 4.10$, $p < 0.05$), whereas *S.* Enteritidis isolates of PT13a were more prevalent among spent hens than they were in other listed sources ($\chi^2 = 73.8$, $p < 0.01$) and *S.* Enteritidis PT28 strains were more frequently isolated from chicken tissues and environment than from chicken ceca and humans ($p < 0.01$ and $p < 0.01$, respectively).

Plasmid Profiles

Of 362 *S.* Enteritidis isolates tested, 299 (83%) had plasmids, but plasmids were not detected in 63 (17%) of the *S.*

Enteritidis isolates. Of 121 *S.* Enteritidis isolates tested from human beings, 113 (88%) had plasmids, and 249 (80%) of 311 isolates from nonhuman sources were found to have plasmids. Analysis of plasmid profiles revealed that more isolates from nonhuman sources had HMW plasmids than did isolates from human beings. Of the 121 isolates from the human beings, 59 (58%) had HMW plasmids, 34 (30%) had a combination of HMW and LMW plasmids, and only seven (6%) had LMW plasmids. LMW plasmids were detected in a significantly higher proportion ($p < 0.05$) of *S.* Enteritidis isolates from chicken ceca than from human beings, eggs, chicken tissues, and the environment. Of 92 cecal isolates, 24 (26%) had HMW plasmids and 18 (20%) had LMW and HMW plasmids. A majority of the isolates from eggs [34 (85%) of 40], chicken tissue [23 (88%) of 26], and the environment

[23 (64%) of 36] had HMW plasmids. Plasmids ranging in size from 16 to 40 kb were not detected among *S.* Enteritidis isolates (Table 16.2).

Salmonella Enteritidis isolates from the different sources were stratified by the classes of plasmids they carried and were tabulated by the phage types (Table 16.3). A total of 104 (74%) of *S.* Enteritidis PT8 strains carried HMW plasmids, whereas 32 (33%) of *S.* Enteritidis PT13a carried LMW plasmids and 37 (39%) of this phage type carried both LMW and HMW plasmids. Among PT8 *S.* Enteritidis isolates from all sources, 30 (21%) did not carry plasmids. Statistical analysis of association between plasmid class carried and phage types of *S.* Enteritidis revealed that strains of PT8 were more commonly found to carry HMW plasmids ($\chi^2 = 38$, $p < 0.01$), and PT13a was more commonly associated with carriage of LMW and HMW plasmids ($\chi^2 = 34$, $p < 0.01$).

A significant proportion ($\chi^2 = 8.32$, $p < 0.05$) of *S.* Enteritidis isolates from human beings that had HMW plasmids were resistant to β-lactam antibiotics and tetracycline. A significant relationship was not detected between size of plasmids and antibiotic resistance among isolates from nonhuman sources.

Plasmids were detected in all human *S.* Enteritidis isolates of PT8 and PT13a except in eight (13%) and one (4%) of the isolates, respectively. These isolates were also found to be sensitive to the antimicrobials. Plasmids were not detected among 49% of *S.* Enteritidis PT8 isolates from chicken cecal samples. However, these isolates were found to express resistance to β-lactam antibiotics and tetracycline. Furthermore, 95% of the egg *S.* Enteritidis isolates of PT8 that were found to carry HMW plasmids were also found to express resistance to β-lactam antibiotics and tetracycline. Statistical analysis of the association between isolates carrying plasmid and expressing resistance to antimicrobials revealed that a significant proportion of *S.* Enteritidis PT8 isolates carrying HMW plasmids in humans were also found to express resistance to a combination of β-lactam antibiotics and tetracycline ($p < 0.05$) when compared with isolates that did not carry plasmids (Table 16.2).

On the other hand, antibiotic resistance profile groups 1 and 2 (resistance to β-lactam and resistance to β-lactams and tetracycline) were more commonly observed among cecal and environmental *S.* Enteritidis PT13a strains. These strains were also found to carry LMW plasmids. Eighteen (37%) of the chicken cecal *S.* Enteritidis isolates and 13 (54%) of the human *S.* Enteritidis isolates of PT13a carried a combination of LMW and HMW (class C) plasmids. Chicken cecal isolates that were found to carry LMW plasmids and to express resistance to β-lactam antibiotics were more likely to be of PT13a ($p < 0.05$). There were small numbers of *S.* Enteritidis isolates of PT23 (two from cecal samples, six from the environment, one isolate each from human and eggs, and two isolates from chicken tissue). *Salmonella* Enteritidis strains of PT34 were observed among isolates from chicken cecal (3%) and human (3%) sources and were found to carry HMW plasmids. Among the 20 phage-untypeable *S.* Enteritidis isolates that were

collected from eggs, 17 (85%) carried HMW (class B) plasmids and were associated with groups 1 and 2 for antibiotic resistance profile. *Salmonella* Enteritidis PT28 and untypeables carried LMW plasmids (6% and 1%, respectively). The majority [21 (88%)] of the untypeable *S.* Enteritidis isolates carried HMW plasmids. Plasmids were not detected in 17% of the isolates from all sources, and some of these isolates were also found to be resistant to the antimicrobial agents.

Plasmids were not detected in 63 (17%) of 362 isolates. Isolates without plasmids were more common ($p < 0.05$) from nonhuman sources than from human beings. Among 121 isolates of *S.* Enteritidis from human beings, 13 (12%) did not have plasmids. Of these 13, three (23%) were found to be resistant to one or more of the antimicrobial agents. In contrast, 50 (11%) of 467 *S.* Enteritidis isolates from nonhuman sources did not have plasmids, and, of these 50, 42 (84%) expressed resistance to one or more of the antimicrobial agents.

A substantial number of *S.* Enteritidis isolates were found to be resistant to β-lactam antibiotics (Table 16.4). In addition, 254 (43%) of 488 isolates were resistant to tetracycline. Few isolates were resistant to aminoglycosides (amikacin and gentamicin), chloramphenicol, ciprofloxacin, or trimethoprim–sulfamethoxazole.

The proportion of isolates that were resistant to each of the β-lactam antibiotics was significantly different ($p < 0.05$) between isolates from human beings and nonhuman sources. The number of *S.* Enteritidis isolates from human beings that was resistant to penicillin was significantly higher ($\chi^2 = 58$, $p < 0.05$) than the number of *S.* Enteritidis isolates from nonhuman sources. *Salmonella* Enteritidis isolates resistant to the other β-lactam antibiotics (ampicillin, amoxicillin, piperacillin, cefotaxime, and cephalothin) other than penicillin were more common from nonhuman sources than from human sources (Table 16.4). Tetracycline-resistant *S.* Enteritidis isolates were more commonly encountered from nonhuman sources than from human sources. Expression of resistance to aminoglycosides (amikacin and gentamicin), chloramphenicol, ciprofloxacin, and trimethoprim–sulfamethoxazole did not differ between *S.* Enteritidis isolates from human beings and nonhuman sources. All of the *S.* Enteritidis isolates from human beings and most of the isolates from nonhuman sources were susceptible to trimethoprim–sulfamethoxazole.

Most of the isolates were resistant to three, four, and five antimicrobial agents (Table 16.5). Of 588 isolates, 478 (81%) were resistant to one or more of the 12 antimicrobials used; however, resistance to multiple antimicrobials was detected in 405 (87%) of 467 isolates from nonhuman sources and in 42 (35%) of 121 isolates from human beings (Table 16.5). Of 121 isolates from human beings, 23 (23%) expressed resistance to β-lactam antibiotics (group 1) and 18 (15%) were resistant to β-lactams and tetracycline (group 2). Only two isolates from human beings were resistant to aminoglycosides, β-lactams, and tetracycline (group 3), but 60 (53%) of 121 isolates from human beings were susceptible to all antimicrobials (group 5). Resistance to β-lactams (group 1) or β-lactams and tetracycline (group 2) was

TABLE 16.2 Plasmid profiles and results of susceptibility testing of *Salmonella* Enteritidis isolates from human beings and nonhuman sources

| Source no. | No. of isolates | Plasmid class[a] | | | | | | | | Antibiotic resistance profile group[b] | | | | | | | | | |
| | | No. without plasmids | (%) | LMW | | HMW | | LMW and HMW | | 1 | | 2 | | 3 | | 4 | | 5 | |
				No.	(%)	No.	(%)	No.	(%)	No.	(%)	No.	(%)	No.	(%)	No.	(%)	No.	(%)
Human beings	101	13	(12)	7	(6)	59	(58)	34	(30)	21	(19)	17	(15)	2	(2)	0		60	(53)
Chickens																			
Ceca	92	28	(31)	22	(24)	24	(26)	18	(20)	32	(35)	43	(47)	6	(7)	3	(3)	1	(1)
Eggs	40	6	(15)	0		34	(85)	0		9	(23)	28	(70)	0		0		1	(3)
Tissue	26	3	(12)	0		23	(88)	0		4	(15)	21	(81)	1	(4)	0		0	
Environment	36	5	(14)	2	(6)	23	(64)	6	(17)	20	(56)	10	(28)	2	(6)	1	(3)	0	
Other	55	8	(15)	2	(4)	36	(65)	9	(16)	7	(13)	7	(13)	1	(2)	1	(2)	34	(62)
Total	362	63	(17)	33	(9)	199	(55)	67	(19)	93	(26)	126	(35)	12	(3)	5	(1)	96	(27)

[a]Low molecular weight (LMW) plasmids, 2–16 kb; HMW plasmids, 40–75 kb.

[b]Group 1, resistant to β-lactam antibiotics; group 2, resistant to β-lactam antibiotics, tetracycline, and aminoglycosides; group 3, resistant to β-lactam antibiotics and tetracycline; group 4, resistant to β-lactam antibiotics and aminoglycosides; group 5, susceptible to all antibiotics tested. Percentages determined on the basis of the total number of isolates from each source.

TABLE 16.3 Relationship of plasmid classes to phage types of *Salmonella* Enteritidis isolates from human and animal sources

Plasmid class[a]	No. (%) of S. Enteritidis isolates of the following phage types				
	8	13a	28	Untypeable	23
A	0	32 (33)	2 (6)	1 (3)	0
B	104 (74)	16 (17)	16 (47)	28 (88)	7 (54)
C	6 (4)	37 (23)	9 (26)	0	1 (8)
D	1 (1)	3 (3)	3 (9)	0	0
NP	30 (21)	8 (8)	4 (12)	3 (9)	5 (38)
Total	141	96	34	32	13

[a]A, single, small plasmid (2–16 kb), low molecular weight (LMW); B, single, large plasmid (40–75 kb), high molecular weight (HMW); C, small and large plasmid, LMW and HMW; D, 3 or more plasmids; NP, no plasmids.

TABLE 16.4 Results of susceptibility testing of 588 isolates of *Salmonella* Enteritidis to antimicrobial agents used in human medicine and comparison of 121 isolates from human beings with 467 isolates from nonhuman sources

Antibiotics	All sources, no. resistant (%)	Human sources, no. resistant (%)	Nonhuman sources, no. resistant (%)	χ^{2a}	p^b
β-Lactams					
Penicillin	271 (46)	93 (77)	178 (38)	58.06	0.00
Amoxicillin	426 (72)	43 (36)	383 (82)	103.99	0.00
Ampicillin	433 (74)	45 (37)	388 (83)	104.27	0.00
Piperacillin	363 (62)	39 (32)	324 (69)	56.14	0.00
Cefotaxime	76 (13)	8 (7)	68 (15)	5.40	0.02
Cephalothin	339 (58)	32 (26)	308 (66)	64.03	0.00
Aminoglycosides					
Amikacin	25 (4)	2 (2)	23 (5)	≠	0.11
Gentamicin	23 (4)	1 (1)	22 (5)	≠	1.00
Tetracycline	254 (43)	27 (22)	227 (49)	27.08	0.00
Chloramphenicol	19 (3)	1 (1)	18 (4)	≠	0.15
Ciprofloxacin	9 (2)	2 (2)	7 (1)	≠	1.00
Sulfamethoxazole	10 (2)	0	10 (2)	≠	0.23

[a]χ^2 value with 1 degree of freedom.
[b]Significance defined as $p < 0.05$; ≠, probability values determined by use of Fisher's exact test.

TABLE 16.5 Results of susceptibility testing indicating resistance to multiple antimicrobial agents among *Salmonella* Enteritidis isolates from human and nonhuman sources

No. of antimicrobials	Human sources (n = 121), no. resistant (%)	Nonhuman sources (n = 467), no. resistant (%)	χ^2	p^b
2	1 (1)	26 (6)		0.02
3	5 (4)	48 (10)	4.43	0.04
4	21 (17)	148 (32)	9.64	0.00
5	12 (10)	123 (26)	14.65	0.00
6	2 (2)	47 (10)	≠	0.00
7	0	8 (2)	≠	0.37
8	1 (1)	3 (1)	≠	1.00
9	0	1 (0)	≠	1.00
10	0	1 (0)	≠	1.00
Total	42 (35)	405 (87)	142.62	0.00

[a]χ^2 value with 1 degree of freedom.
[b]Significance was defined as $p < 0.05$; ≠, probability values determined by use of Fisher's exact test.

expressed by 32 (35%) and 43 (47%) of the 92 chicken cecal isolates, respectively. Six (7%) and three (3%) of the 92 cecal isolates expressed resistance to a combination of aminoglycosides, β-lactams, and tetracycline (group 3) and to a combination of aminoglycosides and β-lactams (group 4), respectively. It is interesting that only a single isolate from chicken ceca was susceptible to all of the antimicrobials (group 5). Among isolates from eggs, resistance was more common to β-lactams and tetracycline (group 2) than to β-lactams alone (group 1). Only one isolate from eggs was sensitive to all antimicrobials (group 5). Of the environmental source isolates, 20 (56%) of 36 expressed resistance to β-lactams (group 1). None of the isolates from the environment was susceptible to all of the antimicrobials (group 5). Of the 26 chicken isolates, 21 (81%) were resistant to β-lactam and tetracycline (group 2). Of 55 S. Enteritidis isolates from other sources, 34 (62%) expressed resistance to β-lactams (group 1) and to β-lactams and tetracycline (group 2) (Table 16.2).

DISCUSSION

The global increase in S. Enteritidis infections in human and poultry populations suggests a new pandemic of the disease (Rodrigue et al., 1990; Altekruse and Swerdlow, 1996). Although the majority of S. Enteritidis infections were related to the consumption of eggs and other poultry products (St. Louis, 1988; Hedberg et al., 1993) the S. Enteritidis organisms could be isolated from an expanding list of food items, such as poultry meat and dairy products, and possibly from human carriers (Buchwald and Blaser, 1984). Therefore, one of the most important goals of epidemiological investigations of foodborne diseases is the identification of major sources of the infection in order to control disease outbreak and to plan for effective prevention programs in human and animal populations.

A broad diversity of phage types, antibiotic resistance, and plasmid profiles has been reported in S. Enteritidis isolates from human and poultry sources (Rodrigue et al., 1992; Poppe et al., 1993; Threlfall et al., 1994). These markers are effective in the identification of common virulence attributes, such as the 38-MDa plasmids, as well as in the identification of certain virulent S. Enteritidis phage types that are commonly associated with the disease. Moreover, the worldwide misuse and abuse of antibiotics during the past half-century have created enormous pressure among microbes for the selection of antibiotic resistance (Davies, 1994; Spratt, 1994), and salmonellae, especially S. Enteritidis, are no exception. Salmonellosis caused by S. Enteritidis in human beings is usually a self-limiting disease, and antibiotic treatment is seldom required (Riley et al., 1984; Tacket et al., 1985; MacDonald et al., 1987; Lee et al., 1994). However, when the infection spreads beyond the intestine or when immunocompromised persons are affected, effective antimicrobial treatment is essential. In such circumstances, knowledge of the resistance to commonly available drugs is of considerable value to clinicians (Tacket et al., 1985; MacDonald et al., 1987).

Resistance to single and multiple antibiotics among salmonella organisms has been increasingly reported during the past decade, especially for serovars S. Typhimurium, S. Heidelberg, and Salmonella Dublin, but resistance to S. Enteritidis was quite infrequent during the past 25 years (Rivera et al., 1991; Lee et al., 1993, 1994).

In 1984, Neu et al. reported that less than a tenth of S. Enteritidis isolates from human beings were resistant to one or more antibiotics. In this report, the distribution of the different phage types, antibiotic resistance, and plasmid profiles among human and nonhuman S. Enteritidis isolates is described.

Humans of all age groups, irrespective of their sex, were infected, but S. Enteritidis organisms were commonly isolated from individuals in the age range of 16–45 years. Since S. Enteritidis infection is perceived as a foodborne disease, the reporting of more infections among individuals in the age range of 16–45 years may have been due to higher exposure frequency than to true biological susceptibility.

Isolation of S. Enteritidis of PT8 was found to decrease with a simultaneous increase in PT13a and PT28 (Fig. 16.2). In addition, we found that PT13a was more prevalent than PT8 in eggs and other poultry tissues in the Midwestern region of the United States. The increase in PT13a among S. Enteritidis may have been due to acquisition of a resistance plasmid (Hickman-Brenner et al., 1991). It was found that isolates of PT13a from chicken ceca were more commonly found to have low molecular weight and also express resistance to β-lactam antibiotics. The increase in the prevalence of PT13a in humans in 1992 was probably due to ingestion of foods contaminated by these strains or exposure to other sources of these organisms or perhaps due to person-to-person spread.

Of 588 of the S. Enteritidis isolates from various sources, 447 (76%) were resistant to two or more antimicrobials commonly used in treating human beings. Resistance to β-lactam antibiotics (group 1) and a combination of β-lactams and tetracycline (group 2) was common among S. Enteritidis isolates from all sources. More S. Enteritidis isolates from human beings were found to be resistant to penicillin than were isolates from nonhuman sources. Increases in resistance to penicillin in bacteria are not surprising considering how frequently this antibiotic has been used in treating human illnesses caused by Gram-negative and Gram-positive microorganisms. Nonclinical infections, with resistant microorganisms, are exacerbated by the use of antimicrobials that reduce competition and promote pathogenesis (Holmberg et al., 1984a; Tacket et al., 1985; Lee et al., 1994).

A greater number of S. Enteritidis isolates from nonhuman sources were resistant to β-lactam antibiotics (with the exception of penicillin) and tetracycline than were isolates from human beings (Table 16.4). Isolates that were found resistant to three, four, and five antimicrobials were more commonly encountered in nonhuman sources than in human beings with salmonellosis (Table 16.5). Nearly half of all antimicrobials produced in the United States are used in food animals and, of these, about nine-tenths are given at subtherapeutic dosages to animals as a prophylactic measure or to promote growth (Holmberg et al., 1984b; Lee et al., 1993). Previous studies also have reported the increase in resistance of salmonellae to tetracycline and attributed the resistance to use of this antibiotic at subtherapeutic concentrations (Neu et al., 1975; Levy et al., 1976; Holmberg et al., 1984b; MacDonald et al., 1987; Georges-Courbot et al., 1990). In the study reported here, it was not ascertained whether the increase in prevalence of resistance to tetracycline among *S.* Enteritidis isolates from animal sources could have been attributed to the routine use of tetracycline and its analogues as feed additives at subtherapeutic concentrations.

Previous studies have reported that although there was an increase in the proportion of salmonellae resistant to ampicillin, the proportion of salmonellae resistant to cephalothin was lower (MacDonald et al., 1987; Bichler et al., 1994). We found that 339 (58%) of 588 *S.* Enteritidis isolates were resistant to cephalothin. The number of isolates resistant to ampicillin in our study [433 (74%) of 588] was almost the same as the 79% reported by Lee et al. (1993). As determined from analysis of results of our study and results from previous reports, the prevalence of resistance to antibiotics, especially penicillin, other β-lactam antibiotics, and tetracycline, has increased during the past 2 decades.

Statistical analysis of the prevalence of antibiotic resistance did not reveal significant differences in the proportion of *S.* Enteritidis isolates that were resistant to β-lactam antibiotics between isolates from eggs and isolates from human beings. A similar pattern of resistance to β-lactams and tetracycline was noticed among isolates from the environment and from human beings, which may be suggestive that there are similarities between isolates from human beings, eggs, and the environment. Several previous studies have documented egg and other poultry products as a potential source for infections in human beings (St. Louis et al., 1988; CDC, 1990, 1993; Hedberg et al., 1993).

Significant differences were not detected between the proportion of isolates from human beings and from nonhuman sources that had both LMW and HMW plasmids. A significant (p < 0.05) proportion of *S.* Enteritidis isolates from human beings had HMW plasmids and expressed resistance to antimicrobials. HMW plasmids have been correlated with virulence and antibiotic resistance among salmonellae, including *S.* Enteritidis and *S.* Typhimurium (Suzuki et al., 1992; Bichler et al., 1994; Threlfall et al., 1994). Data from this study suggest that eggs, chicken tissues, and the environment may represent a major reservoir for *S.* Enteritidis strains with HMW plasmids that subsequently may cause infections in human beings as a result of the consumption of improperly cooked or contaminated eggs, egg-associated products, and other meat and poultry products (Borrego et al., 1992). Current evidence would suggest that being near its target tissue enhances the virulence expression of bacterial pathogens (Finlay et al., 1992; Salyers and Whitt, 1994). In addition, infections of human beings may be enhanced further by selection and reduced enteric competition during treatment of human beings with antibiotics.

Plasmids were not detected in 63 (17%) of 362 isolates. Analysis did not indicate significant differences in the proportion of isolates without plasmids that were obtained from human beings [13 (12%) of 113], eggs [six (15%) of 40], chicken tissue [three (12%) of 26], and the environment [five (14%) of 36], whereas 28 (44%) of 63 isolates from

ceca lacked plasmids (Table 16.2). Analysis of the data reported by Olsen et al. (1994) indicates that plasmid content and implications of the lack of plasmids (lack of virulence or resistance-related plasmids) should be evaluated with caution, because investigators have recently suggested that the potential for plasmid instability exists in salmonellae (Brown et al., 1991). Isolates without plasmids that expressed resistance to the antimicrobials were more common from nonhuman sources [35 (71%) of 50] than from human beings [three (4%) of 13]. In isolates without plasmids, it was likely that resistance to antimicrobials had been encoded by chromosomal genes (Threlfall and Frost, 1990).

Evaluation of gross plasmid analysis indicated that many of our isolates from various sources contained HMW plasmids similar in size to the large virulence-related plasmid (38 MDa, 55 kb) previously identified in *S.* Enteritidis (Nakamura et al., 1985; Suzuki et al., 1989; Rodrigue et al., 1992; Stubbs et al., 1994). Although statistical analysis implicated a phenotypic correlation among isolates from various sources, this assumption cannot be made without use of additional molecular epidemiological techniques to confirm the true prevalence of these isolates.

The prevalence of antimicrobial-resistant strains complicates matters further, especially for people who are seriously ill and are being treated with antimicrobials. Therefore, periodic monitoring of salmonella isolates from animal sources and human beings for their resistance to antimicrobials should be viewed as a prudent practice. In addition, stronger veterinary supervision is required to ensure the responsible use of antibiotics and other antimicrobials in veterinary medicine and food animal production.

REFERENCES

Altekruse, S.F., and Swerdlow, D.L. 1996. The changing epidemiology of food borne diseases. Am. J. Med. Sci. 311:23–29.

Baird-Parker, A.C. 1990. Food-borne illness: food-borne salmonellosis. Lancet 36:1231–1235.

Bichler, L.A., Nagaraja, K.V., and Pomeroy, B.S. 1994. Plasmid diversity in *Salmonella* Enteritidis of animal, poultry, and human origin. J. Food Prot. 57:4–11.

Borrego, J.J., Castro, D., Jimenez-Notario, M., et al. 1992. Comparison of epidemiological markers of *Salmonella* strains isolated from different sources in Spain. J. Clin. Microbiol. 30:3058–3064.

Brown, D.J., Threlfall, E.J., and Row, B. 1991. Instability of multiple drug resistance plasmids in *Salmonella typhimurium* isolated from poultry. Epidemiol. Infect. 106:247–257.

Buchwald, D.S., and Blaser, M.J. 1984. A review of human salmonellosis. II. Duration of excretion following infection with nontyphi *Salmonella*. Rev. Infect. Dis. 6:345–356.

Centers for Disease Control. 1987. Increasing rate of *Salmonella enteritidis* in northeastern United States. MMWR 1:10–11.

Centers for Disease Control Update. 1990. *Salmonella* Enteritidis infections and shell eggs. MMWR 39:909–912.

Centers for Disease Control and Prevention. 1993. Outbreak of *Salmonella enteritidis* gastroenteritis in California. MMWR 42:793–797.

Centers for Disease Control and Prevention. 1996. Outbreaks of *Salmonella* serotype Enteritidis infection associated with consumption of raw shell egg: United States, 1994–1995. MMWR 45:737–742.

Davies, J. 1994. Inactivation of antibiotics and the dissemination of resistance genes. Science 264:375–382.

Finlay, B.B., Leung, K.Y., Rosenshine, I., et al. 1992. *Salmonella* interactions with the epithelial cell. Am. Soc. Microbiol. News 58:486–490.

Georges-Courbot, M.C., Wachsmuth, K., Bouquety, J.C., et al. 1990. Cluster of antibiotic-resistant *Salmonella enteritidis* infections in the Central African Republic. J. Clin. Microbiol. 28:771–773.

Hedberg, C.W., David, J.J., White, K.E., et al. 1993. Role of egg consumption in sporadic *Salmonella enteritidis* and *S. typhimurium* infection in Minnesota. J. Infect. Dis. 176:107–111.

Hickman-Brenner, F.W., Stubbs, A.D., and Farmer, J.J. 1991. Phage typing of *Salmonella enteritidis* in the United States. J. Clin. Microbiol. 29:2817–2823.

Holmberg, S.D., Osterholm, M.T., Senger, K.A., et al. 1984a. Drug-resistant *Salmonella* from animals fed antimicrobials. N. Engl. J. Med. 311:617–622.

Holmberg, S.D., Wachsmuth, I.K., Hickman-Brenner, F., et al. 1984b. Comparison of plasmid profile analysis, phage typing and antimicrobial susceptibility testing in characterizing *Salmonella typhimurium* isolates from outbreaks. J. Clin. Microbiol. 19:100–104.

Holmberg, S.D., Wells, J.G., and Cohen, M.L. 1984c. Animal to man transmission of antimicrobial resistant *Salmonella*: investigation of US outbreaks, 1971–1983. Science 225:833–835.

Lee, L.A., Threatt, V.L., Puhr, N.D., et al. 1993. Antimicrobial-resistant *Salmonella* spp isolated from healthy broiler chickens after slaughter. J. Am. Vet. Med. Assoc. 202:752–755.

Lee, L.A., Puhr, N.D., Maloney, E.K., et al. 1994. Increase in antimicrobial-resistant *Salmonella* infections in the United States, 1989–1990. J. Infect. Dis. 170:128–134.

Levy, S.B., FitzGerald, G.B., and Macone, A.B. 1976. Spread of antibiotic resistance plasmids from chicken to chicken and from chicken to man. Nature 260:40–42.

MacDonald, K.L., Cohen, M.L., Hargrett-Bean, N.T., et al. 1987. Changes in antimicrobial resistance of *Salmonella* isolated from humans in the United States. JAMA 258:1496–1499.

Mishu, B., Koehler, J., Lee, L.A., Rodrigue, D., et al. 1994. Outbreaks of *Salmonella enteritidis* infections in the United States: 1985–1991. J. Infect. Dis. 169:547–552.

Nakamura, M., Sato, S., Ohya, T., et al. 1985. Possible role of 36-megadalton *Salmonella enteritidis* plasmid to virulence in mice. Infect. Immun. 3:831–833.

Neu, C.H., Cherubin, E.C., Lango, D.E., et al. 1975. Antimicrobial resistance and R-factor transfer among isolates of *Salmonella* in the Northeastern United States: a comparison of human and animal isolates. J. Infect. Dis. 132:617–622.

Olsen, J.E., Brown, D.J., Baggesen, D.L., et al. 1994. Stability of plasmids in five strains of *Salmonella* maintained in stab culture at different temperatures. J. Appl. Bacteriol. 77:155–159.

Poppe, C., McFadden, K.A., Brouwer, A.M., and Demczuk, W. 1993. Characterization of *Salmonella enteritidis* strains. Can. J. Vet. Res. 57:176–184.

Riley, L.W., Cohen, M.L., Seals, J.E., et al. 1984. Importance of host factors in human salmonellosis caused by multiresistant strains of salmonella. J. Infect. Dis. 149:878–883.

Rivera, J.M., Rivera, N., Castillo, J., et al. 1991. Molecular and epidemiological study of *Salmonella* clinical isolates. J. Clin. Microbiol. 29:927–932.

Rodrigue, D.C., Tauxe, R.V., and Rowe, B. 1990. International increase in *Salmonella enteritidis*: a new pandemic. Epidemiol. Infect. 105:21–27.

Rodrigue, D.C., Cameron, D.N., Puhr, N.D., et al. 1992. Comparison of plasmid profiles phage types and antimicrobial resistance patterns of *Salmonella enteritidis* isolates in the United States. J. Clin. Microbiol. 4:854–857.

Sahm, D.F., and Washington, J.A. 1991. Antibacterial susceptibility tests: dilution methods. In: Balows, A., Hausler, W.J., Jr., et al., eds. Manual of clinical microbiology, 5th ed. Washington, DC: American Society for Microbiology, pp. 1105–1116.

Salyers, A.A., and Whitt, D.D. 1994. Virulence factors that promote colonization. In: Salyers, A.A., and Whitt, D.D., eds. Bacterial pathogenesis: a molecular approach. Washington, DC: American Society for Microbiology, pp. 30–46.

Sambrook, J., Maniatis, T., and Fritsch, E.F. 1989. Molecular cloning: a laboratory manual. Cold Spring Harbor, NY: Cold Spring Harbor Laboratory.

SAS Institute. 1989. SAS/STA user's guide, version 6, 4th ed., vols. 1 and 2. Cary, NC: SAS Institute.

Spratt, B.G. 1994. Resistance to antibiotics mediated by target alterations. Science 264:388–393.

St. Louis, M.E., Morse, D.L., Potter, M.E., et al. 1988. The emergence of grade A shell eggs as a major source of *Salmonella enteritidis* infection. JAMA 259:2102–2107.

Stubbs, A.D., Hickman-Brenner, F.W., Cameron, D.N., et al. 1994. Differentiation of *Salmonella enteritidis* phage type 8 strains: evaluation of three additional phage typing systems, plasmid profiles, antibiotic susceptibility patterns, and biotyping. J. Clin. Microbiol. 32:199–201.

Suzuki, S., Ohmae, K., Nakamura, M., et al. 1989. Demonstration of the correlation of a 36-megadalton *Salmonella* serovar Enteritidis plasmid to virulence in mice by reintroduction of the plasmid. Jpn. J. Vet. Sci. 51:203–205.

Suzuki, S., Ohisi, K., Takahashi, T., et al. 1992. The role of 36-megadalton plasmid of *Salmonella enteritidis* for the pathogenesis in mice. J. Vet. Med. Sci. 54:845–850.

Tacket, C.O., Dominquez, L.B., Fisher, H.J., et al. 1985. An outbreak of multiple drug resistant *Salmonella enteritidis* from raw milk. JAMA 253:2058–2060.

Threlfall, E.J., and Frost, J.A. 1990. A review: the identification, typing and fingerprinting of *Salmonella*: laboratory aspects and epidemiological applications. J. Appl. Bacteriol. 68:5–16.

Threlfall, E.J., Hampton, M.D., Chart, H., et al. 1994. Identification of a conjugative plasmid carrying antibiotic resistance and *Salmonella* plasmid virulence (*spv*) genes in epidemic strains of *Salmonella typhimurium* phage type 193. Lett. Appl. Microbiol. 18:82–85.

Vatopoulos, C.A., Mainas, E., Balis, E., et al. 1994. Molecular epidemiology of ampicillin-resistant clinical isolates of *Salmonella enteritidis*. J. Clin. Microbiol. 5:1322–1325.

Ward, L.R., De Sa, J.D.H., and Rowe, B. 1994. A phage typing scheme for *Salmonella enteritidis*. Epidemiol. Infect. 112:25–31.

Part III
Virulence and Pathogenesis

17

Virulence of *Salmonella enterica* Serovar Enteritidis

P.A. Barrow

INTRODUCTION

From the point of view of pathogenesis, the *Salmonella* genus can be divided into two major groups. One group typically produces systemic disease and is rarely involved in human food poisoning while the other typically produces food poisoning and only produces systemic disease under special circumstances. A comparison of the biological aspects of the two groups might explain our success in control of the former group and limited success in control of the latter.

The first group consists of a small number of serovars that characteristically produce severe systemic disease, initially involving the reticuloendothelial system in a restricted number of host species. They include *Salmonella* Typhi and *S.* Paratyphi in mice, *S.* Gallinarum and *S.* Pullorum in poultry, *S.* Dublin in cattle, *S.* Choleraesuis in pigs, and a few other serovars. Most experimental work has been carried out on *S.* Typhimurium infection in mice. However, the experimental work with *S.* Gallinarum in chickens, combined with the clinical evidence from cases of human typhoid, indicate that there is no reason to believe that the pathogenesis of the disease is very different in the different hosts.

Infection with these organisms is normally oral. The organisms do not multiply in the alimentary tract to any large extent. The oral median lethal dose of *S.* Gallinarum (virulent) for 3-week-old chickens is about 10^4 colony-forming units. The bacteria are highly invasive. Invasion can be detected microscopically and bacteriologically via enterocytes (Takeuchi, 1967; Turnbull and Richmond, 1978; Popiel and Turnbull, 1985) or via lymphoid tissue (P.A. Barrow, I. Rychlik, and M.A. Lovell, unpublished observations). In the case of *S.* Gallinarum, it is difficult to assess the extent of invasion anterior to the esophagus, although this may occur. In the lower end of the gut, a higher density of the organism can be detected in the cecal tonsils compared with the cecal mucosa. However, the total number of organisms invading via these routes is probably similar. Less invasion occurs via the Peyer's patches (P.A. Barrow, I. Rychlik, and M.A. Lovell, unpublished observations). In mammals, bacteria pass from the submucosa to lymph nodes. Some are trapped at this point, and others reach the circulation probably intracellularly and are removed by the spleen, liver, and bone marrow. If the bacterium is virulent and the host susceptible, multiplication will occur. Parenteral inoculation of virulent organisms results in initial killing of a proportion of the inoculated organisms, followed by multiplication (Hormaeche et al., 1990). There is currently controversy over whether salmonellae are primarily intracellular pathogens. This is the generally accepted opinion, based on microbiological and microscopic evidence for this (Dunlap et al., 1991; Briles et al., 1993). Another school of opinion has developed following studies in which large numbers of *S.* Typhimurium organisms were inoculated intravenously into mice, leading to observations that most of the salmonellae were extracellular, but many people believe that this may be an experimental artifact. Cell death may follow bacterial multiplication followed by host death, or, if a sublethal inoculum was used, the bacterial numbers may reach a plateau before declining. During the early stages of multiplication, organisms are contained within the reticuloendothelial system. In later stages, a bacteremia is evident, and, following infection of the gallbladder (by *S.* Typhi in humans) or the gut (by *S.* Gallinarum in chickens), the organisms are shed in the feces. The amount and duration of shedding is limited, however, and the extent of carcass contamination at slaughter is not great, with the result that these organisms do not regularly enter the human food chain.

These highly invasive organisms can become localized in the genital tract: *S.* Dublin in the bovine cotyledons and *S.* Gallinarum and *S.* Pullorum in the avian ovary. *Salmonella* Gallinarum is a very virulent organism, and although the extent to which this occurs in an infected but not diseased bird is unknown, it may be low. *Salmonella* Pullorum, in contrast, has been shown to persist in the bird from 1 week of age until lay. Contaminated eggs can then be produced for months after (A. Berchieri and P.A. Barrow, unpublished observations). In hosts other than the species in which disease typically occurs, atypical clinical pictures can occur following infection with host-specific serovars (Wilson and Miles, 1964).

The second group of salmonellae, which comprises the remaining 2000 or so serovars, is not restricted to particular host species, and their epidemiology can therefore be complex. Most are able to colonize the alimentary tract of animals without causing disease. Oral infection of newly hatched chickens, which have a very simple gut flora, results in massive bacterial multiplication with extensive fecal shedding that may last for many weeks. After a few weeks of age, the chickens acquire a complex gut flora that is relatively inhibitory for salmonellae so that oral infection results in excretion of smaller numbers of bacteria for a shorter period. Extensive carcass contamination at slaughter can result in salmonella organisms entering the human food chain.

Some strains of particular serovars, most notably *S.* Typhimurium and *S. enterica* serovar Enteritidis (*S.* Enteritidis), are capable of producing clinical disease under certain circumstances. This is particularly the case for very young animals, such as chickens or calves, or during or after a period of physiological stress, such as during lay or in cold, wet weather. In these cases, a systemic disease, again initially involving the reticuloendothelial system, occurs in addition to fecal excretion. The extent of disease and mortality varies according to the strain, but with these serovars there is always some invasion of the intestinal mucosa and reticuloendothelial system.

Due largely to the invasive capacity and ability to colonize the distal alimentary tract of adult hens, serovars such as *S.* Typhimurium and *S.* Enteritidis are capable of being transmitted vertically. This occurs as a result of organisms either becoming localized in the ovary or oviduct after invasion, resulting in contamination of egg contents, or contaminating the egg surface as it passes through the cloaca. In either case, the contents can become contaminated, resulting in the hatching of infected progeny.

HOST SPECIFICITY

It will be apparent from the previous section that infection of poultry by salmonellae takes many forms. Many of the virulence determinants already identified in salmonellae are important for systemic disease but less important for disease-free carriage. Many studies have been carried out using *S.* Typhimurium in mice, and many expressions of virulence may not be terribly relevant to *S.* Enteritidis in chickens. *Salmonella* Enteritidis has many similarities to *S.* Typhimurium in terms of virulence for mice, but infection of chickens is quite different from infection in mice. It will be worthwhile briefly comparing what is known of the host specificity that different serovars have.

Microbiologically, *S.* Enteritidis, *S.* Dublin, and *S.* Gallinarum–*S.* Pullorum have many similarities (Topley and Wilson, 1936; Li et al., 1993). From the point of view of pathogenesis and infection biology (in the latter, where no pathological condition results), they are quite different.

Among the "host specific" serovars producing systemic disease, different degrees of specificity are observed. An experimental comparison (Barrow et al., 1994) of different serovars in mice and 3-week-old chickens showed that *S.* Choleraesuis and *S.* Dublin strains were more virulent for mice than for chickens, whereas *S.* Gallinarum was more virulent for chickens. This was the case whether or not oral or parenteral inoculation was used. Most strains were able to colonize the distal alimentary tract and invade the tissues of mice and chickens. There was, however, a greater difference in the ability to survive and multiply in the liver and spleen once invasion had occurred, and this ability correlated with the virulence for the host species. More recently, some evidence of expression of host specificity between *S.* Typhi and *S.* Typhimurium has been demonstrated to occur at the level of the M cells in mice, but in this case no bacterial quantitation was carried out (Pascopella et al., 1995). *Salmonella* Typhimurium strains vary widely in their virulence for mice. None was found to be virulent for adult chickens, but some produced considerable mortality in newly hatched birds (Barrow et al., 1987, 1994). *Salmonella* Enteritidis strains are similar in this pattern in their virulence for mice and ability to produce severe disease and mortality in newly hatched, but generally not healthy, mature birds (Barrow, 1991; Halavatkar and Barrow, 1993).

Barrow and his coworkers speculated that host specificity might be expressed primarily at the taxonomic level of the class, separating mammals from birds, rather than at the family level, where pigs, cattle, and mice are separated from one another. *Salmonella* Choleraesuis can produce disease in calves, and both this and *S.* Dublin produce typical typhoid in mice, as do *S.* Typhimurium and *S.* Enteritidis. The situation is clearly more complicated, because *S.* Typhi is more host restricted and produces no significant disease in mice whereas *S.* Choleraesuis shows a wider host range.

Although *S.* Dublin, *S.* Typhimurium, *S.* Choleraesuis, and *S.* Enteritidis are important pathogens of cattle, pigs, and chickens, respectively, in agriculture, they generally produce the most severe disease in immunologically compromised animals. It may be that *S.* Typhimurium and *S.* Enteritidis are primarily pathogens of rodents and have entered the food chain as a result of intensification of cattle-, pig-, and poultry-rearing systems.

Nothing is known about the mechanism whereby host specificity is expressed. It seems likely that it is primarily in macrophages (Barrow et al., 1994), but it also seems unlikely that it is related to *Nramp1*-mediated resistance (Vidal et al., 1993).

INTESTINAL COLONIZATION

The ability of salmonellae to colonize relevant parts of the alimentary tract is the first stage of infection, although little is known about this process. The conditions under which salmonellae colonize the gut vary considerably. Conditions in adult gut, possessing a complex, inhibitory intestinal microflora (van der Waaij, 1992) and a mature immune system are very different from those in newly hatched birds. The differences are manifest by the excretion in greater numbers and for greater duration in the feces after oral infection of newly hatched chickens than occurs in older birds (Barrow et al., 1988).

The crop of the adult chickens populated by lactobacilli has a low pH (4–5). This prevents extensive growth of salmonellae or *Escherichia coli* but will allow the development of increased resistance to acidity (Slonczewski and Foster, 1996), which will enhance survival as the organisms pass through the gizzard. The oxygen tension will fall rapidly so that bacteria will be metabolizing primarily anaerobically in the ileum and large intestine. This part of the gut is populated by very high numbers of obligate anaerobic bacteria that prevent massive multiplication of salmonellae. In the ceca, they outnumber salmonellae by 10^3–10^7:1. It is thought that the inhibitory effect of the normal flora on salmonellae is a result of metabolites, such as H_2S and volatile fatty acids, but also results from nutrient depletion (Clarke and Bauchop, 1977; Hentges, 1983; Drasar and Barrow, 1985; van der Waaij, 1992).

This inhibitory effect has been exploited to increase the resistance of newly hatched chickens to oral infection with salmonellae. Very young birds are inoculated orally with cultures of cecal flora obtained from salmonella-free adult birds. Within a few hours, these birds acquire the full resistance of adults. This competitive exclusion has been well studied (Mead and Impey, 1987). It is unlikely that a similar product will become available for use with calves and pigs, because the diet of the adult and young animals are very different. It might be possible to manipulate the flora in a limited way, however, to increase resistance. As a consequence of this inhibitory effect conferred by the gut flora, removal of part of the adult flora with orally administered antibiotics may increase salmonella excretion, indicating the direct relationship between the adult flora and gut colonization (Barrow et al., 1984).

The alimentary tract of the newly hatched bird does not have a complex inhibitory normal microflora and may allow massive multiplication of salmonellae following oral infection. The presence of maternal antibody may reduce this in mammals but hardly does so at all in chickens (P.A. Barrow, unpublished observations; D. Taylor, unpublished observations). It is likely that the nutritional and redox conditions in the gut are also very different from those present in adult birds.

Although many salmonella serovars associated with human food poisoning colonize the gut well when inoculated orally, "typhoid" serovars, such as *S.* Pullorum and *S.* Choleraesuis, colonize the gut poorly under normal conditions. Their colonization may be increased considerably by oral administration of the antibiotic avoparcin (Barrow, 1989), and they colonize newly hatched chickens very well, indicating that they are less able to grow under the conditions imposed by a complete gut flora than are the "food-poisoning nontyphoid" serovars.

Among food-poisoning serovars, some are excreted for longer periods than others (Smith and Tucker, 1980). The reasons for this are not known. Serovars that colonize the chicken gut well are generally isolated more frequently from the ceca and to a lesser extent from the crop (Milner and Shaffer, 1952; Shaffer et al., 1957; Brownell et al., 1969; Snoeyenbos et al., 1982; Barrow et al., 1988). This has been ascribed to the physical attachment of salmonella organisms to the cecal epithelium (Soerjadi et al., 1982). This was suggested by scanning electron microscopy, but the relationship between the numbers of organisms in the cecal contents and those in the epithelium was not investigated in that study. Electron microscopy does not allow preferential adhesion to be distinguished from contamination from a more densely colonized cecal lumen. An alternative explanation for the preferential colonization of these two sites in chickens is that the flow rate of contents is lower in these organs (Smith, 1965). In organs where bacterial multiplication must be under semibatch conditions, there would not seem to be any evolutionary advantage in mucosal adhesion, unlike the situation with enterotoxigenic *E. coli* in the small intestine of pigs.

In support of the hypothesis, in which host factors are probably predominant, was the demonstration of preferential colonization of the ceca, rather than other parts of the gut, by nonenteric organisms: a yeast, a laboratory *E. coli* strain, and *S.* Choleraesuis (Barrow et al., 1988). There is evidence for an association between some salmonella types and the intestinal mucosa. Some strains of *S.* Typhimurium, but not other "nontyphoid" serovars, were isolated from the crop and cecal epithelium in greater numbers than from the lumen, suggesting, in this case, an association resulting from invasion (Barrow et al., 1988). In this study, salmonella organisms present in the cecal epithelium did resist washing off. Thus, even if adhesion to the cecal mucosa is not essential for intestinal colonization, low numbers of organisms embedded in the associated mucous layer would allow fresh chyle to be "inoculated" when the ceca are refilled after emptying. This may be a factor in microbial persistence in this organ.

The microbial characteristics that contribute to the colonizing phenotype are largely unknown. Barrow et al. (1988) produced mutants by nitrosoguanidine mutagenesis. Studying mutants lacking individual major surface antigenic components showed that neither lipopolysaccharide, flagella, nor type-1 fimbriae were essential for colonization by a strain of *S.* Typhimurium or *S.* Infantis; neither was the virulence-associated plasmid of *S.* Typhimurium. One mutant possessing all of these was unable to colonize, suggesting that another chromosomally mediated component was involved. This was studied further by this group, who produced Tn5 mutants and tested them individually for their persistent shedding in the feces. A number of genes have been identified that, when inactivated, reduced this ability (K. Turner,

M.A. Lovell, and P.A. Barrow, unpublished work). Lipopolysaccharide has already been found to be associated with colonization ability (Craven, 1994). In addition, it has been reported that *ompR* mutants have a reduced colonization ability—perhaps by reducing the ability to interact with the environment in the intestine (Dorman et al., 1989). A greater understanding of these genes will enable us to develop live vaccines in a truly nonempirical manner.

As might be expected from the results indicating that host factors play an important role in determining intestinal colonization, the genetic background of the host is able to influence this characteristic. Preliminary experiments with inbred lines (P.A. Barrow, M.A. Lovell, and N. Bumstead, unpublished results) and outbred lines (M. Duchet-Suchaux et al., unpublished results) indicate considerable differences in duration and quantity of fecal excretion of salmonella strains. This is an exciting area of considerable biological and practical significance.

ADHESION

Many members of the Enterobacteriaceae produce fimbriae (pili). Some are common to many genera, whereas others are specific to salmonellae (and other closely related genera, such as *Citrobacter*). These have been reviewed recently (Thorns, 1995).

Historically, they have been classified by their phenotype (Duguid et al., 1966). Thus, some enable attachment to cells or proteins, whereas others may have no apparent adhesive properties at all. The type-1 (SEF21 in *S.* Enteritidis) fimbriae or common pili cause agglutination of blood cells and enable adhesion to a wide variety of eukaryotic cells in vitro, which can be blocked by D-mannose. Their role in disease has been studied for many years, but their significance in infection is still unclear. They are approximately 8 nm long, with a subunit molecular weight of 21 kDa.

Type-2 pili found on *S.* Pullorum and *S.* Gallinarum also are 8 nm long but do not hemagglutinate. These may be derivatives of type-1 pili.

Type-3 pili are found less frequently and, although they bind to type-V collagen, their significance is also unclear.

Thin, aggregative fimbriae from *S.* Enteritidis (SEF17) and other serovars enable binding to fibronectin. They are 3–4 nm long, have a subunit size of 17 kDa, and are produced by the *agfA* gene. They are similar to the "curli" fimbrial antigen of *E. coli.*

SEF14 are thin fimbriae produced by the *sefA* gene in *S.* Enteritidis and a few other obscure, related group-D serovars (Feutrier et al., 1988). They have been studied in depth but seem to contribute little to virulence in *S.* Enteritidis, either from the aspect of systemic disease or intestinal colonization (Thorns et al., 1996). The only detectable difference was an increased rate of phagocytosis of an SEF14⁻ mutant by human polymorphonuclear leukocytes.

SEF18, also found in a wide variety of serovars, is a small (2 nm long) fimbria produced by *sefD* located close to *sefA*. No phenotype has so far been ascribed to it (Clouthier et al., 1994).

Other fimbriae have also been found in *S.* Enteritidis. The gene encoding the bundle-forming pili produced by strains of enteropathogenic *E. coli* has been detected by Southern hybridization in a variety of salmonella serovars. Only one strain of *S.* Enteritidis was tested, but this was positive. A number of host-specific serovars, including *S.* Gallinarum, *S.* Pullorum, and *S.* Dublin also possessed the gene (Sohel et al., 1993). The pili aggregate in groups of 10–100 to form appendages that mediate bacterial aggregation and localized adherence to Hep-2 cells. In enteropathogenic *E. coli* strains, production of the bundle-forming pili is mediated by a 90-kb plasmid. It was unclear whether this was the case with salmonellae, but since many of the serovars tested typically do not possess large plasmids, this seems unlikely.

Salmonella Typhimurium was shown to produce a long polar fimbria produced by the *lpf* operon, which was closely related to the *fim* operon in gene order and amino acid sequence. A gene probe from this region also hybridized with *S.* Enteritidis and *S.* Dublin but not with *S.* Typhi. The function of this fimbria is unknown.

Additional adhesive functions are associated with the virulence-associated plasmids of salmonella serovars that produce systemic disease. Regions outside the *spv* region have been found to be associated with the virulence of *S.* Typhimurium for mice (Sizemore et al., 1991; Pullinger and Lax, 1992). About 20 kb from the *spv* region, fimbrial biosynthesis genes have been identified. These genes have been termed the *pef* genes (plasmid-encoded fimbriae). *PefA* encodes a major fimbrial subunit gene, and other export and assembly genes have homologies with a number of other fimbrial systems. By hybridization, *pefA* has also been shown to be present in *S.* Enteritidis but not in *S.* Dublin or *S.* Gallinarum (Woodward et al., 1996). The *pef* operon has been found to contribute to colonization of the ileal mucosa and to fluid secretion in the mouse gut (Bäumler et al., 1996).

INVASION

Penetration of the intestinal mucosa is a prerequisite for the pathogenesis of systemic infection; this is also thought to be essential for the induction of diarrhea. Thus, the salmonellae invade various cells in the gut (probably epithelial cells and M cells), though their relative importance is unclear (Takeuchi, 1967; Popiel and Turnbull, 1985; Wallis et al., 1986; Pospischil et al., 1990). Other cell types are invaded during the systemic phase of infection (Dunlap et al., 1991). Different mechanisms with distinct gene systems might be involved in these processes. Recent research on adhesion and invasion has been dominated by two features: extensive use of tissue culture systems as models for invasion and identification by mutational analysis of genes involved in this process.

Polarized cell lines, such as Madin-Darby canine kidney (Finlay et al., 1988) and the human intestinal Caco-2 cell (Finlay and Falkow, 1990), have been particularly widely used. These cells maintain epithelial cell structure with tight junctions, a transepithelial potential, and different apical and basolateral surfaces (Simons and Fuller, 1985). Invasion occurs specifically via the apical surface, where within a critical distance from cells, salmonellae induce disruption and elongation of microvilli, which precedes endocytosis. The salmonellae migrate across the cell, appearing at the basolateral face (Finlay et al., 1988).

Invasion is believed to occur by receptor-mediated endocytosis, though receptors have not been identified. Several studies using nonpolar cells have shown that salmonellae subvert eukaryotic signaling pathways to facilitate attachment and uptake, though the molecular events involved are unknown. Thus, it has been shown that, during the invasion process, the epidermal growth factor receptor is phosphorylated (Galan et al., 1992), there is a transient rise in inositol phosphates (Ruschkowski et al., 1992) and intracellular Ca^{2+}, and there is phosphorylation of the mitogen-activated protein kinase (Pace et al., 1993). The inositol phosphate increase probably leads to the rise in Ca^{2+}, which in turn is likely to affect the structural changes around the incoming bacteria. Originally observed by Takeuchi (1967) with enterocytes, several groups have shown with cultured cells that salmonellae induce membrane blebs or ruffles (Ginocchio et al., 1992) caused by rearrangement of cytoskeletal proteins. However, the signaling pathways responsible for mediating ruffling are unclear, since it has been shown to occur in cells lacking the epidermal growth factor receptor and is not blocked by inactivation of the small G proteins usually implicated in this process (Jones et al., 1993). Salmonella interaction with host cells induces transcellular migration of neutrophils and IL-8 secretion (McCormick et al., 1993). The relevance of much of this exciting work to the in vivo situation remains to be proven. The in vitro cultured gut segment model (Worton et al., 1989) and the use of ligated loops in a target animal species provide models connecting cultured cells, which are accessible but of uncertain relevance, and the whole animal, which is of direct relevance but is difficult to understand at the molecular level.

In parallel with this work has been the identification of salmonella genes involved in invasion of cultured cells. Chemotaxis and motility mutants have been shown to have altered invasiveness (Jones et al., 1992), but most work has focused on the invasion loci found on the two recently identified pathogenicity islands (Hacker et al., 1997). These are regions of the chromosome, 40 kb in size, which are not present in nonpathogenic related bacteria (Mills et al., 1995; Shea et al., 1996). The genes in pathogenicity island 1 (SPI-I) are necessary for invasion, whereas pathogenicity island II (SPI-II) seems to contain genes of two-component systems and type-III secretion genes that may be involved in intracellular survival. SPI-I has no significant boundary sequences, whereas SPI-II is located near a recombinational hot spot. SPI-I and SPI-II have been found in all salmonella serovars tested so far.

The invasion genes in salmonellae form a single large locus that has sequence and functional homology with *Shigella* and *Yersinia* invasion genes. Two adjacent operons, *invA-G* and *spaO-S*, together with *prgH-K* form the components of a type-III secretory system involved in exporting invasion genes to the surface of the cell (Galan, 1996). Members of an adjacent operon encoding Sip proteins (*Salmonella* invasion protein) show homology with the invasion protein antigen (Ipa) proteins of *Shigella* and the *Yersinia* outer protein (Yop) proteins. In particular, SipB is homologous to IpaB of *Shigella* and YopB in *Yersinia*. Whereas the function of IpaB is unknown, YopB has been shown to be involved in translocating Yop effectors across the host membrane. These include YopH (tyrosine phosphatase), YopE (cytotoxin), and YpkA (protein kinase) (Cornelis and Wolf-Watz, 1997). It seems likely, therefore, that SipB integrates into the host membrane following close contact between bacterium and cell, allowing translocation of their components into the cell. These are beginning to be identified (Wood et al., 1996).

INTERACTIONS OF SALMONELLAE WITH MACROPHAGES

Although with regard to systemic typhoidlike disease salmonellae have always been regarded as intracellular pathogens, more recent controversial evidence (Hsu, 1989) has suggested that bacterial multiplication may be essentially extracellular, since microscopy had demonstrated large numbers of bacteria outside splenic cells. However, his system involved parenteral inoculation with >10^7 salmonella bacteria, which would overwhelm the phagocytic capacity of Kuppfer's cells.

A number of gene systems whose significance is still unclear have been shown to contribute to virulence by enabling multiplication in macrophages. The two-component regulatory system, *phoP/phoQ* (Miller et al., 1989), acts as an environmental sensor to activate a group of genes involved specifically in intracellular survival in macrophages (Alpuche Aranda et al., 1992). Other novel loci that may play a role in vivo have also been identified (Johnson et al., 1991), and more general analysis of proteins synthesized by salmonellae within the macrophage indicates that this environment triggers substantial differences in expression than that seen in vitro (Abshire and Neidhardt, 1993). More recently, the *slyA* gene, whose function is unclear, has been identified as a putative virulence gene (Libby et al., 1994), but its importance to infection is far from clear. Only when the cell biology associated with intracellular multiplication has been clarified can individual genes be assessed for their roles. This is beginning to happen.

Recently, an interesting phenomenon of cytotoxicity of salmonella cells for macrophages has been studied in greater detail, although similar observations had been observed previously by several authors. Two phenomena may be recognized that have also been found with *Shigella* infection and that are thought to relate to uptake by and destruction of M cells in the intestine and possibly also in the liver and spleen. *Shigella* induces cell death by apoptosis in vitro in the J774 macrophage cell line and the IpaB protein is acquired (Zychlinsky et al., 1992, 1994a,b), inducing release of interleukin-1″ precursor and mature interleukin-1β, which is thought to enhance inflammation. A nonapoptotic lysis that occurs more rapidly has also been observed (Fernandez-Prada et al., 1997). A similar apoptotic cytolysis has also been observed with salmonellae (Chen et al., 1996). Bacterial internalization was not required, but components of SP-1 are involved. *Salmonella* Typhimurium, *S.* Typhi, *S.* Gallinarum, and *S.* Dublin were all toxic for murine macrophages. This is an interesting phenomenon whose significance in the pathogenesis of salmonellosis is, as yet, unclear.

The virulence plasmid (serovar-specific plasmid) found in those serovars capable of producing typhoidlike infections has been studied intensively over the years (Gulig et al., 1993), but the exact mechanism whereby it contributes to virulence is unclear. Their importance differs according to serovar. Thus, *S.* Gallinarum cured of its plasmid is totally avirulent for chickens (a 10^7-fold reduction in virulence). A small plasmid possessed by this serovar does not contribute to virulence (Barrow et al., 1987). The plasmid of *S.* Dublin contributes similarly to the virulence of *S.* Dublin for mice. By contrast, the virulence of *S.* Enteritidis for mice is reduced by 10^4-fold, but not at all for chickens if the plasmid is cured (Halavatkar and Barrow, 1993). The virulence of *S.* Pullorum for chicks and *S.* Typhimurium for mice by parenteral inoculation is reduced only 10-fold if cured of their plasmids (Gulig and Curtiss, 1987; Barrow and Lovell, 1988, 1989). This obviously reflects differences in the pathogenesis of infection in the different host species.

The virulence plasmids vary in size from about 54 to 98 kb and therefore represent up to 2% of the genetic information of the salmonella genome. An 8-kb region common to all the plasmids can restore virulence to cured strains (Lax et al., 1990). Various groups sequenced this region; the sequences from different serovars were very similar and identified six open reading frames encoded on one strand, five of which are believed to form a gene system. A common nomenclature *spv* (salmonella plasmid virulence) has now been agreed upon.

The sequence of SpvR shows homology to proteins of the LysR family of bacterial activator proteins (Pullinger et al., 1989) that bind to DNA. SpvR activates expression of the *spvA* operon (consisting of *spvA*, *spvB*, *spvC*, and probably *spvI*) and of itself (Caldwell and Gulig, 1991). Expression of the *spv* genes is stimulated by starvation in vitro (Fang et al., 1991) and by low-iron conditions (Spink et al., 1992) that probably reflect the intracellular conditions where these genes are required. There is also evidence for control by the cyclic AMP/CRP system (Spink et al., 1992). It has been shown that the *spv* genes are expressed in cultured cells (Fierer et al., 1993).

We have recently found that *spvA* expression negatively regulates *spvR* (Spink et al., 1994) and presumably provides a feedback loop to control *spv* expression. Nonpolar deletions within the *spvB* gene abolish virulence (Williamson et al., 1990), although its mechanism of action is unknown. Although there is good evidence that *spvC* is important for

virulence (Gulig and Chiodo, 1990), deletions near the 3′ end of the gene have variable effects (Roudier et al., 1992), as has also been reported for *spvD*, and no role has been ascribed to either gene.

Other functions ascribed to the salmonella virulence plasmids include loci involved in resistance to serum killing (Vandenbosch et al., 1989). These are not found on plasmids from all serovars, and their role in disease may be of little significance.

SUMMARY

Our understanding of the mechanism whereby salmonellae produce disease in poultry, humans, and other animals is increasing rapidly. However, despite the great deal of in vitro work on invasion and macrophage interactions, we still do not know completely how these findings relate to the situation in vivo. It will be essential to combine the molecular studies with others carried out in vivo to be able to use the information gathered to improve salmonella control.

REFERENCES

Abshire, K.Z., and Neidhardt, F.C. 1993. Analysis of proteins synthesized by *Salmonella typhimurium* during growth within a host macrophage. J. Bacteriol. 175:3734–3743.

Alpuche Aranda, C.M., Swanson, J.A., Loomis, W.P., and Miller, S.I. 1992. *Salmonella typhimurium* activates virulence gene transcription within acidified macrophage phagosomes. Proc. Natl. Acad. Sci. U.S.A. 89:10,079–10,083.

Barrow, P.A. 1989. Further observations on the effect of feeding diets containing avoparcin in the excretion of salmonellas by experimentally infected chickens. Epidemiol. Infect. 102: 239–252.

Barrow, P.A. 1991. Experimental infection of chickens with *Salmonella enteritidis*. Avian Pathol. 20:145–153.

Barrow, P.A., and Lovell, M.A. 1988. The association between a large molecular weight plasmid and virulence in a strain of *Salmonella pullorum*. J. Gen. Microbiol. 134: 307–2316.

Barrow, P.A., and Lovell, M.A. 1989. Functional homology of virulence plasmids in *Salmonella gallinarum*, *S. pullorum* and *S. typhimurium*. Infect. Immun. 57:3136–3141.

Barrow, P.A., Smith, H.W., and Tucker, J.F. 1984. The effect of feeding diets containing avoparcin on the excretion of *Salmonella* by chickens experimentally infected with natural sources of *Salmonella* organisms. J. Hyg. 93:439–444.

Barrow, P.A., Simpson, J.M., Lovell, M.A., and Binns, M.M. 1987. Contribution of *Salmonella gallinarum* large plasmid toward virulence in fowl typhoid. Infect. Immun. 55: 388–392.

Barrow, P.A., Simpson, J.M., and Lovell, M.A. 1988. Intestinal colonization in the chicken of food-poisoning *Salmonella* serotypes: microbial characteristics associated with faecal excretion. Avian Pathol. 17:571–588.

Bäumler, A.J., Tsolis, R.M., Bowe, F.A., Kusters, J.G., Hoffmann, S., and Heffron, F. 1996. The *pef* fimbrial operon of *Salmonella typhimurium* mediates adhesion to murine small intestine and is necessary for fluid accumulation in the infant mouse. Infect. Immun. 64:61–68.

Briles, D.E., Dunlap, N.E., Swords, E., and Benjamin, W.H. 1993. Early events in the pathogenesis of enteric fever in mice. In: Cabello, F., Hormaeche, C., Mastroeni, P., and Bonina, L., eds. The biology of *Salmonella*. NATO ASI Series A245. London: Plenum, pp. 159–167.

Brownell, J.R., Sadler, W.W., and Fanelli, M.J. 1969. Factors influencing the intestinal infection of chickens with *Salmonella typhimurium*. Avian Dis. 4:804–816.

Caldwell, A.L., and Gulig, P.A. 1991. The *Salmonella typhimurium* virulence plasmid encodes a positive regulator of a plasmid-encoded virulence gene. J. Bacteriol. 173:7176–7185.

Chen, L.M., Kanign, K., and Galan, J.E. 1996. *Salmonella* spp. are cytotoxic for cultured macrophages. Mol. Microbiol. 21:1101–1115.

Clarke, R.T.J., and Bauchop, T., eds. 1977. Microbial ecology of the gut. London: Academic.

Clouthier, S.C., Collinson, S.K., and Kay, W.W. 1994. Unique fimbriae-like structures encoded by *sefD* of the SEF14 fimbrial gene cluster of *Salmonella enteritidis*. Mol. Microbiol. 12:893–903.

Cornelis, G.R., and Wolf-Watz, H. 1997. The *Yersinia* Yop virulon: a bacterial system for subverting eukaryotic cells. Mol. Microbiol. 23:861–867.

Craven, S.E. 1994. Altered colonizing ability for the caeca of broiler chicks by lipopolysaccharide-deficient mutants of *Salmonella typhimurium*. Avian Dis. 38:401–408.

Dorman, C.J., Chatfield, S., Higgins, C.F., Hayward, C., and Dougan, G. 1989. Characterization of porin and *ompR* mutants of a virulent strain of *Salmonella typhimurium*: *ompR* mutants are attenuated in vivo. Infect. Immun. 57:2136–2140.

Drasar, B.S., and Barrow, P.A. 1985. Intestinal microbiology. Wokingham, UK: Van Nostrand Reinhold.

Drasar, B.S., and Hill, M.J. 1974. Human intestinal flora. London: Academic.

Duguid, J.P., Anderson, E.S., and Campbell, I. 1966. Fimbriae and adhesive properties in salmonellae. J. Pathol. Bacteriol. 92:107–138.

Dunlap, N.E., Benjamin, W.N., McCall, R.D., Tilden, A.B., and Briles, D.E. 1991. A safe site for *Salmonella typhimurium* is within splenic cells during the early phase of infection in mice. Microb. Pathog. 10:297–310.

Fang, F.C., Krause, M., Roudier, C., Fierer, J., and Guiney, D.G. 1991. Growth regulation of a *Salmonella* plasmid gene essential for virulence. J. Bacteriol. 173:6783–6789.

Fernandez-Prada, C.M., Hoover, D.L., Tall, B.D., Venkatesan, M.M. 1997. Human-monocytes-derived macrophages infected with virulent *Shigella flexneri* in vitro undergo a rapid cytolytic event similar to oncosis but not apoptosis. Infect. Immun. 65:1486–1496.

Feutrier, J., Kay, W.W., and Trust, T.J. 1988. Cloning and expression of a *Salmonella enteritidis* fimbria gene in *Escherichia coli*. J. Bacteriol. 170:4216–4222.

Fierer, J., Eckmann, L., Fang, F., Pfeifer, C., Finlay, B.B., and Guiney, D. 1993. Expression of the *Salmonella* virulence plasmid gene *spvB* in cultured macrophages and non-phagocytic cells. Infect. Immun. 61:5231–5236.

Finlay, B.B., and Falkow, S. 1990. *Salmonella* interactions with polarised human intestinal caco-2 epithelial cells. J. Infect. Dis. 162:1096–1106.

Finlay, B.B., Gumbiner, B., and Falkow, S. 1988. Penetration of *Salmonella* through a polarized Madin-Darby canine kidney epithelial cell monolayer. J. Cell Biol. 107:221–230.

Galan, J.E. 1996. Molecular genetic bases of *Salmonella* entry into host cells. Mol. Microbiol. 20:263–271.

Galan, J.E., Pace, J., and Hayman, M.J. 1992. Involvement of the epidermal growth factor receptor in the invasion of cultured mammalian cells by *Salmonella typhimurium*. Nature 357:588–589.

Ginocchio, C., Pace, J., and Galan, J.E. 1992. Identification and molecular characterization of a *Salmonella typhimurium* gene involved in triggering the internalization of salmonellae into cultured epithelial cells. Proc. Natl. Acad. Sci. U.S.A. 89:5976–5980.

Gulig, P.A., and Chiodo, V.A. 1990. Genetic and DNA sequence analysis of the *Salmonella typhimurium* virulence plasmid gene encoding the 28,000-molecular weight protein. Infect. Immun. 58:2651–2658.

Gulig, P.A., and Curtiss, R. 1987. Plasmid-associated virulence of *Salmonella typhimurium*. Infect. Immun. 55:2891–2901.

Gulig, P.A., Danbara, H., Guiney, D.G., Lax, A.J., Norel, F., and Rhen, M. 1993. Molecular analysis of *spv* virulence genes of the *Salmonella* virulence plasmids. Mol. Microbiol. 7:825–830.

Hacker, J., Blum-Oehler, G., Mühldorfer, I., and Tschäpe, H. 1997. Pathogenicity islands of virulent bacteria: structure, function and impact on microbial evolution. Mol. Microbiol. 23:1089–1097.

Halavatkar, H., and Barrow, P.A. 1993. The role of a 54-kb plasmid in the virulence of strains of *Salmonella enteritidis* of phage type 4 for chickens and mice. J. Med. Microbiol. 38:171–176.

Hentges, D.J., ed. 1983. Human intestinal microflora in health and disease. London: Academic.

Hormaeche, C.E., Mastroeni, P., Arena, A., Uddin, J., and Joysey, H.S. 1990. T cells do not mediate the initial suppression of a *Salmonella* infection in the reticuloendothelial system. Immunology 70:247–250.

Hsu, H.S. 1989. Pathogenesis and immunity in murine salmonellosis. Microbiol. Rev. 53:390–409.

Johnson, K., Charles, I., Dougan, G., Pickard, D., O'Guora, P., Costa, G., Al, T., Miller, I., and Hormaeche, C. 1991. The role of a stress-response protein of *Salmonella typhimurium* virulence. Mol. Microbiol. 5:401–407.

Jones, B.D., Lee, C.A., and Falkow, S. 1992. Invasion by *Salmonella typhimurium* is affected by the direction of flagellar rotation. Infect. Immun. 60:2375–2380.

Jones, B.D., Paterson, H.F., Hall, A., and Falkow, S. 1993. *Salmonella typhimurium* induces membrane ruffling by a growth factor-receptor-independent mechanism. Proc. Natl. Acad. Sci. U.S.A. 90:10,390–10,394.

Lax, A.J., Pullinger, G.D., Baird, G.D., and Williamson, C.M. 1990. The virulence plasmid of *Salmonella dublin*: detailed restriction map and analysis by transposon mutagenesis. J. Gen. Microbiol. 136:1117–1123.

Li, J., Smith, N.H., Nelson, K., Crichton, P.B., Old, D.C., Whittam, T.S., and Selander, R.K. 1993. Evolutionary origin and radiation of the avian-adapted and non-mobile salmonellae. J. Med. Microbiol. 38:129–139.

Libby, S.J., Goebel, W., Ludwig, A., Buchmeier, N., Bowe, F., Fang, F.C., Guiney, D.G., Songer, J.G., and Heffron, F. 1994. A cytolysin encoded by *Salmonella* is required for virulence and survival within macrophages. Proc. Natl. Acad. Sci. U.S.A. 91:489–493.

McCormick, B.A., Colgan, S.P., Delph-Archer, C., Miller, S.I., and Madara, J.L. 1993. *Salmonella typhimurium* attachment to human intestinal epithelial monolayers: transcellular signalling to subepithelial neutrophils. J. Cell Biol. 123:895–907.

Mead, G.C., and Impey, C.S. 1987. The present status of the Nurmi concept for reducing carriage of food-poisoning salmonellae and other pathogens in live poultry. In: Smulders, F.J.M., ed. Elimination of pathogenic organisms from meat and poultry. Amsterdam: Elsevier, pp. 57–77.

Miller, S.I., Kukral, A.M., and Mekalanos, J.J. 1989. A two-component regulatory system (*phoP/phoQ*) controls *Salmonella typhimurium* virulence. Proc. Natl. Acad. Sci. U.S.A. 86:5054–5058.

Mills, D.M., Bajaj, V., and Lee, C.A. 1995. A 40 kb chromosomal fragment encoding *Salmonella typhimurium* invasion genes is absent from the corresponding region of the *Escherichia coli* K12 chromosome. Mol. Microbiol. 15:749–759.

Milner, K.C., and Shaffer, M.F. 1952. Bacteriologic studies of experimental salmonella infections in chicks. J. Infect. Dis. 90:81–96.

Pace, J., Hayman, M.J., and Galan, J.E. 1993. Signal transduction and invasion of epithelial cells by *S. typhimurium*. Cell 72:505–514.

Pascopella, L., Raupach, B., Ghori, N., Monack, D., Falkow, S., and Small, P.L.C. 1995. Host restriction phenotypes of *Salmonella typhi* and *S. gallinarum*. Infect. Immun. 63:4329–4335.

Popiel, I., and Turnbull, P.C.B. 1985. Passage of *Salmonella enteritidis* and *Salmonella thompson* through chick ileocaecal mucosa. Infect. Immun. 47:786–792.

Pospischil, A., Wood, R.L., and Anderson, T.D. 1990. Peroxidase-antiperoxidase and immunogold labelling of *Salmonella typhimurium* and *Salmonella choleraesuis* var *kunzendorf* in tissues of experimentally infected swine. Am. J. Vet. Res. 51:619–624.

Pullinger, G.D., Baird, G.D., Williamson, C.M., and Lax, A.J. 1989. Nucleotide sequence of a plasmid gene involved in the virulence of salmonellas. Nucleic Acids Res. 17:7983.

Pullinger, G.D., and Lax, A.J. 1992. A *Salmonella dublin* virulence plasmid locus that affects bacterial growth under nutrient-limited conditions. Mol. Microbiol. 6:1631–1643.

Roudier, C., Fierer, J., and Guiney, D.G. 1992. Characterization of translation termination mutations in the *spv* operon of the *Salmonella* virulence plasmid pSDL2. J. Bacteriol. 174:6418–6423.

Ruschkowski, S., Rosenshine, I., and Finlay, B.B. 1992. *Salmonella typhimurium* induces an inositol phosphate flux in infected epithelial cells. FEMS Microbiol. Lett. 95:121–126.

Shaffer, M.F., Milner, K.C., Clemmer, D.I., and Bridges, J.F. 1957. Bacteriologic studies of experimental *Salmonella* infections in chicks II. J. Infect. Dis. 100:17–31.

Shea, J.E., Hensel, M., Gleeson, C., and Holden, D.W. 1996. Identification of a virulence locus encoding a second type III secretion system in *Salmonella typhimurium*. Proc. Natl. Acad. Sci. U.S.A. 93:2593–2597.

Simons, K., and Fuller, S.D. 1985. Cell surface polarity in epithelia. Annu. Rev. Cell Biol. 1:243–288.

Sizemore, D.R., Fink, P.S., Ou, J.T., Baron, L., Kopecko, D.J., and Warren, R.L. 1991. Tn5 mutagenesis of the *Salmonella typhimurium* 100 kb plasmid: definition of new virulence regions. Microb. Pathog. 10:493–499.

Slonczewski, J.L., and Foster, J.W. 1996. pH-regulated genes and survival at extreme pH. In: Neidhardt, F.C., ed. in chief. *Escherichia coli* and *Salmonella*, 2nd ed. Washington, DC: American Society for Microbiology, pp. 1539–1549.

Smith, H.W. 1965. Observations on the flora of the alimentary tract of animals and factors affecting its composition. J. Pathol. Bacteriol. 89:95–122.

Smith, H.W., and Tucker, J.F. 1980. The virulence of *Salmonella* strains for chickens: their excretion by infected chickens. J. Hyg. Camb. 84:479–488.

Snoeyenbos, G.H., Soerjadi, A.S., and Weinack, O.M. 1982. Gastrointestinal colonization by *Salmonella* and pathogenic *Escherichia coli* in monoxenic and holoxenic chicks and poults. Avian Dis. 26:566–575.

Soerjadi, A.S., Rufner, R., Snoeyenbos, G.H., and Weinack, O.M. 1982. Adherence of *Salmonella* and natural gut microflora to the gastro-intestinal mucosa of chicks. Avian Dis. 26:576–584.

Sohel, I., Puenti, J.L., Murray, W.J., Vuopio-Varkila, J., and Schoolnik, G.K. 1993. Cloning and characterization of the bundle-forming pilin gene of enteropathogenic *Escherichia coli* and its distribution in *Salmonella* serotypes. Mol. Microbiol. 7:563–575.

Spink, J.M., Wood, M.W., Pullinger, G.D., and Lax, A.J. 1992. Regulation of *Salmonella dublin* virulence-associated plasmid genes. In: Abstracts, 49th symposium, Society for General Microbiology, p. 94.

Spink, J.M., Pullinger, G.D., Wood, M.W., and Lax, A.J. 1994. Regulation of *spvR*, the positive regulatory gene of *Salmonella* plasmid virulence genes. FEMS Microbiol. Lett. 116:113–122.

Takeuchi, A. 1967. Electron microscopic studies of experimental *Salmonella* infection. 1. Penetration into the intestinal epithelium by *Salmonella typhimurium*. Am. J. Pathol. 50:109–136.

Thorns, C.J. 1995. *Salmonella* fimbriae novel antigens in the detection and control of *Salmonella* infections. Br. Vet. J. 151:643–658.

Thorns, C.J., Turcotte, C., Gemmel, C.G., and Woodward, M.J. 1996. Studies on the role of the SEF14 fimbrial antigen in the pathogenesis of *Salmonella enteritidis*. Microb. Pathog. 20:235–246.

Topley, W.W.C., and Wilson, G.S. 1936. Principles of bacteriology and immunity. London: Edward Arnold.

Turnbull, P.C.B., and Richmond, J.E. 1978. A model of *Salmonella enteritidis*: the behaviour of *Salmonella enteritidis* in chick intestine studied by light and electron microscopy. Br. J. Exp. Pathol. 59:64–75.

Vandenbosch, J.L., Rabert, D.K., Kurlandsky, D.R., and Jones, G.W. 1989. Sequence analysis of *rsk*, a portion of the 95-kilobase plasmid of *Salmonella typhimurium* associated with resistance to the bactericidal activity of serum. Infect. Immun. 57:850–857.

Van der Waaij, D. 1992. Mechanisms involved in the development of the intestinal microflora in relation to the host organism: consequences for colonization resistance. In: Hormaeche, C.E., Penn, C.W., and Smyth, C.J., eds. Molecular biology of bacterial infection: 49th symposium of the Society for General Microbiology. London: Cambridge University Press, pp. 1–12.

Vidal, S.M., Malo, D., Vogan, K., Skamene, E., and Gros, P. 1993. Natural resistance to infection with intracellular parasites: isolation of a candidate for *Bcg*. Cell 73:469–485.

Wallis, T.S., Starkey, W.G., Stephen, J., Haddon, S.J., Osborne, M.P., and Candy, D.C.A. 1986. The nature and role of mucosal damage in relation to *Salmonella typhimurium* induced fluid secretion in the rabbit ileum. J. Med. Microbiol. 22:39–49.

Williamson, C.M., Pullinger, G.D., and Lax, A.J. 1990. Identification of proteins expressed by the essential virulence region of the *Salmonella dublin* plasmid. Microb. Pathog. 9:61–66.

Wilson, G.S., and Miles, A.A. 1964. Topley and Wilson's principles of bacteriology and immunity, 5th ed. London: Edward Arnold.

Wood, M.W., Rosqvist, R., Mullan, P.B., Edwards, M.H., and Galyov, E.E. 1996. SopE, a secreted protein of *Salmonella dublin,* is translocated into the target eukaryotic cells via a *sip*-dependent mechanism and promotes bacterial entry. Mol. Microbiol. 22:327–338.

Woodward, M.J., Allen-Vercoe, E., and Redstone, J.S. 1996. Distribution, gene sequence and expression in vivo of the plasmid encoded fimbrial antigen of *Salmonella* serotype Enteritidis. Epidemiol. Infect. 117:17–28.

Worton, K.J., Candy, D.C.A., Wallis, T.S., Clarke, G.J., Osborne, M.P., Haddon, S.J., and Stephen, J. 1989. Studies on early association of *Salmonella typhimurium* with intestinal mucosa in vivo and in vitro: relationship to virulence. J. Med. Microbiol. 29:283–294.

Zychlinsky, A., Prevost, M.C., and Sansonetti, P.J. 1992. *Shigella flexneri* induces apoptosis in infected macrophages. Nature 358:167–168.

Zychlinsky, A., Fitting, C., Cavaillon, J.M., and Sansonetti, P.J. 1994a. Interleukin 1 is released by murine macrophages during apoptosis induced by *Shigella flexneri*. J. Clin. Invest. 94:1328–1332.

Zychlinsky, A., Kenny, B., Menard, R., Prevost, M.C., Holland, I.B., and Sansonetti, P.J. 1994b. IpaB mediates macrophage apoptosis induced by *Shigella flexneri*. Mol. Microbiol. 11:619–627.

18

Contamination of Eggs and Poultry Meat with *Salmonella enterica* Serovar Enteritidis

T.J. Humphrey

INTRODUCTION

The international pandemic of *Salmonella enterica* serovar Enteritidis (*S.* Enteritidis) infection (Rodrigue et al., 1990) began in the mid-1980s and shows no sign of significant reduction. Its root cause was best summarized in a statement made by the Public Health Laboratory Service (PHLS) in evidence to the United Kingdom's (U.K.) House of Commons Agriculture Committee of Enquiry on *Salmonella* in Eggs: The cause is the spread of infection in chickens, and the consequent human *S.* Enteritidis food poisoning comes not only from contaminated chicken carcasses and eggs but also from an important new source, the contents of intact hens' eggs (Anon., 1989).

Thus, *S.* Enteritidis poses both a direct and an indirect threat to public health. The direct threat comes, as just outlined, from the contaminated contents of eggs used for human consumption. The indirect threat is associated with the ability of the bacterium to be transmitted vertically from infected breeder flocks. With broiler breeders, this will lead to the infection of broilers, eventual carcass contamination, and human illness. There are over 50 phage types of *S.* Enteritidis, but most work has been done on phage type 4 (PT4), because this is the most widespread in the U.K. and would seem to be the most important. In this chapter, much of the comment is confined to this bacterium, because its behavior has many similarities to that of other *S.* Enteritidis phage types. Reference will also be made, however, to work on other phage types, where appropriate.

Case-control studies in the United States revealed grade-A shell eggs as important vehicles in cases of *S.* Enteritidis infection (St. Louis et al., 1988). Similar investigations and outbreak analysis in England and Wales (Coyle et al., 1988; Cowden et al., 1989) confirmed an association with dishes containing raw or lightly cooked eggs but also identified chicken meat as important (Cowden et al., 1989; Rampling et al., 1989). This chapter considers the contamination of both eggs and chicken meat.

CONTAMINATION OF CHICKEN MEAT

Discussion in this section is confined to PT4 only. This bacterium is capable of causing infection in both egg-laying and meat-producing (broiler) chickens. The manifestations of infection, however, can be very different in the two groups of birds. Commercial egg layers only rarely show obvious signs of disease when infected with PT4, and they continue to lay and feed normally (see later herein). In contrast, the consequences of PT4 infection in broilers can be profound. Strains of this bacterium can be highly invasive, particularly in young broilers, and studies with naturally infected flocks have revealed increased mortality and stunting (Lister, 1988). Pericarditis and perihepatitis have also been observed in broilers at slaughter (Rampling et al., 1989). Thus, PT4 infection has economic consequences for the poultry-meat industry in addition to major public health implications. The invasive nature of PT4 in broiler chickens means that the infection can be septicemic. If such birds are slaughtered, the bacterium might lodge in the smaller blood vessels when birds are exsanguinated. A small study of chicken carcasses on retail sale in South West England found that muscle tissue of three (7%) of 45 was positive for PT4 (Humphrey, 1991). This study was repeated with essentially similar results in another area of the U.K. (A. Rampling, personal communication).

The pathogenic nature of PT4 in broiler chickens provides a potentially attractive explanation for the isolation of the bacterium from chicken muscle tissues. There is another possible route, however. The intensity of chicken processing provides opportunities for cross-contamination (Mead, 1989). An important site is scalding, where birds are immersed in warm water so that feathers are loosened prior to mechanical plucking. Most scald tanks in the U.K. use a "soft" scalding regimen where the water temperature is 50°–52°C. The scald water becomes heavily contaminated with feces, blood, and other organic matter; the feces will dissociate to form uric acid and ammonium urate in the water, and this provides buffering that maintains the scald water at or around pH 6.0, which maximizes the heat tolerance of salmonellae (Humphrey and Lanning, 1987). As a result, scald water will often contain high numbers of these bacteria (Humphrey and Lanning, 1987). Lillard (1973) demonstrated that *Clostridium perfringens* in scald water can be recovered from the edible parts of chicken carcasses. The mechanisms for such contamination are not fully understood, but there is the possibility that bacteria can enter the body of the chicken through cut blood vessels. It is of interest that case-control studies of sporadic cases of PT4 infection in England and Wales identified hot, cooked, takeout chicken as the second highest risk factor for infection after dishes containing raw eggs (Cowden et al., 1989). Cooked chicken consumed away from the home has also been revealed to be important in cases of *S.* Typhimurium DT104 infection in England and Wales (Wall et al., 1994). There is, of course, the possibility that chickens become contaminated after cooking (Roberts, 1986). Salmonellae are also able to attach to muscle tissue (Dickson and Koohmaraie, 1989; Humphrey et al., 1997), and this has the consequence of markedly increasing heat tolerance (Humphrey et al., 1997). Thus, if chickens are not cooked thoroughly, some cells may survive in muscle tissues. They will be better protected against gastric acidity and may cause infection.

SOURCES OF *SALMONELLA* ENTERITIDIS IN POULTRY-MEAT PRODUCTION

The continuing association between the contamination of poultry carcasses with salmonellae and human infection clearly demands that efforts are made to reduce the threat to the public health. Many of the measures shown to be successful with salmonellae other than *S.* Enteritidis may also be applicable to the control of this bacterium. It is important, however, that control programs recognize that *S.* Enteritidis may have a different epidemiology in broiler production than most other poultry-associated salmonellae. Contaminated poultry feed has long been recognized as an important source of salmonellae in poultry flocks (Williams, 1981). *Salmonella* Enteritidis has also been isolated from poultry feed but at a very low prevalence (Anon., 1995). The bacterium can also be recovered from wild animals, particularly those in the immediate area around a poultry house (Davies and Wray, 1995). While these sources may be involved in the epidemiology of *S.* Enteritidis in poultry-meat production, it would seem that they play only a relatively minor role.

The PHLS Food Microbiology Research Unit has had a long association with the U.K. broiler industry. This has enabled studies on salmonella control. Data from naturally infected broiler flocks revealed that the most important source of PT4 in these chickens was and is infected breeding flocks. Thus, when breeders are infected, so are their progeny (Table 18.1). A collaborative study with a broiler company revealed that when infection was eradicated in parent birds, broilers were also found to be PT4 negative at slaughter (Table 18.1). These data are, perhaps, not surprising, but they do also reveal that, when performed properly, cleansing, disinfection, and vermin control can protect chickens from infection, even with PT4.

In the European Union, an important control measure against *S.* Enteritidis in poultry flocks is the 1992 Zoonoses Directive (Anon., 1992), which requires that all breeding flocks, at any level in the European Poultry Industry, are screened every 14 days for the presence of salmonellae. Those found to be infected with *S.* Enteritidis are killed, with the owners being compensated. In the U.K., the owners of broiler breeder flocks are offered a compromise. They can choose to have their birds slaughtered or they can treat either the breeders or their progeny with antibiotics. The decline of PT4 in Europe, albeit quite slowly, is perhaps an indication that the aforementioned control measures, and others, are having an effect.

CONTAMINATION OF EGGS

Contamination of Eggshells

Although there is little doubt that the continuing pandemic of *S.* Enteritidis infection is associated principally with the contamination of egg contents, this bacterium, and other salmonellae, can also be isolated from eggshells. In fact, the prevalence of eggshell contamination usually exceeds that of egg contents (Humphrey et al., 1989c). It is not unusual for salmonellae on the shell to contaminate egg contents at breaking, and this route was believed to be important in the large number of egg-associated outbreaks in the U.K. and U.S.A. during and immediately after the Second World War. The vehicles in these outbreaks were either spray-dried or bulk liquid eggs. Investigations were

TABLE 18.1   Relationship between *Salmonella* Enteritidis infection in broiler breeder birds and the isolation of the organism from their broiler progeny

Multiple-farm study	
Salmonella status of breeder flocks	No. of broiler flocks positive for *S.* Enteritidis per no. examined[a]
S. Enteritidis positive	13/15
S. Enteritidis negative	1/15

Single-farm study, September 1992–April 1993		
Broiler flock no.	*S.* Enteritidis status of breeder flock supplying chicks	*S.* Enteritidis status of broiler flock
1	+	+
2	+	+
3	+	+
4	−	−
5	−	−

[a]Differences are highly significant, p < 0.0001.

conducted to identify the likely sources of the salmonellae. The examination of eggs taken from processing plants (Solowey et al., 1946) found that approximately 3% of the shells of clean, intact eggs were salmonella positive both before and after washing. The comparative figure for eggs with obvious fecal contamination of the shells was 5%. In another study (Cantor and McFarlane, 1948), either *S.* Montivideo or *S.* Anatum were isolated from the shells of 0.6% of eggs sampled at processing plants. In this latter study, all isolations were from shells with obvious fecal contamination.

Many different salmonella serovars can be isolated from eggshells, and in a study in the U.K. of British and imported eggs (de Louvois, 1993a) the following salmonella serovars were found, among others: *S.* Enteritidis, *S.* Infantis, *S.* Livingstone, *S.* Braenderup, and *S.* Typhimurium.

The aforementioned data are in general accord with data of earlier investigations quoted by Cantor and McFarlane (1948), when a wide range of salmonella serovars, including *S.* Thompson, *S.* Typhimurium, *S.* Borrelei *S.* Oranienberg, *S.* Montivideo, *S.* Tennessee, *S.* Derby *S.* Essen, and *S.* Worthington were recovered from eggshells. With the possible exception of some phage types of *S.* Typhimurium, it is believed that these serovars are not invasive in chickens, and thus the likely source of these bacteria was fecal contamination. With salmonellae other than *S.* Enteritidis, this is probably the most important route. Colonization of the intestine can occur after the consumption of salmonella-positive foodstuffs (Williams, 1981), and many studies over many years have demonstrated that chickens can acquire many salmonella serovars by this route. Poppe et al. (1991), in a study of 295 laying flocks, isolated 35 different salmonella serovars from environmental samples, which included eggshells. Barnhart et al. (1991) investigated laying flocks at slaughter. Of 42 flocks, 32 (76%) were salmonella positive. Although *S.* Heidelberg was the most common isolate, 14 other serovars were also found.

Among the many surveys of eggs in the last few years, some have included examination of eggshells. Perales and Audicana (1989) in Spain examined 372 eggs from laying flocks implicated in cases of human salmonellosis. *Salmonella* Enteritidis PT4 was isolated from four eggs (1.1%). The examination of eggs from flocks not implicated in outbreaks found a lower contamination rate (0.5%). Mawer et al. (1989) in the U.K. did not isolate salmonellae from the shells of any of 360 eggs from a small free-range flock implicated in an outbreak of PT4 salmonellosis even though the bacterium was isolated from egg contents. Birds from this flock were used in subsequent studies (Humphrey et al., 1989b), and *S.* Enteritidis PT4 was recovered from the shells of five (7.4%) of 68 eggs. In other outbreak-associated investigations (Humphrey et al., 1989c), PT4 was recovered from the shells of 5.2% of 194 intact eggs.

The processes behind the contamination of eggshells with *S.* Enteritidis are yet to be fully understood, and there is some dispute over whether intestinal carriage or oviduct infection is the more important. There is no doubt that the presence of *S.* Enteritidis in feces can lead to eggshell contamination. Gast and Beard (1990) reported a correlation between feces positivity in hens artificially infected with *S.* Enteritidis PT13a and eggshell contamination. In a survey of U.K.-produced and imported shell eggs, the presence of visible fecal matter was more frequently reported on eggs contaminated with salmonellae (de Louvois, 1993a). The author did not differentiate between *S.* Enteritidis and other salmonellae, and many serovars were found (de Louvois, 1993b). There is no dispute that PT4 can colonize the intestinal tract and can be isolated from eggshells as a result of fecal contamination. Comparison of the aforementioned data on PT13a (Gast and Beard, 1990) with that on PT4 suggests that there may be differences between phage types. Humphrey et al. (1991b), using artificially infected, specific pathogen-free birds, found that PT4 could be recovered from the shells of intact eggs even when the birds were feces negative for salmonellae. In addition, shell-positive eggs could still be identified over 6 weeks after intestinal carriage of salmonellae had apparently ceased. In this study (Humphrey et al., 1991b), salmonellae were never isolated from the feces of five of the infected birds, but all laid eggs with salmonella-positive shells. These data support the view that infection of the lower reproductive tract may be important with PT4.

In general, salmonellae present on eggshells die rapidly (Baker, 1990), but survival can be enhanced by high relative humidities (Lancaster and Crabb, 1953) and low temperature (Lancaster and Crabb, 1953; Rizk et al., 1966; Baker, 1990). It is also clear that certain isolates of *S.* Enteritidis, and PT4 in particular, can persist for long periods on the shells of eggs stored at ambient temperature, and in a study in the U.K. (de Louvois, 1994) this bacterium was isolated from the shells of eggs that had been stored for over 5 weeks at 20°–21°C. There is very little information on the numbers of salmonellae on eggshells, but the numbers are believed to be low. In one of the few published studies (Baker et al., 1985), duck eggs with obvious fecal contamination were found to be carrying approximately 5×10^5 salmonellae per egg compared with less than 100 cells on eggs that appeared clean.

Contamination of Egg Contents

As with other aspects of the epidemiology of infection with *S.* Enteritidis in both humans and chickens, there is a degree of dispute over the routes of egg-content contamination. It is beyond doubt that *S.* Enteritidis, in common with other salmonellae (Scott, 1930; Brown et al., 1940; Sparks and Board, 1985), if present on the shells of eggs, may be able to contaminate egg contents by migration through the eggshell and membranes. Such a route is facilitated by moist eggshells (Scott, 1930; Brown et al., 1940), storage at ambient temperature (Stokes et al., 1956, Rizk et al., 1960), and shell damage (Vadehra et al., 1969; Humphrey et al., 1989b). It has also been demonstrated that salmonellae are more likely to penetrate eggshells if they are present on the surface of an egg before the cuticle has dried (Sparks and Board, 1985; Padron, 1990). Common sense dictates, however, that if this route was important the *S.* Enteritidis pandemic would not have been unusual, because presumably salmonellae are and always have been regular contaminants of eggshells. *Salmonella* Enteritidis is an important human pathogen because it is able, often with high frequency, to contaminate egg contents as a result of infection of reproductive tissue. Much evidence is accumulating to support this view. Examination of eggs from commercial laying flocks in the U.K. (Humphrey et al., 1989b,c, 1991c; Mawer et al., 1989) could demonstrate no association between contamination of the shell and the presence of *S.* Enteritidis in egg contents. Examination of eggs from birds infected artificially also found no relationship between fecal carriage of *S.* Enteritidis and the presence of the bacterium in egg contents (Gast and Beard, 1990; Humphrey et al., 1991b). It is also possible to isolate *S.* Enteritidis PT4 from the repro-

ductive tissue of naturally infected hens (in these cases, breeder birds), in the absence of intestinal colonization (Lister, 1988; Bygrave and Gallagher, 1989). The aforementioned data are clearly suggestive of the importance of infection of reproductive tissue. Numerous studies on artificially infected hens (Humphrey et al., 1989a, 1991a–c; Barrow and Lovell, 1991; Baskerville et al., 1992; Gast and Beard, 1992; Thiagarajan et al., 1994; Keller et al., 1995) and naturally infected hens (Bygrave and Gallagher, 1989; Cooper et al., 1989; Humphrey et al., 1989b; Hoop and Pospischil, 1993; Corkish et al., 1994) have shown that *S.* Enteritidis can be isolated from reproductive tissues. In many of these studies, but not all, *S.* Enteritidis was also isolated from egg contents.

The size and longevity of the *S.* Enteritidis pandemic, and the widespread nature of PT4 in particular, clearly suggest that this bacterium possesses special properties. Invasion of reproductive tissue may be the most important. Other salmonellae can be recovered from such sites (Snoeyenbos et al., 1969; Barnhart et al., 1991), and Buxton and Gordon (1947) demonstrated that hens infected naturally with *S.* Thompson produced eggs with salmonella-positive shells. The bacterium was also able to penetrate the shells and contaminate the contents of a minority of eggs during incubation at 37°C. Data from studies using hens infected artificially would suggest that such results are unusual. For example, Baker et al. (1980) did not recover *S.* Typhimurium from the contents of eggs following either the oral or intravenous inoculation of either 10^8–10^9 (oral) or 5×10^6 (intravenous) cells of the bacterium. Similarly, *S.* Anatum was not isolated from egg contents even when it was injected into reproductive tissues (Forsythe et al., 1967). It is of interest that in the same study it was possible to recover *S.* Pullorum from egg contents from birds infected with this bacterium.

It would appear that infection of reproductive tissues can occur quite commonly in some commercial flocks. Hoop and Pospischil (1993) examined birds from three small, naturally infected flocks. In six (16%) of 37 birds, ovarian tissue was PT4 positive. The bacterium was also isolated from 10 oviduct tissue samples (27%). Infection with *S.* Enteritidis in commercial laying birds does not cause the often acute and frequently obvious clinical symptoms seen with PT4 in broiler flocks. Birds continue to feed, lay, and behave normally. Examination of reproductive tissues (Lister, 1988; Hoop and Pospischil, 1993), however, has revealed that inflammation may be a common consequence of infection with *S.* Enteritidis. Histopathological findings in the latter study included diffuse and focal inflammation of ovarian tissue with heterophils and focal inflammation and diffuse infiltration with macrophages and plasma cells in the oviduct (Hoop and Pospischil, 1993). Similar findings were reported in a study where point-of-lay pullets were infected with PT4 by an airborne route (Baskerville et al., 1992). In an extensive study of four naturally infected flocks, possible differences between either different breeds of chickens or different PT4 strains were revealed. Thus, while examination of tissues of 20 birds from two broiler breeder flocks found gross pathology in both ovaries and/or oviducts in some birds, all tissues from a commercial layer flock were normal in appearance (Cooper et al., 1989). These data have been supported by later work with *S*. Enteritidis PT4 (Humphrey et al., 1996) and PT13a (Petter, 1993; Keller et al., 1995), which showed that isolates of the same phage type differ in pathogenicity and also that infection of reproductive tissues does not necessarily lead to egg contamination. Petter (1993) demonstrated that different isolates of PT13a contaminated egg contents at very different rates. One isolate, which formed a "lacy" colony on agars incubated at ambient temperatures, contaminated 42% of eggs from birds infected artificially. Such a relationship between colony morphology and increased pathogenicity has also been seen in PT4 (Humphrey et al., 1996). It is not yet known why some isolates of *S*. Enteritidis are better than others at egg contamination, but it is important that this is investigated.

Available scientific data to date suggest that the occasional egg is seeded with a few cells of *S*. Enteritidis while in the reproductive tract. Few studies have looked at this aspect of egg contamination with naturally infected birds, but an investigation by Humphrey et al. (1989b) demonstrated that approximately 1% of the production from 35 hens was content positive, although only 10 of these birds laid positive eggs. These data also revealed that approximately 0.3% of the eggs produced by an individual bird are likely to be positive in the contents for *S*. Enteritidis. Despite the observations on pathological changes in reproductive tissues as a consequence of *S*. Enteritidis infection, it would seem that the great majority of content-positive eggs are normal in appearance. Over the last 10 years, the PHLS Food Microbiology Research Unit in Exeter has examined over 100 eggs with *S*. Enteritidis phage types present in their contents, from naturally and artificially infected hens, and all have appeared normal on superficial examination. It would seem that diseased ova are not recognized by the reproductive system and do not generally become part of fully formed eggs.

The Prevalence of Eggs with Contents Positive for *Salmonella* Enteritidis

The observed prevalences of eggs with salmonella-positive contents can be variable (Table 18.2). This may be due to observed patterns of egg contamination, but it is also important to take into account the impact of different laboratory techniques. The examination of eggs from artificially infected hens (Gast and Beard, 1992) and naturally infected hens (Humphrey and Whitehead, 1992) has shown that, when eggs are pooled for culture, the isolation rate can be increased significantly by extending the culture time from 24 to 48 h or by adding a source of iron, which can help the few cells of a salmonella present overcome the inhibitory mechanisms of egg albumen. The principal site of contamination in eggs would seem to be either the albumen or the outside of the vitelline membrane (Gast and Beard, 1990; Humphrey et al., 1991c). Thus, techniques in which only yolks are examined may also either fail to detect salmonella-positive eggs or underestimate their prevalence. It is also becoming clear, however, that there can be clustering of eggs with salmonella-positive contents. This was first observed during outbreak investigation (Paul and Batchelor, 1988; Humphrey et al., 1989c) and again during studies with naturally infected hens caged individually (Humphrey et al., 1989b). In this latter investigation, 10 of 35 hens produced 11 eggs with contents positive for *S*. Enteritidis. Over one 2-day period, three hens laid contaminated eggs. During another, 6 weeks later, five different hens did so. On 1 day, four (22%) of 18 eggs were positive for salmonellae. Outbreak investigations (Vugia et al., 1993) have also suggested that certain batches can contain many eggs with contaminated contents.

Numbers of *Salmonella* Enteritidis in Egg Contents

It has been indicated that fresh contaminated eggs contain only low numbers of *S*. Enteritidis (Humphrey et al., 1989b,c, 1991c; Mawer et al., 1989; Timoney et al., 1989; Gast and Beard, 1992). The bacterium is capable of growth in a proportion of contaminated eggs, but this is strongly governed by the age of the egg and the conditions under which it is stored (Humphrey et al., 1991c; Humphrey and Whitehead, 1993). In a study using naturally contaminated, intact eggs with shells free from fecal contamination, all content-positive eggs examined within 3 weeks of lay contained fewer than 20 cells of *S*. Enteritidis, whereas six of 13 examined after being stored at 20°C for

TABLE 18.2   Prevalence of *Salmonella* Enteritidis[a] in eggs originating from naturally infected poultry laying flocks

Flock type	No. of flocks	No. of eggs examined	No. of contents positive	%
Commercial layer (free range)	9	2412	24	1.0
Commercial layer (battery)	8	2489	10	0.4
Layer (breeder)	1	1120	1	0.1
Broiler (breeder)	2	1558	10	0.6
Experimental[b]	2	1119	11	1.0
Total	22	8698	56	0.6

[a]All isolates, except one that was PT33 and another that was PT4a, were *S*. Enteritidis PT4.
[b]Two small flocks of naturally infected laying hens were caged individually with each egg laid by each hen examined over a 3-month period.

over 3 weeks contained more than 100 cells. Three eggs were heavily contaminated (Humphrey et al., 1991c; Humphrey and Whitehead, 1993). A PHLS survey on eggs purchased from retail outlets and stored at 20°C for 5 weeks before examination has also found some eggs to be heavily contaminated (de Louvois, 1994).

The observation that S. Enteritidis can grow in the contents of some eggs required that investigations were undertaken to examine the speed of such growth and the parameters that could control it, particularly in countries such as the U.K. where eggs are not usually stored under refrigeration in retail outlets. The relatively low proportion of content-contaminated eggs even from known infected flocks (Humphrey et al., 1989b,c, 1991c; Mawer et al., 1989; Perales and Audicana, 1989) means that the great majority of studies on the growth of S. Enteritidis have been undertaken using artificial methods of contamination. Such investigations have provided valuable data, but it must be recognized that results may not always reflect growth profiles in naturally contaminated egg contents. Different experimental protocols have been developed. Clay and Board (1991, 1992), Dolman and Board (1992), and Lock and Board (1992) inoculated S. Enteritidis onto the inner membrane of the air sac and demonstrated that significant multiplication of the bacteria did not occur until the yolk had made contact with the air-sac membrane. They also found that the addition of either iron (Clay and Board, 1991) or small amounts of fecal material (Clay and Board, 1992) overcame the inhibitory properties of albumen. Other studies have inoculated cells of S. Enteritidis directly into egg contents. When the bacterium is placed into the yolk, growth is rapid and high numbers can be achieved within 24 h at ambient temperature even from a very low inoculum (Humphrey et al., 1989a; Bradshaw et al., 1990). Such studies do not reflect the natural situation, where albumen is the more frequently positive site, and most published work has examined the growth of S. Enteritidis inoculated into the albumen. Two experimental protocols have been adopted. Most investigators inoculated egg contents through the shell with varying numbers of S. Enteritidis. Eggs were then stored under a range of conditions with the salmonellae either being enumerated (Bradshaw et al., 1990; Hammack et al., 1993) or yolk contamination being monitored (Fehlhaber and Braun, 1993; Braun and Fehlhaber, 1995). With inoculation of egg contents through the shell, it can be difficult to be certain about the position of the inoculum. This may be of significance, because the proximity of the bacteria to the yolk may influence observed growth kinetics.

The Exeter Research Group adopted an experimental protocol designed to monitor storage-related changes to egg contents by using intact, uninoculated eggs. Eggs were collected, within 1–2 h of lay, from local commercial farms with salmonella-free flocks. Only eggs with clean, intact shells were used. Eggs were stored under a range of different conditions for varying lengths of time. Irrespective of the storage conditions, the changes that might have influenced the behavior S. Enteritidis were monitored using the same protocol (Humphrey and Whitehead, 1993). Egg contents were removed by using aseptic techniques into sterile containers

chosen so that the egg contents filled them completely. They were inoculated with Ringer's solution containing approximately 500 cells of an isolate of S. Enteritidis PT4 into egg contents under the surface of the albumen next to the intact yolk. Inoculated eggs were held at 20°C for 4 days, and then the numbers of salmonellae counted. The growth rate was expressed as the numbers after 4 days at 20°C (T4) divided by the inoculum (T0). This protocol has the disadvantage of only observing changes in growth rates and not the growth curve of S. Enteritidis in egg contents. It did, however, produce data that appeared to mirror those obtained with naturally contaminated eggs and shows that there is a delay before S. Enteritidis is able to achieve high numbers in egg contents. This is in marked contrast to results obtained in other studies when S. Enteritidis was inoculated through the shell into the albumen. These protocols were presumably used in the belief that they both mirrored what happened in naturally contaminated eggs and that the inoculation of material, often containing nutrients (Braun and Fehlhaber, 1995) and/or high numbers of salmonellae (Hammack et al., 1993; Schoeni et al., 1995), did not disturb the finely balanced interrelationship between egg-content components that controlled the growth of microorganisms. It is of concern that some, but not all, of these investigations produced results on the growth kinetics of S. Enteritidis that did not appear to match those observed with naturally contaminated eggs. In essence, data suggested that growth was very rapid and that yolk invasion occurred within a few days of egg inoculation.

Growth observed in laboratory media can be independent of inoculum levels, especially when salmonella populations are uninjured. This would not appear to be the case when salmonellae are inoculated into egg albumen. This is an iron-restricted environment (Clay and Board, 1991) and when salmonellae are present in low numbers (<10 per egg), as they would be in naturally contaminated eggs, growth is not possible until the bacterial cells can gain access to the iron-rich yolk. This does not seem to take place in fresh eggs (see below). However, if large numbers of salmonellae are inoculated into egg albumen, as the studies of Hammack et al. (1995) used 1.4×10^4 cells per egg and those of Schoeni et al. (1995) used between 5×10^3 and 5×10^5 cells per egg, they may be able to outcompete the albumen for iron in the microenvironment around the inoculum and multiply. Once multiplication has occurred, the larger number of cells will be in a position to extract even more iron, and so on. Recent studies in Exeter (unpublished) have found that observed shelf life is strongly dependent on inoculum size.

When low inoculum (<10 cells per egg) is used, the growth pattern shown in Figure 18.1 is produced. As can be seen, the pattern would appear to have three distinct phases. During the first 24 h after lay, when the pH of the albumen rises from approximately pH 7.0 to approximately pH 9.0, there is about a 10-fold increase in the number of salmonellae. This was confirmed in separate experiments when bacterial numbers were estimated only 1 day after inoculation. The initial growth phase may involve the bacterium using its iron reserves, which appear to be sufficient to support four generations. When iron reserves have been exhausted, cells enter a

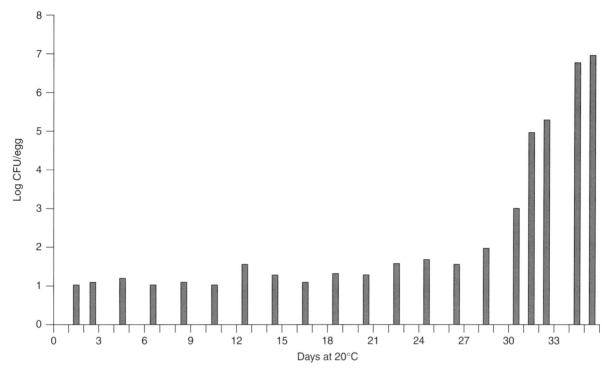

FIGURE 18.1 Growth pattern of an isolate of *Salmonella* Enteritidis PT4 in egg contents. Egg albumen was inoculated, through the shell, with 1–3 cells of PT4. Eggs were held at 20°C for up to 35 days, and then 20 eggs were removed at intervals and salmonellae in egg contents were counted. Each point represents a mean value of the counts in 20 eggs. CFU, colony-forming units.

lag phase where, in the great majority of eggs, there is little or no change in the numbers of salmonellae. The length of this second phase is strongly temperature dependent and, at 20°C, lasts for 3–4 weeks (Fig. 18.1). Exponential growth will then occur in an increasing proportion of the eggs. A possible explanation for the this phenomenon could be as follows. Yolk contents are rich in iron, but cells of *S.* Enteritidis cannot make use of this because the vitelline membrane of fresh eggs does not permit either the ingress of bacteria into yolk contents or the release of iron into the albumen. During storage, the vitelline membrane breaks down (Burley and Vadehra, 1990) and at some point becomes sufficiently permeable to allow salmonellae to enter yolk contents. Once this has taken place, rapid growth is possible (Humphrey et al., 1989d; Bradshaw et al., 1990) and large numbers of salmonellae will be present in both yolk and albumen.

When eggs were stored under conditions where temperatures fluctuated between 18° and 30°C, to simulate those that might be found in kitchens, rapid growth was possible, in the majority of eggs examined, after 6–10 days (Humphrey and Whitehead, 1993).

CONCLUSIONS

The ability of *S.* Enteritidis phage types to contaminate the interior of poultry meat and intact shell eggs presents con-siderable challenges for control. Much has been learned about the epidemiology of *S.* Enteritidis infection in poultry and humans, but much remains to be understood. Phage types of this bacterium would appear to have a predilection for the reproductive tissues of chickens, and PT4 can be isolated from oviduct tissue within 1 h of crop inoculation (Humphrey et al., 1993). The bacterium can also be isolated from the reproductive tissues in the absence of intestinal carriage. This presents problems in routine monitoring, or surveillance, where the examination of either cloacal swabs or feces is commonplace. There is a need for a better understanding of the apparent predilection of *S.* Enteritidis for reproductive tissues, its ability to persist in the farm environment (Davies and Wray, 1994), and the ability of PT4, in particular, to infect adult chickens from a low infective dose particularly by the non-oral route (Baskerville et al., 1992; Humphrey et al., 1992).

REFERENCES

Anonymous. 1989. *Salmonella* in eggs: PHLS evidence to Agriculture Committee. PHLS Microbiol. Digest 6:1–9.

Anonymous. 1992. Council of the European Communities Directive 92/117/EEC, 17 December.

Anonymous. 1995. *Salmonella* in livestock production. London: Veterinary Laboratories Agency and Ministry of Agriculture, Fisheries and Foods.

Baker, R.C. 1990. Survival of *Salmonella enteritidis* on and in shelled eggs, liquid eggs and cooked egg products. Dairy Food Environ. Sanit. 10:273–275.

Baker, R.C., Goff, J.P., and Mulnix, E.J. 1980. Salmonellae recovery following oral and intravenous inoculation of laying hens. Poult. Sci. 59:1067–1072.

Baker, R.C., Qureshi, R.A., Sandhu, T.S., and Timoney, J.F. 1985. The frequency of salmonellae on duck eggs. Poult. Sci. 64:646–652.

Barnhart, H.M., Dreesen, D.W., Bastien, R., and Pancorbo, O.C. 1991. Prevalence of *Salmonella enteritidis* and other serovars in ovaries of layer hens at time of slaughter. J. Food Prot. 54:488–491.

Barrow, P.A., and Lovell, M.A. 1991. Experimental infection of egg-laying hens with *Salmonella enteritidis* phage type 4. Avian Pathol. 20:335–348.

Baskerville, A., Humphrey, T.J., Fitzgeorge, R.B., Cook, R.W., Chart, H., Rowe, B., and Whitehead, A. 1992. Airborne infection of laying hens with *Salmonella enteritidis* phage type 4. Vet. Rec. 130:395–398.

Bradshaw, J.G., Shah, D.B., Forney, E., and Madden, J.M. 1990. Growth of *Salmonella enteritidis* in yolk of shell egg from normal and seropositive hens. J. Food Prot. 53:1033–1036.

Braun, P., and Fehlhaber, K. 1995. Migration of *Salmonella enteritidis* from the albumen into the egg yolk. Int. J. Food Microbiol. 25:95–99.

Brown, E.G., Combs, G.R., and Wright, E. 1940. Food-borne infection with *Salmonella* aertycke. JAMA 114:642–644.

Burley, R.W., and Vadehra, D.V. 1989. The vitelline membrane. In: Burley, R.W., and Vadehra, D.V., eds. The avian egg: chemistry and biology. New York: John Wiley, pp. 147–169.

Buxton, A., and Gordon, R.F. 1947. The epidemiology and control of *Salmonella thompson* infection of fowls. J. Hyg. 45:265–285.

Bygrave, A.C., and Gallagher, J. 1989. Transmission of *Salmonella enteritidis* in poultry. Vet. Rec. 124:333.

Cantor, A., and McFarlane, V.H. 1948. Growth of *Salmonella enteritidis* in artificially contaminated hens' shell eggs. Epidemiol. Infect. 106:271–281.

Clay, C.E., and Board, R.G. 1991. Growth of *Salmonella enteritidis* in artificially contaminated hens shell eggs. Epidemiol. Infect. 106:271–281.

Clay, C.E., and Board, R.G. 1992. Effect of faecal extract on the growth of *Salmonella enteritidis* in artificially contaminated hens' eggs. Br. Poult. Sci. 33:755–760.

Cooper, G.L., Nicholas, R.A., and Bracewell, C.D. 1989. Serological and bacteriological investigations of chickens from flocks naturally infected with *Salmonella enteritidis*. Vet. Rec. 125:567–572.

Corkish, J.D., Davies, R.H., Wray, C., and Nicholas, R.A.J. 1989. Observations on a broiler breeder flock naturally infected with *Salmonella enteritidis* phage type 4. Vet. Rec. 134:591–594.

Cowden, J.M., Lynch, D., Joseph, C.A., O'Mahoney, M., Mawer, S.L., Rowe, B., and Bartlett, C.L.R. 1989. Case-control study of infections with *Salmonella enteritidis* phage type 4 in England. BMJ 299:771–773.

Coyle, E.F., Palmer, S.R., Ribeiro, C.D., Howard, A.J., Jones, H.I., Ward, L., and Rowe, B. 1988. *Salmonella enteritidis* phage type 4 infection: association with hens' eggs. Lancet 2:1295–1297.

Davies, R.H., and Wray, C. 1994. *Salmonella* pollution in poultry units and associated enterprises. In: Dewi, I.A.P., Axford, R.F., Marai, I.F., and Umed, H., eds. Pollution in livestock production systems. Oxon: CAB International, pp. 137–165.

Davies, R.H., and Wray, C. 1995. Mice as carriers of *Salmonella enteritidis* on persistently infected poultry units. Vet. Rec. 137:337–341.

de Louvois, J. 1993a. *Salmonella* contamination of eggs: a potential source of human salmonellosis: a report of the Public Health Laboratory Service survey of imported and home-produced egg. PHLS Microbiol. Digest 10:158–162.

de Louvois, J. 1993b. *Salmonella* contamination of eggs. Lancet 2:366–367.

de Louvois, J. 1994. *Salmonella* contamination of stored hens eggs. PHLS Microbiol. Digest 11:203–205.

Dickson, J.S., and Koohmaraie, M. 1989. Cell surface charge characteristics and their relationship to bacterial attachment to meat surfaces. Appl. Environ. Microbiol. 55:832–836.

Dolman, J., and Board, R.G. 1992. The influence of temperature on the behaviour of mixed bacterial contamination of the shell membrane of hens' eggs. Epidemiol. Infect. 108:115–121.

Fehlhaber, K., and Braun, P. 1993. Untersuchungen zum Eindringen von *Salmonella enteritidis* aus dem Eiklar in das Dotter von Hühnereiern und zur Hitzeinaktivierung beim Kochen und Braten. Arch. Lebensmittelhyg. 44:57–80.

Forsythe, R.H., Ross, W.J., and Ayres, J.C. 1967. Salmonellae recovery following gastro-intestinal and ovarian inoculation in the domestic fowl. Poult. Sci. 46:849–855.

Gast, R.K., and Beard, C.W. 1990. Isolation of *Salmonella enteritidis* from internal organs of experimentally infected hens. Avian Dis. 34:991–993.

Gast, R.K., and Beard, C.W. 1992. Detection and enumeration of *Salmonella enteritidis* in fresh and stored eggs laid by experimentally infected hens. J. Food Prot. 55:152–156.

Hammack, T.S., Sherrod, P.S., Verneal, R., Bruce, G.A., Satchell, F.B., and Andrews, W.H. 1993. Growth of *Salmonella enteritidis* in grade A eggs during prolonged storage. Poult. Sci. 72:373–377.

Hoop, R.K., and Pospischil, A. 1993. Bacteriological, serological, histological and immuno-histochemical findings in laying hens with naturally acquired *Salmonella enteritidis* phage type 4 infection. Vet. Rec. 133:391–393.

Humphrey, T.J. 1991. Food poisoning: a change in patterns? Vet. Annu. 31:32–37.

Humphrey, T.J., Baskerville, A., Chart, H., and Rowe, B. 1989a. Infection of egg-laying hens with *Salmonella enteritidis* by oral inoculation. Vet. Rec. 125:531–532.

Humphrey, T.J., Baskerville, A., Chart, H., Rowe, B., and Whitehead, A. 1992. Infection of laying hens with *Salmonella enteritidis* PT4 by conjunctival challenge. Vet. Rec. 131:386–388.

Humphrey, T.J., Baskerville, A., Chart, H., Rowe, B., and Whitehead, A. 1991a. *Salmonella enteritidis* PT4 infection in specific pathogen-free hens: influence of infecting dose. Vet. Rec. 129:482–485.

Humphrey, T.J., Baskerville, A., Mawer, S.L., Rowe, B., and Hopper, S. 1989b. *Salmonella enteritidis* PT4 from the contents of intact eggs: a study involving naturally infected hens. Epidemiol. Infect. 103:415–423.

Humphrey, T.J., Baskerville, A., Whitehead, A., Rowe, B., and Henley, A. 1993. Influence of feeding patterns on the artificial infection of laying hens with *Salmonella enteritidis* phage type 4. Vet. Rec. 132:407–409.

Humphrey, T.J., Chart, H., Baskerville, A., and Rowe, B. 1991b. The influence of age on the response of SPF hens to infection with *Salmonella enteritidis* PT4. Epidemiol. Infect. 106:33–43.

Humphrey, T.J., Cruickshank, J.G., and Rowe, B. 1989c. *Salmonella enteritidis* PT4 and hens' eggs. Lancet 1:281.

Humphrey, T.J., and Lanning, D.G. 1987. *Salmonella* and *Campylobacter* contamination of broiler chickens and scald water: the influence of water pH. J. Appl. Bacteriol. 63:21–25.

Humphrey, T.J., Greenwood, M., Gilbert, R.J., Rowe, B., and Chapman, P.A. 1989d. The survival of salmonellas in shell eggs cooked under simulated domestic conditions. Epidemiol. Infect. 103:35–45.

Humphrey, T.J., and Whitehead, A. 1992. Techniques for the isolation of salmonellas from eggs. Br. Poult. Sci. 33:761–768.

Humphrey, T.J., and Whitehead, A. 1993. Egg age and the growth of *Salmonella enteritidis* in egg contents. Epidemiol. Infect. 111:209–219.

Humphrey, T.J., Whitehead, A., Gawler, A.H.L., Henley, A., and Rowe, B. 1991c. Numbers of *Salmonella enteritidis* in the contents of naturally contaminated hens' eggs. Epidemiol. Infect. 106:489–496.

Humphrey, T.J., Wilde, S.J., and Rowbury, R.J. 1997. Heat tolerance of *Salmonella typhimurium* DT104 isolates attached to muscle tissue. Lett. Appl. Microbiol. 25:265–268.

Humphrey, T.J., Williams, A., McAlpine, K., Lever, S., Guard-Petter, J., and Cox, J.M. 1996. Isolates of *Salmonella enterica* Enteritidis PT4 with enhanced heat and acid tolerance are more virulent in mice and more invasive in chickens. Epidemiol. Infect. 117:79–88.

Keller, L.H., Benson, C.E., Krotec, K., and Eckroade, R.J. 1995. *Salmonella enteritidis* colonisation of the reproductive tract and forming and freshly laid eggs of chickens. Infect. Immun. 63:2443–2449.

Lancaster, J.E., and Crabb, W.E. 1953. Studies on disinfection of eggs and incubators. Br. Vet. J. 109:139–148.

Lillard, H.S. 1973. Contamination of blood system and edible parts of poultry with *Clostridium perfringens* during water scalding. J. Food Sci. 38:151–154.

Lister, S.A. 1988. *Salmonella enteritidis* infection in broilers and broiler breeders. Vet. Rec. 123:350.

Lock, J.L., and Board, R.G. 1992. Persistence of contamination of hens' egg albumen in vitro with *Salmonella* serotypes. Epidemiol. Infect. 108:389–396.

Mawer, S.L., Spain, G.E., and Rowe, B. 1989. *Salmonella enteritidis* phage type 4 and hens' eggs. Lancet 1:280–281.

Mead, G.C. 1989. Hygiene problems and control of process contamination. In: Mead, G.C., ed. Processing of poultry. London: Elsevier, pp. 183–220.

Padron, M. 1990. *Salmonella typhimurium* penetration through the eggshell of hatching eggs. Avian Dis. 34:463–465.

Paul, J., and Batchelor, B. 1988. *Salmonella enteritidis* phage type 4 and hens' eggs. Lancet 2:1421.

Perales, I., and Audicana, A. 1989. The role of hens' eggs in outbreaks of salmonellosis in north Spain. Int. J. Food Microbiol. 8:175–180.

Petter, J.G. 1993. Detection of two smooth colony phenotypes in a *Salmonella enteritidis* isolate which vary in their ability to contaminate eggs. Appl. Environ. Microbiol. 59:2884–2890.

Poppe, C., Irwin, R.J., Forsberg, C.M., Clark, R.C., and Oggel, J. 1991. The prevalence of *Salmonella enteritidis* and other *Salmonella* spp. among Canadian registered commercial layer flocks. Epidemiol. Infect. 106:259–270.

Rampling, A., Anderson, J.R., Upson, R., Peters, E., Ward, L., and Rowe, B. 1989. *Salmonella enteritidis* phage type 4 infection of broiler chickens: a hazard to public health. Lancet 2:436–438.

Rizk, S.S., Ayres, J.C., and Craft, A.A. 1966. Effect of holding condition on the development of salmonellae in artificially inoculated hens' eggs. Poult. Sci. 45:823–829.

Roberts, D. 1986. Factors contributing to outbreaks of foodborne infection and intoxication in England and Wales 1970–1982. In: Proceedings of the second world congress of foodborne infections and intoxications, vol. 1. Berlin: Institute of Veterinary Medicine/Robert von Ostertag Institute, pp. 157–158.

Rodrigue, D.C., Tauxe, R.V., and Rowe, B. 1990. International increase in *Salmonella enteritidis*: a new pandemic? Epidemiol. Infect. 105:21–27.

Schoeni, J.L., Glass, K.A., McDermott, J.L., and Wong, A.C.L. 1995. Growth and penetration of *Salmonella enteritidis*, *Salmonella heidelberg* and *Salmonella typhimurium* in eggs. Int. J. Food Microbiol. 24:385–396.

Scott, W.M. 1930. Food poisoning due to eggs. BMJ 11:56–58.

Snoeyenbos, G.H., Smyser, C.F., and van Roekel, H. 1969. *Salmonella* infections of the ovary and peritoneum of chickens. Avian Dis. 13:668–670.

Solowey, M., Spaulding, E.H., and Goresline, H.E. 1946. An investigation of a source and mode of entry of *Salmonella* organisms in spray-dried whole egg powder. Food Res. 5:380–390.

Sparks, N.H.C., and Board, R.G. 1985. Bacterial penetration of the recently oviposited shell of hens' eggs. Aust. Vet. J. 62:169–170.

St. Louis, M.E., Morse, D.L., Potter, M.E., DeMelfi, T.M., Guzewich, J.J., Tauxe, R.V., Blake, P.A., and the *Salmonella enteritidis* Working Group. 1988. The emergence of grade A eggs as a major source of *Salmonella enteritidis* infection. JAMA 259:2102–2107.

Stokes, J.L., Osborne, W.W., and Bayne, H.G. 1956. Penetration and growth of *Salmonella* in shell eggs. Food Res. 21:510–518.

Thiagarajan, D., Saeed, A.M., and Asem, E.K. 1994. Mechanism of transovarian transmission of *Salmonella enteritidis* in laying hens. Poult. Sci. 73:89–98.

Timoney, J.F., Shivaprasad, H.L., Baker, R.C., and Rowe, B. 1989. Egg transmission after infection of hens with *Salmonella enteritidis* phage type 4. Vet. Rec. 125:600–601.

Vadehra, D.V., Baker, R.C., and Naylor, H.B. 1969. *Salmonella* infection of cracked eggs. Poult. Sci. 48:954–957.

Vugia, D.J., Bishu, B., Smith, M., Tavris, D.R., Hickman-Brenner, F.W., and Tauxe, R.V. 1993. *Salmonella enteritidis* outbreak in a restaurant chain: the continuing challenges of prevention. Epidemiol. Infect. 110:49–61.

Wall, P.G., Morgan, D., Lamden, K., et al. 1994. A case control study of infection with an epidemic strain of multiresistant *Salmonella typhimurium* DT104 in England and Wales. Communicable Dis. Rep. Rev. 4:R130.

Williams, J.E. 1981. Salmonellae in poultry foods: a worldwide review. Part 1. Worlds Poult. Sci. J. 37:16–19.

19

Mechanism of Transovarian Transmission of *Salmonella enterica* Serovar Enteritidis in Laying Hens

A.M. Saeed, D. Thiagarajan, and E. Asem

INTRODUCTION

During the last decade, *Salmonella enterica* serovar Enteritidis (*S.* Enteritidis) became a major cause of food poisoning (Coyle et al., 1988; Lin et al., 1988; St. Louis et al., 1988; Cowden et al., 1989a,b). Grade-A shell eggs contaminated with *S.* Enteritidis have been implicated as an important cause of such foodborne infections in the United States [Centers for Disease Control (CDC), 1988, 1990; St. Louis et al., 1988; Hedberg et al., 1993] and throughout the world (Cowden et al., 1989a; Rodrigue et al., 1990; Altekruse and Swerdlow, 1996). Adult laying hens infected with *S.* Enteritidis may carry the organism in their large intestines and shed it in their feces, which may lead to contamination of the eggshell surface. Penetration of the eggshell by the organism during storage abuse will lead to contamination of the egg contents (Coyle et al., 1988). Alternatively, contamination of the laid egg may occur in vivo through the dissemination of the organism to the ovaries following localization and colonization of the large intestine by *S.* Enteritidis, that is, by transovarian transmission (Anon., 1989; Timoney et al., 1989; Shivaprasad et al., 1990). This view has gained a lot of acceptance because (a) contamination is unlikely to occur through properly sanitized grade-A shell eggs, and (b) *S.* Enteritidis can be isolated from the ovaries and other internal organs of experimentally inoculated adult laying hens (CDC, 1990; Gast and Beard, 1990a,b, 1992). Ovarian infections of *S.* Enteritidis will result not only in the laying of contaminated eggs but also infected chicks hatched from the contaminated eggs. These infected chicks will grow up to become pullets and subsequently lay contaminated eggs (Hopper and Mawer, 1988; Lister, 1988; O'Brien, 1988). A preovulatory follicle consists of a central yolk mass surrounded by a perivitelline layer, a granulosa cell layer, a basement membrane, and the thecal cell layers in that order from inside out. The mechanism(s) by which transovarian transmission occurs is not known. The possibility remains that *S.* Enteritidis invades and passes through the walls of the follicle and enters the yolk. Alternatively, *S.* Enteritidis attaches to certain components of the follicular wall that enables it to be carried into the oviduct following ovulation. For transovarian transmission to occur, the bacteria have to interact with the cellular component(s) of the preovulatory follicle of the chicken. The aim of the present study was to describe the interaction of *S.* Enteritidis with the laying hen's ovary and determine the growth stage of the preovulatory follicles that interact with *S.* Enteritidis. Additionally, the in vitro attachment patterns of different phage types of *S.* Enteritidis to ovarian granulosa cells and the role of adhesive proteins in the attachment process were examined.

MATERIALS AND METHODS

Animals

Single-comb white leghorn hens in their first year of reproductive activity were obtained from a local farm known by serological testing to be free of S. Enteritidis infections. The birds were housed in individual cages in a windowless, air-conditioned room with a 14 h light–10 h dark cycle. They had unlimited access to a commercial layer ration and tap water.

Bacteria

A total of 83 S. Enteritidis isolates serotyped and phage typed at the National Veterinary Laboratory Services (Ames, IA) were used to study the attachment to granulosa and HEp-2 cells. The sources and phage types of the S. Enteritidis isolates are listed in Table 19.1. The isolates were maintained in tryptic soy agar slants at room temperature. The organisms were grown overnight in brain-heart infusion broth (BHI) with or without 1% D-mannose in static, aerated cultures at 37°C. For quantitative attachment assay, an S. Enteritidis phage type 8 (PT8) strain (AE9) was used. The organism was radiolabeled by growing in colonization-factor broth containing 80 mCi of ^{14}C in the form of sodium acetate. The specific unit of radioactivity per colony-forming unit (CFU) was established at $1 \times$ to 2×10^2 cpm.

Experimental Infection of Laying Hens with *Salmonella* Enteritidis Phage Type 8 Isolates

A total of 140 laying hens were divided into four random groups and orally inoculated with four different isolates of S. Enteritidis by using the procedure of Lindell et al. (1994). Five randomly selected birds from each group were killed at weekly intervals by placement into a CO_2 chamber before cervical dislocation. The largest (F1, 30–35 mm in diameter), second largest (F2, 15–20 mm in diameter), and third largest (F3, 6–15 mm in diameter) preovulatory follicles (Fig. 19.1, Plate I) were removed aseptically and placed in ice-cold Hanks' balanced salt solution (HBSS). The follicles were classified according to the criteria of Robinson and Etches (1986). The follicles were punctured with a sterile pair of scissors, and the yolk was allowed to fall into a sterile, plastic bag. The follicular wall (granulosa and thecal layers) was collected in a separate sterile, plastic bag. Tetrathionate broth

(20 ml) was added to the bags, and the contents were minced using a laboratory blender. After incubation at 37°C for 18–24 h, a loopful of the contents was streaked on to xylose-lysine-tergitol 4 (XLT4) agar plates (Miller and Tate, 1991), which were then incubated for 24–48 h at 37°C, and salmonella-like colonies were picked and transferred to triple-sugar iron-agar slants. These colonies were subsequently identified as S. Enteritidis by standard serological and biochemical tests (Edwards and Ewing, 1986). Throughout the infectivity trial, eggs were collected daily, and each shell surface was sanitized immediately with Betadine (povidone-iodine) diluted 1:3 with 70% ethanol. The eggs were cracked open, and the egg white and yolk were collected in separate, sterile plastic bags and cultured for isolation of S. Enteritidis, as in the case of preovulatory follicles.

Chemicals

Cell culture medium 199 (M199) containing Hanks' salts, fetal calf serum, and HBSS were obtained from Gibco (Gaithersburg, MD). Minimum essential medium, collagenase, and fibronectin inhibitory factor (Arg-Gly-Asp-Ser) were from Sigma Chemical Company (St. Louis, MO). BHI was purchased from Difco (Detroit, MI). Electrophoretic reagents were obtained from AT Biochem (Malvern, PA). Anti-chicken fibronectin antiserum raised in rabbit was obtained from Chemicon International (Temecula, CA). This antiserum blocks cell adhesion to fibronectin (Yamada, 1983). The synthetic peptide Arg-Gly-Asp-Ser (RGDS) and bovine plasma fibronectin were obtained from Sigma. M199 and the oligopeptides Gly-Arg-Gly-Asp-Asn-Pro (GRGD) and Gly-Arg-Ala-Asp-Ser-Pro (GRAD) were from Life Technologies (Gaithersburg).

Isolation of Hen Ovarian Granulosa Cells

Granulosa layers of the F1, F2, and F3 preovulatory follicles were separated from the thecal layer as previously described by Gilbert et al. (1977), and the cells were dissociated in collagenase containing M199 (Novero and Asem, 1993a). Cell viability, determined by the trypan-blue exclusion method, was routinely greater than 95%. The dispersed cells were suspended in M199 supplemented with 5% fetal calf serum and 100 U/ml penicillin G and 100 mg/ml of streptomycin sulfate. Ovarian granulosa were grown overnight at 37°C under 5% CO_2 atmosphere in 24-well or 96-well tissue culture plates.

TABLE 19.1   Phage types and sources of *Salmonella* Enteritidis isolates used in this study

S. Enteritidis phage type	Source
8 (n = 47)	Chicken ceca and other organs, egg yolk, and environment
23 (n = 13)	Chicken ceca, egg yolk, and environment
28 (n = 6)	Egg yolk
13 (n = 5)	Chicken ceca and environment
Untypeable (n = 12)	Egg yolk

In Vitro Attachment Assays to Granulosa Cells

Salmonella Enteritidis PT8 strain (AE9) labeled with ^{14}C was added at a density of 2×10^7 CFU/ml. In all of the in vitro attachment assays described below, radiolabeled bacteria were added to tissue culture wells without granulosa cells, and the recovered radioactivity after 1 h of incubation at 37°C (background) was subtracted from the test wells. For inhibition of attachment using antifibronectin antibodies, granulosa cells were incubated for 30 min at 37°C with various dilutions of antiserum before addition of radiolabeled bacteria. Control wells were incubated with 0.01% (wt/vol) of bovine gamma globulin. Each dilution was tested in triplicate, and the experiment was repeated three times. Following incubation with bacteria for 1 h at 37°C, the wells were washed three times with HBSS, and the granulosa cells along with the attached bacteria were removed by using 100 μl of 0.02 N NaOH. The mixture from each well was taken in separate scintillation vials (Ecolite, ICN Pharmaceuticals, Costa Mesa, CA), and the radioactivity was measured in a Beckman scintillation counter (Fullerton, CA). Radioactivity obtained from test wells was expressed as percentage of controls for each dilution of antibody tested.

In the case of inhibition experiments using 14-kDa fimbrial protein, the granulosa cells were incubated with various concentrations of the protein (0, 2.5, 5, 10, and 20 μg/well) for 1 h at 37°C before radiolabeled bacteria were added. Control wells were incubated with M199 containing 0.1% (wt/vol) of bovine serum albumin (BSA). The attachment inhibition was measured as previously described.

For attachment assays involving synthetic peptides, various concentrations of the peptides (500, 250, and 125 μg/ml) were incubated end over end with 2×10^7 CFU bacteria/ml for 1 h at room temperature in the presence of 0.01% (vol/vol) Tween 80 before the granulosa cells were inoculated. Bacterial suspensions for control wells were incubated with 0.1% BSA in M199 or 0.01% (vol/vol) Tween 80 (polysorbate) in M199. Concentrations for each peptide (RGD, GRGD, and GRAD) were tested in triplicate. The attachment inhibition was measured as just described. The experiments were repeated three times, and the radioactivity recovered from each test well was expressed as percentage of control.

Invasion of Granulosa Cells by *Salmonella* Enteritidis

Invasion experiments were carried out essentially as described before (Mehlman et al., 1977). Chicken ovarian granulosa cells were grown on glass coverslips in 24-well tissue culture plates at a concentration of 5×10^5 cells/ml. The cells were inoculated with 2×10^7 CFU/ml of *S.* Enteritidis strain AE9 grown overnight in BHI broth under static, aerated conditions. After 2 h incubation at 37°C the cells were washed once with M199, and intracellular growth medium consisting of M199, 2% fetal bovine serum, and 100 μg/ml of gentamicin was added. Following incubation at 37°C, the medium was replaced every hour with intracellular growth medium containing 10 μg/ml of gentamicin to suppress extracellular multiplication of bacteria. Coverslips were removed for examination after 3 h of incubation at 37°C. The coverslips were washed five times with phosphate-buffered saline (PBS). For light-microscopic observations, the coverslips were fixed with methanol and stained with 10% Giemsa. For electron-microscopic observations, the cover slips were fixed with phosphate-buffered 3% glutaraldehyde.

Purification of 14-kDa Fimbrial Protein

The 14-kDa fimbrial protein was purified from *S.* Enteritidis as described previously (Feutrier et al., 1986).

Protein Determination

Protein determinations were done using the bicinchoninic acid (BCA) method (Pierce Chemical Company, Rockford, IL). BSA was used as the standard protein.

SDS-PAGE Gels for Separation of Proteins

To analyze fimbrial protein preparations, a 16×14 vertical slab gel system was used. A gel slab consisted of 4.5% stacking gel and 15% separation gel. Electrophoresis was performed according to the method of Laemmli (1970). The molecular weight of the fimbrial protein was estimated by plotting a standard curve based on migration distances of the marker proteins (Chart, 1994).

Electron Microscopy

The coverslips were further fixed with 1% osmium tetroxide–1.5% potassium ferrocyanide, dehydrated by passing through graded ethanol and rinsed twice in propylene oxide before being embedded in epoxy resin. The glass coverslip was removed either by heat or by treatment with hydrofluoric acid. Thin sections were stained with uranyl acetate and lead citrate and viewed in a Jeol JEM-100 CX electron microscope.

Immunohistochemical Identification of *Salmonella* Enteritidis in Tissues of Experimentally Infected Hens

For immunohistochemical identification, thin sections were obtained from paraffin-embedded ovarian and cecal tissue samples. The sections were passed through xylene and graded ethanol before they were immersed in PBS containing 0.5% gelatin. The primary antibody was a monoclonal antibody used for detection of *S.* Enteritidis (a generous gift from Dr. Richard Goldspy, Department of Animal Science, University of Massachusetts, Amherst). The tissue sections were incubated with primary antibody for 1 h, immersed in PBS for 5 min to wash away unbound antibody, and secondary antibody from goat–anti-mouse immunoglobulin

G conjugated with peroxidase enzyme was added. Specific antibody binding was detected by using a color development solution containing 3-diaminobenzidine as the substrate. Hematoxylin was used for background staining of the tissue sections, which were then mounted using a water-based mounting solution and observed with a light microscope.

Statistical Analysis

The differences between the number of isolates showing positive attachment on HEp-2 cells and granulosa cells were compared using a χ^2 contingency table (Fleiss, 1981).

RESULTS

Isolation of *Salmonella* Enteritidis from the Preovulatory Follicle Membranes during Experimental Infection of Layer Birds

After experimental infection of laying hens with *S.* Enteritidis, the organisms were isolated, at weekly intervals, from the preovulatory follicle wall and yolk for up to 35 days. The yolk and follicle wall were cultured separately, and *S.* Enteritidis was isolated from the follicle wall alone in 10 (7.14%) of 140 birds tested, whereas *S.* Enteritidis was isolated from the preovulatory follicle yolk in four (2.86%) of 140 birds tested ($p < 0.05$). In addition, *S.* Enteritidis was isolated mostly from the yolk but not the white of 13 eggs laid by experimentally infected hens and positively cultured for *S.* Enteritidis (Table 19.2).

Attachment Patterns of *Salmonella* Enteritidis on Granulosa Cells

Three different attachment patterns (local, diffuse, and aggregative) (Nataro et al., 1987) were observed with different isolates of *S.* Enteritidis belonging to the various phage types that were used in this study. The local attachment was seen as a cluster or a microcolony of organisms at one end of the cell (Fig. 19.2A, Plate II). The diffuse attachment was seen as the cell surface was mostly covered by the attaching bacteria (Fig. 19.2B, Plate II), whereas the aggregative type of attachment was seen as bacteria around the periphery of the cells as well as between the cells (Fig. 19.2C, Plate III). The mannose-resistant local attachment was the predominant pattern observed for the *S.* Enteritidis isolates tested: 56.6% of the isolates tested demonstrated this pattern (Table 19.3). Of the PT8 isolates, 15% demonstrated mannose-resistant diffuse attachment, as did 8% of PT23. The mannose-resistant aggregative attachment pattern was observed with 4% of PT8 and 31% of PT23 (Table 19.4). Of the isolates belonging to the untypeable category, 25% also showed mannose-resistant aggregative attachment on granulosa cells. The different patterns of attachment shown by *S.* Enteritidis on granulosa cells and HEp-2 cells were compared for each phage type by using χ^2 analyses. A significantly higher number of *S.* Enteritidis PT8 isolates showed mannose-resistant local attachment on

granulosa cells than on HEp-2 cells ($p < 0.05$) (Table 19.2). None of the *S.* Enteritidis isolates tested demonstrated diffuse or aggregative attachment on HEp-2 cells. The total number of *S.* Enteritidis isolates that demonstrated any pattern of attachment on granulosa cells was significantly higher than on HEp-2 cells ($p < 0.00005$).

To determine the influence of stage of follicular maturation on the *S.* Enteritidis attachment pattern, granulosa cells isolated from three different developmental stages—F1, F2, and F3 (Fig. 19.1, Plate I)—were used in a separate set of experiments. Attachment assays were conducted using several *S.* Enteritidis isolates of PT8, and the results were compared for each isolate on granulosa cells obtained from F1, F2, and F3 follicles. Similar attachment patterns were demonstrated by the *S.* Enteritidis isolates on granulosa cells derived from F1, F2, and F3 follicles.

Attachment Patterns of *Salmonella* Enteritidis on HEp-2 Cells

When attachment assays were done using HEp-2 cells, only a local attachment pattern was observed (Fig. 19.2A, Plate II). Except for PT13, *S.* Enteritidis isolates belonging to the other phage types showed mannose-resistant local attachment in varying proportions (Table 19.2), including several isolates belonging to the untypeable category. Of the PT8 isolates, 4% demonstrated local attachment only in the absence of 1% mannose, and hence they were classified as isolates possessing a mannose-sensitive local attachment pattern.

Purification of 14-kDa Fimbrial Protein and Amino Acid Composition Analysis

The purified fimbrial protein preparation showed a single protein band in SDS-PAGE gel, with an approximate molecular weight of 14,000 Daltons. The amino acid composition analysis was similar to the one reported earlier (Feutrier et al., 1986), with differences in the percentage of some amino acids. The estimated molecular weight based on the amino acid composition analysis was 14,400 Daltons.

Inhibition of *Salmonella* Enteritidis Attachment to Granulosa Cells

The attachment of *S.* Enteritidis to granulosa cells could be inhibited by preincubation of the cells with anti-chicken fibronectin antiserum. Preincubation of granulosa cells with 1/10 dilution of the antiserum resulted in nearly 80% inhibition of *S.* Enteritidis attachment compared with control wells in which cells were preincubated with 0.01% bovine gamma globulin (Fig. 19.3). Higher dilutions of the antiserum resulted in reduction in the inhibition of attachment. At the highest dilution tested in this study (1/10,000), nearly 20% inhibition of attachment was observed.

The purified fimbrial protein (14 kDa) was also used to inhibit the attachment of *S.* Enteritidis to granulosa cells by preincubation of the granulosa cells with various

TABLE 19.2 Distribution of *Salmonella* Enteritidis in the preovulatory follicles and eggs of experimentally infected chickens

S. Enteritidis phage type	Preovulatory follicle (n = 14)[b]			Laid eggs (n = 11)[c]		
	Membrane[a]	Yolk[a]	p[d]	Yolk[a]	White[a]	p[d]
8	8 (57.0)	3 (21.0)		7 (64.0)	3 (27.0)	
28	2 (14.0)	1 (7.0)		1 (9.0)	0	
Total	10 (71.0)	4 (28.0)	0.057	8 (72.0)	3 (27.0)	0.086

[a]Number positive (percentage).
[b]S. Enteritidis was isolated from both follicle membrane and yolk in an additional two birds.
[c]S. Enteritidis was isolated from both egg yolk and white in one additional bird.
[d]Fisher's exact two-tailed test.

TABLE 19.3 Number of *Salmonella* Enteritidis isolates of different phage types that demonstrated mannose-resistant local attachment on HEp-2 cells and hen ovarian granulosa cells

S. Enteritidis phage type	HEp-2 cells[a]	Granulosa cells[a]	χ^2 value (df = 1)	p
8 (n = 47)	20 (43)	29 (62)	3.45	0.0631
23 (n = 13)	4 (31)	7 (61)	1.41	0.2337
28 (n = 6)	2 (33)	1 (17)	0.44	0.5049
13 (n = 5)	0	4 (80)	5.38	0.0202
Untypeable (n = 12)	6 (50)	6 (50)	0	1.0000
Total (n = 83)	32 (39)	47 (57)	5.43	0.0197

[a]Number positive (percentage).

TABLE 19.4 Number of *Salmonella* Enteritidis isolates that demonstrated mannose-resistant diffuse attachment and mannose-resistant aggregative attachment on hen granulosa cells

S. Enteritidis phage type	Mannose-resistant diffuse attachment[a]	Mannose-resistant aggregative attachment[a]
8 (n = 47)	7 (15)	2 (4)
23 (n = 13)	1 (8)	4 (31)
28 (n = 6)	0	0
13 (n = 5)	0	0
Untypeable (n = 12)	0	3 (25)
Total (n = 83)	8 (10)	9 (11)

[a]Number positive (percentage).

concentrations of the fimbrial protein. When granulosa cells were preincubated with 20 µg of fimbrial protein, the radioactivity recovered from the test wells indicated an approximate 70% inhibition of attachment (Fig. 19.4).

Solid-Phase Protein Binding by *Salmonella* Enteritidis

To determine differences in the binding of S. Enteritidis to various extracellular matrix proteins, the binding of the organism to fibronectin, laminin, and collagen IV that were used to coat 96-well tissue culture wells was examined. The binding was greater with fibronectin at all concentrations tested (Fig. 19.5). The affinity of S. Enteritidis strain AE9 to the matrix proteins can be ranked as fibronectin > laminin > collagen IV.

Immunohistochemistry

Salmonella Enteritidis was identified by the monoclonal antibody and peroxidase-antiperoxidase technique along the villous border and, in some instances, in the submucosa (Fig. 19.6, Plate IV). In tissue sections obtained from preovulatory follicles of infected hens, rod-shaped organisms were apparent in the central yolk mass and also along the perivitelline membrane (Fig. 19.7, Plate IV). Bacteriological culture of these membranes yielded the same strain of S. Enteritidis that was used in the experimental infection of the laying hens.

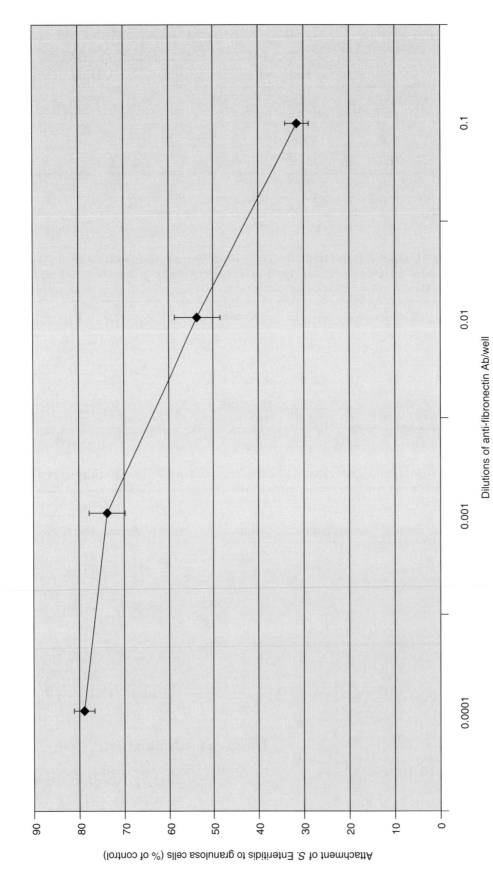

FIGURE 19.3 Inhibition of in vitro attachment of *Salmonella* Enteritidis to chicken ovarian granulosa cells, using rabbit anti-chicken fibronectin antibody (Ab).

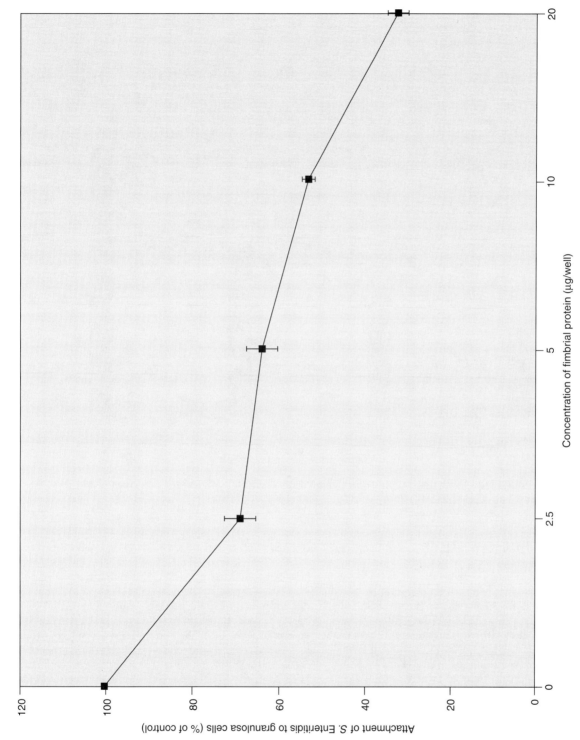

FIGURE 19.4 Inhibition of in vitro attachment of *Salmonella* Enteritidis to chicken ovarian granulosa cells, using a 14-kDa fimbrial protein isolated from strain AE9.

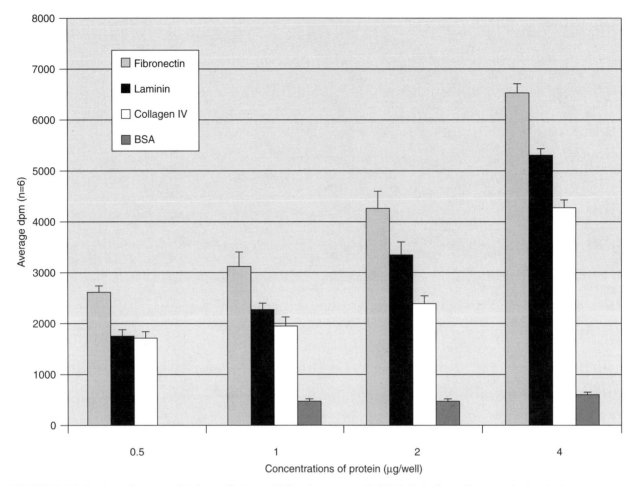

FIGURE 19.5   Attachment of *Salmonella* Enteritidis phage type 8 (^{14}C-labeled) to fibronectin-laminin-mouse-collagen IV- and bovine-serum-albumin-coated ELISA plates.

Invasion of Granulosa Cells by *Salmonella* Enteritidis

Microscopic examination of Giemsa-stained granulosa cell preparation revealed that the salmonella organisms invaded the cells and some multiplication inside the cells may be apparent (Fig. 19.2D, Plate III). In transmission electron micrographs, the organisms can be seen surrounded by a membrane and as free organisms as well (Fig. 19.8A). In some micrographs, a microcolony of bacteria with dividing bacterial cells can be seen, indicating that the organism is capable of multiplying with in the granulosa cells (Fig. 19.8B).

DISCUSSION

The dynamics of *S.* Enteritidis dissemination within the host body is not clear at present, although existing evidence points to transport of the organisms in macrophages from the gut (Popiel and Turnbull, 1985). During experimental infections of layer birds with *S.* Enteritidis, organisms were

isolated from the ovaries and from egg yolks (Shivaprasad et al., 1990; Barrow and Lovell, 1991). Previous reports have suggested the possibility of contamination of yolk in vivo either through a hematogenous spread or colonization of peritoneum by the organism (Timoney et al., 1989; Shivaprasad et al., 1990). In the present study, after oral inoculations of layer birds, *S.* Enteritidis were isolated from the membranes of the preovulatory follicles during the first few weeks of infection. The fact that *S.* Enteritidis could be isolated from the follicular wall but not from the yolk in the majority of the cultured follicles of the infected hens may indicate that the organism interacts with a cellular component of these follicles. Gast and Beard (1990a,b, 1992) reported that *S.* Enteritidis could be isolated from egg yolk membranes but not from the yolk of eggs laid by experimentally infected hens. It is conceivable that after transovarian transmission the *S.* Enteritidis organisms remain attached to the egg-yolk membranes and could most frequently be isolated from this part of the egg. Isolates of *S.* Enteritidis representing the major phage types obtained from human and animal sources were tested for their attachment on hen ovarian granulosa cells. The attachment

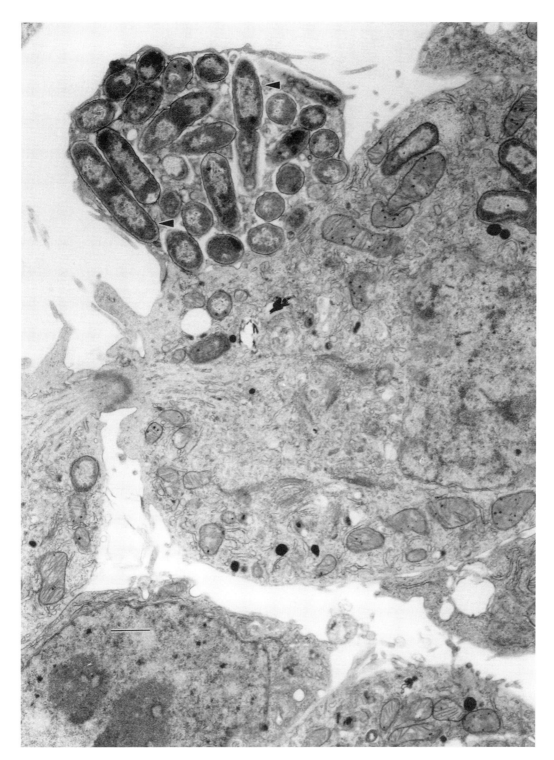

FIGURE 19.8A   Transmission electron micrographs of granulosa cells invaded by *Salmonella* Enteritidis. Organisms found within the cytoplasm of the granulosa cells (*arrowheads*) 5 h after inoculation. Bar = 1 μ.

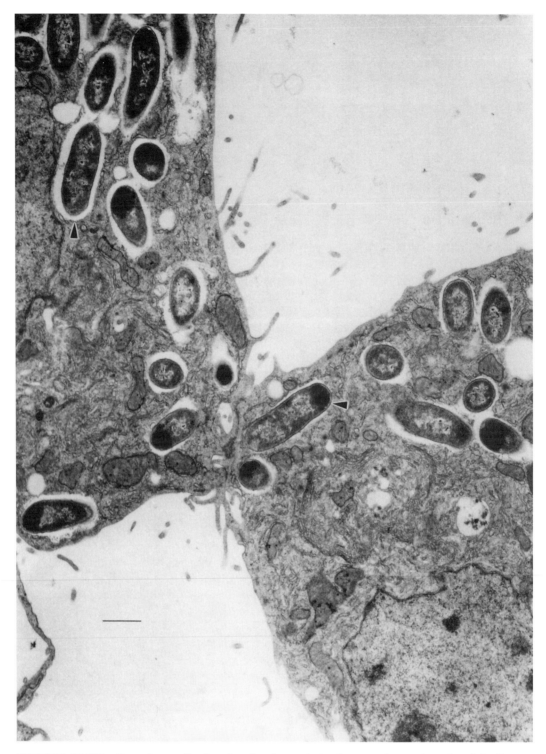

FIGURE 19.8B Granulosa cells showing free bacteria in the cytoplasm. *Arrowheads* indicate the halo surrounding the bacteria. Bar = 1 μ.

of these isolates to HEp-2 cells was also studied in order to compare the attachment patterns obtained with the granulosa cell system. *Salmonella* Enteritidis of various phage types demonstrated local, diffuse, and aggregative patterns of attachment to hen ovarian granulosa cells.

Attachment of a microbial pathogen to its host cell surface is the first step during the pathogenesis of many bacterial diseases (Finlay and Falkow, 1989; Gomes et al., 1989; Knutton et al., 1992). Enteropathogenic *Escherichia coli* in human beings have been classified according to their patterns of attachment to HEp-2 cells and HeLa cells (Cravioto et al., 1979; Nataro et al., 1985; Gomes et al., 1989). These attachment patterns are mediated by distinct fimbrial structures on the bacterial surface and are coded by genes on plasmids or on the chromosome (Nataro et al., 1985; Gomes et al., 1989).

There was no relationship between any specific pattern of attachment on the granulosa cells and the phage types of the *S.* Enteritidis strains tested. This interpretation is supported by the fact that *S.* Enteritidis isolates that did not belong to any phage type (untypeable) demonstrated mannose-resistant local attachment on both HEp-2 cells and granulosa cells. In this regard, attachment patterns can be used to classify *S.* Enteritidis isolates that were obtained from various sources. *Salmonella* Enteritidis strains screened for attachment on granulosa cells obtained from F1, F2, and F3 follicles demonstrated similar patterns on all of these cells. It is conceivable that the granulosa cells isolated from these three developmental stages carry certain structures on their surface that mediate the attachment of *S.* Enteritidis during ovarian infection with these organisms. When HEp-2 cells were used in attachment assays, only local attachment patterns were recorded with the *S.* Enteritidis isolates that were used in this study. Whether local attachment is the only attachment pattern that could be demonstrated on HEp-2 cells by *S.* Enteritidis or whether other attachment patterns are possible by testing larger number of isolates needs further investigation. The total number of *S.* Enteritidis that demonstrated any pattern of attachment was greater on the hen ovary granulosa cells than on the HEp-2 cells (p < 0.00005). Additionally, diffuse and aggregative patterns of attachment by *S.* Enteritidis were demonstrated only on granulosa cells. These findings may suggest that the hen ovary granulosa cells have a diversity of surface structures that mediate the expression of the different patterns of attachment by the salmonella strains. Data from this study support the value of using granulosa cells from hen ovary for more sensitive detection of attaching salmonella organisms. If a relationship is established between attachment patterns on the granulosa cells and the infectivity of the salmonella strains tested, this new test can be used to establish a new pathotypic system for salmonella strains that are isolated from different sources. The currently available phage-typing system is useful but is a cumbersome procedure that takes over a week to complete. Based on these results, it is conceivable that *S.* Enteritidis contaminates the yolk in vivo by invading the granulosa cells, residing at this site, and when the follicle ruptures during ovulation, some of the granulosa cells carrying the organism may slough off and contaminate the egg.

In certain instances, the attachment of bacteria to cells requires the presence of adhesive proteins, such as fibronectin, on cell surface. It has been shown that the interaction of a number of bacteria with tissue cells is mediated by peptide sequences that contain the arg-gly-asp (RGD) motif that is a part of the extracellular matrix of the cell (Pierschbacher and Ruoslahti, 1984a,b; Ruoslahti and Pierschbacher, 1986).

The phenomenon of transovarian transmission by *S.* Enteritidis is an intriguing aspect of the pathogenesis of this organism in chickens. The organism does not cause overt clinical infections in adult laying hens but leads to laying of contaminated eggs after oral inoculation (Gast and Beard, 1990b; Lindell et al., 1994). Invasion of intestinal walls by *S.* Enteritidis leads to systemic spread of the organism (Timoney et al., 1989; Gast and Beard, 1990a,b; Shivaprasad et al., 1990; Barrow and Lovell, 1991). Previous studies indicated that, after invasion of intestinal epithelial cells, *S.* Enteritidis were found in macrophages in the lamina propria (Popiel and Turnbull, 1985). The colonization of preovulatory follicles by bloodborne *S.* Enteritidis from the gut would possibly involve interactions with the cellular components in the follicular wall (Thiagarajan et al., 1994). The follicular membrane is a highly vascularized structure, with vessels of increased permeability (Griffin et al., 1984), and this anatomical feature may facilitate the transport of the organism from the blood to the developing follicle (Barrow and Lovell, 1991). In this study, it was possible to demonstrate the presence of the *S.* Enteritidis organisms stained with peroxidase-antiperoxidase *S.* Enteritidis-specific monoclonal antibody at the cecal tonsils. Bloodborne organisms may be deposited near the basement membrane itself, since many of the vessels terminate right beneath the membrane. From this locus, bacteria may penetrate the basement membrane and enter the yolk by invading the granulosa cells or by migrating between the cells. It has been reported that *S.* Enteritidis attaches to granulosa cells and that this may be one of the ways in which the egg may become contaminated in vivo (Thiagarajan et al., 1994). In that study, positive antibody binding was demonstrated along the villus border and, in some instances, in the submucosa (Fig. 19.6). Additionally, the *S.* Enteritidis organisms were demonstrated at the granulosa cell layer of the preovulatory follicles isolated from the experimentally infected birds (Fig. 19.7). The present study was conducted to identify some of the molecular components involved in the attachment of *S.* Enteritidis to granulosa cells.

The in vitro attachment of *S.* Enteritidis to chicken ovarian granulosa cells could be inhibited using anti-chicken fibronectin antiserum, indicating that fibronectin may be a major component in the attachment process. It has been shown that *S.* Enteritidis binds to fibronectin (Baloda, 1988) and that fibronectin binding may be involved in the *S.* Enteritidis attachment phenomenon observed in vitro (Baloda et al., 1988). The polyclonal antibody preparation used in this study recognizes fibronectin secreted by granulosa cells cultured in vitro, as evidenced by positive fluorescence when fluorescein-conjugated secondary antibody was used (data not shown). The anti-chicken fibronectin antiserum may recognize several different epitopes in the fibronectin molecule that are involved in the binding of *S.* Enteritidis to granulosa cells. In the present study, the inhibition may involve regions in the fibronectin molecule that contain the cell-binding domain, because the polyclonal antibody preparation used in this study is capable of blocking cell adhesion to fibronectin (Yamada, 1983). It is tempting to speculate that attachment of *S.* Enteritidis to granulosa cells may involve sites other than the cell-binding domain, because a higher degree of inhibition was achieved with fibronectin antiserum than with the RGD peptide (Figs. 19.4, 19.9). However, binding studies using proteolytic fragments of the fibronectin molecule would reveal the presence of other sites and their respective affinities.

To determine the significance of the cell-binding domain of the fibronectin molecule in the attachment process, the synthetic peptide RGD was used to inhibit the attachment of *S.* Enteritidis to granulosa cells. Two other peptides—GRGD and GRAD—were used as controls. GRGD is a strong inhibitor of fibronectin but a weak inhibitor of vitronectin (Pierschbacher and Ruoslahti, 1987). GRAD is an inactive control that does not block binding of fibroblasts to fibronectin (Pierschbacher and Ruoslahti, 1984b). It has been shown that RGD can abrogate attachment of *S.* Enteritidis to granulosa cells grown on coverslips (Thiagarajan et al., 1994). Using radioactively labeled bacteria, the present study has shown that RGD can inhibit *S.* Enteritidis attachment to granulosa cells at 500-µg/ml, 250-µg/ml, and 125-µg/ml concentrations. When the peptide GRGD was used, the pattern of inhibition was similar, suggesting that fibronectin was the major molecule involved in the attachment process. Although the amount of inhibition by GRGD at the 250-µg/ml concentration appears to be lower than that of RGD, the significance of this difference is questionable. In contrast, the inactive control GRAD did not have a significant role in the inhibition of attachment (about 10%–20% inhibition at both concentrations tested). At the maximum concentration tested in this study (500 µg/ml), both RGD and GRGD were effective in inhibiting 60% of *S.* Enteritidis strain AE9 attachment to granulosa cells. The factors that contribute to the rest of the attachment to the granulosa cells remain to be determined. Baloda et al. (1988) examined attachment of several strains of *S.* Enteritidis to human intestinal cells and concluded that attachment may involve binding of fibronectin. Additionally, they reported that some strains bound the 29-kDa amino-terminal fragment, whereas other strains did not. However, the latter class bound the whole fibronectin molecule, indicating that sites other than the those at the amino-terminal domain may also be involved in fibronectin binding (Baloda et al., 1988). The results of the present study indicated that the cell-binding domain alone can not account for the entire attachment activity.

Chicken ovarian granulosa cells have been shown to deposit fibronectin in vitro, and this deposition can be modulated by hormones (Ansem et al., 1992, 1994; Novero and Asem, 1993a,b). The expression of fibronectin seems to vary between different developmental stages of the follicles, with maximal expression appearing at the F1 (most mature) follicle stage. It is not clear at present as to how this may affect the in vivo interactions of *S.* Enteritidis with granulosa cells. However, it has been shown that granulosa cells are obtained from the three most developed follicular structures (F1, F2, and F3).

Salmonella Enteritidis strains have been shown to express several different types of fimbriae. These fimbriae are involved in the agglutination of red blood cells from various animal species (Duguid, 1966) and adherence to mouse intestinal cells (Aslanzadeh and Paulissen, 1992). In the present study, in vitro attachment of *S.* Enteritidis to granulosa cells was inhibited by preincubating the cells with purified fimbrial preparation. Nearly 70% inhibition was achieved when cells were preincubated with 20 µg of the purified 14-kDa fimbrial protein, suggesting a major role for this fimbrial protein in the attachment process. Although the 14-kDa fimbrial protein may be involved in the attachment of *S.* Enteritidis strain AE9 to granulosa cells, the role of other fimbrial types and their relative contributions to the attachment process remain to be examined.

Another set of experiments examined the binding of *S.* Enteritidis to fibonectin, laminin, and collagen IV coated on tissue culture wells. Four different concentrations of each protein were tested. Compared with control wells coated with BSA, there was significant binding by strain AE9 to all of the proteins tested (Fig. 19.5). It appears that fimbrial structure(s) on *S.* Enteritidis may provide binding sites to a variety of extracellular matrix proteins (Baloda, 1988; Collinson et al., 1991; Kukkonen et al., 1993). The present study has demonstrated that strain AE9 can bind fibronectin, laminin, and collagen IV. It remains to be seen whether the binding involves the 14-kDa fimbrial protein or other fimbrial structures on the bacterial surface. Binding to laminin and collagen IV may be relevant because in vivo access to granulosa cells would involve binding to the basement membrane, which is rich in collagen IV and laminin.

Salmonella Enteritidis not only attaches to granulosa cells but also invades them, as shown in this study. This implies that ovarian granulosa cells may be one type of target cell involved in the transovarian transmission of the organism. In transmission electron micrographs, it is possible to see organisms surrounded by a membrane and, in some instances, as free bacteria in the cytoplasm (Fig. 19.8). The presence of a membrane would suggest that the organisms may have been endocytosed by invagination of the granulosa cellular membrane. A detailed study of the kinetics of the invasion process would reveal the steps involved in the invasive process. The free bacteria found in the cytoplasm of granulosa cells are often surrounded by a halo (Fig. 19.8B). The authors speculate that they may represent areas within the cytoplasm that have been lysed by bacterial toxins or enzymes. The cytopathic effect of *S.* Enteritidis on granulosa cells and its significance in vivo requires further examination. The present study has shown that some of the bacterial cells in membrane-surrounded vacuoles are dividing, which suggests that *S.* Enteritidis is capable of multiplying in the granulosa cells (Fig. 19.8B), as has been

PLATE I

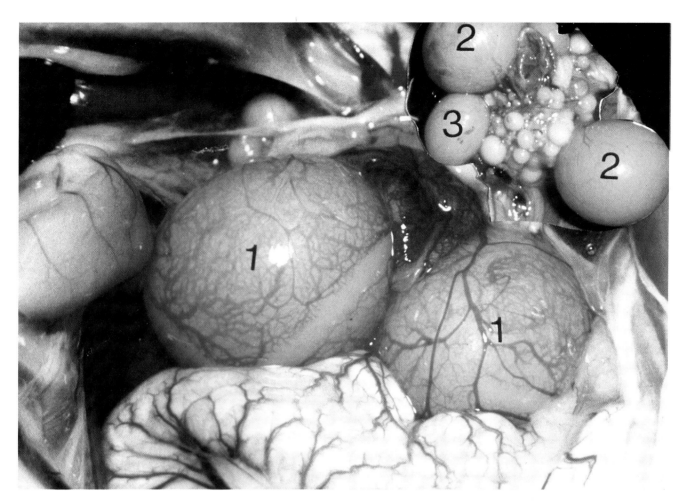

FIGURE 19.1 The follicular hierachy in the ovary of an adult laying hen. Numbers indicate the three largest preovulatory follicles: (1) F1 preovulatory follicle (diameter, 35 mm), (2) F2 preovulatory follicle (diameter, 15–30 mm), and (3) F3 preovulatory follicle (diameter, 6–15 mm).

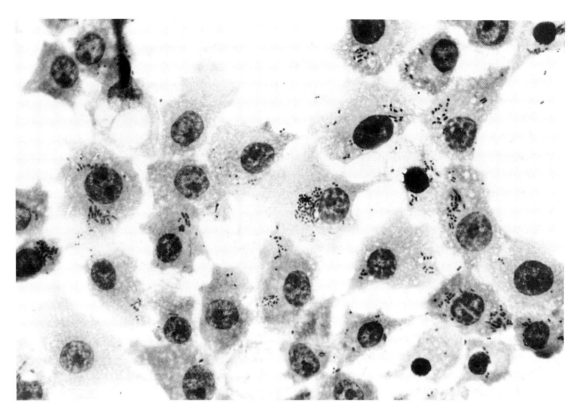

FIGURE 19.2A   Light micrograph of in vitro local attachment of *Salmonella* Enteritidis to chicken ovarian granulosa cells. The organisms were found on discrete sites on the cell surface.

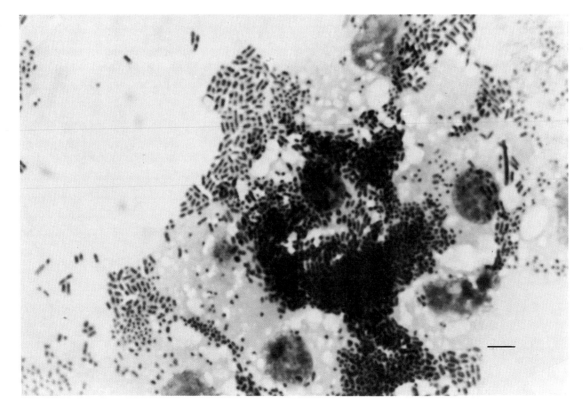

FIGURE 19.2B   Light micrograph of in vitro diffuse attachment of *Salmonella* Enteritidis to chicken ovarian granulosa cells. Bacteria were found covering most of the cell surface. Bar = 10 μ.

PLATE III 207

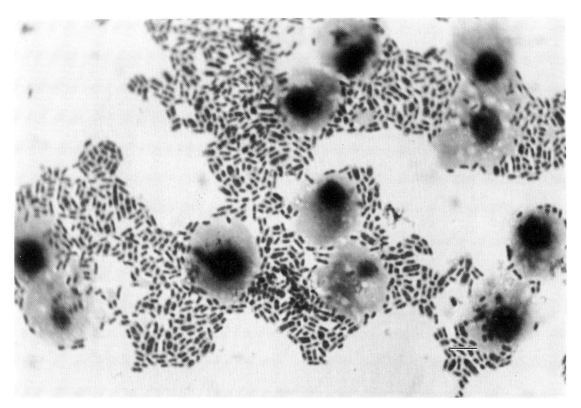

FIGURE 19.2C Light micrograph of in vitro aggregative attachment of *Salmonella* Enteritidis to chicken ovarian granulosa cells. Bacteria were found surrounding the cell membrane. Bar = 10 μ.

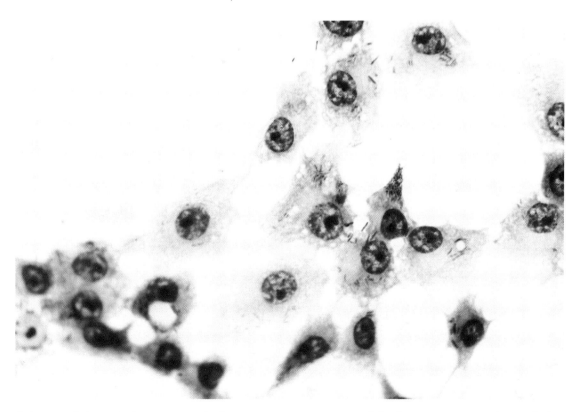

FIGURE 19.2D Light micrograph showing in vitro invasion of chicken ovarian granulosa cells by *Salmonella* Enteritidis AE9. Granulosa cells grown on coverslips were inoculated with *S.* Enteritidis. Giemsa stain.

PLATE IV

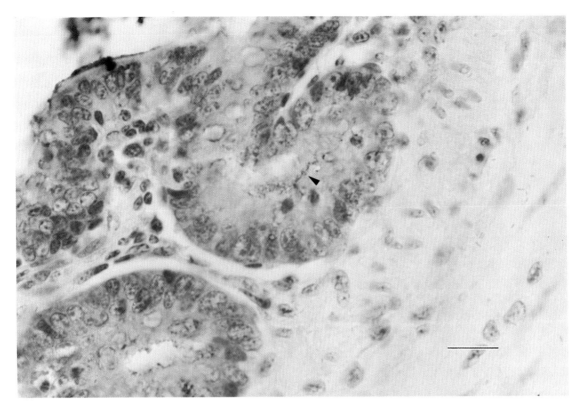

FIGURE 19.6 Light micrographs of cecal tonsil section obtained from an adult laying hen 2 weeks after oral inoculation of *Salmonella* Enteritidis. The presence of *S.* Enteritidis was identified by using a specific monoclonal antibody and a peroxidase-antiperoxidase detection system. The brown precipitate (*arrow*) indicates positive binding of primary antibody. Bar = 5 μ.

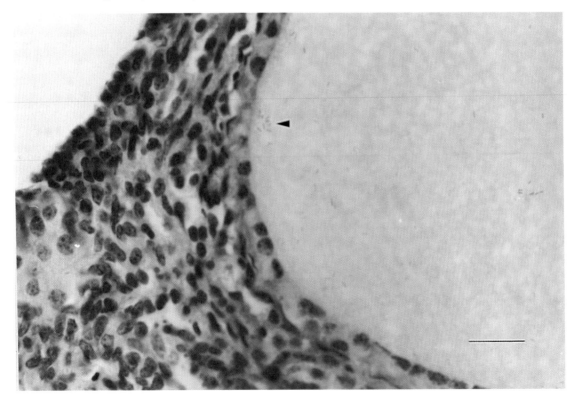

FIGURE 19.7 Light micrographs of cecal tonsil section obtained from an adult laying hen 2 weeks after oral inoculation of *Salmonella* Enteritidis. Several rod-shaped organisms were visible (*arrowhead*) in the central yolk and along the granulosa cell layer. Bar = 5 μ.

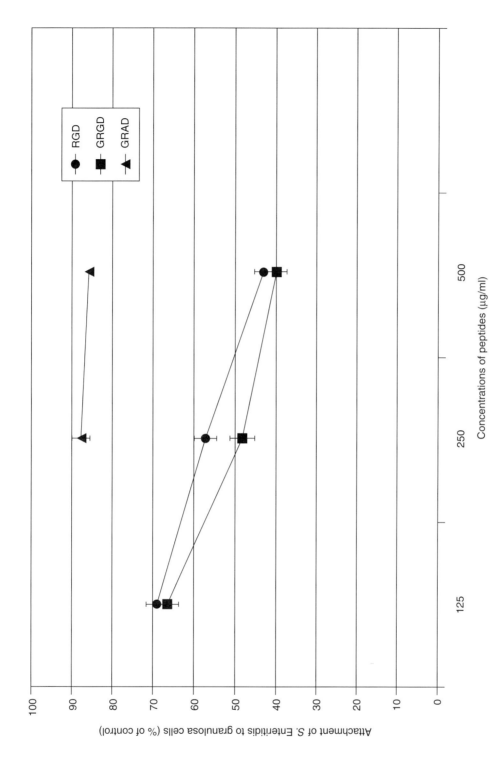

FIGURE 19.9 Inhibition of in virto attachment of S. Enteritidis to chicken ovarian granulosa cells following preincubation of the bacteria with the synthetic peptides Arg-Gly-Asp-Ser (RGD, ●), Gly-Arg-Gly-Asp-Asn-pro (GRGD, ■), and Gly-Arg-Ala-Asp-Ser-pro (GRAD, ▲). Bars indicate standard errors of means (n = 9 wells, 3 experiments).

described for other cell types. It would be interesting to study whether invasion followed by multiplication is an essential prerequisite for transovarian transmission of the organism. The results presented in this study indicate that *S.* Enteritidis interacts with granulosa cells in a specific manner and that it invades the granulosa cells. This pathway may be a possible mechanism by which eggs are contaminated in vivo.

ACKNOWLEDGMENTS

This research was supported by the Crossroads Project of Purdue University Agricultural Research Programs and by the Purdue University Showalter Fund.

REFERENCES

Altekruse, S.F., and Swerdlow, D.L. 1996. The changing epidemiology of food borne diseases. Am. J. Med. Sci. 344:23–29.

Anonymous. Salmonella in eggs. 1989. PHLS Laboratory evidence to Agriculture Committee. PHLS Microbiol. Digest 6:1–9.

Asem, E.K., Carnegie, J.A., and Tsang, B.K. 1992. Fibronectin production by chicken granulosa cells in vitro: effect of follicular development. Acta Endocrinol. 127:466–470.

Asem, E.K., Conkright, M.D., and Novero, R.P. 1994. Progesterone stimulates fibronectin production by chicken granulosa cells in vitro. Eur. J. Endocrinol. 130:159–165.

Aslanzadeh, J., and Paulissen, L.J. 1992. Role of type 1 and type 2 fimbriae in the adherence and pathogenesis of *Salmonella enteritidis* in mice. Microbiol. Immunol. 36:351–359.

Baloda, S.B. 1988. Characterization of fibronectin binding to *Salmonella enteritidis* strain 27655R. FEMS Microbiol. Lett. 49:483–488.

Baloda, S.B., Faris, A., and Krovacek, K. 1988. Cell surface properties of enterotoxigenic and cytotoxic *Salmonella enteritidis* and *Salmonella typhimurium*: studies on hemagglutination, cell-surface hydrophobicity, attachment to human intestinal cells and fibronectin binding. Microbiol. Immunol. 32:447–459.

Barrow, P.A., and Lovell, M.A. 1991. Experimental infection of egg laying hens with *Salmonella enteritidis* phage type 4. Avian Pathol. 20:335–348.

Centers for Disease Control. 1988. Update: *Salmonella enteritidis* infections and grade A shell eggs: United States. MMWR 37:490–496.

Centers for Disease Control. 1990. Update: *Salmonella enteritidis* infections and shell eggs in the United States. MMWR 39:909–912.

Chart, H. 1994. Sodium dodecyl sulfate–polyacrylamide gel electrophoresis for separation and resolution of bacterial components. In: Chart, H., ed. Methods in practical laboratory bacteriology. Boca Raton, FL: CRC, pp. 21–33.

Collinson, S.K., Emody, L., Muller, K., Trust, T.J., and Kay, W.W. 1991. Purification and characterization of thin, aggregative fimbriae from *Salmonella enteritidis*. J. Bacteriol. 173:4773–4781.

Cowden, J.M., Chishom, D., O'Mahoney, M., Lynch, D., Mawer, S.L., Spain, G.E., Ward, L., and Rowe, B. 1989a. Two outbreaks of *Salmonella enteritidis* phage type 4 infection associated with the consumption of fresh shell-egg products. Epidemiol. Infect. 103:47–52.

Cowden, J.M., Lynch, D., Joseph, C.A., O'Mahoney, M., Mawer, S.L., Rowe, B., and Bartlett, C.L.R. 1989b. Case-control study of infections with *Salmonella enteritidis* phage type 4 in England. BMJ 299:771–773.

Coyle, E.F., Ribiero, C.D., Howard, A.J., Palmer, S.R., Jones, H.I., Ward, L., and Rowe, B. 1988. *Salmonella enteritidis* phage type 4 infection: association with hens' eggs. Lancet 2:1295–1297.

Cravioto, A., Gross, R.J., Scotland, S.M., and Rowe, B. 1979. An adhesive factor found in strains of *Escherichia coli* belonging to the traditional infantile enteropathogenic serotypes. Curr. Microbiol. 3:95–99.

Duguid, J.P., Anderson, E.S., and Campbell, I. 1966. Fimbriae and adhesive properties in salmonellae. J. Pathol. Bacterial. 92:107–138.

Edwards, P.R., and Ewing, W.H. 1986. Identification of Enterobacteriaceae, 4th ed. New York: Elsevier Science.

Feutrier, J., Kay, W.W., and Trust, T.J. 1986. Purification and characterization of fimbriae from *Salmonella enteritidis*. J. Bacteriol. 168:221–227.

Finlay, B.B., and Falkow, S. 1989. Common themes in microbial pathogenicity. Microbiol. Rev. 53:210–230.

Fleiss, J.L. 1981. Statistical methods for rates and proportions, 2nd ed. New York: John Wiley.

Gast, R.K., and Beard, C.W. 1990a. Isolation of *Salmonella enteritidis* from internal organs of experimentally infected hens. Avian Dis. 34:991–993.

Gast, R.K., and Beard, C.W. 1990b. Production of *Salmonella enteritidis* contaminated eggs by experimentally infected hens. Avian Dis. 34:438–446.

Gast, R.K., and Beard, C.W. 1992. Detection and enumeration of *Salmonella enteritidis* in fresh and stored eggs laid by experimentally infected hens. J. Food. Prot. 55:152–156.

Gilbert, A.B., Evans, A.J., Perry, M.M., and Davidson, M.H. 1979. A method for separating the granulosa cells, the basal lamina and the theca of the pre-ovulatory ovarian follicle of the domestic fowl: *Gallus domesticus*. J. Reprod. Fertil. 50:179–181.

Gomes, T.T., Blake, P.A., and Trabulsi, L.R. 1989. Prevalence of *Escherichia coli* strains with localized, diffuse and aggregative adherence to HeLa cells in infants with diarrhoea and matched controls. J. Clin. Microbiol. 27:266–269.

Griffin, H.D., Perry, M.M., and Gilbert, A.B. 1984. Yolk formation. In: Freeman, B.M., ed. Physiology and biochemistry of the domestic fowl. New York: Academic, pp. 345–378.

Hedberg, C.W., David, J.J., White, K.E., MacDonald, K.L., and Osterholm, M.T. 1993. Role of egg consumption in sporadic *S. enteritidis* and *S. typhimurium* infection in Minnesota. J. Infect. Dis. 176:107–111.

Hopper, S.A., and Mawer, S. 1988. *Salmonella enteritidis* in a commercial layer flock. Vet. Rec. 123:351.

Knutton, S., Shaw, R.K., Bhan, M.K., Smith, H.R., McConnell, M.M., Cheasty, T., Williams, P.H., and Baldwin, T.J. 1992. Ability of enteroaggregative *Escherichia coli* strains to adhere in vitro to human intestinal mucosa. Infect. Immun. 60:2083–2091.

Kukkonen, M., Raunio, T., Virkola, R., Lahteenmaki, K., Makela, P.H., Klemm, P., Clegg, S., and Korhonen, T.K. 1993. Basement membrane carbohydrate as a target for bacterial adhesion: binding of type 1 fimbriae of *Salmonella enterica* and *Escherichia coli* to laminin. Mol. Microbiol. 7:229–237.

Laemmli, U.K. 1970. Cleavage of structural protein during the assembly of the head of bacteriophage T4. Nature 227:680–685.

Lin, F.-Y.C., Morris, J.G., Jr., Trump, D., Tilghman, D., Wood, P.K., Jackman, N., Israel, E., and Libonati, J.P. 1988. Investigation of an outbreak of *Salmonella enteritidis* gastroenteritis associated with consumption of eggs in a restaurant chain in Maryland. Am. J. Epidemiol. 128:839–844.

Lindell, K.A., Saeed, A.M., and McCabe, G.P. 1994. Evaluation of resistance of four strains of commercial laying hens to experimental infection with *Salmonella enteritidis* phage type eight. Poult. Sci. 73:757–762.

Lister, S.A. 1988. *Salmonella enteritidis* infection in broilers and broiler breeders. Vet. Rec. 123:351.

Mehlman, I.J., Eide, E.L., Sanders, A.C., Fishbein, M., and Aulisio, C.C.G. 1977. Methodology for recognition of invasive potential of *Escherichia coli*. J. AOAC 60:546–562.

Miller, R.G., and Tate, C.R. 1991. Xylose-lysine-tergitol 4: an improved selective agar medium for the isolation of *Salmonella*. Poult. Sci. 70:2429–2432.

Nataro, J.P., Scaletesky, I.C.A., Kaper, J.B., Levine, M.M., and Trabulsi, L.R. 1985. Plasmid-mediated factors conferring diffuse and localized adherence of enteropathogenic *E. coli*. Infect. Immun. 48:378–383.

Nataro, J.P., Kaper, J.B., Robins-Browne, R., Prado, V., Vial, P., and Levine, M.M. 1987. Patterns of adherence of diarrhoeagenic *Escherichia coli* to HEp-2 cells. Pediatr. Infect. Dis. J. 6:829–831.

Novero, R.P., and Asem, E.K. 1993a. Follicle-stimulating hormone-enhanced fibronectin production by chicken granulosa cells is influenced by follicular development. Poult. Sci. 72:709–729.

Novero, R.P., and Asem, E.K. 1993b. Chicken gonadotropin-releasing hormones enhance soluble and insoluble fibronectin production by granulosa cells of the domestic fowl in vitro. Poult. Sci. 72:1961–1971.

O'Brien, J.D.P. 1988. *Salmonella enteritidis* infection in broiler chickens. Vet. Rec. 123:214.

Pierschbacher, M.D., and Ruoslahti, E. 1984a. Variants of the cell recognition site of fibronectin that retain attachment promoting activity. Proc. Natl. Acad. Sci. USA 81:5985–5988.

Pierschbacher, M.D., and Ruoslahti, E. 1984b. The cell attachment activity of fibronectin can be duplicated by small synthetic fragments of the molecule. Nature 309:30–33.

Pierschbacher, M.D., and Ruoslahti, E. 1987. Influence of stereochemistry of the sequence Arg-Gly-Asp-Xaa on binding specificity in cell adhesion. J. Biol. Chem. 262:17,294–17,298.

Popiel, I., and Turnbull, P.C.B. 1985. Passage of *Salmonella enteritidis* and *Salmonella thompson* through chick ileocecal mucosa. Infect. Immun. 47:786–792.

Robinson, F.E., and Etches, R.J. 1986. Ovarian steroidogenesis during follicular maturation in the domestic fowl (*Gallus domesticus*). Biol. Reprod. 35:1096–1105.

Rodrigue, D.C., Taux, R.V., and Rowe, B. 1990. International increase in *Salmonella enteritidis*: a new pandemic? Epidemiol. Infect. 105:21–27.

Ruoslahti, E., and Pierschbacher, M.D. 1986. Arg-Gly-Asp: a versatile cell recognition signal. Cell 44:517–518.

Shivaprasad, H.L., Timoney, J.F., Morales, S., Lucio, B., and Baker, R.C. 1990. Pathogenesis of *Salmonella enteritidis* infection in laying chickens. I. Studies on egg transmission, clinical signs, fecal shedding, and serologic responses. Avian Dis. 34:548–557.

St. Louis, M.E., Morse, D.L., Potter, M.E., DeMelfi, T.M., Guzewich, J.J., Tauxe, R.V., and Blake, P.A. 1988. The emergence of grade A eggs as a major source of *Salmonella enteritidis* infections: new implications for the control of salmonellosis. JAMA 259:2103–2107.

Thiagarajan, D., Saeed, A.M., and Asem, E.K. 1994. Mechanism of transovarian transmission of *Salmonella enteritidis* in laying hens. Poult. Sci. 73:89–98.

Thomas, D.D., Baseman, J.B., and Alderete, J.F. 1985. Fibronectin mediates *Treponema pallidum* cytoadherence through recognition of fibronectin cell-binding domain. J. Exp. Med. 161:514–525.

Timoney, J.F., Shivaprasad, H.L., Baker, R.C., and Rowe, B. 1989. Egg transmission after infection of hens with *Salmonella enteritidis* phage type IV. Vet. Rec. 125:600–601.

Yamada, K.M. 1983. Cell surface interactions with extracellular materials. Annu. Rev. Biochem. 52:761–799.

20

Characterization of Chicken Ovarian Infection with *Salmonella enterica* Serovar Enteritidis

C.E. Benson and L.H. Keller

INTRODUCTION

This topic may seem strange to those who have not lived through the events that have led us to the appreciation that *Salmonella enterica* serovar Enteritidis (*S.* Enteritidis) may well mimic *S.* Pullorum in the colonization of the ovarian tissues and subsequent deposition of the pathogen in the forming egg. Little hints presented in the scientific literature provide perspective to the problem and to the experiments performed to gain the additional insight into the problem. There is much more to be done. Perhaps the following discussion will stimulate an interest to complete the work we have begun.

Our laboratory initially became involved with the possibility of vertical transmission of *S.* Enteritidis when we were invited by scientists at the Centers for Disease Control and Prevention and the U.S. Department of Agriculture to evaluate the microbiological status of ovaries collected from hens implicated via an epidemiological study of suspected eggborne salmonellosis in humans. We successfully isolated *S.* Enteritidis from nearly two-thirds (383) of 555 ovaries (Benson and Eckroade, 1991). Who would have expected such a high rate of isolation of a pathogen previously not shown to have any tissue or host specificity? Agglutination with group-specific antisera established that the isolates were salmonella group D. By using biochemical and motility assays, we quickly confirmed that the isolate was not *S.* Pullorum or *S.* Galli-

narum. A number of possible sources of the pathogen, including contamination of the ovaries during the acquisition of these specimens at the site of collection (a processing plant), could have explained these isolation rates. Despite our suspicions about the elevated rate of association of *S.* Enteritidis with the ovaries, we were convinced that some number of the ovaries had been colonized.

We were later provided with the opportunity to evaluate some of these hens' eggs, which had been held at refrigeration temperature storage in New York City. Upon arrival at our facility, the eggs were placed at 4°C prior to culture. Within 36 h after arrival, all of the eggs had been placed in culture. The eggs were surface sterilized by soaking in 95% ethanol for 30 min, and then they were carefully removed with sterile forceps and allowed to air dry in a biosafety cabinet. The eggs were then aseptically cracked, and the albumen fraction was carefully collected in one sterile container while the yolk component (along with some closely associated albumen material that is virtually inseparable from the yolk) was placed into a second container. The albumen fraction was supplemented with $Fe(NH_4)_2(SO_4)_2$ before both containers were incubated overnight at 37°C (Board and Halls, 1973). Aliquots were streaked onto selective differential media and incubated overnight at 37°C. Fractions of over 600 eggs were cultured in this fashion before the technique was modified to the pooling of the separated components in pools representative of 10 eggs (until the rest of the 1500 eggs had been evaluated). Cracked or spoiled eggs were discarded from the sampling process. Only 15 egg yolks were found to carry *S.* Enteritidis, whereas all albumen cultures were negative, thus implying, we speculated, contamination of the yolk portion of the egg from an interior source rather than by passage of the pathogen through the eggshell after the egg had been laid. We concluded that transovarian transmission of the pathogen had probably occurred, although we had expected a higher rate of *S.* Enteritidis associated with the eggs since the rate of isolation from the ovary tissue had been so high. Our deduction, in a small part, provided several research directions and was supported by the conclusion provided by St. Louis et al. (1988) in their discussion of grade-A eggs as the major source of *S.* Enteritidis. Thus, we were not alone in arriving at the possibility of ovarian transmission.

HISTORICAL REVIEW

The inference of transovarial transmission had been introduced long ago. In 1942, it was reported, without specific scientific references, that the frequency of isolation of salmonellae from ovaries indicates that the infection is probably transmitted though the egg (Bunyea, 1942). A subsequent article appeared several years later in an epidemiological report that carried the subject closer to present-day analytical methodology (Watt, 1945). The report concerned an American merchant vessel that had arrived in a New Orleans port approximately 12 h after an outbreak of acute diarrheal disease. An epidemiological and microbiological evaluation of the food consumed by the patients implicated *S.* Montevideo. Systematic elimination of possible sources implicated either eggs or pork chops as the primary carriers of the microbe. On microbiological examination, the pork chops were not found to contain any microbes. Candling of the eggs revealed only slight shrinkage or other signs of deterioration. Tetrathionate enrichment of the yolks from a case of eggs resulted in the isolation of *S.* Montevideo in 11 of 14 flasks (pools). When the eggshell was sterilized prior to cracking the egg, several additional *S.* Montevideo were isolated. The eggs were traced back to specific packing plants in Iowa and then to the farms providing eggs to the packing plants. These farms were surveyed by (a) culturing fresh chicken droppings and (b) acquiring eggs for culture from the packing plants. [We found these survey techniques interesting because they are quite similar to the techniques employed by the *S.* Enteritidis Pilot Project (1995) and currently by Pennsylvania Egg Quality Assurance Program (unpublished).] *Salmonella* Montevideo was not found in either type of the sample, but *S.* Derby (one of 143 farms) and *S.* Pullorum (12 of 143 farms) were present in the fecal specimens. *Salmonella* Pullorum and *S.* Gallinarum were frequently found in the shell eggs along with *S.* Derby and *S.* Choleraesuis (var. Kunzendorf). Although the author (Watt, 1945) could not confirm the presence of *S.* Montevideo in the fecal or egg specimens from the farms, he concluded that this was the first report implicating "outbreaks of salmonellosis in man to chickens or shell eggs."

The two aforementioned reports that first led to the suggestion that transovarial transmission of salmonellae was possible were based on the interpretation of data about eggs laid by naturally infected laying hens. Although the presence of *S.* Pullorum in the reproductive tissues of laying hens was universally accepted (Snoeyenbos et al., 1969), the suggestion that other serovars of salmonellae might also gain entrance into the ovaries and/or the oviduct was a startling notion. Thus, there is no surprise in finding a series of experimental studies in the literature evaluating the suggestion that transovarial transmission of salmonellae occurred for serovars other than *S.* Pullorum. Shortly after Watts reported his findings, Gibbons and Moore (1945) reported the results of the inoculation of four pullorum-positive hens via per os feeding with *S.* Bareilly. Two additional hens were used as uninoculated controls. The inoculation was repeated three times during 13 days. The eggs were collected twice daily and *S.* Bareilly was found on the shell of three eggs while *S.* Pullorum was present in the "meat" of one of 63 eggs. The intestine was readily colonized by *S.* Bareilly, but only *S.* Pullorum was present in the ovaries, oviduct, and ova. The authors concluded that the localization of *S.* Bareilly in the intestine could result in eggs being contaminated via contact with *S.* Bareilly-contaminated feces. The essence of the report was that the longer the hen carries the pathogen, the higher is the likelihood that the egg will become contaminated. Thus, the isolation of salmonellae from egg contents could be interpreted as representative of two different modes of entry by the pathogen: (a) deposition of contaminated feces onto the eggshell with subsequent penetration of the shell by the pathogen or (b) as the result of transovarial infection. Review of this topic revealed the intensity of the controversy over the issue of transovarial transmission. However, Forsythe et al. (1967) notes that "Those who accept the theory that eggs can contain salmonellae at the time of lay conclude that an ovarian infection must exist." This line served to introduce their study of per os and direct ovarian inoculation to determine the physiological mechanisms required for colonization of the reproductive tissue with consequential internal deposition of viable organisms into the contents of an egg. The inoculum was either *S.* Lexington or *S.* Anatum and was fed, to individual hens, in gelatin capsules containing lyophilized bacteria in quantities ranging from 10^5 to 10^{11} organisms per dose. The organisms were recovered in the feces, the surface of the shell, and (only when *S.* Anatum was the inoculum) the intestines. Neither serovar was recovered from the ovaries or the oviduct. The contents of one of 519 eggs did contain *S.* Lexington. Although the authors concluded that the low incidence observed during the per os inoculation was probably not the cause of egg-content contamination, they also concluded that the content isolation could not be evidence of eggshell penetration, because the time between lay and collection of eggs for culture was too short (several hours) for penetration to occur. In the absence of the colonization of the reproductive tissues, such a conclusion is difficult to understand. There were, however, six isolations of the inoculum (one *S.* Lexington and five *S.* Anatum) from the eggshell following the per os inoculation.

In another set of experiments, the direct ovarian inoculation was performed with only *S.* Anatum, while *S.* Pullorum, an organism with recognized ability to infect reproductive tissue, thus providing recoverable organism in the egg contents, was used as the control. One chicken, inoculated with a large dose of 10^{11} *S.* Anatum, died of massive invasion of all tissues. The eggs laid by other two chickens inoculated with 10^3 *S.* Anatum did not contain *S.* Anatum, nor was the ovarian tissue positive when the birds were necropsied. In the control, six chickens were individually inoculated by placing 10^5 *S.* Pullorum into the ovarian tissue. Four hens produced eggs containing *S.* Pullorum, and this organism was subsequently also isolated from the ovarian tissues collected at necropsy (16–28 days after inoculation). Two of the inoculated controls produced no eggs, and *S.* Pullorum was absent from the ovarian tissue at necropsy. The authors concluded that (a) *S.* Pullorum could be recovered from eggs of chickens with active ovarian infections, (b) the establishment of an infection of the ovarian tissue by other salmonellae following per os inoculation was unlikely, (c) direct inoculation of the ovary with *S.* Anatum did not result in the establishment of an infection, (d) cleaning the surface of eggs was essential quality control to reduce the salmonellae on eggs, and (e) the role of feed as the source of a salmonellae inoculum for chickens had been overemphasized. These conclusions conflict with the initial aforementioned statement purporting to introduce a study to define the physiological mechanisms necessary for infected hens to lay salmonella-contaminated eggs. One must also wonder about the decision process followed to select the specific serovars used to evaluate the possibility of transovarial transmission.

Based on current experience, there would appear to be no justification for the use of some of these strains. Whatever the process, such research served only to collect partial data, giving miscues and confusing the issues involved in the isolation of salmonella serovars from the contents of chicken eggs. Evaluation of the reports from earlier studies of egg-associated salmonellae, in eggs presumed to have been laid by naturally infected chickens, highlighted only certain strains of salmonellae to have a host preference for avian species. At the same time, one should note that these strains were discovered only because they maintained the capability (virulence factors?) of producing the disease state in humans. These earlier lessons were again emphasized by the work of Snoeyenbos et al. (1969), who provided insights for future evaluations. They summarized the results of the necropsy studies of 1050 chickens (collected during a period of 18 years). The data were purposefully screened to exclude those chickens shown to be infected with *S.* Pullorum or *S.* Gallinarum and to include in the analysis the data on all chickens that appeared to be infected, as determined by positive pullorum-testing methods, but were negative for *S.* Pullorum or *S.* Gallinarum. This selection criterion reduced the number of files to be reviewed to 121 semimature or mature chickens. The operating protocol utilized to necropsy and collect specimens from the 1050 chickens during the original 18-year period necessitated a detailed bacteriological evaluation of any chicken with a suspicious type of agglutination. This protocol included aseptic entrance into the peritoneal cavity and swabbing of the cavity before removing organs for individual culture. The meticulous approach used in the original work greatly facilitated the subsequent compilation of the data described here. The serovars found associated with the ovaries, the peritoneal cavity, or both sites were *S.* Enteritidis, *S.* Heidelberg, *S.* Typhimurium, and *S.* Typhimurium var. copenhagen. All of these serovars shared agglutinins with *S.* Pullorum. An additional 58 chickens had other salmonellae isolated from diverse sites, though most frequently the intestine. The authors noted that peritoneal infection might lead to contamination of the ovary and hence could contribute to an infected egg. However, there were more positive ovary cultures than either the total of positive peritoneal cavities or when both sites were positive. Infection of the peritoneal cavity or the ovary could lead to contamination of the egg prior to shell formation. Since the data studied were selected on only chickens positive by the pullorum test, the data could have been biased, because there remained the possibility of having missed those serovars of salmonellae that do not cross-react in the pullorum test but could colonize the ovary. Such a possibility, however remote, should not be ignored. Nevertheless, the data provided by Snoeyenbos et al. (1969) suggested that there may be a possibility that "true egg transmission may play a significant role in the epizoology of salmonellosis in chickens" and, we would add, in humans. This short report provided insights that have never been pursued.

Studies of naturally infected hens are inherently difficult because one must search for positive flocks by using a variety of assay procedures (testing for antibodies or the presence of salmonellae on cloacal swabs, in the environment, or in eggs) to find a pathogen in asymptomatic chickens. A number of negative cultures is the usual experience. Thus, the move toward experimental inoculations is a reasonable and reproducible approach to provide insight into the nature and magnitude of the problem. In addition, an experimental inoculation designed to mimic the presumed natural course of infection would enable the host response associated with ovarian colonization to be tracked.

CURRENT RESEARCH

O'Brien (1988) reported that chickens could acquire *S.* Enteritidis as a result of transovarial transmission from infected parent flocks, and Hinton et al. (1989) demonstrated that young chicks could acquire *S.* Enteritidis from contaminated feed. Humphrey et al. (1989) carried these observations further by inoculating two sets of chickens (one group was 52 weeks old, whereas the other was 18 weeks old) per os with *S.* Enteritidis phage type 4 (PT4). The liver, spleen, ovary, and oviduct of six of 25 chickens (including one of the control birds) in the first set were positive for *S.* Enteritidis PT4, whereas the organism was isolated from only one bird (from a total of 30) in the second experiment. None of the infected or control birds exhibited any signs of illness, and there was no evidence of macroscopic or significant microscopic lesions in the viscera. However, only the eggs from the younger inoculated set produced eggs containing *S.* Enteritidis (four of 375 laid). This experiment demonstrated that oral inoculation could lead to colonization of internal organs and the production of eggs containing salmonellae. Humphrey and colleagues also noted that the possibility remained that naturally infected hens acquire *S.* Enteritidis by some route other than oral. These studies mimic situations seen among naturally infected hens where organs are positive but all of the eggs are negative or where very few birds are culture positive but the eggs are culture positive for salmonellae. The absence of lesions is not unusual.

Shivaprasad et al. (1990) looked at egg transmission of *S.* Enteritidis in chickens infected by oral or intravenous inoculation. Infection was documented by fecal shedding, and the chickens exhibited a variety of symptoms ranging from depression, drop in egg production, and diarrhea to apparent clinically normal behavior. The most severely symptomatic birds were inoculated with an isolate obtained from an infected human, and no culture-positive eggs were found. Inoculation of chickens with two different strains (Y8P2, an egg isolate; and 27A, an ovarian isolate) individually initiated infections that resulted in the production of eggs containing *S.* Enteritidis in the albumen or in the yolk. Several of the control birds became serologically positive for *S.* Enteritidis and produced positive eggshell cultures. Transmission to the control hens probably represented a naturally acquired inoculation via an aerosol (Snoeyenbos et al., 1969). Gast and Beard (1989) also established that experimentally inoculated hens produced eggs containing *S.* Enteritidis and that the ovaries and oviduct were colonized with the inoculated organism (Gast and Beard, 1990). There was no record of illness among the chickens nor the presence of obvious lesions observed during necropsy. The studies by Shivaprasad et al. and by Gast and Beard provide the insight that strains of *S.* Enteritidis may express differing characteristics leading to invasion and colonization of the reproductive tissue, resulting in the production of *S.* Enteritidis-contaminated eggs. Shivarasad and colleagues used *S.* Enteritidis PT8 strains in their studies, whereas Gast and Beard used an *S.* Enteritidis PT 13a isolate. It is tempting to hypothesize a potential role for phage type of a strain as just one variable (virulence) factor of the pathogenic mechanism of *S.* Enteritidis in chickens.

In a different approach, Lindell et al. (1994) found that different strains of hens seem to vary slightly in the colonization of the reproductive tissues. During the first 2 weeks after infection, one strain of hens had a higher rate of production of eggs with internalized *S.* Enteritidis than did the other three strains of chickens. During the 10-week experiment, these differences disappeared. The mechanism of these variations is presumed to be differences in the major histocompatibility antigens. In our laboratories, we have noted differences in the multiplicity of infection in chicks with genetic differences in the major histocompatibility antigens (Keller et al., 1995, 1997). There is, then, the suggestion that strains of chickens vary in their susceptibility (or resistance) to infection by *S.* Enteritidis, as well as the aforementioned: that different strains of the pathogen vary in the capabilities to colonize their avian host.

We have studied the colonization of the reproductive tract of chickens, with special attention to the location of *S.* Enteritidis in reproductive tissues and in forming and freshly laid eggs (Keller et al., 1995). Two experiments were performed using commercial white leghorn laying hens between the ages of 23 and 25 weeks. *Salmonella* Enteritidis strains 575 (PT8) served as the inoculum in a preliminary study to determine whether immunohistochemistry could reveal the mechanism of egg contamination. The chickens were inoculated per os, and 2 to 3 hens were randomly selected and killed daily (days 1–21 and 32–40). The tissues collected for evaluation were (a) the ovary; (b) sections of the oviduct (the infundibulum, upper magnum, lower magnum, isthmus, uterus, vagina, and cloaca); (c) an organ pool comprised of the liver, spleen, gallbladder, and heart; and (d) an intestinal pool including the small intestine and the cecum with contents. The histochemical preparation incorporated the specificity of a monoclonal antibody to show highly positive reactions in all tissues between days 2 and 4, with a decrease in positivity by days 5–8, in all tissues except the ovary and isthmus. This finding coincided with the appearance of a culture-positive egg pool on day 5. On days 17–21, the pool from three birds became positive for *S.* Enteritidis and remained so for 3 days. The cloaca, organ pool, and intestinal pool remained strongly positive for the samples taken on days 9–12, after which the number of positive tissues gradually decreased to the end of the study. At no time were all specimens from these sites uniformly negative. The incidence of positive cloaca had dropped nearly 50% by the end of the study. More dramatic decreases in the incidence of salmonella positivity were observed in the ovary, infundibulum, vagina, organ pool, and intestinal pool; other specimens were negative after day 8 after infection.

Histochemical staining revealed very few *S.* Enteritidis bacteria in the tissues, with the exception of oviductal tissues collected with four forming eggs. Two of these forming eggs were in the upper or lower magnum, and antigen staining was seen in, and associated with, the goblet cells of the mucosal epithelium extending into the albumen of the lumen. This staining extended from the peritoneal epithelial layer to the lumen. Positive staining of the lower magnum section and in the isthmus section associated with the other two forming eggs appeared as few bacterial aggregates associated with the peritoneal epithelium. Several areas of staining were observed in the ciliated epithelium in the lumen of the infundibulum and the isthmus, in the peritoneal epithelium of the vagina, and in the stratified squamous epithelium of the vent portion of the cloaca. There was staining in a few interstitial cells in the medulla of the ovary and, in one case, diffuse staining in the cortical stromal tissue of an atretic follicle. This experiment suggested that the oviductal tissues were highly colonized, and this region became the focus for the next two experiments.

The next experiment used SE6-E21 (PT13a), which had been shown to be shed into freshly laid eggs with high frequency after experimental inoculation of mature laying hens (Petter, 1993). The tissues were evaluated by microbiological methods to determine the presence of salmonellae. During this experiment, the tissues of the control birds became culture positive despite being housed in an isolation facility separate from the inoculated hens. The experiment was continued because the forming eggs of the inoculated birds became positive during the 2- to 4-day evaluation and 50% were positive on sampling days 9–12 and 13–16, dropping to 38% positive by days 17–20. All positive samples, except for the last specimen, came from broken yolks. In addition, the lower magnum had a higher colonization rate than observed in experiment 1. An interesting observation is that, despite the high level of salmonella-positive forming eggs, none of the control or infected birds laid a positive egg (among 870 eggs examined).

The third study was basically a repeat of the second study, with the following modifications: (a) the inoculum was strain 575 (PT8), (b) the experimental chicken was a brown laying hen, and (c) no tissues were examined for histological changes. High levels of colonization of the intestine, organ pool, and cloaca were maintained throughout the experiment. Half of the ovary and vaginal tissues were positive by day 2, a colonization rate maintained throughout the experiment. The incidence of infected tissue from the upper oviduct was consistently low. Tissues from the control birds were uniformly culture negative throughout the experiment. From the infected hens, 11 forming eggs were positive for S. Enteritidis from days 2 through 20, and the pathogen was cultured from the ovaries of eight of the hens carrying the forming eggs. It is noteworthy that six of these forming eggs were found in the uterus, another one in the infundibulum, and the eighth egg in the upper magnum. There was one positive egg in the upper magnum when the ovarian tissue was negative, and two positive eggs were obtained from the uterine tissue when only the cloacal and vaginal tissues were positive. The conclusion proposed regarding these last two eggs is that the infection was ascending to the uterus from the cloaca or vagina. Evaluation of freshly laid eggs indicated that five were positive for S. Enteritidis. The culture status of the five birds laying these eggs indicated that two hens had a positive ovary and cloaca, one had a negative ovary but a positive cloaca, and one had a positive ovary and a negative cloaca, whereas the fifth had a culture-negative ovary and cloaca but a positive organ pool. These results were interpreted as implying that ascending, descending, and lateral infections of the eggs are possible. The intestines of all but one hen were culture positive. In this hen, the only positive sample was the organ pool (heart, spleen, liver, and gallbladder).

Throughout these studies, clinical signs of an infection and noticeable lesions in the tissue were absent. Microscopic evaluation of stained tissue indicated some signs of inflammatory response in the uterus and several follicles. The nonspecific responses were not dramatic nor consistent among the tissue specimens. Interpretation of the results of these three experiments requires a brief summary of the progress of the ovum through the reproductive tissues to be deposited as a fully formed, intact egg. Greater detail may be found in the book by Johnson (1976). The maturing ovum is collected by the infundibulum, where it resides for approximately 18 min and where the first layer of the albumen is produced. Coincidentally, the ovum may also be fertilized under the appropriate conditions. The developing egg then migrates from the infundibulum into the upper magnum and then into the lower magnum for the next 2–3 h. A majority of the albumen is formed in the magnum. Ovotransferrin, ovomucoid, and avidin are also produced here and added to the forming egg. In addition, a large amount of calcium is secreted by the magnum. Moving through the muscular structure of the magnum via a peristaltic mechanism, the forming egg enters the isthmus, which is a thick circular layer of muscle containing glandular tissue that is less developed than in magnum. In this site, the egg gains the inner and outer shell membranes during the 1- to 2-h passage through this portion of the oviduct. Finally, the forming egg enters a tubular structure (called the "shell gland" or uterus) characterized by a prominent longitudinal muscle layer with both tubular and unicellular goblet cells. The egg takes up salt and approximately 15 g of water into the albumen from the tubular glands. The forming egg remains associated with this portion of the reproductive organ for 20–26 h. It is here that calcification is initiated during 15 h of the approximate 20-h residence in this site. Shell pigmentation is formed during the final 5 h in the uterus. The vagina is separated from the uterus by a sphincter muscle and terminates at the cloaca. The vagina has no role in the formation of the egg but functions in coordination with the uterus to expel the fully formed egg.

Thus, our interpretation of the aforementioned experiments is that colonization of eggs in the reproductive tract by S. Enteritidis can occur via colonization of the ovarian membrane or in the infundibulum during deposition of the albumen around the yolk or in the ascent from the cloaca. Other sites along the oviduct would contain many antibacterial inhibitors to colonization, and microbial resistance to the action of such factors by some unknown mechanism(s) could enable survival of the pathogen in eggs after oviposition.

Turnbull and Snoeyenbos (1973) have reported on the apparent ease whereby S. Enteritidis can colonize along any point in the intestine, with the crop apparently serving as the reservoir of a persisting infection. Persistence without observable proliferation was evident in all age groups studied (1-day-old, 2-week-old, and 6- and 9-month-old chicks). The incidence of entry fell rapidly with increasing age. The number of bacteria observed in these sites decreased with the age of the bird. Unfortunately, the reproductive organs of the older birds were not evaluated by microscopic or microbiological techniques. Later, by light-microscopic and electron-microscopic techniques, Turnbull and Richmond (1978) demonstrated the behavior of S. Enteritidis when injected into isolated "loops" of duodenum, midgut, and ileoceca in anesthetized 1-day-old chicks. The microbes were found to be able to proliferate and invade the mucosa at any point via evagination of cells in the luminal surface of the epithelium. The bacteria appeared to be enclosed in a membrane-bound vacuole and passed unharmed through the cell. Salmonellae could be found free and within cells in the lamina propria.

Coupling the studies performed by Turnbull and Snoeyenbos (1973) with our evaluation of the reproductive tissue, the salmonellae could be acquired by ingestion or possibly by inhalation. In the latter instance, one might expect to find the microbe rapidly phagocytosed by the alveolar macrophages and destroyed or, alternatively, transported by macrophages to other sites, possibly leading to colonization of other sites. Dissemination from these sites could occur via the hematogenous route. The ingestion of the microbe requires that the organism successfully pass through the stomach into the intestine, where the organism readily gains entrance into the intestinal epithelial cells. The organism passes into the lamina propria and will probably colonize the diffuse lymphoid tissue of the intestine. Cell-associated or cell-free bacteria can then move through the body of the host and colonize other sites, including the ovary and upper portion (upper magnum) of the oviduct.

FUTURE CHALLENGES

We wish we could say the rest of the story is history, but the problem remains. Certainly much of the inoculum is probably destroyed by the antibacterial activities of the host. We do not know how many bacteria are present in the ovary and upper portions of the oviduct, nor do we know how many bacteria need to be deposited in association with the forming egg so that it becomes a contaminated egg. In fact, speculation leads us to state that we do not know how many bacteria survive the deposition process or coexist with all of the antibacterial components in the albumen around the yolk in the egg-forming process. Considering the aforementioned number of positive ovaries and oviducts found by the investigators, one could infer that many of the organisms are destroyed/killed during egg development. If one considers our experience with strain SE6-E21, the absence of positive eggs despite the presence of culture-positive organisms in the forming eggs might imply that the salmonellae *are* killed during the approximate 26-h egg-development period. Consider also that the genetic strain of chicken may significantly affect the susceptibility of the chicken to colonization by *S.* Enteritidis and the pathological lesions that may occur as a consequence of the developing infection.

We challenge the readers to consider and evaluate experimentally the following questions:

- What is the true multiplicity of infection of the pathogen required to colonize the reproductive tissues to contribute to the laying of contaminated eggs?
- What is the biochemical nature of the *S.* Enteritidis that escape the antibacterial factors of the host?

- What determines the survival of the pathogen in a laid egg?
- What role does the phage type of the pathogen play relative to the nature of the infection within the host?
- What impact does the genetic constitution of the chicken have on the role of pathogenesis of *S.* Enteritidis?

These are only a few of the questions one could raise concerning the relationship of *S.* Enteritidis to the chicken and the egg. There are, unfortunately, a growing list of such questions to challenge us.

REFERENCES

Benson, C.E., and Eckroade, R.J. 1991. Virulence of *Salmonella enteritidis* isolates. In: Blankenship, L.C., ed. Colonization control of human bacterial enteropathogens in poultry. San Diego, CA: Academic, pp. 149–160.

Board, R.G., and Halls, N.A. 1973. The effect of iron on the growth of *Escherichia coli* in albumen taken from the hen's egg. Br. Poult. Sci. 14:359–371.

Bunyea, H. 1942. Miscellaneous diseases of poultry. Washington, DC: USDA Yearbook of Agriculture, p. 994.

Forsythe, R.H., Ross, W.J., and Ayres, J.C. 1967. Salmonellae recovery following gastro-intestinal and ovarian inoculation in the domestic fowl. Poult. Sci. 46:849–855.

Gast, R.K., and Beard, C.W. 1989. Production of *Salmonella enteritidis*-contaminated eggs by experimentally infected hens. Avian Dis. 34:438–446.

Gast, R.K., and Beard, C.W. 1990. Isolation of *Salmonella enteritidis* from internal organs of experimentally infected hens. Avian Dis. 34:991–993.

Gibbons, N.E., and Moore, R.L. 1945. A note on artificially infected fowl as carriers of *Salmonella*. Poult. Sci. 25:115–118.

Hinton, M., Pearson, G.R., Threlfall, E.J., Rowe, B., Woodward, M., and Wray, C. 1989. Experimental *Salmonella enteritidis* infection in chicks. Vet. Rec. 124:223.

Humphrey, T.J., Baskerville, A., Chart, H., and Rowe, B. 1989. Infection of egg-laying hens with *Salmonella enteritidis* PT4 by oral inoculation. Vet. Rec. 125:531–532.

Johnson, A.L. 1976. Reproduction in the female. In: Sturkie, P.D., ed. Avian physiology. New York: Springer-Verlag.

Keller, L.H., Benson, C.E., Krotec, K., and Eckroade, R.J. 1995. *Salmonella enteritidis* colonization of the reproductive tract and forming and freshly laid eggs of chickens. Infect. Immun. 63:2443–2449.

Keller, L.H., Schifferli, D.M., Benson, C.E., Aslam, S., and Eckroade, R.J. 1997. Invasion of chicken reproductive tissues and forming eggs is not unique to *Salmonella enteritidis*. Avian Dis. 41:535–539.

Lindell, K.A., Saeed, A.M., and McCabe, G.P. 1994. Evaluation of resistance of four strains of commercial laying hens to experimental infection with *Salmonella enteritidis* phage type eight. Poult. Sci. 73:757–762.

O'Brien, J.D.P. 1988. *Salmonella enteritidis* infection in broiler chickens. Vet. Rec. 122:214.

Petter, J.G. 1993. Detection of two smooth colony phenotypes in a *Salmonella enteritidis* isolate which vary in their
ability to contaminate eggs. Appl. Environ. Microbiol.
59:2884–2890.

S. Enteritidis Pilot Project Progress Report. USDA/FSIS,
22 May 1995.

Shivaprasad, H.L., Timoney, J.F., Morales, S., Lucio, B., and
Baker, R.C. 1990. Pathogenesis of *Salmonella enteritidis*
infection in laying chickens. I. Studies on egg transmission,
clinical signs, fecal shedding, and serologic response. Avian
Dis. 34:548–557.

Snoeyenbos, G.H., Smyser, C.F., and Van Roekel, H. 1969.
Salmonella infections of the ovary and peritoneum of chickens. Avian Dis. 13:668–670.

St. Louis, M.E., Morse, D.L., Potter, M.E., DeMelfi, T.M.,
Guzewich, J.J., Tauxe, R.V., and Blake, P.A. 1988. The
emergence of grade A eggs as a major source of *Salmonella
enteritidis* infections: new implications for the control of
salmonellosis. JAMA 259:2103–2107.

Turnbull, P.C.B., and Richmond, J.E. 1978. A model of *Salmonella enteritidis:* the behavior of *Salmonella enteritidis* in
chick intestine studied by light and electron microscopy. Br.
J. Exp. Pathol. 59:64–75.

Turnbull, P.C.B., and Snoeyenbos, G.H. 1973. Experimental
salmonellosis in the chicken. 1. Fate and host response in
alimentary canal, liver, and spleen. Avian Dis. 18:153–177.

Watt, J. 1945. An outbreak of *Salmonella* infection in man from
infected chicken eggs. U.S. Public Health Rep. 60:835–839.

21

Phage Type and Other Outer-Membrane Characteristics of *Salmonella enterica* Serovar Enteritidis Associated with Virulence

J. Guard-Petter

INTRODUCTION

Salmonella enterica serovar Enteritidis (*S.* Enteritidis) infection in humans was associated with consumption of eggs contaminated with this pathogen (St. Louis et al., 1988; Humphrey et al., 1991; Threlfall et al., 1992; Altecruse et al., 1993; Ebel et al., 1993; Caffer and Eiguer, 1994; Fantasia and Filetici, 1994; Glosnicka and Kunikowska, 1994; Mishu et al., 1994; Poppe, 1994; Schroeter et al., 1994). Several epidemiological markers are used for the differentiation between *S.* Enteritidis isolates. Phage typing has been among the common tools used for this purpose. Bacteriophages are viruses that infect susceptible host bacteria. These viruses, or phages, can be used to generate typing patterns that divide a single bacterial species into phage-resistant or phage-sensitive variants. Phage typing usually follows identification of an organism as *S.* Enteritidis by biochemical and serological analysis (Kauffman, 1966; Selander and Musser, 1990; Li et al., 1993; Sanderson et al., 1996). Ideally, we would like to use phage typing to identify virulent *S.* Enteritidis isolates, to trace the source of an outbreak, to make decisions about how best to interrupt the pathogen's spread, and, ultimately, to protect the food supply from bacterial contamination. However, indiscriminate use of phage typing with-

out understanding its limitations will, at best, fail to exploit the technique fully and, at worst, lead to wrong decisions about how the information should be applied.

Controversy about the meaning of *S.* Enteritidis phage type has increased concomitantly with the number of phage-type designations in use. Identification of multiple phage types at the very least indicates that *S.* Enteritidis surface structure is pleiotropic, whereas analysis of DNA from strains from around the world indicates that all *S.* Enteritidis strains are closely related, as shown by a limited number of clonal types (Stanley et al., 1992a,b; Katouli et al., 1993; Murase et al., 1995, 1996). This inverse relationship detected by two different epidemiological approaches suggests that relatively minor genetic differences account for the different *S.* Enteritidis phage types. Subtle genetic variations that change cell-surface properties by altering gene expression are commonplace in bacteria and can be reversible (Silverman and Simon, 1983; Citti and Wise, 1995; Gunn et al., 1996; Matsushita et al., 1996; Theiss et al., 1996; Belland et al., 1997; Jishage and Ishihama, 1997). Since phage-type diversity should be expected to occur in pathogenic bacteria that must adapt to and survive in a wide range of in vivo and in vitro environments, development of a phage-typing system should be coupled with analysis of molecules that are receptors.

Here, an attempt is made to present the strengths as well as pitfalls of using bacteriophages to arrive at conclusions about the epidemiology of *S*. Enteritidis.

The *S*. Enteritidis phage-typing scheme was developed at the Central Public Health Laboratory in London, England, in collaboration with the World Health Organization (WHO) (Ward et al., 1987). In the United States, phage typing is performed by the Centers for Disease Control (CDC), in Atlanta, Georgia, or by the National Veterinary Services Laboratory (NVSL), in Ames, Iowa (Hickman-Brenner et al., 1991; Ebel et al., 1993). Comments herein are directed toward the WHO method because of the prodigious amount of information generated from this scheme of phage typing. The original scheme used 10 bacteriophages (typing phages) to classify *S*. Enteritidis into 27 different phage types. Since 1987, the scheme has become more complex by the addition of more typing phages, but additional information is still unavailable for review (F. Hickmann-Brenner, personal communication). In-depth reviews of basic questions about how a virus infects its host, the biology of bacteriophage, or how infection results in lysogeny versus lysis have been previously published (Susskind and Botstein, 1978; Mathews et al., 1983; Aoyama and Hayashi, 1986; Hausmann, 1988; Mosig and Eiserling, 1988; Geiduschek, 1991; Ptashne, 1992; Young, 1992; Campbell, 1996). This chapter reviews the biology of *S*. Enteritidis and the characteristics of bacteriophages that limit our ability to use phage typing with the certainty that medical microbiologists desire for epidemiological investigations. In particular, the limitations of the scheme for detection of changes in the outer membrane that are associated with heightened virulence of *S*. Enteritidis are discussed.

CHARACTERISTICS OF A MODEL PHAGE-TYPING SCHEME

To develop a typing scheme, a set of bacterial strains must be maintained as hosts for assay of environmental samples that might contain infectious phage. These strains should differ from each other in their ability to produce outer-membrane molecules that are potentially phage receptors. Indeed, a phage-typing scheme used to investigate the outer-membrane properties of *Salmonella* Typhimurium incorporated intentionally mutagenized strains for its fullest development (Lilleengen, 1948; Boyd, 1950; Zinder and Lederberg, 1952; Sanderson et al., 1996). Simple techniques aided investigation of bacteriophage interactions with host cells (Adams, 1950). For example, inhibition of lysis indicated that certain outer-membrane fractions from wild-type strains contained receptor molecules. Advances in molecular genetics enabled receptors to be identified by restoring function to mutants with plasmids carrying intact genes (complementation). This basic research approach had great impact on the development of modern molecular biology, microbiology, and genetics (Lindberg, 1973, 1977;

Berget and Poteete, 1980; Morona et al., 1984; Nikaido, 1992, 1996). Consequently, the *Salmonella* Typhimurium phage-typing scheme remains the "gold standard" for use of bacteriophages in characterizing the Gram-negative bacteria outer membrane.

As an aid to readers, a model *S*. Enteritidis phage-typing scheme is depicted that incorporates the use of hypothetical typing phages a–h to divide *S*. Enteritidis into several phage types (Table 21.1). Numerical designations are assigned to these phage types that are similar to those of the *S*. Enteritidis typing scheme, indicating how *S*. Enteritidis strains are classified (Ward et al., 1987). The model incorporates ideal characteristics of host and virus that would be required to eliminate some of the uncertainty of using phage typing as an epidemiological tool. Problems associated with conducting phage typing are discussed in comparison to the model throughout this chapter. The model includes two hypothetical typing phages (a and b) that bind two different unknown outer-membrane molecules. These unknown receptors (A and B) are stringently regulated but are constitutively produced by some *S*. Enteritidis strains, one of which produces both molecules at the same time. These molecules could be porins, proteins associated with invasion, or stringently regulated modifications to a surface carbohydrate or a protein. The other six typing phages bind different lipopolysaccharide (LPS) structures (Fig. 21.1), and more detail about LPS heterogeneity of *S*. Enteritidis is presented later in this chapter. Three phages (c, d, and e) bind the O-chain region of LPS but recognize different sugar residues within the O chain. Strains that produce an O-chain region, usually composed of 5–28 repeating units, are smooth phenotypes (Fig. 21.1). Three phages (f–h) bind different sugars within the core region of LPS and thus continue to infect strains lacking O chain. Strains lacking O chain have a rough phenotype. A "semismooth" LPS, containing fewer than five O-chain repeating units, is also hypothesized. Semismooth strains lose the ability to bind phages c and d but continue to bind phage e. It is hoped that by providing a framework for explaining how phage types are determined, insight will be obtained into the complex nature of the outer membrane of *S*. Enteritidis.

PROPERTIES OF BACTERIOPHAGES THAT AFFECT PHAGE TYPE

Infection of the bacterial cell by a bacteriophage has two outcomes: lysis of the host cell or integration into its chromosome (lysogeny). Lytic phage is best suited for epidemiological studies, because distinctions made between strains on the basis of optical characteristics are more apparent from clear plaques than from the turbid plaques of lysogenic phage (Delbruck, 1945; Anderson and Roth, 1978; Koch, 1996). If bacterial strains are classified as different phage types based on patterns of incomplete lysis, then at some point one will be studying the characteristics of the

TABLE 21.1 A model scheme for phage typing *Salmonella enterica* serovar Enteritidis

	Identifying cell-surface characteristics of the host strain							
Model phage type	Unknown A	Unknown B	Smooth LPS	Smooth LPS	Semismooth LPS, one repeat unit	Rough LPS, Ra core	Rough LPS, Ra core	PT4 lineage core
			Typing phage					
	(a)	(b)	(c)	(d)	(e)	(f)	(g)	(h)
Untypeable A	–	–	–	–	–	–	–	–
3	+	–	+	+	–	–	–	–
1	+	+	+	+	+	+	+	+
2	+	–	+	+	+	+	+	–
4	–	+	+	+	+	+	+	+
8	+	–	+	+	+	+	+	–
6	–	–	+	+	+	+	+	+
13a	–	–	+	+	+	+	+	–
24	–	–	–	wk	wk	wk	+	wk
13	–	–	–	–	+	+	+	+
6a	–	–	–	–	+	+	+	–
23	–	–	–	–	–	+	+	+
7	–	–	–	–	–	+	+	+
Untypeable B	–	–	–	–	–	–	–	–

PT4, phage type 4; LPS, lipopolysaccharide; wk, weak reaction.

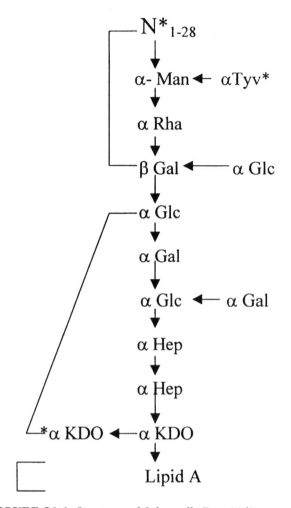

FIGURE 21.1 Structure of *Salmonella* Enteritidis lipopolysaccharide (LPS). The three major regions of LPS are *bracketed*. Linkages of sugars to each other are alpha (α) or beta (β). Nonstoichiometric modifications that have been identified as important to *S.* Enteritidis outer-membrane heterogeneity and phage type are indicated by an *asterisk*. See reviews on LPS structure for more detail about linkages and other known nonstoichiometric modifications (Schnaitman and Klena, 1993; Reeves, 1994; Raetz, 1996). Man, mannose; Tyv, tyvelose; Rha, rhamnose; Gal, galactose; Glc, glucose; Hep, heptose; KDO, 2-keto-3-deoxyoctulosonic acid.

bacteriophage in addition to those of the host cell (Adams, 1950; Wilkinson et al., 1972; Iwashita and Kanegasaki, 1973; Goldberg et al., 1974; Koch, 1996). Therefore, the model scheme reports results only as positive or negative, and makes no distinction between semiclear, opaque, or other possible forms of incomplete lysis (Table 21.1). Thus, in the development of a typing scheme, some ambiguity

can be resolved by isolating phages that are only lytic by screening for clear plaque mutants (Iwashita and Kanegasaki, 1973; Goldberg et al., 1974). The *S.* Enteritidis phage-typing scheme incorporates several phages that produce incomplete lysis, which is often used as a basis to differentiate phage types.

An additional outcome of infection is that prophage lysogenized into the host chromosome may cause resistance to subsequent infection (superimmunity) by other phages or the initially infecting phage. Resistance to infection often occurs when genes encoded by prophage modify host cell molecules that function as receptors (Pugsley and Schnaitman, 1978; Campbell et al., 1990; Schnaitman and Klena, 1993). Superinfection immunity can also impart new biological properties to the host cell that can alter the immunological properties of the outer membrane (Campbell, 1988; Barondess and Beckwith, 1990; Campbell et al., 1990). It is likely that some of the diversity of *S.* Enteritidis phage types results from the evolutionary interplay between different phages and the host. However, although there appear to be two major groupings of *S.* Enteritidis phage types, which will be discussed, a prophage has not been identified as the cause of division in clonal lineages. Form variation due to prophage modification of LPS occurs within the salmonellae that changes the α1,4 glucose linkage to galactose of O chain to α1,6 (Fig. 21.1) (Makela and Stocker, 1969; Plosila and Makela, 1972; Schnaitman and Klena, 1993). Chemical and immunological analyses of *S.* Enteritidis O chain obtained from naturally infected mice have never revealed this prophage-encoded linkage (J. Guard-Petter, unpublished data; Guard-Petter et al., 1997).

The *S.* Enteritidis phage-typing scheme also makes distinctions on the basis of efficiency of plating, and, currently, four categories ranging from very weak lysis (+/−) to complete lysis (4+) are routinely reported. As in the case of incomplete lysis, there are problems associated with assigning a new phage type based on evidence that viral heterogeneity exists (Koch, 1996). For example, cells might be infected by the virus, but the virus remains lysogenized for reasons associated more with the characteristics of the virus than with differences between host cell-surface properties. Since lysis is an outcome that is the last event in an infectious process that begins by recognition of a receptor by a viral particle, the presence of a few plaques is as indicative of successful infection as are many plaques. Thus, in the model scheme (Table 21.1), no distinctions are made on the basis of efficiency of plating.

There is information that could be derived from phage typing that is not reported by the *S.* Enteritidis typing scheme. Binding by phage to a receptor is often a cooperative process, where several receptors on the host cell are bound by several tail-fiber proteins of a single phage particle (Berget and Poteete, 1980; Goldenberg and King, 1982). If the amount of receptor produced by the host is below a threshold amount, binding is unstable, and cells remain uninfected. Since receptors on host cells are sometimes important virulence factors, kinetic binding studies with lytic phages could yield important insight about outer-membrane heterogeneity of *S.* Enteritidis. However, strains that constitutively hyperproduce receptors will not be differentiated from those that produce threshold amounts, because an excess of receptor does not contribute more to the outcome of an infection. These details of phage binding are particularly relevant when applied to the analysis of the *S.* Enteritidis outer membrane, because strains that readily increase production of certain outer-membrane structures above a threshold level are possibly more efficient at producing contaminated eggs (Guard-Petter, 1997; Guard-Petter et al., 1997).

LIPOPOLYSACCHARIDE AND PORE-FORMING PROTEINS ARE COMMON PHAGE RECEPTORS

Bacteriophages are most useful for epidemiological purposes if they provide information similar to the specificity achieved, for example, with monoclonal antibodies, thus providing unequivocal information about the presence of specific epitopes on the bacterial cell surface. Fortunately, bacteriophages bind with the same specificity as monoclonal antibodies (Iwashita and Kanegasaki, 1973; Goldberg et al., 1974; Gross et al., 1977). As with a monoclonal antibody, a typing phage is more informative if its receptor has been identified. The *S.* Typhimurium scheme revealed that LPS was a cell-surface molecule that commonly functioned as a bacteriophage receptor (Yarmolinsky and Sternberg, 1988; Berg and Howe, 1989; Casadesus and Roth, 1989; Campbell, 1996). Other common phage receptors are the F pilus, outer-membrane porins, transport proteins, and capsules (Hershey and Rotman, 1949; Adams and Park, 1952; Gross et al., 1977; Rieger-Hug and Stirm, 1981; Model and Russell, 1988; van Duin, 1988; Campbell, 1996). Surprisingly, some complex outer-membrane structures, for example, flagellin and attachment fimbria, are not often observed to be phage receptors. In addition, none of the more recently identified invasion proteins appear to be common phage receptors (Galan and Curtiss, 1989; Mahan et al., 1995). Thus, medical microbiologists should recognize that phage typing provides only partial information about the outer membrane, and that dramatic changes occur in molecules that are not receptors for typing phages but that are important virulence factors nonetheless.

Why bacteriophages evolve to bind certain molecules is not clear, but some differences between a frequent phage receptor, LPS, and an infrequent one, flagellin, can be described. LPS O antigen is a flexible polymer with many identical repeating epitopes separated by only a few sugars, and thus several tail fibers can bind to one LPS molecule. Also, LPS molecules are crowded together, which again increases the overall density of binding sites for phages that can bind as many as six receptors at once. For example, the LPS galactose residue of *S.* Enteritidis is repeated every fourth sugar, and the total molecular weight for one com-

plete subunit is about 720 atomic mass units. In contrast, the repeating epitopes of proteins composed of subunits are separated by a much greater interunit distance. A single H1 flagellin subunit of *S.* Enteritidis has 504 amino acids and a molecular weight of 52,855 kDa (Joys, 1985; Li et al., 1993). Thus, flagellin has numerous antigenic epitopes, but binding-site density of any one epitope is low. Also, the intermolecular distance between each flagellum is large in comparison to that between LPS molecules. However, not all phages use a cooperative binding process, and the presence of one molecule in the outer membrane can be sufficient for infection to occur (Model and Russell, 1988). These receptors allow direct access of the phage into the host cell, and some phages evolved to take advantage of these conduits. Flagellin also has a central conduit for multimeric assembly, but if flagellin monomers are not flowing out of the cell, the channel is either not yet completely formed or is sealed (Hughes et al., 1993; MacNab, 1996).

THE STRUCTURE OF LPS HAS MACROHETEROGENEITY AND MICROHETEROGENEITY

Two characteristics of LPS make it particularly attractive as a phage receptor. First, it is the most prevalent single molecule in the outer membrane of Gram-negative organisms and, secondly, it has a complex structure that may be greatly altered between strains. A complete LPS molecule is composed of lipid A, core oligosaccharide, and O antigen (Fig. 21.1) (Schnaitman and Klena, 1993; Reeves, 1994; Raetz, 1996). Incomplete molecules lacking O chain are commonly produced by some "rough" strains, which have a cobblestone appearance on agar (Naide et al., 1965). Major changes in *S.* Enteritidis LPS structure are easily detectable by techniques such as phage typing, polyacrylamide-gel electrophoresis (PAGE), colony immunoblotting, slide agglutination, or other immunoassays. Rough phenotypes of *S.* Enteritidis always lack slide-agglutination immunoreactivity with D1-typing antisera that detect O antigen, although traces of O antigen can be detected by the more sensitive PAGE techniques and compositional analyses (Petter, 1993; Guard-Petter et al., 1995, 1996). The core region of rough strains can sometimes be linked to other complex carbohydrates, such as enterobacterial common antigen, which can impart unique immunogenicity and the deceptive appearance of an O chain by PAGE to some rough strains (Kiss et al., 1978; Kuhn et al., 1988; Rick and Silver, 1996). The absence of an entire region such as O chain is an example of LPS macroheterogeneity.

For epidemiologists, the association of phage type with a complete LPS molecule is a first step at arriving at conclusions about the nature of a bacterial population involved in an epidemic. This knowledge is especially important for salmonellae because the absence of O chain profoundly affects the ability of these organisms to cause disease (Roantree, 1967; Joiner, 1988; Goldman and Hunt, 1990; Cox and Woolcock, 1994). Little information is available about the *S.* Enteritidis host strains that were used to develop the original phage-typing system, although this relationship can be reconstructed from the available data (Table 21.1). Assuming that typing phages c and d bind the typical *S.* Enteritidis O-chain structure that has more than five repeating units, then phage types (PTs) 1, 2, 3, 4, 6, 8, and 13a all produce an O-chain region, whereas PT7 and PT23 do not (Table 21.1). The typing characteristics of PT6a, PT13, and PT24 suggest that there are strains that produce O chain with a less frequently encountered "semismooth" structure, which might completely lack glucosylation and fail to produce more than trace amounts of O chain (Fig. 21.1; Table 21.1). Actual phage typing indicates that PT7 is a rough phenotype of PT4, and that rough PT23 is derived from PT13a and PT8 (Chart et al., 1991, 1993; Powell et al., 1995; Guard-Petter et al., 1996; Baggesen et al., 1997).

Although it is more common to recover strains with O chain from infected animals, rough strains might still be important to the overall epidemiological problem of egg contamination by *S.* Enteritidis. Indeed, investigations revealed that strains lacking O chain are quickly generated from virulent ones (Guard-Petter et al., 1995, 1996, 1997). Under defined growth conditions, some rough *S.* Enteritidis strains can revert to smooth (Guard-Petter, 1997), although most evidence indicates that the generation of rough or semismooth phenotypes from smooth is much more frequent (Guard-Petter et al., 1996). Apparently, the rough and semismooth phenotypes emerge when growth conditions provide limited access to nutrients and metabolites that are essential for cell differentiation and survival (Guard-Petter et al., 1996; Guard-Petter, 1997). LPS core is often divided into an inner-core region and outer-core region, in part because heptose and 2-keto-3-deoxyoctulosonic acid comprising the inner-core region are unique to bacteria (Fig. 21.1). Strains that produce complete core regions (Ra core chemotype) grow well and are stable in the environment, whereas those lacking core components are infrequently observed (Makela and Stocker, 1984; Schnaitman and Klena, 1993; Vaara, 1993). Lack of core components (Fig. 21.1) has a marked effect on the ability of cells to bind bacteriophage for possibly two reasons (Lindberg, 1977). First, loss of core constituents removes sugar moieties that might be receptors, and, second, protein composition of the outer membrane changes as the structure of LPS changes (Ames et al., 1974; Pugsley, 1993; Schulz, 1993; Stanley et al., 1993). The model typing phages f, g, and h are depicted as interacting with the common constituents of LPS core (Table 21.1). It is possible to propose this binding pattern, because a strain designated as "reacts but does not conform (RDNC)" was generated and further characterized by PAGE and chemical analyses (Guard-Petter et al., 1995). Results indicated that this strain produced a defective core LPS compared with wild-type or rough strains with a complete Ra core region. Since changes in core contribute to phage resistance, it is likely that some isolates classified as untypeable produce deep rough cores and fail to produce many of the receptors normally encountered in strains that produce a complete core region with or without O chain.

PHAGE TYPING DETECTS SOME, BUT NOT ALL, LPS MICROHETEROGENEITY

LPS microheterogeneity occurs when strains modify the basic structure of a complete LPS molecule by the addition of R-group substituents (Fig. 21.1) (Schnaitman and Klena, 1993; Reeves, 1994; Raetz, 1996). Stoichiometric substituents do not vary in amount within the regions of LPS, an example of which is that one repeating unit of O chain has one tyvelose residue (Fig. 21.1). Nonstoichiometric LPS substituents are sometimes referred to as "decorations," or modifications that vary considerably between strains from a single serovar. In comparison to having one tyvelose per repeating unit of O chain, linkage of glucose to galactose is nonstoichiometric and might occur in only a fraction of the total repeating units on a cell surface (Fig. 21.1). Nonstoichiometric changes to the structure of an "average" LPS molecule can be numerous and are of interest to molecular biologists, since the changes alter immunogenicity and attributes of LPS that have biological consequences, including the ability to serve as receptors for phages.

Strains that yield significantly different amounts of nonstoichiometric substituents compared with wild-type *S.* Enteritidis are distinct phenotypes. For example, most *S.* Enteritidis field isolates produce a low amount of high molecular weight (HMW) O chain, where the number of LPS molecules with more than 10 repeating units is probably fewer than 10% of all LPS molecules (Fig. 21.1) (Rahman et al., 1997). Thus, approximately 90% of O-chain molecules from these strains are of low molecular weight (LMW) and have an average of five repeating units, whereas a few molecules have as many as 28 repeating units. Conversely, the occasional *S.* Enteritidis isolate produces greater than 50% HMW O chain, and some fresh isolates produce close to 100% HMW LPS (Guard-Petter et al., 1996, 1997; Rahman et al., 1997). O-chain variation between strains is not detectable by phage typing, since all strains with even a few O-chain molecules greater than five repeating units produce a threshold level of receptor. Quantitative PAGE and immunoblotting techniques for assessing this type of variation in the *S.* Enteritidis O chain have been described (Guard-Petter et al., 1996). Research also indicates that epidemiologically important phage types that have a smooth LPS (such as PT4, PT8, and PT13a) can all be subdivided into different populations on the basis of O-chain structure (Guard-Petter et al., 1995, 1996; Humphrey et al., 1996). HMW LPS is more frequently glucosylated than is LMW LPS, and when total yields of O-chain glucose are a log higher than the wild-type structure, *S.* Enteritidis LPS structure resembles that produced by *S.* Typhi (Hellerqvist et al., 1969; Rahman et al., 1997). Glucosylation of HMW LPS might be a type of microheterogeneity that occurs in other salmonellae (Helander et al., 1992).

Recently, another example of how LPS microheterogeneity is associated with a biological consequence has come to light. Namely, lipid A in the phospholipid bilayer of the outer membrane was found to have an alternative structure, which altered the ability of bacterial cells to stimulate cytokines and to behave as an endotoxin (Takada and Kotani, 1992; Raetz, 1996; Guo et al., 1997). Bacteriophages are unable to use lipid A as a receptor because its location in the outer membrane makes it inaccessible to phage attachment organelles. These examples of microheterogeneity of LPS that do not change *S.* Enteritidis phage type further illustrate that phage typing is limited as a technique for describing strain variability associated with changing patterns of virulence.

OTHER COMPLEX CARBOHYDRATES BESIDES LPS AFFECT *SALMONELLA* ENTERITIDIS PHAGE TYPE

During an on-farm investigation of rodent populations naturally infected with invasive *S.* Enteritidis, the surface characteristics of strains obtained directly from spleens of mice indicated that HMW LPS could be recovered in unexpectedly high amounts (Guard-Petter et al., 1997). However, one additional in vitro passage required for phage typing resulted in classification of the six strains under investigation as "*Salmonella*, phage type untypeable." This phage-type designation occurred in concert with a drastic change in colony morphology of strains to a mucoid phenotype. Indeed, the mucoid strains were not lysed by bacteriophage P22, indicating the absence or inaccessibility of O chain. Chemical analyses revealed that these six isolates lacked O chain and, in addition, were producing fucose-rich colanic acid (M.M. Rahman, personal communication). Colanic acid is a group IA (LPS-like) capsule produced by many bacterial species at non-physiological temperatures to protect cells against desiccation, osmotic stress, and oxidative stress (Gottesman and Stout, 1991; Keenlyside et al., 1993; Whitfield and Valvano, 1993). Thus, conversion of *S.* Enteritidis that produced copious amounts of both O and H antigens to a mucoid salmonella that could not be serotyped or phage typed is another indication that part of the important biology of *S.* Enteritidis is its ability to adapt quickly to a number of environments by altering its cell-surface characteristics. Although capsules often bind phage, there has been no evidence that any of the *S.* Enteritidis typing phages use colanic acid as a receptor (Adams and Park, 1952; Gross et al., 1977; Silver and Vimr, 1990). Thinning of capsule was associated with emergence of new phage types, represented in the model scheme as PT3, and such strains are identified by their binding O-chain phages c and d without binding core-specific phages e–h (Table 21.1). Apparently then, there are two kinds of untypeable salmonellae that can occur in *S.* Enteritidis populations: the first kind, untypeable A, has phage receptors masked by colanic acid, whereas untypeable B strains lack phage receptors due to loss of core constituents (Fig. 21.1) (Table 21.1).

PLASMIDS CAN SOMETIMES AFFECT PHAGE TYPE

PT4 is converted to PT6a after transformation with a naturally isolated ampicillin resistance plasmid belonging to incompatibility (Inc) group X (Frost et al., 1989; Vatopoulos et al., 1994; Ridley et al., 1996). This same plasmid also converts PT8 to PT13 (Ridley et al., 1996). Strains transformed with this plasmid are no longer resistant to complement, suggesting that the acquisition of plasmids other than the commonly encountered virulence plasmid of *S.* Enteritidis is associated with attenuation (Chart et al., 1996). Loss of complement resistance often occurs when the structure of LPS lacks O chain, but characterization of PT6a and 13 yielded a banding pattern suggestive of O chain in silver-stained polyacrylamide gels. However, no confirmatory analyses of LPS were performed to determine whether the ratio of O chain to core (O/C ratio) had not been significantly decreased, or whether O chain had been replaced by other carbohydrates. If loss or diminution of O/C ratios had occurred, then it is possible PT6a and PT13 lost phage receptors for O-chain phages c and d but not e (Table 21.1). Although plasmids are involved in generating tetracycline resistance, no correlation with phage type could be established (Son et al., 1995). Therefore, the preponderance of evidence indicates that plasmids occasionally alter phage type, and when they do, strains have a tendency to become attenuated. Although plasmids are involved in generating tetracycline resistance, no correlation with phage type can be established (Ward et al., 1990; Son et al., 1995).

PHAGE TYPE 4 *SALMONELLA* ENTERITIDIS IS UNIQUE

The WHO phage-typing scheme does detect one phage type that historical evidence suggests is of epidemiological significance. The emergence of PT4 has been associated with an increased incidence of human illness in those countries where it becomes the predominant phage type (Rampling et al., 1989; Katouli et al., 1993; Caffer and Eiguer, 1994; Cox and Woolcock, 1994; Glosnicka and Kunikowska, 1994; Schroeter et al., 1994; Boyce et al., 1996; Humphrey et al., 1996; Irino et al., 1996). Recent comparison of LPS samples from 18 unrelated PT4 *S.* Enteritidis with those from 31 non-PT4 *S.* Enteritidis indicates that the LPS of PT4 differs in structure from that of PT23, PT13a, and PT8, with a probability (p value) of less than 0.001 that LPS from PT4 and LPS from non-PT4 *S.* Enteritidis are the same (Asokan, 1997; J. Guard-Petter, manuscript in preparation). These findings provide strong biological evidence that there are two distinct lineages of *S.* Enteritidis distinguishable by phage typing. Using the model typing scheme depicted in Table 21.1, typing phage h distinguishes between PT4 and non-PT4 lineages. Those phage types that are sensitive to infection by typing phage h are members of the PT4 lineage, and include PT1, PT6, PT24, PT6a, and PT7, in addition to PT4 (Table 21.1)

(Ward et al., 1987; Threlfall et al., 1993, 1994; Baggesen et al., 1997). Those phage types that are resistant to infection by typing phage h form the non-PT4 lineage, and include PT2, PT8, PT13a, PT13, and PT23 (Table 21.1) (Ward et al., 1987). It is not possible to group phage types that are producing colanic acid (untypeable A and PT3) or those that have lost core constituents (untypeable B) into either lineage, because the receptor for h is either masked or missing. Further investigation is in progress to define the unique structural details of PT4 LPS, and it has been determined that the change occurs in LPS core. Other investigators have produced evidence that a PT4 family exists. For example, there is evidence that some PT23 strains might be a common reservoir from which both families originate, because transformation of plasmid pDEP44 from a PT23 strain into PT8 and PT4 strains resulted in conversion of both strains to PT24 (Threlfall et al., 1993).

There is additional evidence that PT4 has unique biological capabilities. *Salmonella* Enteritidis typically produces only H1 flagella (Kauffman, 1966; Li et al., 1993). However, induction of biphasic flagellation by *S.* Enteritidis on specialized media has recently been described (Guard-Petter, 1997). Under these conditions, *S.* Enteritidis phage types other than PT4 have immunoreactivity to H2 flagella typing antisera. Thus, PT4 *S.* Enteritidis is more likely than other *S.* Enteritidis to remain in the H1 phase. The H1 gene product of *S.* Enteritidis is FliC, and hyperproduction of this type of flagella is associated with the enhanced ability of some Gram-negative bacteria to migrate across surfaces (Allison et al., 1994). A unique feature of *S.* Enteritidis biology in comparison to other swarming Gram-negative pathogens is that its ability to undergo migration across inhibitory agar surfaces has been associated with the production of glucosylated HMW LPS (Guard-Petter et al., 1996, 1997; Guard-Petter, 1997).

FUTURE IMPROVEMENTS SUGGESTED FOR *SALMONELLA* ENTERITIDIS MOLECULAR TYPING

The *S.* Enteritidis WHO phage-typing scheme successfully distinguishes PT4 and non-PT4 lineages, and there is historical evidence that emergence of PT4 *S.* Enteritidis is associated with increased incidence of salmonellosis in people. Therefore, an assay to detect the unique PT4 LPS structure is being developed as a rapid method to screen large numbers of isolates. This assay will not replace phage typing, and if a suspect PT4 is detected, confirmation by one of the two U.S. laboratories approved to do *S.* Enteritidis phage typing would be required. Neither will it replace routine surveillance of a portion of *S.* Enteritidis isolates within the United States for the presence of PT4 strains. However, a rapid method is needed so that routine culturing required to do hazard analysis of critical control points (HACCPs) will yield information that enables initial classification of an isolate as PT4 or non-PT4.

Research also indicates that strains do not have to be PT4 to be highly virulent (Petter, 1993; Guard-Petter et al., 1995). Conversely, classification of a strain simply as PT4 is not necessarily an indicator of virulence (Gast and Benson, 1996; Humphrey et al., 1996). Therefore, there are avirulent and virulent PT4 strains, as well as avirulent and virulent non-PT4 strains. Perhaps the unique biology of PT4 helps it to survive and spread in the environment of the henhouse, to survive within the egg for longer periods, or to overgrow bacterial floras present in the bird or henhouse (Selander and Musser, 1990). Thus, a virulence assay is needed as part of an early warning system for public health agencies that strains have emerged that are likely to be highly invasive. No data conflict with several studies that indicate unusual structures of LPS O chain are predictors of enhanced virulence of *S.* Enteritidis for poultry and rodents that inhabit poultry houses. Rapid methods for subtyping O-chain structure have been described (Guard-Petter et al., 1995, 1996). By combining a simple assay for phage type with assays for O-chain structure, *S.* Enteritidis can be classified into four groups that can be tracked and investigated for their role in propagating human salmonellosis associated with the consumption of contaminated eggs (Fig. 21.2). Strains that are from a PT4 lineage and producing HMW LPS would be of most concern within the United States, because they are complement resistant, more invasive in chickens, and historically associated with increased salmonellosis in people. However, detection of any *S.* Enteritidis that could possibly be PT4 would be valuable information that could help us make decisions about how any one flock of birds should be handled.

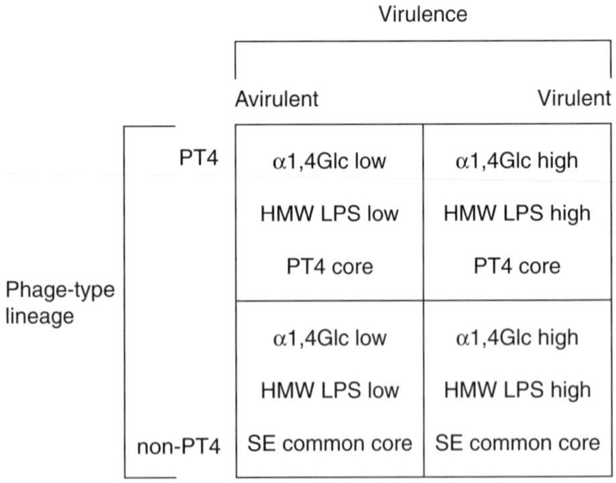

	Virulence	
	Avirulent	Virulent
PT4	α1,4Glc low HMW LPS low PT4 core	α1,4Glc high HMW LPS high PT4 core
non-PT4	α1,4Glc low HMW LPS low SE common core	α1,4Glc high HMW LPS high SE common core

Phage-type lineage

FIGURE 21.2 Hazard analysis of *Salmonella* Enteritidis (SE) by rapid assay of lipopolysaccharide (LPS) structure. Levels of glucosylation (α1,4Glc) and high molecular weight (HMW) LPS are reported relative to wild-type *S.* Enteritidis LPS structure (Hellerqvist et al., 1969). The core of phage type 4 (PT4) is reported as present or absent. SE, *S.* Enteritidis.

DISCUSSION

The United States is at a critical juncture in regard to controlling *S.* Enteritidis contamination of eggs. Information about the epidemiology of *S.* Enteritidis associated with human salmonellosis and phage type has been collected for a decade, and rigorous application of the WHO phage-typing scheme has generated a large part of this knowledge. Certainly this information has guided research efforts intended to prevent egg contamination, yet it appears that this pathogen remains pervasive and successful. If *S.* Enteritidis PT4 begins spontaneously and stably to produce virulence factors such as glucosylated HMW LPS, it is possible we will be faced with controlling a formidable organism that research indicates is efficient at spreading, invading the reproductive tracts of hens and internal organs of animal reservoirs such as mice, and producing cell-surface molecules that might improve its ability to infect people. We can now see that phage type is but part of the story of how this pathogen emerged to be the threat to food safety that it is today. The good news is that additional information about virulent *S.* Enteritidis could indicate that it has an Achilles' heel hidden within its biology. As we are facing *S.* Enteritidis as an emerging pathogen in the United States, it is time to take the best lessons learned from a decade of studying *S.* Enteritidis phage type and combine them with the strengths of alternative typing methods.

REFERENCES

Adams, M.H. 1950. Method of study of bacterial viruses. In: Methods in medical research 7.

Adams, M.H., and Park, B.H. 1952. An enzyme produced by a phage-host cell system. II. The properties of the polysaccharide depolymerase. Virology 2:719–736.

Allison, C., Emody, L., Coleman, N., and Hughes, C. 1994. The role of swarm cell differentiation and multicellular migration in the uropathogenicity of *Proteus mirabilis*. J. Infect. Dis. 169:1155–1158.

Altecruse, S., Koehler, J., Hickman-Brenner, F., Tauxe, R.V., and Ferris, K. 1993. A comparison of *Salmonella enteritidis* phage types from egg associated outbreaks and implicated laying flocks. Epidemiol. Infect. 110:17–22.

Ames, G.-F., Spudich, E.N., and Nikaido, H. 1974. Protein composition of the outer membrane of *Salmonella typhimurium*: effect of lipopolysaccharide mutations. J. Bacteriol. 117:406–416.

Anderson, R.P., and Roth, J.R. 1987. Tandem genetic duplications in phage and bacteria. Annu. Rev. Microbiol. 31:473–505.

Aoyama, A., and Hayashi, M. 1986. Synthesis of bacteriophage fX174 in vitro: mechanism of switch from DNA replication to DNA packaging. Cell 47:99–106.

Asokan, K. 1997. Isolation, characterization and structural analysis of capsular- and lipo-polysaccharides from pathogenic strains of *Salmonella enteritidis*, *Proteus vulgaris* and *Proteus mirabilis* [Thesis]. Athens: University of Georgia.

Baggesen, D.L., Wegener, H.C., and Madsen, M. 1997. Correlation of conversion of *Salmonella enterica* serovar Enteritidis phage type 1, 4, or 6 to phage type 7 with loss of lipopolysaccharide. J. Clin. Microbiol. 35:330–333.

Barondess, J.J., and Beckwith, J. 1990. A bacterial virulence determinant encoded by lysogenic coliphage lambda. Nature (London) 346:871–874.

Belland, R.J., Morrison, S.G., Carlson, J.H., and Hogan, D.M. 1997. Promoter strength influences phase variation of neisserial opa genes. Mol. Microbiol. 23:123–135.

Berg, D.E., and Howe, M.M., eds. 1989. Mobile DNA. Washington, DC: American Society for Microbiology.

Berget, P.T., and Poteete, A.R. 1980. Structure and function of the bacteriophage P22 tail protein. J. Virol. 34:234–243.

Boyce, T.G., Koo, D., Swerdlow, D.L., Gomez, T.M., Serrano, B., Nickey, L.N., Hickman-Brenner, F.W., Malcolm, G.B., and Griffin, P.M. 1996. Recurrent outbreaks of *Salmonella enteritidis* infections in a Texas restaurant: phage type 4 arrives in the United States. Epidemiol. Infect. 117:29–34.

Boyd, J.S.K. 1950. The symbiotic bacteriophages of *Salmonella typhimurium*. J. Pathol. Bacteriol. 62:501–517.

Caffer, M.I., and Eiguer, T. 1994. *Salmonella enteritidis* in Argentina. Int. J. Food Microbiol. 21:15–19.

Campbell, A. 1988. Phage evolution and speciation. In: Calendar, R., ed. The bacteriophages. New York: Plenum, pp. 1–14.

Campbell, A., Kim-Ha, J., Limberger, R.J., and Schneider, S.J. 1990. Bacteriophage evolution and population structure. In: Clegg, M.T., and O'Brien, S.J., eds. Molecular evolution. New York: Wiley-Liss, pp. 191–199.

Campbell, A.M. 1996. Bacteriophages. In: Neidhardt, F.C., et al., eds. *Escherichia coli* and *Salmonella*: cellular and molecular biology. Washington, DC: American Society for Microbiology, pp. 2325–2338.

Casadesus, J., and Roth, J.R. 1989. Transcriptional occlusion of transposon targets. Mol. Gen. Genet. 216:204–209.

Chart, H., Ward, L.R., and Rowe, B. 1991. Expression of lipopolysaccharide by phage types of *Salmonella enteritidis*. Lett. Appl. Microbiol. 13:39–41.

Chart, H., Threlfall, E.J., Ward, L.R., and Rowe, B. 1993. Unusual expression of lipopolysaccharide by strains of *Salmonella enteritidis* phage type 30. Lett. Appl. Microbiol. 16:87–90.

Chart, H., Threlfall, E.J., Powell, N.G., and Rowe, B. 1996. Serum survival and plasmid possession by strains of *Salmonella enteritidis*, *Salm. typhimurium* and *Salm. virchow*. J. Appl. Microbiol. 80:31–36.

Citti, C., and Wise, K.S. 1995. *Mycoplasma hyorhinis* vlp gene transcription: critical role in phase variation and expression of surface lipoproteins. Mol. Microbiol. 18:649–660.

Cox, J.M., and Woolcock, J.B. 1994. Lipopolysaccharide expression and virulence in mice of Australian isolates of *Salmonella enteritidis*. Lett. Appl. Microbiol. 19:95–98.

Delbruck, M. 1945. The burst size distribution in the growth of bacterial viruses (bacteriophages). J. Bacteriol. 50:131–135.

Ebel, E.D., Mason, J., Thomas, L.A., Ferris, K.E., Beckman, M.G., Cummins, D.R., Schroeder-Tucker, L., Sutherlin, W.D., Glasshoff, R.L., and Smithhisler, N.M. 1993. Occurrence of *Salmonella enteritidis* in unpasteurized liquid egg in the United States. Avian Dis. 37:135–142.

Frost, J.A., Ward, L.R., and Rowe, B. 1989. Acquisition of a drug resistance plasmid converts *Salmonella enteritidis* phage type 4 to phage type 24. Epidemiol. Infect. 103:243–248.

Galan, J.E., and Curtiss III, R. 1989. Cloning and molecular characterization of genes whose products allow *Salmonella typhimurium* to penetrate tissue culture cells. Proc. Natl. Acad. Sci. U.S.A. 86:6383–6387.

Gast, R.K., and Benson, S.T. 1996. Intestinal colonization and organ invasion in chicks experimentally infected with *Salmonella enteritidis* phage type 4 and other phage types isolated from poultry in the United States. Avian Dis. 40:853–857.

Geiduschek, E.P. 1991. Regulation of expression of the late genes of bacteriophage T3. Annu. Rev. Genet. 25:437–460.

Glosnicka, R., and Kunikowska, D. 1994. The epidemiological situation of *Salmonella enteritidis* in Poland. Int. J. Food Microbiol. 21:21–30.

Goldberg, R.B., Bender, R.A., and Streicher, S.L. 1974. Direct selection for P1-sensitive mutants of enteric bacteria. J. Bacteriol. 118:810–814.

Goldenberg, D., and King, J. 1982. Trimeric intermediate in the in vivo folding and subunit assembly of the tail spike endorhamnosidase of bacteriophage P22. Proc. Natl. Acad. Sci. U.S.A. 79:3403.

Goldman, R.C., and Hunt, F. 1990. Mechanism of O-antigen distribution in lipopolysaccharide. J. Bacteriol. 172:5352–5359.

Gottesman, S., and Stout, V. 1991. Regulation of capsular polysaccharide synthesis in *Escherichia coli* K-12. Mol. Microbiol. 5:1599–1606.

Gross, R.J., Cheasty, T., and Rowe, B. 1977. Isolation of bacteriophage specific for the K1 polysaccharide antigen of *Escherichia coli*. J. Clin. Microbiol. 6:548–550.

Guard-Petter, J. 1997. Induction of flagellation and a novel agar-penetrating flagellar structure in *Salmonella enterica* grown on solid media: possible consequences for serological identification. FEMS Microbiol. Lett. 149:173–180.

Guard-Petter, J., Lakshmi, B., Carlson, R., and Ingram, K. 1995. Characterization of lipopolysaccharide heterogeneity in *Salmonella enteritidis* by an improved gel electrophoresis method. Appl. Environ. Microbiol. 61:2845–2851.

Guard-Petter, J., Keller, L.H., Rahman, M.M., Carlson, R.W., and Silvers, S. 1996. A novel relationship between O-antigen variation, matrix formation, and invasiveness of *Salmonella enteritidis*. Epidemiol. Infect. 117:219–231.

Guard-Petter, J., Henzler, D.J., Rahman, M.M., and Carlson, R.W. 1997. On-farm monitoring of mouse-invasive *Salmonella enterica* serovar Enteritidis and a model for its association with the production of contaminated eggs. Appl. Environ. Microbiol. 63:1588–1593.

Gunn, J.S., Hohmann, E.L., and Miller, S.I. 1996. Transcriptional regulation of *Salmonella* virulence: a PhoQ periplasmic domain mutation results in increased net phosphotransfer to PhoP. J. Bacteriol. 178:6369–6373.

Guo, L., Lim, K.B., Gunn, J.S., Bainbridge, B., Darveau, R.P., Hackett, M., and Miller, S.I. 1997. Regulation of lipid A modifications by *Salmonella typhimurium* virulence genes phoP-phoQ. Science 276:250–253.

Hausmann, R. 1988. The T7 group. In: Calendar, R., ed. The bacteriophages, vol. 1. New York: Plenum, pp. 259–290.

Helander, I.M., Moran, A.P., and Makela, P.H. 1992. Separation of two lipopolysaccharide populations with different contents of O-antigen factor 122 in *Salmonella enterica* serovar Typhimurium. Mol. Microbiol. 6:2857–2862.

Hellerqvist, C.G., Lindberg, B., Svensson, S., Holme, T., and Lindberg, A.A. 1969. Structural studies on the O-specific side chains of the cell wall lipopolysaccharides from *Salmonella typhi* and *Salmonella enteritidis*. Acta Chem. Scand. 23:1588–1596.

Hershey, A.D., and Rotman, R. 1949. Genetic recombination between host-range and plaque-type mutants of bacteriophage in single bacterial cells. Genetics 34:44–71.

Hickman-Brenner, F.W., Stubbs, A.D., and Farmer III, J.J. 1991. Phage typing of *Salmonella enteritidis* in the United States. J. Clin. Microbiol. 29:2817–2823.

Hughes, K.T., Gillen, K.L., Semon, M.J., and Karlinsky, J.E. 1993. Sensing structural intermediates in bacterial flagellar assembly by export of a negative regulator. Science 262:1277–1280.

Humphrey, T.J., Whitehead, A., Gawler, A.H.L., Henley, A., and Rowe, B. 1991. Numbers of *Salmonella enteritidis* in the contents of naturally contaminated hens' eggs. Epidemiol. Infect. 106:489–496.

Humphrey, T.J., Williams, A., McAlpine, K., Lever, S., Guard-Petter, J., and Cox, J.M. 1996. Isolates of *Salmonella enteritidis* PT4 with enhanced heat and acid tolerance are more virulent in mice and more invasive in chickens. Epidemiol. Infect. 117:79–88.

Irino, K., Fernandes, S.A., Tavechio, A.T., Neves, B.C., and Dias, A.M.G. 1996. Progression of *Salmonella enteritidis* phage type 4 strains in Sao Paulo State, Brazil. Rev. Inst. Med. Trop. Sao Paulo 38:193–196.

Iwashita, S., and Kanegasaki, S. 1973. Smooth specific phage adsorption: endorhamnosidase activity of tail parts of P22. Biochem. Biophys. Res. Commun. 55:403–409.

Jishage, M., and Ishihama, A. 1997. Variation in RNA polymerase sigma subunit composition within different stocks of *Escherichia coli* W3110. J. Bacteriol. 179:959–963.

Joiner, K.A. 1988. Complement evasion by bacteria and parasites. Annu. Rev. Microbiol. 42:201–230.

Joys, T.M. 1985. The covalent structure of the phase-1 flagellar filament protein of *Salmonella typhimurium* and its comparison to other flagellins. J. Biol. Chem. 260:15,758–15,761.

Katouli, M., Seuffer, R.H., Wollin, R., Kuhn, I., and Mollby, R. 1993. Variations in biochemical phenotypes and phage types of *Salmonella enteritidis* in Germany, 1980–1992. Epidemiol. Infect. 111:199–207.

Kauffman, F. 1966. The bacteriology of Enterobacteriaceae. Copenhagen: Munksgaard.

Keenleyside, W., Bronner, D., Jann, K., Jann, B., and Whitfield, C. 1993. Coexpression of colanic acid and serotype-specific capsular polysaccharides in *Escherichia coli* strains with group II K antigens. J. Bacteriol. 175:6725–6730.

Kiss, P., Rinno, J., Schmidt, G., and Mayer, H. 1978. Structural studies on the immunogenic form of the enterobacterial common antigen. Eur. J. Biochem. 88:211–218.

Koch, A.L. 1996. Similarities and differences of individual bacteria within a clone. In: Neidhardt, F.C., et al., eds. *Escherichia coli* and *Salmonella*: cellular and molecular biology. Washington, DC: American Society for Microbiology, pp. 1640–1651.

Kuhn, H.M., Neter, E., and Mayer, H. 1988. ECA, the enterobacterial common antigen. FEMS Microbiol. Rev. 54:195–222.

Li, J., Smith, N.H., Nelson, K., Crichton, P.B., Old, D.C., Whittam, T.S., and Selander, R.K. 1993. Evolutionary origin and radiation of the avian-adapted non-motile salmonellae. J. Med. Microbiol. 38:129–139.

Lilleengen, K. 1948. Typing *Salmonella typhimurium* by means of bacteriophage. Acta Pathol. Microbiol. Scand. Suppl. 77:11–125.

Lindberg, A.A. 1973. Bacteriophage receptors. Annu. Rev. Microbiol. 27:205–241.

Lindberg, A.A. 1977. Bacterial surface carbohydrates and bacteriophage absorption. In: Sutherland, I., ed. Surface carbohydrates of the procaryotic cell. New York: Academic, pp. 289–356.

MacNab, R.M. 1996. Flagella and motility. In: Neidhardt, F.C., et al., eds. *Escherichia coli* and *Salmonella*: cellular and molecular biology, 2nd ed. Washington, DC: American Society for Microbiology, pp. 123–145.

Mahan, M.J., Slauch, J.M., and Mekalanos, J.J. 1995. Environmental regulation of virulence gene expression in *Escherichia*, *Salmonella* and *Shigella*. In: Neidhardt, F.C., et al., eds. *Escherichia coli* and *Salmonella*: cellular and molecular biology, 2nd ed. Washington, DC: American Society for Microbiology, pp. 2803–2815.

Makela, P.H., and Stocker, B.A.D. 1969. Genetics of the bacterial cell surface. Symp. Soc. Gen. Microbiol. 31:219–264.

Makela, P.H., and Stocker, B.A.D. 1984. Genetics of lipopolysaccharide. In: Rietschel, E.T., ed. Handbook of endotoxin, vol. 1: chemistry of endotoxin. Amsterdam: Elsevier/North-Holland Biomedical, pp. 59–137.

Mathews, C.K., Kutter, E.M., Mosig, G., and Berget, P.B., eds. 1983. Bacteriophage T4. Washington, DC: American Society for Microbiology.

Matsushita, C., Matsushita, O., Katayama, S., Minami, J., Takai, K., and Okabe, A. 1996. An upstream activating sequence containing curved DNA involved in activation of the *Clostridium perfringens* plc promoter. Microbiology (Reading) 142:2561–2566.

Mishu, B., Koehier, J., Lee, L.A., Rodriguez, D., Brenner, F.H., and Tauxe, R.V. 1994. Outbreaks of *Salmonella enteritidis* infections in the United States, 1985–1991. J. Infect. Dis. 169:547–552.

Model, P., and Russell, M. 1988. Filamentous bacteriophage. In: Calendar, R., ed. The bacteriophages, vol. 2. New York: Plenum, pp. 375–456.

Morona, R., Klose, M., and Henning, U. 1984. *Escherichia coli* K-12 outer membrane protein (OmpA) as a bacteriophage receptor: analysis of mutant genes expressing altered proteins. J. Bacteriol. 159:570–578.

Mosig, G., and Eiserling, F. 1988. Phage T4 structure and metabolism. In: Calendar, R., ed. The bacteriophages, vol. 2. New York: Plenum, pp. 521–606.

Murase, T., Okitsu, T., Suzuki, R., Morozumi, H., Matsushima, A., Nakamura, A., and Yamai, S. 1995. Evaluation of DNA fingerprinting by PFGE as an epidemiologic tool for *Salmonella* infections. Microbiol. Immunol. 39:673–676.

Murase, T., Nakamura, A., Matsushima, A., and Yamai, S. 1996. An epidemiological study of *Salmonella enteritidis* by pulsed-field gel electrophoresis (PFGE): several PFGE patterns observed in isolates from a food poisoning outbreak. Microbiol. Immunol. 40:873–875.

Naide, Y., Nikaido, H., Makela, P.H., Wilkinson, R.G., and Stocker, B.A.D. 1965. Semirough strains of *Salmonella*. Proc. Natl. Acad. Sci. U.S.A. 53:147–153.

Nikaido, H. 1992. Porins and specific channels of bacterial outer membranes. Mol. Microbiol. 6:435–442.

Nikaido, H. 1996. Outer membrane. In: Neidhardt, F.C., et al., eds. *Escherichia coli* and *Salmonella*: cellular and molecular biology. Washington, DC: American Society for Microbiology, pp. 29–47.

Petter, J. 1993. Detection of two smooth colony phenotypes in a *Salmonella enteritidis* isolate which vary in their ability to contaminate eggs. Appl. Environ. Microbiol. 59:2884–2890.

Plosila, M., and Makela, P.H. 1972. Mapping of a gene *oaf*A determining antigen 1 in *Salmonella* of group E4. Scand. J. Clin. Lab. Invest. 29(Suppl. 122):55.

Poppe, C. 1994. *Salmonella enteritidis* in Canada. Int. J. Food Microbiol. 21:1–5.

Powell, N.G., Threlfall, E.J., Chart, H., Schofield, S.L., and Rowe, B. 1995. Correlation of change in phage type with pulsed field profile and 16S rrn profile in *Salmonella enteritidis* phage types 4, 7 and 9a. Epidemiol. Infect. 114:403–411.

Ptashne, M. 1992. A genetic switch: phage lambda and higher organisms, 2nd ed. Cambridge, MA: Blackwell Scientific.

Pugsley, A.P. 1993. The complete general secretory pathway in gram-negative bacteria. Microbiol. Rev. 57:50–108.

Pugsley, A.P., and Schnaitman, C.A. 1978. Identification of three genes controlling production of new outer membrane pore proteins in *Escherichia coli* K-12. J. Bacteriol. 135:1118–1129.

Raetz, C.R.H. 1996. Bacterial lipopolysaccharides: a remarkable family of bioactive macroamphiphiles. In: Neidhardt, F.C., et al., eds. *Escherichia coli* and *Salmonella*: cellular and molecular biology. Washington, DC: American Society for Microbiology, pp. 1035–1063.

Rahman, M.M., Guard-Petter, J., and Carlson, R.W. 1997. A virulent isolate of Salmonella enteritidis produces a *Salmonella typhi*-like lipopolysaccharide. J. Bacteriol. 179:2126–2131.

Rampling, A., Anderson, J.R., Upson, R., Peters, E., Ward, L.R., and Rowe, B. 1989. *Salmonella enteritidis* phage type 4 infection of broiler chickens: a hazard to public health. Lancet 2:436–438.

Reeves, P. 1994. Biosynthesis and assembly of lipopolysaccharide. In: Ghysen, J.M., and Hakenbeck, R., eds. Bacterial cell wall. New York: Elsevier, pp. 281–317.

Rick, P.D., and Silver, R.P. 1996. Enterobacterial common antigen and capsular polysaccharides. In: Neidhardt, F.C., ed. *Escherichia coli* and *Salmonella*: cellular and molecular biology. Washington, DC: American Society for Microbiology, pp. 104–122.

Ridley, A.M., Punia, P., Ward, L.R., and Rowe, B. 1996. Plasmid characterization and pulsed-field electrophoretic analysis demonstrate that ampicillin-resistant strains of *Salmonella enteritidis* phage type 6a are derived from *S. enteritidis* phage type 4. J. Appl. Bacteriol. 81:613–618.

Rieger-Hug, D., and Stirm, S. 1981. Comparative study of host capsule depolymerases associated with *Klebsiella* bacteriophages. Virology 173:363–378.

Roantree, R.J. 1967. *Salmonella* O antigen and virulence. Annu. Rev. Microbiol. 21:443–466.

Sanderson, K.E., Hessel, A., and Stocker, B.A.D. 1996. Strains of *Salmonella typhimurium* and other *Salmonella* species used in genetic analysis. In: Neidhardt, F.C., et al., eds. *Escherichia coli* and *Salmonella*: cellular and molecular biology. Washington, DC: American Society for Microbiology, pp. 2496–2503.

Schnaitman, C.A., and Klena, J.D. 1993. Genetics of lipopolysaccharide biosynthesis in enteric bacteria. Microbiol. Rev. 57:655–682.

Schroeter, A., Ward, L.R., Rowe, B., Protz, D., Hartung, M., and Helmuth, R. 1994. *Salmonella enteritidis* phage types in Germany. Eur. J. Epidemiol. 10:645–648.

Schulz, G.E. 1993. Bacterial porins: structure and function. Curr. Opin. Cell Biol. 5:701–707.

Selander, R.K., and Musser, J.M. 1990. Population genetics of bacterial pathogenesis. In: Iglewski, B.H., and Clark, V.L., eds. The bacteria, vol. 11: molecular basis of bacterial pathogenesis. San Diego, CA: Academic, pp. 11–36.

Silver, R.P., and Vimr, E.R. 1990. Polysialic acid capsule of *Escherichia coli* K1. In: Iglewski, B., and Clark, V., eds. The bacteria, vol. 11: molecular basis of bacterial pathogenesis. New York: Academic, pp. 39–60.

Silverman, M., and Simon, M. 1983. Phase variation and related systems. In: Shapiro, J.A., ed. Mobile genetic elements. Orlando, FL: Academic, pp. 537–557.

Son, R., Ansary, A., Salmah, I., and Maznah, A. 1995. Survey of plasmids and resistance factors among veterinary isolates of *Salmonella enteritidis* in Malaysia. World J. Microbiol. Biotechnol. 11:315–318.

Stanley, J., Burnens, A.P., Threlfall, E.J., Chowdry, N., and Goldsworthy, M. 1992a. Genetic relationships among strains of *Salmonella enteritidis* in a national epidemic in Switzerland. Epidemiol. Infect. 108:213–220.

Stanley, J., Goldsworthy, M., and Threlfall, E.J. 1992b. Molecular phylogenetic typing of pandemic isolates of *Salmonella enteritidis*. FEMS Microbiol. Lett. 90:153–160.

Stanley, P., Koronakis, V., and Hughes, C. 1993. Loss of secreted hemolysin activity caused by a lesion in the rfaP gene required for lipopolysaccharide assembly. Mol. Microbiol. 10:781–788.

St. Louis, M.E., Morse, D.L., Potter, M.E., DeMelfi, T.M., Guzewuch, J.J., Tauxe, V., and Blake, P.A. 1988. The emergence of grade A eggs as a major source of *Salmonella enteritidis* infections: new implications for the control of salmonellosis. JAMA 259:2103–2109.

Susskind, M.M., and Botstein, D. 1978. Molecular genetics of bacteriophage P22. Microbiol. Rev. 42:385–413.

Takada, H., and S. Kotani. 1992. Structure-function relationships of lipid A. In: Morrison, D.C., and Ryan, J.L., eds. Bacterial endotoxic lipopolysaccharides, vol. 1: molecular biochemistry and cellular biology. Boca Raton, FL: CRC, pp. 107–134.

Theiss, P., Karpas, A., and Wise, K.S. 1996. Antigenic topology of the P29 surface lipoprotein of *Mycoplasma fermentans*: differential display of epitopes results in high-frequency phase variation. Infect. Immun. 64:1800–1809.

Threlfall, E.J., Hall, M.L.M., and Rowe, B. 1992. *Salmonella* bacteraemia in England and Wales 1981–1990. J. Clin. Pathol. 45:34–36.

Threlfall, E.J., Chart, H., Ward, L.R., De Sa, J.D.H., and Rowe, B. 1993. Interrelationships between strains of *Salmonella enteritidis* belonging to phage types 4, 7, 7a, 8, 13, 13a, 23, 24, and 30. J. Appl. Bacteriol. 75:43–48.

Threlfall, E.J., Hampton, M.D., Chart, H., and Rowe, B. 1994. Use of plasmid profile typing for surveillance of *Salmonella enteritidis* phage type 4 from humans, poultry and eggs. Epidemiol. Infect. 112:25–31.

Vaara, M. 1993. Antibiotic-supersusceptible mutants of *Escherichia coli* and *Salmonella typhimurium*. Antimicrob. Agents Chemother. 37:2255–2260.

van Duin, J. 1988. The single-stranded RNA bacteriophages. In: Calendar, R., ed. The bacteriophages, vol. 1. New York: Plenum, pp. 117–168.

Vatopoulos, A.C., Mainas, E., Balis, E., Threlfall, E.J., Kanelopoulou, M., Kalapothaki, V., Malamou-Lada, H., and Legakis, N.J. 1994. Molecular epidemiology of ampicillin-resistant clinical isolates of *Salmonella enteritidis*. J. Clin. Microbiol. 32:1322–1325.

Ward, L.R., De Sa, J.D.H., and Rowe, B. 1987. A phage typing scheme for *Salmonella enteritidis*. Epidemiol. Infect. 99:291–294.

Ward, L.R., Threlfall, E.J., and Rowe, B. 1990. Multiple drug resistance in salmonellae in England and Wales, UK: a comparison between 1981 and 1988. J. Clin. Pathol. 43:563–566.

Whitfield, C., and Valvano, M.A. 1993. Biosynthesis and expression of cell-surface polysaccharides in gram-negative bacteria. Adv. Microb. Physiol. 35:135–246.

Wilkenson, R.G., Gemski, P., Jr., and Stocker, B.A.D. 1972. Non-smooth mutants of *Salmonella typhimurium*: differentiation by phage sensitivity and genetic mapping. J. Gen. Microbiol. 70:527–554.

Yarmolinsky, M.R., and Sternberg, N.A. 1988. Bacteriophage P1. In: Calendar, R., ed. The bacteriophages, vol. 1. New York: Plenum, pp. 291–438.

Young, R. 1992. Bacteriophage lysis: mechanism and regulation. Microbiol. Rev. 56:430–481.

Zinder, N.D., and Lederberg, J. 1952. Genetic exchange in *Salmonella*. J. Bacteriol. 64:679–699.

22

Applying Experimental Infection Models to Understand the Pathogenesis, Detection, and Control of *Salmonella enterica* Serovar Enteritidis in Poultry

R.K. Gast

INTRODUCTION

The important role of eggs in the transmission of *Salmonella enterica* serovar Enteritidis (*S.* Enteritidis) to humans has stimulated considerable interest in *S.* Enteritidis infections of chickens. Surveys of the incidence and distribution of *S.* Enteritidis in commercial laying flocks have provided information essential to the formulation of effective control strategies. However, because field studies usually involve many undefined and uncontrolled variables, clear and applicable conclusions are often rather elusive. Biosecurity and confidentiality concerns further complicate the collection and compilation of field data. Accordingly, experimental models have often been employed to obtain valuable information under carefully controlled conditions. Although the degree of correlation between experimental and natural infections is not always entirely certain, experimental infection studies have been of vital significance in providing dependable answers to numerous specific questions posed by regulatory agencies and the poultry industry. Experimental *S.* Enteritidis infections in chickens have been studied or applied to help understand how infection can lead to egg contamination, to explain the transmission and persistence of infection, to investigate factors that affect susceptibility to infection, to evaluate virulence properties of *S.* Enteritidis isolates, to test methods for detecting infected flocks, and to assess the efficacy of treatments for diminishing the incidence of *S.* Enteritidis infection in laying flocks.

PATHOGENESIS AND CLINICAL EFFECTS

Intestinal Colonization and Organ Invasion

The course of experimental *S.* Enteritidis infection in both young and mature chickens has generally been observed to be consistent with patterns characteristically associated with paratyphoid salmonellae. Extensive initial colonization of the gastrointestinal tract is often followed by invasion through mucosal epithelial cells and dissemination to a variety of internal organs. The crop and ceca have been identified as principal sites of translocation of *S.* Enteritidis from the gut lumen to internal tissues of orally infected chicks (Turnbull and Snoeyenbos, 1974). One week after oral inoculation of hens with 10^9 *S.* Enteritidis cells, 83% of cloacal swabs were positive for *S.* Enteritidis (Gast and Beard, 1990a). During the first 5 weeks after these hens were inoculated, *S.* Enteritidis was recovered from 53% of the sampled livers, 49% of the spleens, 19% of the ovaries, and 17% of the oviducts (Gast and Beard, 1990c). Thiagarajan et al. (1994) isolated *S.* Enteritidis from preovulatory follicles of experimentally infected hens. Humphrey et al. (1993) noted that *S.* Enteritidis could sometimes be recovered from various internal tissues, including the oviduct, within 1 h after laying hens were orally inoculated.

Clinical Effects

Like most other paratyphoid salmonellae, *S.* Enteritidis can cause significant morbidity and mortality in highly susceptible young chicks. Gorham et al. (1994) reported thickened abdominal air sacs and pericardia and enlarged, firm yolk sacs in chicks inoculated at 1 day of age. Oral inoculation of newly hatched chicks with large doses of a variety of *S.* Enteritidis strains has been found to cause a high incidence of mortality (Gast and Beard, 1992b; Gast and Benson, 1995). However, *S.* Enteritidis infection has not been consistently associated with severe clinical responses in mature chickens. Although Timoney et al. (1989) isolated *S.* Enteritidis from the majority of sampled ovules and oviducts during the first week after inoculation of laying hens, total egg production by these birds was not affected. Oral doses of 10^6 cells of *S.* Enteritidis strains phage type 4 (PT4) (Humphrey et al., 1989) or PT8 (Shivaprasad et al., 1990) produced no signs of illness or lesions in orally infected hens, but oral or intravenous inoculation with 10^8 cells resulted in depression, anorexia, diarrhea, reduced egg production, and a few deaths (Shivaprasad et al., 1990). Aerosol administration of as few as 10^5 *S.* Enteritidis cells was reported by Baskerville et al. (1992) to produce diarrhea, anorexia, and some mortality. Barrow and Lovell (1991) saw egg production drop by about 10% (and remain at lower levels for 4 weeks) after intravenous inoculation with 10^5 cells of *S.* Enteritidis. Gast and Beard (1990a) administered oral doses of 10^9 *S.* Enteritidis cells to hens ranging in age from 27 to 62 weeks and observed egg production decreases of 10%–30% for several weeks in all age groups.

Egg Contamination

The ability of *S.* Enteritidis to be deposited in eggs produced by infected laying hens is the distinctive characteristic that has made this serovar the focus of so much attention. Because of its epidemiological significance, egg contamination has been the subject of extensive experimental investigation. In some studies, experimentally infected hens have laid very few internally contaminated eggs. For example, after Barrow and Lovell (1991) administered oral doses of 10^8 *S.* Enteritidis cells to laying hens, they found *S.* Enteritidis in 6% of sampled whole eggs (shells plus contents) but in just 0.3% of the eggs when only the contents were sampled. Because *S.* Enteritidis was isolated from the ovaries of 30% of the hens sampled in this study, the authors concluded that shell contamination was likely the principal route of egg contamination. Other studies have similarly shown a higher incidence of shell contamination than of content contamination following oral inoculation of hens (Methner et al., 1995a; Bichler et al., 1996). Timoney et al. (1989) detected *S.* Enteritidis at a frequency just above 1% in the albumens and yolks of eggs laid during the first 2 weeks after hens were infected orally with 10^6 *S.* Enteritidis cells. However, other investigators have observed experimentally infected hens to lay substantial numbers of internally contaminated eggs, although generally for only a short period of time after inoculation. Gast and Beard (1990a) found *S.* Enteritidis in 19% of the albumens and 16% of the yolks, but on only 10% of the shells, of eggs laid during the first 4 weeks after hens were orally inoculated (the last contaminated egg was laid 23 days after inoculation). This indicated that internal contamination of eggs sometimes occurs prior to oviposition and is not always the consequence of deposition on the shell. Keller et al. (1995) noted that forming eggs removed from the oviduct were contaminated by *S.* Enteritidis much more often than were freshly laid eggs.

TRANSMISSION AND PERSISTENCE OF INFECTION

Route of Exposure

The consequences of experimental *S.* Enteritidis infections have been found to vary considerably, depending on the route of inoculation. Shivaprasad et al. (1990) observed that intravenous doses of up to 10^8 *S.* Enteritidis caused more severe clinical effects, induced detectable antibody titers more frequently, and were more likely to persist for many weeks in the peritoneum, liver, and spleen of inoculated hens than were similar doses given orally or intracloacally. Nakamura et al. (1993a) reported no reduction in total egg production and a 1.5% incidence of egg-content contamination during the first month after oral administration of 10^{10} *S.* Enteritidis to a group of hens, whereas intramuscular administration of 10^9 *S.* Enteritidis to another group of hens led to a significant drop in egg production for 3 weeks and an 8% incidence of egg contamination. Porter and Curtiss (1997) determined that *S.* Enteritidis strains can be fully virulent when administered intraperitoneally, even if they carry mutations in genes that are essential for virulence following oral inoculation. The route of inoculation can also influence the pattern of systemic dissemination of *S.* Enteritidis. After Barrow and Lovell (1991) gave an intravenous dose of 10^5 *S.* Enteritidis to one group of hens and an oral dose of 10^8 *S.* Enteritidis to another group, they detected *S.* Enteritidis far more often in the ceca of the orally infected group, but the frequency of *S.* Enteritidis isolation from internal organs of the two groups was similar. Both intestinal colonization and systemic infection have been demonstrated following experimental intratracheal (Nakamura et al., 1995) or conjunctival (Humphrey et al., 1992) administration of *S.* Enteritidis, although conjunctival challenge has been reported to elicit only a very weak antibody response (Chart et al., 1992). After the administration of aerosol doses of 10^2–10^5 cells to hens by Baskerville et al. (1992), *S.* Enteritidis was excreted intermittently in the feces for 28 days and was found in lungs, crops, ovaries, oviducts, spleens, kidneys, and eggshells (but not egg contents). Aerosol exposure of hens to 10^2 or 10^3 has been found to elicit a detectable immunoglobulin G (IgG) response to *S.* Enteritidis lipopolysaccharide (LPS) (Chart et al., 1992).

Infecting Dose

The consequences of experimental *S.* Enteritidis infection are also influenced by the inoculum dose administered. After giving hens oral doses of 10^3, 10^6, or 10^8 cells of *S.* Enteritidis, Humphrey et al. (1991a) found that fecal shedding of *S.* Enteritidis and the antibody response to infection, but not the production of contaminated eggs, were dose dependent (the only contaminated eggs detected were laid by a hen given a dose of 10^3 *S.* Enteritidis). The incidence and severity of clinical signs associated with both oral (Shivaprasad et al., 1990) and aerosol (Baskerville et al., 1992) inoculation have been found to vary directly with the administered dose of *S.* Enteritidis. Following oral challenge with 10^4 cells of *S.* Enteritidis, Gast (1993) noted that very few hens excreted *S.* Enteritidis in their feces, laid contaminated eggs, seroconverted, or showed evidence of systemic dissemination. However, most hens given an oral dose of 10^6 *S.* Enteritidis in the same study shed *S.* Enteritidis in their feces, and nearly half produced contaminated eggs, had detectable levels of serum antibodies, or harbored *S.* Enteritidis in their internal organs. Chart et al. (1992) determined that aerosol levels of 10^3 or less stimulated an antibody response that was principally IgG, but a dose of 10^5 *S.* Enteritidis stimulated a response that was predominantly IgM.

Mode of Transmission

Experimental infections have been widely applied for investigating various potential modes of transmission of *S.* Enteritidis between chicks and hens. When Gast and Beard (1990a) exposed laying hens to *S.* Enteritidis by contact with orally inoculated birds in adjacent cages, 43% of ceca, 36% of livers, 36% of spleens, 21% of oviducts, and 7% of ovaries sampled from the contact-exposed hens were positive for *S.* Enteritidis during the first 5 weeks after exposure. Intestinal colonization persisted for more than 4 months in about 6% of these contact-exposed hens. Although contact-exposed hens became seropositive more slowly than did orally inoculated hens, antibody titers from inoculated and contact-exposed hens had become similar within 3 weeks after inoculation (Gast and Beard,

1990b). Experimental *S.* Enteritidis infections have also been transmitted horizontally by contaminated feed (Hinton et al., 1989) and water (Nakamura et al., 1994a). Lever and Williams (1996) noted the movement of *S.* Enteritidis infection between groups of chicks housed in the same room, apparently by airborne transmission. As would be expected from the production of internally contaminated eggs, vertical transmission of *S.* Enteritidis infection has also been demonstrated experimentally. Although the injection of *S.* Enteritidis into the yolk of fertile eggs at 5–7 days of incubation was usually lethal, the injection of a dose of about 10^3 *S.* Enteritidis cells into the albumen of such eggs resulted in the hatching of infected chicks (Methner et al., 1995b). After Reiber et al. (1995) inseminated hens with contaminated semen, *S.* Enteritidis was found in feces, ovaries, oviducts, and eggshells from these hens.

Persistence of Infection

Experimental *S.* Enteritidis infections have sometimes been observed to be highly persistent. The administration of doses of 10^6–10^8 *S.* Enteritidis cells by Shivaprasad et al. (1990) led to fecal shedding for 21 days after oral inoculation and 42 days after intravenous inoculation. Timoney et al. (1989) were able to find *S.* Enteritidis in the ceca, peritoneum, and liver of hens for up to 42 days after oral inoculation. Humphrey et al. (1989) found *S.* Enteritidis in the liver and spleen of one hen at 70 days following oral inoculation. Although the frequency of intestinal colonization declined steadily after oral infection of hens with a large *S.* Enteritidis dose (Gast and Beard, 1990a), 11% of these hens were still *S.* Enteritidis positive at 18 weeks after inoculation. Among the same birds, *S.* Enteritidis was recovered at a low frequency from several internal organs at up to 22 weeks after inoculation (Gast and Beard, 1990c). Nakamura et al. (1993b) reported that horizontal contact exposure of newly hatched chicks led to intermittent fecal shedding that persisted for up to 28 weeks. About half of the chicks infected orally at 2 days of age by Phillips and Opitz (1995) were still shedding *S.* Enteritidis in their feces at 34 weeks of age, and some of these birds remained colonized for up to 64 weeks.

SUSCEPTIBILITY TO INFECTION

Effect of Age

The susceptibility of chickens to the most severe consequences of *S.* Enteritidis infection decreases very rapidly during the first week after hatching. Administration of large doses of some *S.* Enteritidis strains can cause a high incidence of mortality in newly hatched chicks but will seldom be lethal for chicks after the first few days of life (Gast and Benson, 1995, 1996). Gorham et al. (1991) found that oral inoculation of day-old chicks with 10^7 *S.* Enteritidis cells led to the subsequent isolation of *S.* Enteritidis from most intestinal and organ samples for 42 days, but similar inoculation of week-old chicks resulted in a much lower frequency of *S.* Enteritidis recovery. Duchet-Suchaux et al. (1995) established persistent *S.* Enteritidis colonization of the ceca and internal organs by oral inoculation of 1-week-old chicks, but 1-day-old chicks often succumbed to the lethal effects of infection and 3-week-old chicks were relatively resistant to infection. Age has also sometimes been shown to be a factor affecting the susceptibility of hens to *S.* Enteritidis infection. When Humphrey et al. (1991b) administered 10^6 *S.* Enteritidis orally to 20-week-old hens, the hens responded with a high level of serum antibodies and no clinical signs were observed, whereas similar inoculation of 1-year-old hens elicited a negligible antibody response and caused septicemia and death of a significant proportion of the birds. In another study, oral inoculation of 52-week-old hens with 10^6 *S.* Enteritidis cells did not lead to the production of any internally contaminated eggs, but similar inoculation of 18-week-old hens resulted in the production of contaminated eggs over a period of 30 days at a 1% incidence.

Induced Molting

Induced molting by feed deprivation, often employed to extend the productive life of commercial laying hens, has been extensively investigated for its effects on susceptibility to *S.* Enteritidis infection. Feed deprivation has been reported to increase both the incidence and level of fecal shedding of *S.* Enteritidis by orally infected hens (Holt and Porter, 1992; Nakamura et al., 1994a). Induced molting has been shown to reduce the oral dose of *S.* Enteritidis needed to establish intestinal colonization (Holt, 1993) and to increase the severity of intestinal lesions associated with *S.* Enteritidis infection (Porter and Holt, 1993), the invasion of *S.* Enteritidis to internal organs (Holt et al., 1995), the incidence of horizontal transmission of *S.* Enteritidis (Holt, 1995), and the likelihood of recurrence of previous *S.* Enteritidis infections (Holt and Porter, 1993). Feed deprivation has also been reported to increase the susceptibility of chickens to intratracheal administration of *S.* Enteritidis (Nakamura et al., 1995). However, susceptibility to *S.* Enteritidis infection was not increased when molting was induced by the use of a special diet formulation instead of by feed deprivation (Holt et al., 1994).

Other Infectious Agents and Immunosuppressive Drugs

Secondary infections with various viral and protozoan agents have been reported to exert significant effects on the course of *S.* Enteritidis infections in chickens. Phillips and Opitz (1995) found that although *S.* Enteritidis infection persisted until maturity in many chickens inoculated at 2 days of age, only birds that were also exposed to infectious bursal disease virus at 1 day of age eventually laid eggs contaminated by *S.* Enteritidis. Concurrent *Eimeria tenella* infection can increase intestinal colonization by *S.* Enteritidis and promote the recrudescence of previous *S.* Enteritidis infections, but does not affect the frequency of isolation of *S.* Enteritidis from internal organs or egg contents (Qin et al., 1995a,b, 1996). Especially at high-exposure

doses, coccidial infection may increase the thickness of the lamina propria and thus increase resistance to the invasion of *S.* Enteritidis to internal organs (Tellez et al., 1994a). Immunosuppressive drugs were observed to increase the intestinal shed rate of *S.* Enteritidis but did not affect dissemination of *S.* Enteritidis to the spleen (Arnold and Holt, 1995). Chemical depletion of heterophils decreased the intravenous dose of *S.* Enteritidis necessary to cause organ invasion and lesions (Kogut et al., 1994).

Genetic Factors

Several genetically based differences in the susceptibility of lines of chickens to *S.* Enteritidis infection have been identified by experimental infection studies. Guillot et al. (1995) determined that lines of day-old chicks varied in their susceptibility to organ invasion and lethality following intramuscular or oral infection with *S.* Enteritidis and that meat-type lines were more resistant than egg-type lines. An assortment of *S.* Enteritidis isolates of various phage types was found to be generally less virulent for a meat-type line of chicks than for an egg-type line (Gast and Benson, 1995). Beaumont et al. (1994) reported that lines of chickens differed in their susceptibility to lethality, organ invasion, and egg contamination following *S.* Enteritidis inoculation. Of four lines of chickens infected experimentally by Protais et al. (1996), a commercial egg-type line laid the most eggs with contaminated yolks and had the highest incidence of organ and intestinal infection. Similarly, Lindell et al. (1994) associated a higher incidence of fecal shedding and egg-yolk contamination with one of four experimentally inoculated lines. Bumstead and Barrow (1988) observed that the relative resistance of inbred lines of chickens was similar for a variety of salmonella serovars, suggesting a common mechanism of resistance.

VIRULENCE PROPERTIES

Virulence Mechanisms

Experimental infection models have played a vital role in identifying and characterizing the various bacterial properties responsible for the unique virulence behavior of *S.* Enteritidis. Chart et al. (1991) observed that virulent strains of several *S.* Enteritidis phage types expressed long-chain LPS and carried a 38-MDa plasmid. A 54-kb plasmid, found by Halavatkar and Barrow (1993) to be essential for virulence in mice, appeared to have very little effect on virulence in chicks or hens. Thiagarajan et al. (1996) reported that an *S.* Enteritidis strain lacking fimbria was less often isolated from ceca or shed in the feces than were fimbriated strains. However, Thorns et al. (1996b) noted that mutant *S.* Enteritidis strains lacking fimbria had virulence properties similar to those of wild-type strains in chicks and hens. Humphrey et al. (1996) determined that an *S.* Enteritidis isolate with high inherent tolerance to heat and acid was more invasive in hens (especially to reproductive tissue) than a less tolerant isolate, although no difference in virulence for chicks was observed for these two strains.

Differences between Isolates and Phage Type

Experimental infection models have often been applied in an attempt to explain the extent of, or basis for, differences between particular *S.* Enteritidis strains or isolates. Some discriminating characteristics are useful for establishing epidemiological relationships between isolates from different sources, and others have been applied for identifying highly virulent strains. The incidence at which experimentally infected hens lay contaminated eggs has been found to vary considerably according to the inoculum strain used, even among isolates of the same phage type (Shivaprasad et al., 1990). Gast and Beard (1992b) administered large doses of eight different *S.* Enteritidis strains to laying hens and reported that the incidence of egg-content contamination during the first 3 weeks after inoculation ranged from 0% to 8% for the various *S.* Enteritidis strains, although no differences between strains were observed in regard to intestinal colonization, invasion to internal organs, or elicitation of a serum antibody response. The eight isolates also differed in their effects on total egg production by infected hens. When these investigators inoculated groups of day-old chicks with large oral doses of these same eight *S.* Enteritidis isolates, mortality during the following week ranged from 15% to 90% for the various groups. The disparities between strains observed in this study were not related to their phage types, and the lethality of particular isolates for chicks was apparently unrelated to the propensity of these isolates to be deposited in eggs. Experimental infection studies have associated the elevated expression of flagellar proteins and high-molecular-weight LPS with invasion to internal organs in chicks (Guard-Petter et al., 1996) and egg contamination in laying hens (Petter, 1993).

One especially consequential observation of experimental infection studies is that PT4 *S.* Enteritidis isolates have sometimes been associated with an unusually high level of invasiveness and virulence. When administered to day-old chicks in their feed, a PT4 strain was more often recovered from livers than were isolates of several other phage types (Hinton et al. 1990). When Barrow (1991) administered large oral doses of various *S.* Enteritidis isolates to day-old chicks, higher mortality was associated with PT4 isolates than with other isolates. However, noticeable variation in virulence is also often evident between PT4 strains. A PT4 *S.* Enteritidis isolate obtained from a human source in the United Kingdom was found to be more virulent in orally inoculated day-old chicks and more invasive in laying hens than was a PT4 isolate obtained from a Canadian poultry source (Poppe et al., 1993). Gast and Benson (1995) determined that some, but not all, PT4 *S.* Enteritidis strains were more virulent for orally infected chicks than were strains of *S.* Enteritidis phage types found more often in U.S. poultry, although some significant differences in virulence were also observed within the set of PT4 strains tested. In another study, significant differences were sometimes observed between individual *S.* Enteritidis isolates in the frequencies at which they colonized the intestinal tracts and invaded the spleens of inoculated 5-day-old chicks, but no consistent overall pattern differentiated PT4 isolates from isolates of other phage types (Gast and Benson, 1996).

DETECTION

Detection of *Salmonella* Enteritidis in Chickens and Eggs

Experimental infection models have also been widely applied for assessing the effectiveness of various methods for detecting *S.* Enteritidis in chickens, eggs, and environmental samples. For example, newly developed methods such as enzyme immunoassays (Desmidt et al., 1994) and DNA hybridization assays (Cotter et al., 1995) have been tested in experimentally infected groups of chickens and found to be capable of detecting *S.* Enteritidis in the feces or environment with a sensitivity comparable to that of traditional culture methods. Because egg contamination occurs infrequently and usually involves relatively small numbers of *S.* Enteritidis cells (Gast and Beard, 1992a), the development of effective and practical methods for detecting *S.* Enteritidis in egg contents has been the specific focus of much research. Gast (1993) determined that traditional enrichment culturing methods could be successfully applied to detect *S.* Enteritidis in pooled samples of egg contents from experimentally infected hens if the egg pools were allowed to incubate before culturing to promote the expansion of very small numbers of *S.* Enteritidis contaminants to detectable levels. However, more sensitive and longer-lasting detection of infected hens was provided by sampling for *S.* Enteritidis in voided feces or by testing for serum antibodies. A method that combined concentration by centrifugation and detection by polymerase chain reaction identified *S.* Enteritidis contamination in eggs from experimentally inoculated hens with a sensitivity comparable to that of enrichment culturing (McElroy et al., 1996).

Detection of Specific Antibodies in Serum and Eggs

Experimental *S.* Enteritidis infections in mature chickens have generally been associated with the production of high titers of specific serum antibodies. Gast and Beard (1990b) reported that, after laying hens were infected with large oral doses of *S.* Enteritidis, serum antibody titers to *S.* Enteritidis rose to peak levels within 2 weeks after inoculation and often remained at detectable levels for several months. Barrow and Lovell (1991) detected high IgG titers to *S.* Enteritidis LPS for at least 27 weeks after oral inoculation. However, Desmidt et al. (1992) observed a significant degree of cross-reactivity when an enzyme immunoassay using *S.* Enteritidis LPS was applied to sera from chickens infected with other salmonella serovars. Experimentally infected chickens have likewise been used to compare and validate the application of enzyme immunoassays using outer-membrane proteins (Kim et al., 1991; Charles et al., 1996), flagellar proteins (Timoney et al., 1990; Zijderveld et al., 1992), and fimbrial proteins (Cooper and Thorns, 1996; Thorns et al., 1996a) as antigens for detecting antibodies to *S.* Enteritidis.

Gast and Beard (1991) showed that specific antibodies could be detected in the yolks of eggs from orally infected hens, by using an agglutination assay with a whole cell antigen, as early as 9 days after inoculation. These egg-yolk antibody titers peaked at 3–5 weeks after inoculation and remained at high levels for several months. Desmidt et al. (1996) reported that an enzyme immunoassay using *S.* Enteritidis LPS could similarly detect antibodies in egg yolks from experimentally infected hens. Egg-yolk antibody testing is potentially advantageous because samples can be collected with minimal labor and without posing flock biosecurity or occupational safety hazards. However, the relevance of egg-yolk antibody testing for predicting the public health threat posed by laying flocks has sometimes been questioned. Gast et al. (1997) determined that testing for egg-yolk antibodies (by enzyme immunoassay with a flagellar antigen) was at least as effective as culturing voided feces for predicting the likelihood that experimentally infected hens would lay eggs internally contaminated by *S.* Enteritidis. These two parameters followed opposite patterns over time, with fecal shedding peaking early and then gradually declining while egg-yolk antibody titers slowly and steadily climbed.

OPTIONS FOR CONTROLLING *SALMONELLA* ENTERITIDIS INFECTION

Vaccination

Experimentally infected chickens have been used to evaluate the protective efficacy of a variety of vaccine preparations. Gast et al. (1992) administered an acetone-killed oil-emulsion vaccine to laying hens and found that the bacterin provided significant (but not complete) protection against invasion of *S.* Enteritidis to internal organs and the production of contaminated eggs following oral challenge. In another study (Gast et al., 1993), two different bacterin preparations were both able to reduce the incidence of intestinal colonization and the mean number of *S.* Enteritidis cells shed in the feces of orally challenged laying hens. However, the degree of protection afforded by vaccination was again only partial, as more than half of the vaccinated hens still shed substantial numbers of *S.* Enteritidis in their feces. Barbour et al. (1993) similarly observed a reduction in fecal shedding of *S.* Enteritidis associated with the use of a killed vaccine. A bacterin administered by Timms et al. (1990) reduced mortality and lesions following intramuscular or intravenous challenge with *S.* Enteritidis. Another potentially useful outcome of vaccination was reported by Holt et al. (1996), who noted that antibodies in eggs from vaccinated hens temporarily inhibited the growth of inoculated *S.* Enteritidis. Adjuvanted subunit vaccines have also demonstrated protective efficacy against *S.* Enteritidis infection (Charles et al., 1994). However, the effectiveness of vaccines can be compromised by stressors such as feed or water deprivation (Nakamura et al., 1994b).

Several live attenuated vaccine preparations have also been tested in experimentally infected chickens. Cooper et al. (1990, 1992) determined that oral administration of an aromatic-dependent (aroA) *S.* Enteritidis mutant reduced fecal shedding and organ invasion after subsequent oral challenge with virulent *S.* Enteritidis, even though a significant serum antibody response was not evident. This live vaccine also reduced the horizontal spread of *S.* Enteritidis from infected chickens (Cooper et al., 1993) and organ dissemination after intravenous challenge (Cooper et al., 1994) but did not provide effective cross-protection against challenge with *Salmonella* Typhimurium. However, Lumsden et al. (1991) achieved effective protection against *S.* Enteritidis challenge following vaccination with an attenuated mutant of *S.* Typhimurium. A live *Salmonella* Gallinarum vaccine (the rough mutant strain, 9R) has also significantly reduced organ invasion and egg contamination associated with experimental *S.* Enteritidis infection (Barrow et al., 1990, 1991). Nassar et al. (1994) found that the combined administration of both the 9R vaccine and an *S.* Enteritidis bacterin provided better protection against fecal shedding and egg contamination following oral challenge than did either single vaccine treatment. The elicitation of humoral antibodies did not correlate with protection in this study.

Immunoprophylaxis

The prophylactic administration of lymphokines from experimentally infected chickens has been shown to provide protection against organ invasion after challenge with *S.* Enteritidis (Tellez et al., 1994b). This effect is apparently mediated by the phagocytosis and destruction of *S.* Enteritidis following an influx of inflammatory heterophils (Kogut et al., 1995a,b). Protection can be conferred by cytokines from T cells, but not from macrophages, and can be achieved only when the lymphokines are administered before *S.* Enteritidis infection (McGruder et al., 1993, 1995a). Administration of protective lymphokines in ovo resulted in improved resistance to organ invasion when chicks were later challenged with *S.* Enteritidis (McGruder et al., 1995b). Lymphokines from immunized chickens or turkeys can be cross-protective against *S.* Enteritidis infection in the other species (Ziprin et al., 1996).

Colonization Control

Experimental challenge studies have also been important in establishing the usefulness of colonization control treatments for protecting chickens against *S.* Enteritidis infection. The administration of undefined competitive exclusion cultures has reduced the incidence of fecal shedding, the number of *S.* Enteritidis shed in feces, and the incidence of organ invasion after challenge with *S.* Enteritidis (Bolder et al., 1992; Cameron and Carter, 1992; Nuotio et al., 1992). The provision of dietary lactose has been reported to increase resistance to *S.* Enteritidis organ invasion by increasing organic acid concentrations in the intestinal tract (Tellez et al., 1993a) and to thereby diminish the heightened susceptibility of force-molted hens to *S.* Enteritidis infection (Corrier et al., 1997). Combined administration of dietary lactose and anaerobic cultures of protective cecal microflora can reduce intestinal colonization, organ invasion, seroconversion, and horizontal transmission following *S.* Enteritidis challenge (Corrier et al., 1991). Administration of defined mixtures of cecal bacteria (Corrier et al., 1994), single cultures of *Lactobacillus acidophilus* (Qin et al., 1995c) or *Escherichia coli* (Behling and Wong, 1994), and used poultry litter (Corrier et al., 1993) have variously been found to provide protection against experimental *S.* Enteritidis infection when used in concert with dietary lactose.

Drugs and Chemical Treatments

Experimental infection models have also offered an opportunity to test the efficacy of various chemical therapeutic or prophylactic agents. Administration of the antibiotics polymyxin B and trimethoprim to chickens was seen both to prevent and to remove intestinal colonization by *S.* Enteritidis (Goodnough and Johnson, 1991). However, prior antibiotic treatment (with nitrofurazone or novobiocin) has also been associated with increased susceptibility to *S.* Enteritidis, perhaps as a consequence of interference with bacterial flora that produce inhibitory volatile fatty acids (Manning et al., 1992). Antibiotic treatment can also interfere with the protective effect of some competitive exclusion cultures (Manning et al., 1994). Dietary administration of capsaicin (a pungent and vasoactive compound found in certain peppers) to chickens reduced both intestinal colonization and organ invasion following *S.* Enteritidis challenge (Tellez et al., 1993b; McElroy et al., 1994). The addition of organic acids to feed has not generally been associated with consistent protection against experimental challenge with *S.* Enteritidis (Hinton et al., 1991; Opitz et al., 1993).

CONCLUSION

Although field studies are indispensable for supplying relevant answers to many important questions about *S.* Enteritidis infections in commercial poultry flocks, experimental models afford opportunities to investigate very specific issues under precisely defined conditions. Experimental infection studies have provided particularly useful information about the efficacy of proposed methods for protecting chickens against *S.* Enteritidis infection or for detecting *S.* Enteritidis in chickens, eggs, and the poultry-house environment. In these contexts, experimentally infected chickens have facilitated cost-effective assessment of the probable effectiveness of proposed control strategies. The coordinated implementation of experimental and field studies enables ideas generated under controlled laboratory conditions to be validated under commercial conditions and vice versa, ensuring the development of control strategies for *S.* Enteritidis that are both dependable and practical.

REFERENCES

Arnold, J.W., and Holt, P.S. 1995. Response to *Salmonella enteritidis* infection by the immunocompromised avian host. Poult. Sci. 74:656–665.

Barbour, E.K., Frerichs, W.M., Nabbut, N.H., Poss, P.E., and Brinton, M.K. 1993. Evaluation of bacterins containing three predominant phage types of *Salmonella enteritidis* for prevention of infection in egg-laying chickens. Am. J. Vet. Res. 54:1306–1309.

Barrow, P.A. 1991. Experimental infection of chickens with *Salmonella enteritidis*. Avian Pathol. 20:145–153.

Barrow, P.A., and Lovell, M.A. 1991. Experimental infection of egg-laying hens with *Salmonella enteritidis* phage type 4. Avian Pathol. 20:335–348.

Barrow, P.A., Lovell, M.A., and Berchieri, A. 1990. Immunisation of laying hens against *Salmonella enteritidis* with live attenuated vaccines. Vet. Rec. 126:241–242.

Barrow, P.A., Lovell, M.A., and Berchieri, A. 1991. The use of two live attenuated vaccines to immunize egg-laying hens against *Salmonella enteritidis* phage type 4. Avian Pathol. 20:681–692.

Baskerville, A., Humphrey, T.J., Fitzgeorge, R.B., Cook, R.W., Chart, H., Rowe, B., and Whitehead, A. 1992. Airborne infection of laying hens with *Salmonella enteritidis* phage type 4. Vet. Rec. 130:395–398.

Beaumont, C., Trotais, J., Colin, P., Guillot, J.F., Ballatif, F., Mouline, C., Lantier, F., Lantier, I., Girard, O., and Pardon, P. 1994. Comparison of resistance of different poultry lines to intramuscular or oral inoculation by *Salmonella enteritidis*. Vet. Res. 25:412.

Behling, R.G., and Wong, A.C.L. 1994. Competitive exclusion of *Salmonella enteritidis* in chicks by treatment with a single culture plus dietary lactose. Int. J. Food Microbiol. 22:1–9.

Bichler, L.A., Nagaraja, K.V., and Halvorson, D.A. 1996. *Salmonella enteritidis* in eggs, cloacal swab specimens, and internal organs of experimentally infected white leghorn chickens. Am. J. Vet. Res. 57:489–495.

Bolder, N.M., van Lith, L.A.J.T., Putirulan, F.F., Jacobs-Reitsma, W.F., and Mulder, R.W.A.W. 1992. Prevention of colonization by *Salmonella enteritidis* PT4 in broiler chickens. Int. J. Food Microbiol. 15:313–317.

Bumstead, N., and Barrow, P.A. 1988. Genetics of resistance to *Salmonella typhimurium* in newly hatched chicks. Br. Poult. Sci. 29:521–529.

Cameron, D.M., and Carter, J.N. 1992. Evaluation of the efficacy of Broilact® in preventing infection of broiler chicks with *Salmonella enteritidis* PT4. Int. J. Food Microbiol. 15:319–326.

Charles, S.D., Hussain, I., Choi, C.-U., Nagaraja, K.V., and Sivanandan, V. 1994. Adjuvanted subunit vaccines for the control of *Salmonella enteritidis* infection in turkeys. Am. J. Vet. Res. 55:636–642.

Charles, S.D., Sreevatsan, S., Bey, R.F., Sivanandan, V., Halvorson, D.A., and Nagaraja, K.V. 1996. A dot immunobinding assay (dot-ELISA) for the rapid serodiagnosis of *Salmonella enteritidis* infection in chickens. J. Vet. Diagn. Invest. 8:310–314.

Chart, H., Threlfall, E.J., and Rowe, B. 1991. Virulence studies of *Salmonella enteritidis* phage types. Lett. Appl. Microbiol. 12:188–191.

Chart, H., Baskerville, A., Humphrey, T.J., and Rowe, B. 1992. Serological responses of chickens experimentally infected with *Salmonella enteritidis* PT4 by different routes. Epidemiol. Infect. 109:297–302.

Cooper, G.L., and Thorns, C.J. 1996. Evaluation of SEF14 fimbrial dot blot and flagellar Western blot tests as indicators of *Salmonella enteritidis* infection in chickens. Vet. Rec. 138:149–153.

Cooper, G.L., Nicholas, R.A.J., Cullen, G.A., and Hormaeche, C.E. 1990. Vaccination of chickens with a *Salmonella enteritidis* aro A live oral salmonella vaccine. Microb. Pathog. 9:255–265.

Cooper, G.L., Venables, L.M., Nicholas, R.A.J., Cullen, G.A., and Hormaeche, C.E. 1992. Vaccination of chickens with chicken-derived *Salmonella enteritidis* phage tye 4 aro A live oral salmonella vaccines. Vaccine 10:247–254.

Cooper, G.L., Venables, L.M., Nicholas, R.A.J., Cullen, G.A., and Hormaeche, C.E. 1993. Further studies of the application of live *Salmonella enteritidis aro*A vaccines in chickens. Vet. Rec. 133:31–36.

Cooper, G.L., Venables, L.M., Woodward, M.J., and Hormaeche, C.E. 1994. Vaccination of chickens with strain CVL30, a genetically defined *Salmonella enteritidis aroA* live oral vaccine candidate. Infect. Immun. 62:4747–4754.

Corrier, D.E., B. Hargis, Hinton, A., Jr., Lindsey, D., Caldwell, D., Manning, J., and DeLoach, J. 1991. Effect of anaerobic cecal microflora and dietary lactose on colonization resistance of layer chicks to invasive *Salmonella enteritidis*. Avian Dis. 35:337–343.

Corrier, D.E., Hargis, B.M., Hinton, A., Jr., and DeLoach, J.R. 1993. Protective effect of used poultry litter and lactose in the feed ration on *Salmonella enteritidis* colonization of leghorn chicks and hens. Avian Dis. 37:47–52.

Corrier, D.E., Nisbet, D.J., Scanlan, C.M., Tellez, G., Hargis, B.M., and DeLoach, J.R. 1994. Inhibition of *Salmonella enteritidis* cecal and organ colonization in leghorn chicks by a defined culture of cecal bacteria and dietary lactose. J. Food Prot. 56:377–381.

Corrier, D.E., Nisbet, D.J., Hargis, B.M., Holt, P.S., and DeLoach, J.R. 1997. Provision of lactose to molting hens enhances resistance to *Salmonella enteritidis* colonization. J. Food Prot. 60:10–15.

Cotter, P.F., Murphy, J.E., Klinger, J.D., and Taylor, R.L., Jr. 1995. Identification of *Salmonella enteritidis* from experimentally infected hens using a colorimetric DNA hybridization method. Avian Dis. 39:873–878.

Desmidt, M., De Groot, P.A., Haesebrouck, F., and Ducatelle, R. 1992. Development of a lipopolysaccharide based ELISA for the detection of antibodies to *Salmonella enteritidis* phage type 4 in poultry. Med. Fac. Landbouww. Univ. Gent. 57:1851–1854.

Desmidt, M., Haesebrouck, F., and Ducatelle, R. 1994. Comparison of the Salmonella-Tek ELISA to culture methods for detection of *Salmonella enteritidis* in litter and cloacal swabs of poultry. J. Vet. Med. [B] 41:523–528.

Desmidt, M., Ducatelle, R., Haesebrouck, F., De Groot, P.A., Verlinden, M., Wijffels, R., Hinton, M., Bale, J.A., and Allen, V.M. 1996. Detection of antibodies to *Salmonella enteritidis* in sera and yolks from experimentally and naturally infected chickens. Vet. Rec. 138:223–226.

Duchet-Suchaux, M., Léchopier, P., Marly, J., Bernardet, P., Delaunay, R., and Pardon, P. 1995. Quantification of experimental *Salmonella enteritidis* carrier state in B13 leghorn chicks. Avian Dis. 39:796–803.

Gast, R.K. 1993. Detection of *Salmonella enteritidi*s in experimentally infected laying hens by culturing pools of egg contents. Poult. Sci. 72:267–274.

Gast, R.K., and Beard, C.W. 1990a. Production of *Salmonella enteritidis*-contaminated eggs by experimentally infected hens. Avian Dis. 34:438–446.

Gast, R.K., and Beard, C.W. 1990b. Serological detection of experimental *Salmonella enteritidis* infections in laying hens. Avian Dis. 34:721–728.

Gast, R.K., and Beard, C.W. 1990c. Isolation of *Salmonella enteritidis* from internal organs of experimentally infected hens. Avian Dis. 34:991–993.

Gast, R.K., and Beard, C.W. 1991. Detection of *Salmonella* serogroup D-specific antibodies in the yolks of eggs laid by hens infected with *Salmonella enteritidis*. Poult. Sci. 70:1273–1276.

Gast, R.K., and Beard, C.W. 1992a. Detection and enumeration of *Salmonella enteritidis* in fresh and stored eggs laid by experimentally infected hens. J. Food Prot. 55:152–156.

Gast, R.K., and Beard, C.W. 1992b. Evaluation of a chick mortality model for predicting the consequences of *Salmonella enteritidis* infections in laying hens. Poult. Sci. 71:281–287.

Gast, R.K., and Benson, S.T. 1995. The comparative virulence for chicks of *Salmonella enteritidis* phage type 4 isolates and isolates of phage types commonly found in poultry in the United States. Avian Dis. 39:567–574.

Gast, R.K., and Benson, S.T. 1996. Intestinal colonization and organ invasion in chicks experimentally infected with *Salmonella enteritidis* phage type 4 and other phage types isolated from poultry in the United States. Avian Dis. 40:853–857.

Gast, R.K., Stone, H.D., Holt, P.S., and Beard, C.W. 1992. Evaluation of the efficacy of an oil-emulsion bacterin for protecting chickens against *Salmonella enteritidis*. Avian Dis. 36:992–999.

Gast, R.K., Stone, H.D., and Holt, P.S. 1993. Evaluation of the efficacy of oil-emulsion bacterins for reducing fecal shedding of *Salmonella enteritidis* by laying hens. Avian Dis. 37:1085–1091.

Gast, R.K., Porter, R.E., Jr., and Holt, P.S. 1997. Applying tests for specific yolk antibodies to predict contamination by *Salmonella enteritidis* in eggs from experimentally infected laying hens. Avian Dis. 41:195–202.

Goodnough, M.C., and Johnson, E.A. 1991. Control of *Salmonella enteritidis* infections in poultry by polymyxin B and trimethoprim. Appl. Environ. Microbiol. 57:785–788.

Gorham, S.L., Kadavil, K., Lambert, H., Vaughan, E., Pert, B., and Abel, J. 1991. Persistence of *Salmonella enteritidis* in young chickens. Avian Pathol. 20:433–437.

Gorham, S.L., Kadavil, K., Vaughan, E., Lambert, H., Abel, J., and Pert, B. 1994. Gross and microscopic lesions in young chickens experimentally infected with *Salmonella enteritidis*. Avian Dis. 38:816–821.

Guard-Petter, J., Keller, L.H., Rahman, M.M., Carlson, R.W., and Silvers, S. 1996. A novel relationship between O-antigen variation, matrix formation, and invasiveness of *Salmonella enteritidis*. Epidemiol. Infect. 117:219–231.

Guillot, J.F., Beaumont, C., Bellatif, F., Mouline, C., Lantier, F., Colin, P., and Protais, J. 1995. Comparison of resistance of various poultry lines to infection by *Salmonella enteritidis*. Vet. Res. 26:81–86.

Halavatkar, H., and Barrow, P.A. 1993. The role of a 54-kb plasmid in the virulence of strains of *Salmonella enteritidis* of phage type 4 for chickens and mice. J. Med. Microbiol. 38:171–176.

Hinton, M., Pearson, G.R., Threlfall, E.J., Rowe, B., Woodward, M., and Wray, C. 1989. Experimental *Salmonella enteritidis* infection in chicks. Vet. Rec. 124:223.

Hinton, M., Threlfall, E.J., and Rowe, B. 1990. The invasive potential of *Salmonella enteritidis* phage types for young chickens. Lett. Appl. Microbiol. 10:237–239.

Hinton, M., Mead, G.C., and Impey, C.S. 1991. Protection of chicks against environmental challenge with *Salmonella enteritidis* by "competitive exclusion" and acid-treated feed. Lett. Appl. Microbiol. 12:69–71.

Holt, P.S. 1993. Effect of induced molting on the susceptibility of white leghorn hens to *Salmonella enteritidis* infection. Avian Dis. 37:412–417.

Holt, P.S. 1995. Horizontal transmission of *Salmonella enteritidis* in molted and unmolted laying chickens. Avian Dis. 39:239–249.

Holt, P.S., and Porter, R.E., Jr. 1992. Microbiological and histopathological effects of an induced-molt fasting procedure on a *Salmonella enteritidis* infection in chickens. Avian Dis. 36:610–618.

Holt, P.S., and Porter, R.E., Jr. 1993. Effect of induced molting on the recurrence of a previous *Salmonella enteritidis* infection. Poult. Sci. 72:2069–2078.

Holt, P.S., Buhr, R.J., Cunningham, D.L., and Porter, R.E., Jr. 1994. Effect of two different molting procedures on a *Salmonella enteritidis* infection. Poult. Sci. 73:1267–1275.

Holt, P.S., Macri, N.P., and Porter, R.E., Jr. 1995. Microbiological analysis of the early *Salmonella enteritidis* infection in molted and unmolted hens. Avian Dis. 39:55–63.

Holt, P.S., Stone, H.D., Gast, R.K., and Porter, R.E., Jr. 1996. Growth of *Salmonella enteritidis* (SE) in egg contents from hens vaccinated with an *S.* Enteritidis bacterin. Food Microbiol. 13:417–426.

Humphrey, T.J., Baskerville, A., Chart, H., and Rowe, B. 1989. Infection of egg-laying hens with *Salmonella enteritidis* PT4 by oral inoculation. Vet. Rec. 125:531–532.

Humphrey, T.J., Baskerville, A., Chart, H., Rowe, B., and Whitehead, A. 1991a. *Salmonella enteritidis* PT4 infection in specific pathogen free hens: influence of infecting dose. Vet. Rec. 129:482–485.

Humphrey, T.J., Chart, H., Baskerville, A., and Rowe, B. 1991b. The influence of age on the response of SPF hens to infection with *Salmonella enteritidis* PT4. Epidemiol. Infect. 106:33–43.

Humphrey, T.J., Baskerville, A., Chart, H., Rowe, B., and Whitehead, A. 1992. Infection of laying hens with *Salmonella enteritidis* PT4 by conjunctival challenge. Vet. Rec. 131:386–388.

Humphrey, T.J., Baskerville, A., Whitehead, A., Rowe, B., and A. Henley. 1993. Influence of feeding patterns on the artificial infection of laying hens with *Salmonella enteritidis* phage type 4. Vet. Rec. 132:407–409.

Humphrey, T.J., Williams, A., McAlpine, K., Lever, M.S., Guard-Petter, J., and Cox, J.M. 1996. Isolates of *Salmonella enterica* Enteritidis PT4 with enhanced heat and acid tolerance are more virulent in mice and more invasive in chickens. Epidemiol. Infect. 117:79–98.

Keller, L.H., Benson, C.E., Krotec, K., and Eckroade, R.J. 1995. *Salmonella enteritidis* colonization of the reproductive tract and forming and freshly laid eggs of chickens. Infect. Immun. 63:2443–2449.

Kim, C.J., Nagaraja, K.V., and Pomeroy, B.S. 1991. Enzyme-linked immunosorbent assay for the detection of *Salmonella enteritidis* infection in chickens. Am. J. Vet. Res. 52:1069–1074.

Kogut, M.H., Tellez, G.I., McGruder, E.D., Hargis, B.M., Williams, J.D., Corrier, D.E., and DeLoach, J.R. 1994. Heterophils are decisive components in the early responses of chickens to *Salmonella enteritidis* infections. Microb. Pathog. 16:141–151.

Kogut, M.H., McGruder, E.D., Hargis, B.M., Corrier, D.E., and DeLoach, J.R. 1995a. Characterization of the pattern of inflammatory cell influx in chicks following the intraperitoneal administration of live *Salmonella enteritidis* and *Salmonella enteritidis*-immune lymphokines. Poult. Sci. 74:8–18.

Kogut, M.H., McGruder, E.D., Hargis, B.M., Corrier, D.E., and DeLoach, J.R. 1995b. In vivo activation of heterophil function in chickens following injection with *Salmonella enteritidis*-immune lymphokines. J. Leukoc. Biol. 57:56–62.

Lever, M.S., and Williams, A. 1996. Cross-infection of chicks by airborne transmission of *Salmonella enteritidis* PT4. Lett. Appl. Microbiol. 23:347–349.

Lindell, K.A., Saeed, A.M., and McCabe, G.P. 1994. Evaluation of resistance of four strains of commercial laying hens to experimental infection with *Salmonella enteritidis* phage type eight. Poult. Sci. 73:757–762.

Lumsden, J.S., Wilkie, B.N., and Clarke, R.C. 1991. Resistance to fecal shedding of salmonellae in pigs and chickens vaccinated with an aromatic-dependent mutant of *Salmonella typhimurium*. Am. J. Vet. Res. 52:1784–1787.

Manning, J.G., Hargis, B.M., Hinton, A., Jr., Corrier, D.E., DeLoach, J.R., and Creger, C.R. 1992. Effect of nitrofurazone or novobiocin on *Salmonella enteritidis* cecal colonization and organ invasion in leghorn hens. Avian Dis. 36:334–340.

Manning, J.G., Hargis, B.M., Hinton, A., Jr., Corrier, D.E., DeLoach, J.R., and Creger, C.R. 1994. Effect of selected antibiotics and anticoccidials on *Salmonella enteritidis* cecal colonization and organ invasion in leghorn chicks. Avian Dis. 38:256–261.

McElroy, A.P., Manning, J.G., Jaeger, L.A., Taub, M., Williams, J.D., and Hargis, B.M. 1994. Effect of prolonged administration of dietary capsaicin on broiler growth and *Salmonella enteritidis* susceptibility. Avian Dis. 38:329–333.

McElroy, A.P., Cohen, N.D., and Hargis, B.M. 1996. Evaluation of the polymerase chain reaction for the detection of *Salmonella enteritidis* in experimentally inoculated eggs and eggs from experimentally challenged hens. J. Food Prot. 59:1273–1278.

McGruder, E.D., Ray, P.M., Tellez, G.I., Kogut, M.H., Corrier, D.E., DeLoach, J.R., and Hargis, B.M. 1993. *Salmonella enteritidis* immune leukocyte-stimulated soluble factors: effects on increased resistance to *Salmonella* organ invasion in day-old leghorn chicks. Poult. Sci. 72:2264–2271.

McGruder, E.D., Kogut, M.H., Corrier, D.E., DeLoach, J.R., and Hargis, B.M. 1995a. Comparison of prophylactic and therapeutic efficacy of *Salmonella enteritidis*-immune lymphokines against *Salmonella enteritidis* organ invasion in neonatal leghorn chicks. Avian Dis. 39:21–27.

McGruder, E.D., Ramirez, G.A., Kogut, M.H., Moore, R.W., Corrier, D.E., DeLoach, J.R., and Hargis, B.M. 1995b. In ovo administration of *Salmonella enteritidis*-immune lymphokines confers protection to neonatal chicks against *Salmonella enteritidis* organ infectivity. Poult. Sci. 74:18–25.

Methner, U., Al-Shabibi, S., and Meyer, H. 1995a. Experimental oral infection of specific pathogen-free laying hens and cocks with *Salmonella enteritidis* strains. J. Vet. Med. [B] 42:459–469.

Methner, U., Al-Shabibi, S., and Meyer, H. 1995b. Infection model for hatching chicks infected with *Salmonella enteritidis*. J. Vet. Med. [B] 42:471–480.

Nakamura, M., Nagamine, N., Norimatsu, M., Suzuki, S., Ohishi, K., Kijima, M., Tamura, Y., and Sato, S. 1993a. The ability of *Salmonella enteritidis* isolated from chicks imported from England to cause transovarian infection. J. Vet. Med. Sci. 55:135–136.

Nakamura, M., Nagamine, N., Suzuki, S., Norimatsu, M., Ohishi, K., Kijima, M., Tamura, Y., and Sato, S. 1993b. Long-term shedding of *Salmonella enteritidis* in chickens which received a contact exposure within 24 hrs of hatching. J. Vet. Med. Sci. 55:649–653.

Nakamura, M., Nagamine, N., Takahashi, T., Suzuki, S., Kijima, M., Tamura, Y., and Sato, S. 1994a. Horizontal transmission of *Salmonella enteritidis* and effect of stress on shedding in laying hens. Avian Dis. 38:282–288.

Nakamura, M., Nagamine, N., Takahashi, T., Suzuki, S., and Sato, S. 1994b. Evaluation of the efficacy of a bacterin against *Salmonella enteritidis* infection and the effect of stress after vaccination. Avian Dis. 38:717–724.

Nakamura, M., Nagamine, N., Takahashi, T., Norimatsu, M., Suzuki, S., and Sato, S. 1995. Intratracheal infection of chickens with *Salmonella enteritidis* and the effect of feed and water deprivation. Avian Dis. 39:853–858.

Nassar, T.J., Al-Nakhli, H.M., and Al-Ogaily, Z.H. 1994. Use of live and inactivated *Salmonella enteritidis* phage type 4 vaccines to immunise laying hens against experimental infection. Rev. Sci. Tech. OIE 13:855–867.

Nuotio, L., Schneitz, C., Halonen, U., and Nurmi, E. 1992. Use of competitive exclusion to protect newly-hatched chicks against intestinal colonisation and invasion by *Salmonella enteritidis* PT4. Br. Poult. Sci. 33:775–779.

Opitz, H.M., El-Begearmi, M., Flegg, P., and Beane, D. 1993. Effectiveness of five feed additives in chicks infected with *Salmonella enteritidis* phage type 13a. J. Appl. Poult. Res. 2:147–153.

Petter, J.G. 1993. Detection of two smooth colony phenotypes in a *Salmonella enteritidis* isolate which vary in their ability to contaminate eggs. Appl. Environ. Microbiol. 59:2884–2890.

Phillips, R.A., and Opitz, H.M. 1995. Pathogenicity and persistence of *Salmonella enteritidis* and egg contamination in normal and infectious bursal disease virus–infected leghorn chicks. Avian Dis. 39:778–787.

Poppe, C., Demczuk, W., McFadden, K., and Johnson, R.P. 1993. Virulence of *Salmonella enteritidis* phage types 4, 8, and 13 and other *Salmonella* spp. for day-old chicks, hens and mice. Can. J. Vet. Res. 57:281–287.

Porter, S.B., and Curtiss III, R. 1997. Effect of inv mutations on *Salmonella* virulence and colonization in 1-day-old white leghorn chicks. Avian Dis. 41:45–57.

Porter, R.E., Jr., and Holt, P.S. 1993. Effect of induced molting on the severity of intestinal lesions caused by *Salmonella enteritidis* infection in chickens. Avian Dis. 37:1009–1016.

Protais, J., Colin, P., Beaumont, C., Guillot, J.F., Lantier, F., Pardon, P., and Bennejean, G. 1996. Line differences in resistance to *Salmonella enteritidis* PT4 infection. Br. Poult. Sci. 37:329–339.

Qin, Z.R., Arakawa, A., Baba, E., Fukata, T., Miyamoto, T., Sasai, K., and Withanage, G.S.K. 1995a. *Eimeria tenella* infection induces recrudescence of previous *Salmonella enteritidis* infection in chickens. Poult. Sci. 74:1786–1792.

Qin, Z.R., Fukata, T., Baba, E., and Arakawa, A. 1995b. Effect of *Eimeria tenella* infection on *Salmonella enteritidis* infection in chickens. Poult. Sci. 74:1–7.

Qin, Z.R., Fukata, T., Baba, E., and Arakawa, A. 1995c. Effect of lactose and *Lactobacillus acidophilus* on the colonization of *Salmonella enteritidis* in chicks concurrently infected with *Eimeria tenella*. Avian Dis. 39:548–553.

Qin, Z.R., Arakawa, A., Baba, E., Fukata, T., and Sasai, K. 1996. Effect of *Eimeria tenella* infection on the production of *Salmonella enteritidis*-contaminated eggs and susceptibility of laying hens to *S. enteritidis* infection. Avian Dis. 40:361–367.

Reiber, M.A., Conner, D.E., and Bilgili, S.F. 1995. Salmonella colonization and shedding patterns of hens inoculated via semen. Avian Dis. 39:317–322.

Shivaprasad, H.L., Timoney, J.F., Morales, S., Lucio, B., and Baker, R.C. 1990. Pathogenesis of *Salmonella enteritidis* infection in laying chickens. I. Studies on egg transmission, clinical signs, fecal shedding, and serologic responses. Avian Dis. 34:548–557.

Tellez, G., Dean, C.E., Corrier, D.E., DeLoach, J.R., Jaeger, L., and Hargis, B.M. 1993a. Effect of dietary lactose on cecal morphology, pH, organic acids, and *Salmonella enteritidis* organ invasion in leghorn chicks. Avian Dis. 72:636–642.

Tellez, G.I., Jaeger, L., Dean, C.E., Corrier, D.E., DeLoach, J.R., Williams, J.D., and Hargis, B.M. 1993b. Effect of prolonged administration of dietary capsaicin on *Salmonella enteritidis* infection in leghorn chicks. Avian Dis. 37:143–148.

Tellez, G.I., Kogut, M.H., and Hargis, B.M. 1994a. *Eimeria tenella* or *Eimeria adenoeides*: induction of morphological changes and increased resistance to *Salmonella enteritidis* infection in leghorn chicks. Poult. Sci. 73:396–401.

Tellez, G.I., Kogut, M.H., and Hargis, B.M. 1994b. Immunoprophylaxis of *Salmonella enteritidis* infection by lymphokines in leghorn chicks. Avian Dis. 37:1062–1070.

Thiagarajan, D., Saeed, A.M., and Asem, E.K. 1994. Mechanism of transovarian transmission of *Salmonella enteritidis* in laying hens. Poult. Sci. 73:89–98.

Thiagarajan, D., Thacker, H.L., and Saeed, A.M. 1996. Experimental infection of laying hens with *Salmonella enteritidis* strains that express different types of fimbriae. Poult. Sci. 75:1365–1372.

Thorns, C.J., Bell, M.M., Sojka, M.G., and Nicholas, R.A. 1996a. Development and application of enzyme-linked immunosorbent assay for specific detection of *Salmonella enteritidis* infections in chickens based on antibodies to SEF14 fimbrial antigen. J. Clin. Microbiol. 34:792–797.

Thorns, C.J., Turcotte, C., Gemmell, C.G., and Woodward, M.J. 1996b. Studies into the role of the SEF14 fimbrial antigen in the pathogenesis of *Salmonella enteritidis*. Microb. Pathog. 20:235–246.

Timms, L.M., Marshall, R.N., and Breslin, M.F. 1990. Laboratory assessment of protection given by an experimental *Salmonella enteritidis* PT4 inactivated, adjuvant vaccine. Vet. Rec. 127:611–614.

Timoney, J.F., Shivaprasad, H.L., Baker, R.C., and Rowe, B. 1989. Egg transmission after infection of hens with *Salmonella enteritidis* phage type 4. Vet. Rec. 125:600–601.

Timoney, J.F., Sikora, N., Shivaprasad, H.L., and Opitz, M. 1990. Detection of antibody to *Salmonella enteritidis* by a gm flagellin-based ELISA. Vet. Rec. 127:168–169.

Turnbull, P.C.B., and Snoeyenbos, G.H. 1974. Experimental salmonellosis in the chicken. 1. Fate and host response in alimentary canal, liver, and spleen. Avian Dis. 18:153–177.

Zijderveld, F.G. van, Zijderveld-van Bemmel, A.M. van, and Anakotta, J. 1992. Comparison of four different enzyme-linked immunosorbent assays for serological diagnosis of *Salmonella enteritidis* infections in experimentally infected chickens. J. Clin. Microbiol. 30:2560–2566.

Ziprin, R.L., Kogut, M.H., McGruder, E.D., Hargis, B.M., and DeLoach, H.R. 1996. Efficacy of *Salmonella enteritidis* (SE)-immune lymphokines from chickens and turkeys on SE liver invasion in one-day-old chicks and turkey poults. Avian Dis. 40:186–192.

23

Experimental Infection of Four Strains of Commercial Laying Hens with *Salmonella enterica* Serovar Enteritidis Phage Type 8

A.M. Saeed, K.A. Lindell, and H.L. Thacker

INTRODUCTION

Foodborne illness is a major cause of morbidity in the United States and throughout the world. In recent years there has been an important rise in the number of outbreaks of human food poisoning caused by *Salmonella enterica* serovar Enteritidis (*S.* Enteritidis), and in the majority of these outbreaks the source has been linked to food that was prepared from whole shell eggs infected with *S.* Enteritidis (Lin et al., 1988; St. Louis et al., 1988; Cowden et al., 1989a,b; Perales and Audican, 1989; Hedberg et al., 1993).

It is well known that selection for disease resistance in poultry stocks can be an effective strategy for the prevention and control of several important infectious diseases affecting these animals (Gross and Siegel, 1975; Hall and Gross, 1975; Gross, 1976; Gross et al., 1980). It has been suggested that some strains of chickens are more genetically susceptible or resistant to infection with *S.* Enteritidis than are others (Benjamin et al., 1991). Strain differences in genetic responses to bacterial and viral antigens have been suggested for many years, and the theory has been used to explain variations in the effectiveness of vaccination programs between different farms (Gyles et al., 1986). Sheep red blood cells have been used as a cellular antigen by many researchers (Gross et al., 1980; Gyles et al., 1986) to evaluate the immune responsiveness of different strains of chickens. Research work done by Martin et al. (1989) and Dunnington et al. (1991) points to inheritance of the genotype at the major histocompatibility locus as a major determining factor for disease resistance.

This study attempted to identify variations that may exist among different strains of white leghorn chickens in regard to their susceptibility and responses to experimental infection with *S.* Enteritidis phage type 8 (PT8). This was accomplished by orally infecting four popular strains of white leghorns with *S.* Enteritidis and monitoring several variables for variations in response. These parameters included: (a) *S.* Enteritidis colonization of internal organs (liver, spleen, ovary, and cecum), (b) contamination with *S.* Enteritidis of the content of eggs laid by the infected hens, (c) *S.* Enteritidis fecal shedding, and (d) *S.* Enteritidis-specific antibody response in serum and egg yolk. These parameters were monitored for 10 weeks after *S.* Enteritidis infection.

MATERIALS AND METHODS

Experimental Chickens

A total of 300 commercial laying hens of white leghorn stock were obtained from commercial vendors. Four different strains (A, B, C, and D) of commonly used laying hens were included (75 from each), and all birds were approximately 45 weeks old. This sample size was selected to enable the observation of organ colonization at 10-day intervals for at least 2 months after infection by killing 10 birds from each strain while serological immune response and egg-yolk antibody could be monitored for the same duration. This experiment was conducted in two back-to-back trials using 150 birds at a time. Each trial was composed of an equal number of birds from each strain. All birds were randomized to individual cages throughout two identical rooms (75 birds per room), identified with a leg band, and housed for 2 weeks to assure acclimatization. Each cage was a standard wire-mesh construction measuring $30 \times 20 \times 25$ cm, with a common feed trough in front and one water cup per two birds. All environmental variables (temperature, feed, water, light, and so on) were maintained at constant levels throughout the experiment.

Collection and Processing of Serum and Egg-Yolk Samples

Each hen was bled at 10-day intervals by brachial vein venipuncture: 2–3 ml of blood were collected, allowed to clot, and centrifuged at 3000 g for 10 min. Sera were collected and stored at –20°C. Egg-yolk samples were collected in volumes of 0.5–1.0 ml from the weekly pools before they were cultured during the infectivity experiment. Yolk samples were diluted 1:10 in sterile normal saline before they were stored at –20°C. Sera and egg-yolk samples from 140 hens were tested using enzyme-linked immunosorbent assay (ELISA). Bacteriological data, used for evaluation of the ELISA, came from the same group of birds.

ELISA Protocol

An indirect ELISA protocol was used that was designed to measure the immunoglobulin G (IgG) antibody levels in egg yolk and sera of laying hens (Lindell et al., 1995).

Inoculation of Chickens with *Salmonella* Enteritidis

A culture of *S.* Enteritidis PT8 (isolated from naturally infected laying hens) was grown overnight in Mueller-Hinton broth. Serial dilutions and plate counts were performed using standard techniques. *Salmonella* Enteritidis PT8 was used in this infectivity experiment because it is the most common *S.* Enteritidis phage type isolated from sporadic and outbreak cases of human and poultry salmonellosis. Each bird was inoculated with 1×10^8 colony-forming units suspended in 0.5 ml of sterile solution. This inoculum was introduced orally into the crop of each bird by using a tuberculin syringe and a curved, bulbed 10-cm needle.

Bacteriological Analysis of Collected Samples

Eggs were collected daily, stored at 4°C, and each bird's weekly production was pooled for bacteriological analysis.

Each egg was soaked for 5 min in a 10% bleach solution, dried, cracked, and the white separated from the yolk by hand technique. The yolks from each bird's weekly production were pooled in a Whirl-Pak bag (Nasco, Fort Atkinson, WI) and stomached to homogeneity by a laboratory Stomacher (Stomacher 400; Tekmar, Cincinnati, OH). Each sample was then incubated at 37°C overnight. A total of 100 ml of tetrathionate broth was then added to each sample, and these were again incubated overnight at 37°C. A loopful from each sample was then inoculated onto xylose-lysine-tergitol 4 (XLT4) plates (Miller et al., 1991). After 48 h, suspect colonies were subbed onto triple-sugar iron slants and eventually further confirmed by serotyping with salmonella O antiserum (group D) by using slide agglutination.

Egg whites that had been separated from the yolks were also cultured initially for a 3-week period by the same aforementioned technique. This was done to determine whether any *S.* Enteritidis could be recovered from the whites and to assure that positive samples would not be missed by culturing the yolks only.

Feces were cultured in a similar manner. Each bird's fecal production was collected weekly on a disposable tray beneath the bird's cage. A uniform mixture of the feces was made and 10 g was collected and placed in a Whirl-Pak bag. A total of 100 ml of tetrathionate broth was added to each sample, and these were incubated at 42°C overnight. A loopful from each sample was then inoculated onto XLT4 plates and processed as for the yolks. Yolk and fecal samples from one weekly pool from each bird were cultured prior to *S.* Enteritidis inoculation to ensure the freedom of the hens from natural *S.* Enteritidis infection

To assess organ carriage, 10 birds from each strain (five per trial) were randomly selected every 10 days after infection and killed using CO_2 chamber and cervical dislocation. The birds were posted and inspected for gross pathology, and samples were collected with a sterile technique for bacteriological analysis. Organs cultured included liver and spleen (cultured together), large developing follicles, ovarian tissue, and ceca. Organ samples were placed in Whirl-Pak bags and stomached for 30 s. A total of 100 ml of tetrathionate was added, and these were then incubated overnight at 37°C. Subsequently, a loopful was streaked onto XLT4 plates and processed as for the yolks.

These procedures were followed for 10 weeks until all birds had been killed. Egg production was recorded prior to inoculation to obtain a baseline production level and then monitored throughout the experiment.

Statistical Analysis

Logistic regression was used to model the probability of a positive culture result from the bird's organs. To test for an association between positive bacteriological results and layer strains the chi-squared test was used. All analyses were performed using SAS software (SAS Institute, 1989). Serological data were analyzed using Epi Info software. Analysis of variance was used and F statistics and probability (p) values were reported at $\alpha = 0.05$ in comparing the means of serum and egg-yolk IgG titers when the means were homogeneous and normally distributed. However, where Bartlett's test indicated lack of homogeneity of the variances of the means of some samples, a nonparametric test (Kruskal-Wallis H) was applied and chi-squared values were reported. These exceptions are noted in the tables.

RESULTS

Organ Colonization of *Salmonella* Enteritidis in the Different Hen Strains

All baseline bacteriological results of fecal and egg cultures were negative for recovery of S. Enteritidis. The egg-white samples that were cultured for an initial 3-week period after infection were also all negative. Therefore, the culturing of egg white was discontinued.

Isolation rates of S. Enteritidis from liver and spleen pools, ovarian tissue, cecal tissues, and egg yolk did not differ among the four different strains of hens during the first and second halves of the infectivity experiment: liver and spleen, $\chi^2 = 2.036$ (p < 0.565); ovarian tissue, $\chi^2 = 0.707$ (p < 0.872); cecal tissues, $\chi^2 = 0.512$ (p < 0.916); and egg yolks, $\chi^2 = 0.787$ (p < 0.853). There were no significant differences in the isolation rates of S. Enteritidis from the fecal samples in three of the four different strains of hens during the first and the second halves of the infectivity

experiment. However, it was more likely to isolate S. Enteritidis from the fecal samples of strain-D hens than strain-A hens during the first half of the experiment, $\chi^2 = 4.31$ (p < 0.05), whereas isolation rates of the organisms were more frequent from the fecal samples of strain-A hens than strain-D hens during the second half of the experiment; $\chi^2 = 4.88$ (p < 0.05). The data of the two halves of the experiment were combined for further analysis. Table 23.1 depicts the combined bacteriological data from the organ cultures of both trials. This table shows the number of birds from each strain from which S. Enteritidis was recovered at 10-day intervals (10 birds killed per strain). There is a clear trend of decreasing positive culture results by days after infection. This was true for all organs, and all strains showed very similar trends of decreasing probability of S. Enteritidis-positive bacteriological cultures.

A summary of the logistic regression analysis of the positive isolation of S. Enteritidis from the organs of the four different strains of chickens is presented in Table 23.2. Strain, days, and strain by days of interaction were used as explanatory variables. There was no statistically significant difference among hen strains in regard to the positive isolation of S. Enteritidis from internal organs (Table 23.2). Likewise, no days-by-strain interactions were evident; no strain shows an increased probability of positive isolation of S. Enteritidis from internal organs for a significantly shorter or longer period after infection than another strain. However, as mentioned previously, all hen strains show a strong days' effect.

TABLE 23.1   Isolation of *Salmonella* Enteritidis phage type 8 from organs of four strains of laying hens experimentally infected with the organism

| | No. of hens of each strain (A, B, C, and D) with S. Enteritidis-positive organ cultures (n = 10 birds per strain that were killed at 10-day intervals) | | | | | | | | | | | |
| | Liver and spleen | | | | Ovary | | | | Ceca | | | |
Days after infection	A	B	C	D	A	B	C	D	A	B	C	D
10	8	7	6	9	6	5	3	5	6	5	6	8
20	2	1	5	6	0	4	4	0	1	2	1	4
30	1	2	3	2	0	0	1	0	0	0	1	0
40	1	0	2	0	0	0	0	0	0	0	0	0
50	3	1	2	3	0	0	0	1	0	0	0	1
60	1	0	1	1	1	0	0	0	0	0	0	0
70	0	1	1	1	0	0	0	0	0	0	0	0

TABLE 23.2   Summary of logistic regression analysis of positive bacterial isolation from organs of four different strains of egg-laying hens experimentally infected with *Salmonella* Enteritidis phage type 8

| | Liver and spleen | | | Ovary | | | Ceca | | |
Variables	χ^2	df	p	χ^2	df	p	χ^2	df	p
Strain	1.6	3	0.66	1.5	3	0.68	0.52	3	0.90
Days	39.8	3	0.00	26.91	3	0.00	25.83	3	0.00
Days × strain	0.95	3	0.81	0.89	3	0.83	1.37	3	0.71

Contamination of Eggs with *Salmonella* Enteritidis and Fecal Shedding of the Organisms

Results of bacteriological analysis of yolk and fecal cultures are presented in Table 23.3. As with organ cultures, there was a distinct trend of decreasing *S.* Enteritidis-positive cultures by days after infection that was observed in all four strains. Chi-square tests (2 × 4 contingency tables) were used to test for statistical significance of variations between strains for the percentage of positive yolk-pool culture results. At 7 and 14 days after infection, the chi-square values and p values derived from the contingency tables were 20.072 (p < 0.001) and 22.593 (p < 0.001), respectively (Table 23.4). The data in Table 23.3 suggest that weekly egg pools from strain A were more likely to yield a positive culture result for *S.* Enteritidis than were egg pools from the other hen strains. By 21 days after infection, no differences were evident among the four different strains of laying hens.

The same methods (2 × 4 contingency tables) were used to test for statistical significance of variations in the percentage of *S.* Enteritidis-positive fecal cultures that were obtained from the four different hen strains (Table 23.4). As with yolk pools, at 7 days after infection there was a significant variation among the four hen strains in the percentage of *S.* Enteritidis-positive culture results. Referring again to Table 23.3, the data suggest that *S.* Enteritidis is more likely to be isolated from the egg and fecal samples of strain-A hens than from the other hen strains. At 14 and 21 days after infection, this variation in *S.* Enteritidis-positive fecal cultures was no longer seen. Note that the number of birds of each strain decreases by 10 for each 10 days after infection. A consequence is that the power of detecting strain differences decreases with increasing number of days after infection.

A slight rise in the recovery rates of *S.* Enteritidis from the internal organs and the fecal samples of all the hen strains was noted at approximately 50 days after infection (Tables 23.1 and 23.3).

Relationship between Serum and Egg-Yolk IgG Titers and Isolation Rates of *Salmonella* Enteritidis from Liver and Spleen Pools

Figure 23.1 shows the mean IgG titers of serum *S.* Enteritidis-specific antibody of the four hen strains during the 10

TABLE 23.3 Isolation of *Salmonella* Enteritidis phage type 8 from yolk and fecal samples collected from four different strains of laying hens experimentally infected with the organism

| | No. (%) of hens that laid *S.* Enteritidis-positive eggs | | | | No. (%) of hens with *S.* Enteritidis-positive fecal cultures | | | |
| | Hen strain | | | | Hen strain | | | |
Days after infection	A	B	C	D	A	B	C	D
7	35 (50)	13 (19)	23 (33)	15 (21)	36 (51)	21 (30)	21 (30)	28 (40)
14	12 (20)	11 (18)	1 (2)	0 (0)	25 (42)	21 (35)	17 (28)	15 (25)
21	5 (10)	7 (14)	6 (12)	5 (10)	6 (12)	8 (16)	7 (14)	14 (28)
28	1 (3)	3 (8)	1 (3)	0 (0)	1 (2)	0 (0)	0 (0)	0 (0)
35	0 (0)	0 (0)	0 (0)	0 (0)	0 (0)	0 (0)	2 (5)	1 (2)
42	0 (0)	0 (0)	0 (0)	0 (0)	0 (0)	0 (0)	0 (0)	0 (0)
49	0 (0)	0 (0)	0 (0)	0 (0)	1 (3)	2 (6)	0 (0)	1 (3)
56	0 (0)	0 (0)	0 (0)	0 (0)	0 (0)	0 (0)	0 (0)	0 (0)
63	0 (0)	0 (0)	0 (0)	0 (0)	0 (0)	0 (0)	0 (0)	0 (0)

TABLE 23.4 Statistical analysis of results from bacteriological testing of egg-yolk and fecal samples collected from four different strains of laying hens that were experimentally infected with *Salmonella* Enteritidis phage type 8 and followed for 10 weeks after infection (frequency of isolation at 7, 14, and 21 days)

| | Days after infection | | | | | | | | |
| | 7 | | | 14 | | | 21 | | |
Sample	χ^2	df	p	χ^2	df	p	χ^2	df	p
Yolk	20.027	3	0.00	22.593	3	0.00	0.54	3	0.00
Feces	9.291	3	0.03	4.482	3	0.21	5.368	3	0.15

weeks of observation. It must be noted that 10 birds from each of the four hen strains were killed at 10-day intervals to study *S.* Enteritidis organ invasion rate in each strain. Therefore, with smaller sample size, the power of detecting significant differences among the four hen strains decreases toward the end of the experiment.

Figures 23.2 and 23.3 show the mean serum and egg-yolk IgG titers, respectively, in hens classified on the basis of liver and spleen pool culture results for *S.* Enteritidis. Hens were classified based on whether or not *S.* Enteritidis was recovered from their liver and spleen pool at the time of necropsy, and all titers measured at 10-day intervals for each hen were included. The percentage of hens with *S.* Enteritidis-positive liver and spleen pools at each 10-day interval is also provided in Figure 23.1 for comparison.

A clear trend of higher mean IgG titers is seen in both sera and yolks (Figure 23.4) 1 month after infection for those hens having positive liver and spleen pool culture results at the time of necropsy. Statistical analyses showed significantly higher mean serum IgG titers in birds with positive liver and spleen pools at 40 days after infection (F = 11.96, p < 0.001) and at 50 days after infection (F = 9.00, p < 0.004). Similarly, the mean egg-yolk IgG

titers were higher at 35 days after infection (F = 7.36, p < 0.009), 42 days after infection (F = 4.65, p <0.032), 49 days after infection (F = 6.10, p < 0.016), 56 days after infection (F = 7.11, p < 0.010), and at 71 days after infection (F = 5.35, p < 0.034) (Tables 23.4–23.8). Due to this apparent association between high serum and egg-yolk IgG titers and positive liver and spleen pool culture results, analyses were performed to test for a concurrent association between positive liver and spleen pool culture results and the duration of postinfection recovery of *S.* Enteritidis from egg yolks. There was no association between birds that produced eggs contaminated with *S.* Enteritidis for longer than 2 weeks after infection and birds with positive liver and spleen pool culture results (Mantel Haenszel χ^2= 0.79, p < 0.374).

DISCUSSION

Several researchers have shown good evidence to suggest that immune responsiveness and susceptibility to diseases among different strains or lines of egg-laying strains of hens may be genetically related (Dunnington et al., 1991).

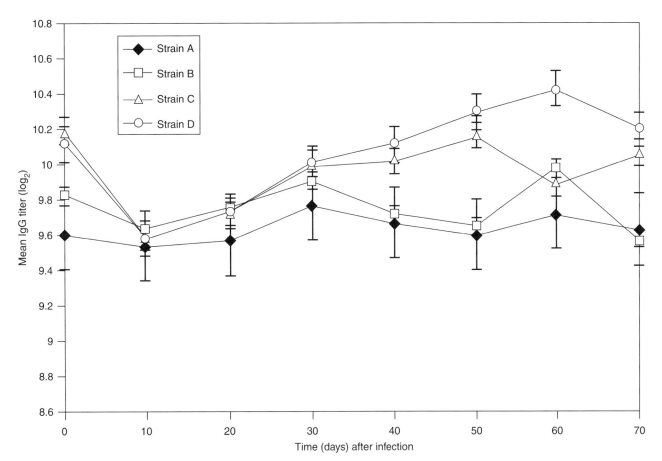

FIGURE 23.1   Mean immunoglobulin G (IgG) titers (with standard error bars) of serum *Salmonella* Enteritidis-specific antibody of the four hen strains experimentally infected with *S.* Enteritidis phage type 8 and monitored for 10 weeks

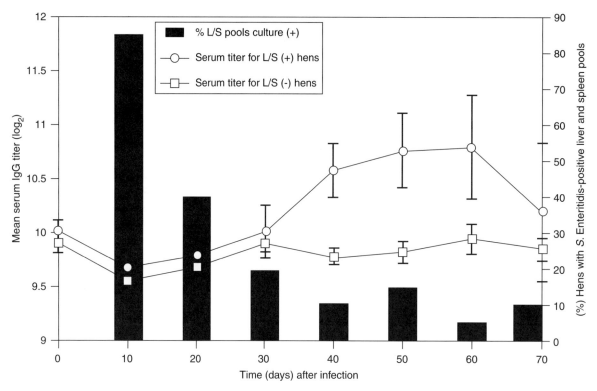

FIGURE 23.2   Mean immunoglobulin G (IgG) titers (with standard error bars) of serum *Salmonella* Enteritidis-specific antibody of the four hen strains grouped on the basis of liver-pool and spleen-pool culture results at the time of necropsy compared with the percent of hens with positive liver and spleen (L/S) pools.

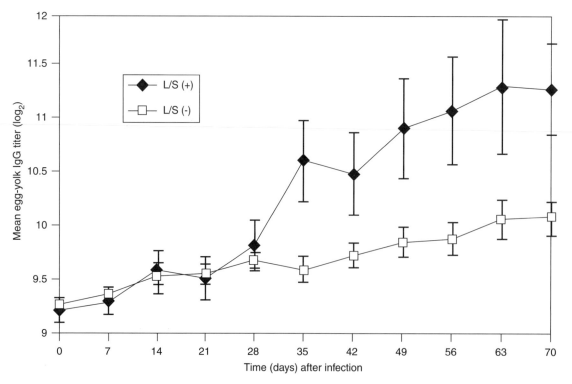

FIGURE 23.3   Mean immunoglobulin G (IgG) titers (with standard error bars) of egg-yolk *Salmonella* Enteritidis-specific antibody of the four hen strains grouped on the basis of liver-pool and spleen-pool (L/S) culture results at the time of necropsy.

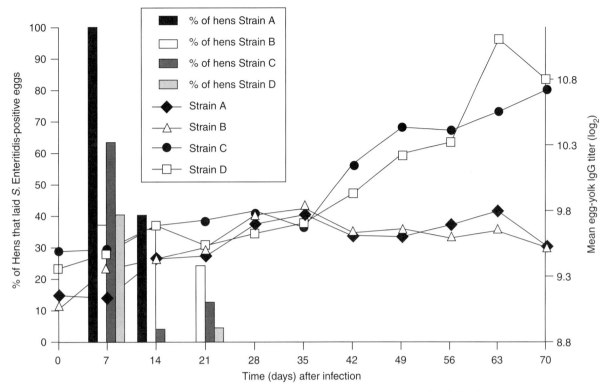

FIGURE 23.4   Isolation rates of *Salmonella* Enteritidis from weekly egg pools of the four hen strains compared with the mean egg-yolk immunoglobulin G (IgG) titer of each strain over the duration of the trial.

TABLE 23.5   Geometrical mean titers of *Salmonella* Enteritidis-specific immunoglobulin G in sera from strain-A hens compared with three other strains of hens followed for 10 weeks after infection with *S.* Enteritidis phage type 8

Days after infection[a]	Strain B			Strain C			Strain D		
	F	df	p	F	df	p	F	df	p
0	3.85	1	0.051	22.2	1	0.000	9.05[b]	1	0.003
10	2.56[b]	1	0.176	0.18	1	0.680	0.116	1	0.734
20	1.70[b]	1	0.193	0.11[b]	1	0.737	1.20[b]	1	0.237
30	0.75	1	0.865	1.34	1	0.251	1.254	1	0.268
40	0.05	1	0.817	2.36	1	0.129	4.20	1	0.045
50	0.04	1	0.831	3.99	1	0.053	5.50	1	0.025
60	0.36	1	0.564	0.22	1	0.647	3.19	1	0.089
70	0.03	1	0.862	1.96	1	0.189	2.48	1	0.152

[a]There is a decreasing number of birds by days after infection: 20 birds (five from each strain) were killed every 10 days. There were 35 birds per strain at 0 days after infection. Five birds remained from each strain at 70 days after infection.
[b]Kruskal-Wallis chi-squared value reported due to lack of homogeneity of variances of the compared means.

TABLE 23.6 Geometrical mean titers of *Salmonella* Enteritidis-specific immunoglobulin G in sera of strain-B hens compared with strain-C and strain-D laying hens monitored for 10 weeks after infection with *S.* Enteritidis phage type 8

Days after infection[a]	Strain C			Strain D		
	F	df	p	F	df	p
0	9.00	1	0.004	1.66[b]	1	0.198
10	0.18	1	0.679	0.22	1	0.644
20	0.02	1	0.964	0.01	1	0.933
30	0.06[b]	1	0.804	0.21[b]	1	0.649
40	1.15[b]	1	0.283	4.68	1	0.035
50	4.22	1	0.047	5.86	1	0.021
60	0.05	1	0.824	1.37	1	0.256
70	2.46	1	0.145	2.93	1	0.123

[a]There is a decreasing number of birds by days after infection: 20 birds (five from each strain) were killed every 10 days. There were 35 birds per strain at 0 days after infection. Five birds remained from each strain at 70 days after infection.
[b]Kruskal-Wallis chi-square value reported due to lack of homogeneity of variances of the compared means.

TABLE 23.7 Geometrical mean titers of *Salmonella* Enteritidis-specific immunoglobulin G in egg-yolk samples of strain-A hens compared with three other strains of laying hens monitored for 10 weeks after infection with *S.* Enteritidis phage type 8

Days after infection[a]	Strain B			Strain C			Strain D		
	F	df	p	F	df	p	F	df	p
0	0.33	1	0.573	4.90	1	0.029	3.85[b]	1	0.050
7	3.70	1	0.056	4.70[b]	1	0.030	5.72	1	0.017
14	0.00	1	0.982	1.73	1	0.190	1.43	1	0.235
21	0.14	1	0.714	1.38	1	0.243	0.08	1	0.770
28	0.15	1	0.699	0.17	1	0.684	0.19[b]	1	0.659
35	0.02	1	0.872	0.07	1	0.795	0.04	1	0.836
42	1.35[b]	1	0.245	2.30	1	0.135	0.97	1	0.667
49	1.28[b]	1	0.259	4.45	1	0.042	1.93	1	0.174
56	0.03	1	0.861	3.43	1	0.072	1.66	1	0.207
63	0.09	1	0.770	2.06	1	0.168	5.19	1	0.035
70	0.00	1	0.980	6.86	1	0.033	24.8	1	0.003

[a]There is a decreasing number of birds by days after infection: 20 birds (five from each strain) were killed every 10 days. There were 35 birds per strain at 0 days after infection. Five birds remained from each strain at 70 days after infection.
[b]Kruskal-Wallis chi-square value reported due to lack of homogeneity of variances of the compared means.

Although the results of this study revealed no significant statistical difference among the four strains of birds with regard to organ colonization and the window of opportunity for positive *S.* Enteritidis organ cultures (Table 23.2), the data provide useful information about some variations in the probability of *S.* Enteritidis-positive organ culture from these different birds. These data may be used in the prediction of the duration of *S.* Enteritidis organ carriage after an *S.* Enteritidis infection and provide a base for the proper timing of bird sampling for organ culture during surveys on the disease in layer houses. On the other hand, significant differences were revealed between the different bird strains in regard to *S.* Enteritidis fecal shedding and the production of *S.* Enteritidis-contaminated eggs; birds of strain A showed the highest rates of *S.* Enteritidis isolation in yolk pools by 7 and 14 days after infection and also the highest rate of *S.* Enteritidis isolation from fecal samples by 7 days after infection. These differences were statistically

significant ($p < 0.02$) (Table 23.4). Egg contamination with *S.* Enteritidis and fecal shedding of these organisms have the greatest impact on the egg-layer industry and public health. Data from this study suggest the existence of variability in the resistance of different strains of egg layers to *S.* Enteritidis infection. Additionally, data from a recent survey conducted by the authors on the prevalence of *S.* Enteritidis in nest run eggs from laying flocks in the Midwestern states (data not shown) supported the findings of this experimental work. This resistance could be measured by the ability of some laying strains to produce relatively fewer *S.* Enteritidis-contaminated eggs in the face of infection and to be less frequent fecal shedders of these organisms. These features may be of significant advantage toward reduction in the number of laid *S.* Enteritidis-contaminated eggs, which is the focus of current public health concern, and the reduction in *S.* Enteritidis environmental contamination resulting from the fecal shedding,

TABLE 23.8   Geometrical mean titers of *Salmonella* Enteritidis-specific immunoglobulin G in egg-yolk samples of strain-B hens compared with strain-C and strain-D laying hens monitored for 10 weeks after infection with *S.* Enteritidis phage type 8

Days after infection[a]	Strain C			Strain D		
	F	df	p	F	df	p
0	7.99	1	0.006	4.63[b]	1	0.031
7	1.01	1	0.320	0.75	1	0.386
14	1.57	1	0.213	1.30	1	0.258
21	0.76	1	0.607	0.00	1	0.966
28	0.01	1	0.913	0.03	1	0.869
35	0.17	1	0.690	0.12	1	0.729
42	3.15[b]	1	0.076	2.24	1	0.135
49	3.63[b]	1	0.057	3.84	1	0.050
56	3.63[b]	1	0.057	4.13	1	0.042
63	6.41	1	0.020	12.5	1	0.003
70	9.53	1	0.015	34.8	1	0.001

[a]There is a decreasing number of birds by days after infection: 20 birds (five from each strain) were killed every 10 days. There were 35 birds per strain at 0 days after infection. Five birds remained from each strain at 70 days after infection.
[b]Kruskal-Wallis chi-square value reported due to lack of homogeneity of variances of the compared means.

which is a common means of horizontal transmission of the infection throughout the flock and therefore affects the safety of poultry-house workers.

There are two possible explanations for the increased *S.* Enteritidis isolation rates from layers noted at approximately 50 days after infection. Reinfection of the birds might have occurred either through horizontal transmission or some outside source (for example, feed). This can be avoided through the design of the facilities in which the birds were housed and the care taken to prevent such an occurrence. Increased *S.* Enteritidis isolation rates were seen during both trials. It is unlikely that both groups were reinfected at the same time during each trial. A more plausible scenario is that a "reawakening" or superinfection occurred within some birds at a point in time at which the primary immune response was tapering off to a level that allowed a resurgence and recolonization of some bacteria that had been previously suppressed or sequestered without being killed. Adding credence to this theory is our observation of a concurrent rise in the antibody titer as measured by ELISA (A.M. Saeed et al., unpublished data) that parallels these increased isolation rates.

There is presently some controversy as to the main route of infection for eggs that are found to be culture positive for salmonella. Ongoing research from the author's laboratory (unpublished data) leads to the conclusion that a transovarian infection could be a main route from which eggs become infected. This lends support to the theory that genetic responsiveness or the lack of an appropriate response plays a role in the variabilities noted between strains. Data from this study suggest that there may be inherent differences between popular layer strains in regard to the probability of the production of eggs that are culture positive for *S.* Enteritidis after experimental infection.

The serum and egg-yolk IgG titers did differ significantly in regard to baseline titers (0 days after infection). This is particularly evident in strains C and D, which showed relatively high baseline serum IgG titers that dramatically decreased by

10 days after infection. It is unlikely that these high serum baseline titers were due to laboratory or experimental error, because of the large sample size (35 hens per strain) and the observation that this phenomenon is much more prominent in strains C and D. To ensure comparability, serum and yolk samples from the four hen strains were included on each ELISA plate along with serum and yolk from specific pathogen-free (SPF) hens as negative controls. In addition, a repeat of the serum ELISAs revealed the same trend.

Although all birds were negative for the recovery of *S.* Enteritidis based on yolk and fecal cultures prior to inoculation, these hens were not SPF stock and were likely exposed to other Gram-negative organisms that share partial antigenic similarity with the *S.* Enteritidis organism. It has been suggested that the use of lipopolysaccharide (LPS) as a coating antigen may result in some amount of cross-reactivity with other antigenically related organisms, and several studies have shown that other capture antigens, such as flagella, may be more specific than LPS (van Zijderveld et al., 1992; Baay and Huis in 't Veld, 1993). Recently however, it has been reported that "*Salmonella* serology using LPS antigens is highly O antigen specific and predictable" (Konrad et al., 1994).

All hen strains showed some decrease in serum IgG titers between days 0 and 10 after infection. This is likely the manifestation of some amount of immunosuppression induced by a high oral dose of *S.* Enteritidis. This temporary immunosuppression is consistent among the four hen strains in that there is no significant difference in mean IgG titers between strains at 10 days after infection. Virulent *Salmonella* Typhimurium has been shown to induce lymphocyte depletion and immunosuppression in chickens (Hassan and Curtiss, 1994). It has also been suggested that massive bacteremia can remove specific IgG from circulation (Barrow et al., 1991).

A comparison of the IgG response of the four hen strains revealed that strain A had significantly lower mean IgG levels in both sera and yolk at several points in time. Similarly, hen strain B had significantly lower IgG titers in comparison with strains C and D at the same testing times (Tables 23.5–23.8). The significance of these observations is that not only does there appear to be inherent genetic differences in regard to immune responsiveness, but these differences can be linked to bacteriological data. It was observed that at 7 days after infection *S. Enteritidis* was more likely to be isolated from the fecal samples of hens of strain A than from the other hen strains. These findings suggest an inverse relationship between the immunological response, as measured by serum and egg-yolk IgG, and the probability of the production of eggs contaminated with *S. Enteritidis*.

Genetic selection and breeding for disease resistance will ultimately play a role in reducing the incidence of animal and human salmonellosis.

REFERENCES

Baay, M.F.D., and Huis in 't Veld, J.H.J. 1993. Alternative antigens reduce cross-reactions in an ELISA for the detection of *Salmonella enteritidis* in poultry. J. Appl. Bacteriol. 74:243–247.

Barrow, P.A., Berchieri, A., Jr., and Al-Haddad, O. 1991. Serological response of chickens to immunosorbent assay. Avian Dis. 35:227–236.

Benjamin, W.H., Jr., Briles, W.E., Waltman, W.D., and Briles, D.E. 1991. Effects of genetics and prior *S. enteritidis* infection on the ability of chickens to be infected with *S. enteritidis*. In: Blankenship, L.C., ed. Colonization control of human bacterial enteropathogens in poultry. New York: Academic, pp. 365–369.

Cowden, J.M., Chisholm, D., O'Mahoney, M., Mawer, S.L., Spain, G.E., Ward, L., and Rowe, B. 1989a. Two outbreaks of *S. enteritidis* phage type 4 infection associated with the consumption of fresh shell-egg products. Epidemiol. Infect. 103:47–52.

Cowden, J.M., Lynch, D., Joseph, C.A., O'Mahoney, M., Mawer, S.L., Rowe, B., and Bartlett, C.L.R. 1989b. Case-control study of infections with *S. enteritidis* phage type 4 in England. BMJ 299:771–773.

Dunnington, E.A., Siegel, P.B., and Gross, W.B. 1991. *Escherichia coli* challenge in chickens selected for high or low antibody response and differing in haplotypes at the major histocompatibility complex. Avian Dis. 35:937–940.

Gross, W.B. 1976. Plasma steroid tendency, social environment and *Eimeria necatrix* infection. Poult. Sci. 55:1508–1512.

Gross, W.B., and Siegel, P.B. 1975. Immune response to *Escherichia coli*. Am. J. Vet. Res. 36:568–571.

Gross, W.G., Siegel, P.B., Hall, W.R., Domermuth, C.H., and Duboise, R.T. 1980. Production and persistence of antibodies in chickens to sheep erythrocytes. 2. Resistance to infectious diseases. Poult. Sci. 59:205–210.

Gyles, N.R., Fallah-Moghddam, H., Patterson, L.T., Skeeles, J.K., Whitfill, C.E., and Johnson, L.W. 1986. Genetic aspects of antibody responses in chickens to different classes of antigens. Poult. Sci. 65:223–232.

Hall, R.D., and Gross, W.B. 1975. Effect of social stress and inherited plasma corticosteroid levels in chickens on populations of northern fowl mites, *Ornithonyssus sylviarum*. J. Parasitol. 61:1096–1100.

Hassan, J.O., and Curtis III, R. 1994. Virulent *Salmonella typhimurium*-induced lymphocyte depletion and immunosuppression in chickens. Infect. Immun. 62:2027–2036.

Hedberg, C.W., David, J.J., White, K.E., MacDonald, K.L., and Osterholm, M.T. 1993. Role of egg consumption in sporadic *Salmonella enteritidis* and *S. typhimurium* infection in Minnesota. J. Infect. Dis. 176:107–111.

Konrad, H., Smith, B.P., Dilling, G.W., and House, J.K. 1994. Production of *Salmonella* serogroup D(O9)-specific enzyme-linked immunosorbent assay antigen. Am. J. Vet. Res. 55:1647–1651.

Lin, F.Y.C., Morris, J.G., Jr., Trump, D., Tilgham, D., Wood, P.K., Jackman, N., Israel, E., and Libonati, J.P. 1988. Investigation of an outbreak of *S. enteritidis* gastroenteritis associated with consumption of eggs in a restaurant chain in Maryland. Am. J. Epidemiol. 128:839–844.

Lindell, K.A., Saeed, A.M., and Thacker, H.L. 1995. Optimization and evaluation of serum and egg yolk ELISA for monitoring *S. enteritidis* infection in laying hens. In: Proceedings of the symposium on the diagnosis of salmonella infections, October 31, Reno, Nevada, pp. 15–32.

Martin, A., Dunnington, E.A., Briles, W.E., Briles, R.W., and Siegel, P.B. 1989. Marek's disease and major histocompatibility complex haplotypes in chickens selected for high or low antibody response. Anim. Genet. 20:407–414.

Miller, R.G., Tate, C.R., Mallinson, E.T., and Scherre, J.A. 1991. Xylose-lysine-tergitol 4: an improved agar medium for the isolation of *Salmonella*. Poult. Sci. 70:2429–2432.

Perales, I., and Audican, A. 1989. The role of hens eggs in outbreaks of salmonellosis in north Spain. Int. J. Food Microbiol. 8:175–180.

SAS Institute. 1989. SAS/STATR users guide, version 6, 4th ed., vols. 1 and 2. Cary, NC: SAS Institute.

St. Louis, M.E., Morse, D.L., Potter, M.E., DeMelfi, T.M., Guzewich, J.J., Tauxe, R.V., and Blake, P.A. 1988. The emergence of grade A eggs as a major source of *S. enteritidis* infections: new implications for the control of salmonellosis. JAMA 259:2103–2107.

van Zijderveld, F.G., van Zijderveld-van Bemmel, A.M., and Anakutta, J. 1992. Comparison of four different enzyme-linked immunosorbent assays for serological diagnosis of *Salmonella enteritidis* infections in experimentally infected chickens. J. Clin. Microbiol. 30:2560–2566.

24

Role of Fimbriae of *Salmonella enterica* Serovar Enteritidis in the Pathogenesis of the Disease in Experimentally Infected Laying Hens

A.M. Saeed, D. Thiagarajan, and H.L. Thacker

INTRODUCTION

Salmonella enterica serovar Enteritidis (*S.* Enteritidis) is a major cause of gastroenteritis in humans and is associated with consumption of contaminated, raw, or undercooked eggs and other food products (Coyle et al., 1988; Lin et al., 1988; St. Louis et al., 1988; Cowden et al., 1989a,b; Hedberg et al., 1993). The disease is especially severe in infants, elderly people, and immunocompromised patients. Incidence of this disease has shown a steady increase during the past few years (Centers for Disease Control, 1988, 1990; St. Louis et al., 1988). In infected laying hens, *S.* Enteritidis colonizes the ceca and causes contamination of the eggshell surface when the laid egg comes in contact with fecal material. However, sanitation of eggshell surface following collection suggests that this route for egg contamination with the organism is unlikely (St. Louis et al., 1988). Alternatively, due to dissemination of the organism from the alimentary tract to various internal organs, the organism may enter egg yolk during its formation in the hen's body. Colonization of the ovaries may also result in transovarian transmission of *S.* Enteritidis (Coyle et al.,

1988; Bygrave and Gallagher, 1989; Timoney et al., 1989; Gast and Beard, 1990a; Thiagarajan et al., 1994). Although several reports describe the natural and experimental infection of chickens with *S.* Enteritidis (Hopper and Mawer, 1988; Lister, 1988; Gast and Beard, 1990b; Shivaprasad et al., 1990; Barrow and Lovell, 1991), the characteristics of *S.* Enteritidis that influence the mechanism of the disease in hens are largely unknown.

Fimbriae are rod-shaped structures on the surface of bacteria that are involved in the attachment of the organism to the eukaryotic cells' surface and may thus contribute to disease pathogenesis (Finlay and Falkow, 1989; Muller et al., 1991). Although the correlation between possession of fimbriae and virulence is not clearly established, attachment of salmonellae to eukaryotic cells in vitro has been attributed to the presence of fimbriae. Duguid et al. (1966) have shown that the ability of salmonella serovars to agglutinate erythrocytes is related to the possession of fimbriae. Similarly, attachment of *S.* Enteritidis to human intestinal epithelial cells is mediated by fimbriae (Baloda et al., 1988). The ability of "rough" strains of *S.* Enteritidis to attach in significantly higher numbers than "smooth" strains was related to the dense expression of fimbriae by the "rough" strains (Baloda et al., 1988). Binding of *S*. Enteritidis to extracellular matrix proteins such as fibronectin involves fimbriae expressed on the bacterial surface (Baloda, 1988; Baloda et al., 1988). In studies of adherence and pathogenesis of *S*. Enteritidis in mice, Aslanzadeh and Paulissen (1992) reported that adherence of *S*. Enteritidis to mouse intestinal cells involves two types of fimbriae and that they are important in the pathogenesis of the disease in mice. In addition, mice can be passively immunized against *S*. Enteritidis by the administration of egg-yolk antibodies to a 14-kDa fimbrial protein of *S*. Enteritidis (Peralta et al., 1994), suggesting the important role of fimbriae in the disease process.

It is not clear at present whether the expression of fimbriae by *S*. Enteritidis is correlated with their pathogenicity in laying hens. In an attempt to correlate fimbrial expression to pathogenicity, three *S*. Enteritidis strains with different types of fimbrial expression were used in experimental infections of laying hens. The main objectives of this study included the comparison of three *S*. Enteritidis phage type 8 (PT8) strains, which expressed different attachment patterns on avian ovary granulosa cells, for their pathogenicity in laying hens. Pathogenicity is measured by cecal colonization, fecal shedding, egg contamination, and serum antibody levels following oral inoculation. Additionally, the role of membrane-associated structures in the humoral immune response to experimental *S*. Enteritidis infection in chickens was examined.

MATERIALS AND METHODS

Experimental Hens

Single-comb white leghorn hens (30 weeks old) were obtained from a local farm known by serological testing to be free of *S*. Enteritidis infection. This was further confirmed by killing randomly selected hens and culturing their visceral organs (ceca, liver, spleen, and ovaries) for *S*. Enteritidis isolation. The hens were housed in individual, wire-mesh cages in a windowless, air-conditioned room with a 16-h-light–8-h-dark cycle. They had unlimited access to tap water and a commercial layer ration with crude protein and metabolizable energy content that exceeded the National Research Council requirements.

Media, Chemicals, and Equipment

Bacteriological media and agar were obtained from Difco Laboratories (Detroit, MI). Medium 199 and prestained molecular-weight markers for immunoblot were obtained from Life Technologies Corporation (Gaithersburg, MD). *Salmonella* Enteritidis-specific lipopolysaccharide (LPS), rabbit anti-chicken immunoglobulin G (IgG) conjugated with alkaline phosphatase, rabbit anti-chicken IgG conjugated with peroxidase, Fast DAB system as substrate for peroxidase enzyme, and Tween 20 were from Sigma Chemical Company (St. Louis, MO). For sodium dodecyl sulfate–polyacrylamide-

gel electrophoresis (SDS-PAGE) analysis, the Penguin electrophoresis system and Joey gel-casting system obtained from AT Biochem (Malvern, PA) were used. For transfer of electrophoresed proteins in the immunoblot protocol, Protean transfer blot cell, nitrocellulose membranes, and prestained molecular-weight proteins were obtained from Bio-Rad (Hercules, CA).

Preparation of Membrane-Associated Proteins from *Salmonella* Enteritidis

Membrane-associated proteins were extracted from bacterial cells as described previously (Chart, 1994). Briefly, each *S*. Enteritidis strain was grown in 100 ml of colonization factor antigen broth at 37°C in static, aerated cultures for 24 h. The culture was spun down (3000 *g*, 20 min, 20°C) and resuspended in 15 ml of phosphate-buffered saline. The suspension was then incubated at 60°C for 30 min. After the suspension was allowed to cool to room temperature, it was spun down (3000 *g*, 20 min, 20°C) to sediment bacterial cells and cellular debris. The supernatant was collected, and the protein concentration was determined by the bicinchoninic acid method using bovine serum albumin (BSA) as the standard protein. The bicinchoninic acid assay kit was obtained from Pierce Chemical Company (Rockford, IL). The supernatant was then lyophilized and stored at –20°C. The 14-kDa fimbrial protein expressed by strain 9 was purified to homogeneity according to the procedure described by Feutrier et al. (1986), and LPS from the same strain was isolated using the method described by Konrad et al. (1994).

SDS-PAGE Analysis of Bacterial Proteins

Membrane-associated proteins, purified LPS, and purified 14-kDa fimbrial protein were analyzed according to the method of Laemmli (1970). A 16×14 vertical slab gel consisting of 4.5% stacking gel and 15% separation gel was used. The protein preparations were electrophoresed at 200 V for 2 h, and the separated protein bands were stained using 0.025% Coomassie brilliant blue. The molecular weight of the fimbrial proteins was estimated by plotting a standard curve based on migration distances of the marker proteins (Chart, 1994).

Experimental Infection of Laying Hens with *Salmonella* Enteritidis

Three *S*. Enteritidis strains designated numbers 9, 21, and 30 were used in this study. They were serotyped and phage typed at the National Veterinary Service Laboratories (Ames, IA). They belong to the PT8 group but demonstrated different patterns of attachment to chicken ovarian granulosa cells. Strain 9 exhibited mannose-resistant local attachment, whereas strain 30 exhibited mannose-sensitive local attachment. Strain 21 demonstrated mannose-resistant diffuse attachment on granulosa cells. Adult laying hens were randomly allotted to three treatment groups (35 hens per group). Each group received a single strain of *S*. Enteritidis by oral inoculation. For inoculation of hens, these strains were grown in brain-heart infusion broth in static, aerated cultures at 37°C. The inoculum (1×10^8 colony-forming units per hen) was introduced orally into the crop by using a tuberculin syringe fitted with a curved, bulbed 10-cm needle (Lindell et al., 1994). Five randomly selected hens from each group were killed at weekly intervals by placing them in a CO_2 chamber followed by cervical dislocation.

Collection of Specimens for Bacteriological Examination

ORGANS
Cecum, oviduct, and ovaries were removed aseptically and placed in separate, sterile, plastic bags. Similarly, portions of liver (5 g) and whole spleen were collected in a single bag. Tetrathionate broth (50 ml) was added to the plastic bags, and the contents were homogenized using a laboratory blender (Stomacher 400; Tekmar, Cincinnati, OH). After incubation at 37°C for 18–24 h, a loopful of the contents was streaked on to xylose-lysine-tergitol 4 agar plates (Miller and Tate, 1991). The plates were incubated for 24–48 h at 37°C. Black colonies (indicative of salmonellae) were picked and transferred to triple-sugar iron agar slants, and the colonies were identified by using standard serological and biochemical tests (Edwards and Ewing, 1986).

EGGS
Eggs were collected daily, and the shell surface was sanitized immediately using Betadine (povidone-iodine) (Purdue Fredrick, Norwalk, CT) diluted 1:3 with 70% ethanol. The eggs were cracked open, and the egg contents were collected in sterile, plastic bags and cultured for isolation of *S.* Enteritidis as described for organs.

FECES
A disposable tray was kept beneath each cage for the collection of feces. At the end of each week, fecal material was mixed and 5 g was transferred to a sterile, plastic bag. The trays were discarded every week after sample collection. Tetrathionate broth (50 ml) was added to each bag, and the contents were mixed well, incubated at 37°C for 24 h, and streaked on to xylose-lysine-tergitol 4 plates as just described.

Measurement of Serum Immune Response against *Salmonella* Enteritidis

Blood was collected by brachial vein puncture at weekly intervals and by cardiac puncture before the hens were killed. Sera were tested for *S.* Enteritidis LPS-specific antibodies by using an indirect ELISA (Cooper et al., 1989).

Immunoblot of Membrane-Associated Proteins

Immunoblot to identify the components involved in the immune response to *S.* Enteritidis was performed essentially as described previously (Towbin, 1984). The membrane-associated proteins along with a 14-kDa fimbrial protein

and the LPS obtained from strain 9 were electrophoresed and used in an immunoblot. Prestained molecular-weight marker proteins ranging in size from 14.3 to 97.4 kDa were included in the electrophoretic run. A blot sandwich was prepared by placing the gel on a blotting paper soaked with transfer buffer (165 mM Tris and 20% methanol). The equilibrated nitrocellulose membrane was then carefully placed on top of the gel, taking care to avoid any air bubbles between the gel and the membrane. The membrane was then covered by another blotting paper soaked with transfer buffer, and the blot sandwich was placed between two sponges presoaked in transfer buffer. The whole transfer blot was then placed in a transfer tank with the membrane at the anode. Electrophoresed proteins were transferred electrically (100 V for 45 min). After transfer, the nitrocellulose membrane was removed from the blot sandwich and 3% BSA was used to block unoccupied sites. This was accomplished by incubating the membrane along with 3% BSA in a shaker at room temperature for 30 min. The blocking solution was replaced with 0.03% BSA solution to which was added 90 ml of antiserum obtained from one of the hens inoculated with strain 9. The antiserum was allowed to react for 2 h at room temperature. After washing the membrane three times with phosphate-buffered saline, fresh BSA solution (0.03%) was applied on the blot. Secondary antibody in the form of anti-chicken IgG raised in rabbit conjugated with horseradish peroxidase was added at a final concentration of 1:10,000. The incubation was continued for 1 h at room temperature. Positive reaction was identified by applying a color development solution containing diaminobenzidine and hydrogen peroxide per the manufacturer's recommendations.

Immunogold Electron Microscopy

Immunogold electron microscopy of bacteria was conducted to reveal the presence of the fimbrial protein (14 kDa) on the outer surface of *S.* Enteritidis following the method of Van Tuinen and Riezman (1987) using monoclonal antibody against fimbrial protein (14 kDa), which was a generous gift from Dr. C.J. Thorns (Central Veterinary Laboratory, New Haw, Addleston, Surrey, U.K.) (Thorns et al., 1992).

Statistical Analysis

Differences between proportions of hens with positive *S.* Enteritidis isolation were compared using 2×2 contingency tables or Fisher's exact tests (SAS Institute, 1989).

RESULTS

SDS-PAGE Analysis of Membrane-Associated Proteins Isolated from *Salmonella* Enteritidis Strains

Membrane-associated proteins extracted from the three strains of *S.* Enteritidis were analyzed using SDS-PAGE. The analysis revealed a 14-kDa structure in the case of strain 9 and a 21-kDa structure in the case of strain 30. No protein bands indicative of fimbriae were seen on SDS-PAGE separation of heat-extracted proteins obtained from strain 21 (Fig. 24.1).

Isolation of *Salmonella* Enteritidis from Various Organs of Experimentally Inoculated Hens

Hens inoculated with *S.* Enteritidis were killed at weekly intervals, and the visceral organs were collected for bacteriological examination. The results are shown in Table 24.1. *Salmonella* Enteritidis was isolated from all of the organs tested, indicating that the isolates used in this study are invasive. Because of the absence of a clear trend in terms of positive organ isolation between weeks, comparisons were made based on total number of positive isolations over the 10-week period. The number of hens positive for cecal colonization in the group inoculated with strain 21 was significantly lower than that of the group inoculated with strain 9 ($p < 0.05$) (Table 24.1). The isolation of *S.* Enteritidis

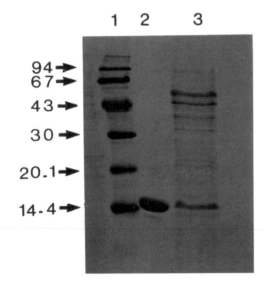

FIGURE 24.1 SDS-PAGE analysis of fimbrial proteins heat extracted from three strains of *Salmonella* Enteritidis that demonstrated different patterns of attachment to chicken ovarian granulosa cells: lane 1, molecular-weight markers [phosphorylase b (94,000), albumin (67,000), ovalbumin (43,000), carbonic anhydrase (30,000), trypsin inhibitor (20,100), and α-lactalbumin (14,400)]; and lanes 2–4, membrane-associated proteins obtained from *S.* Enteritidis strains 9, 21, and 30, respectively, *Arrows* show 14-kDa fimbrial protein and 21-kDa fimbrial protein. From Thiagarajan et al. (1996).

from the reproductive organs and the reticuloendothelial organs did not differ between the groups.

Isolation of *Salmonella* Enteritidis from Fecal Samples and Egg Contents

The frequency of *S.* Enteritidis isolation from fecal samples showed a steady decline with progression of time (Table 24.2). At the end of week 1, a significantly lower proportion of hens in the group inoculated with *S.* Enteritidis strain 21 were responsible for fecal shedding than were the groups inoculated with strain 9 ($p < 0.05$) and strain 30 ($p < 0.05$). Hens inoculated with strain 30 showed a remarkable decline in fecal shedding at the end of week 2. However, one hen in this group was found to excrete the organism until the end of week 4 (Table 24.2).

Eggs were collected daily, and egg contents were examined for the presence of *S.* Enteritidis. Since the objective was to estimate the number of eggs that were contaminated in vivo, the shell surface was sanitized immediately upon collection of eggs. Although the frequency of *S.* Enteritidis-contaminated eggs was sporadic, except for one instance, all positive isolations occurred during weeks 2 and 3 after inoculation (data not shown). No correlation was evident with regard to the type of strain used for inoculation and the number of hens that laid contaminated eggs (Table 24.2).

Serum Immune Responses against *Salmonella* Enteritidis

The LPS-specific antibody levels in hens of all three groups increased at the end of week 2. However, differences were apparent between the experimental groups during the following weeks. The differences between the antibody levels were compared using an F test, and the results are presented in Table 24.3. The serum IgG level of hens inoculated with strain 21 was lower than those of the other two groups at the end of 3 weeks after inoculation ($F = 6.52$ and 9.02, and $p = 0.04$ and 0.02, when compared with groups inoculated with strains 9 and 30, respectively). However, differences were not significant at the end of 5 and 7 weeks after inoculation (Table 24.3). At the end of 9 weeks, serum antibody levels rose again in the groups inoculated with strains 9 and 30 but not in the group inoculated with strain 21.

Immunoblot of Membrane-Associated Proteins

Outer-membrane structures obtained from *S.* Enteritidis strain 9 and the antiserum collected from a hen inoculated with strain 9 were used. The antiserum recognized the major membrane-associated proteins, the 14-kDa fimbrial protein, and the LPS isolated from *S.* Enteritidis strain 9 (Fig. 24.2).

Immunogold Microscopy of *Salmonella* Enteritidis Strains

The distribution of fimbrial protein (14 kDa) on the surface of *S.* Enteritidis strain 9 is depicted in Figure 24.3.

TABLE 24.1   Isolation of *Salmonella* Enteritidis from the internal organs of laying hens orally inoculated with three different strains (1 x 10⁸ CFU per hen).

S. Enteritidis strain no.	Liver and spleen	Ceca	Reproductive organs
	No. positive/no. tested (% positive)[a]		
9	10/35 (28.6)*	8/35 (22.9)*	10/35 (28.6)*
21	5/35 (14.3)*	2/35 (5.7)†	6/35 (17.1)*
30	8/35 (22.9)*	6/35 (17.1)*	7/35 (20)*

[a]Numbers with different symbols (*, †) in the same column are significantly different (p < 0.05).

TABLE 24.2   Fecal shedding and laying of contaminated eggs by hens orally inoculated with three *Salmonella* Enteritidis strains (1 x 10⁸ CFU per hen)

S. Enteritidis strain no.	Fecal shedding week after inoculation				Total number of hens that laid contaminated eggs (%)[a]
	1	2	3	4–10	
	No. of hens positive (%)				
9	22 (62.9)[a]	4 (13.3)	0 (0)	0 (0)	3 (8.6)
21	6 (17.1)[a]	2 (6.6)	0 (0)	0 (0)	4 (11.4)
30	13 (37.1)[a]	1 (3.3)	1 (4)	1 (5)	4 (11.4)

[a]Numbers with different symbols in the same column are significantly different (p < 0.05).

TABLE 24.3   Comparison between geometrical mean serum antibody titers of hens orally inoculated with three different *Salmonella* Enteritidis strains[a] and followed for 10 weeks after inoculation: mean titers of hens inoculated with strain 21 were compared with titers of hens inoculated with strain 9 (column 2) and strain 30 (column 3)

Strain 21	Strain 9		Strain 30	
Time (week) after inoculation	F[a]	p (one-tailed)	F[a]	p (one-tailed)
1	1.11	0.46	2.49	0.19
2	2.20	0.23	1.00	0.49
3	6.52	0.04	9.02	0.02
5	2.41	0.20	5.54	0.06
7	1.91	0.27	2.03	0.25
9	385.60	0.00002	85.92	0.0003
10	4.85	0.077	1.72	0.31

[a]Mean titers were compared using an F test.

Fimbriae are clearly expressed as a fussy surface structure that was amplified by the immunogold technique.

DISCUSSION

Food poisoning caused by *S.* Enteritidis is a major concern for the poultry industry. To formulate efficient control and prevention measures, a clear understanding of the disease process in poultry is necessary. *Salmonella* Enteritidis isolates have been traditionally classified based on two major characteristics: susceptibility to phages and plasmid profiles. As a result, studies on the pathogenesis and virulence of the organism have largely depended on comparing isolates of various phage types (Hinton et al., 1990a; Barrow, 1991; Gast and Beard, 1991) and plasmid carriage (Chart, et al., 1989, 1991). However, studies have shown that strains within the same phage type may differ in their ability to invade internal organs of chickens (Hinton et al., 1990b). These studies have also shown that virulence was not associated with possession of a 38-MDa plasmid. Similarly, Halavatkar and Barrow (1993) have reported that although the presence of a 54-kb plasmid is essential for virulence of PT4 in mice, it is not necessary in young chickens and laying

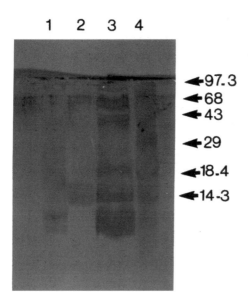

FIGURE 24.2 Immunoblot of outer-membrane structures obtained from *Salmonella* Enteritidis strain 9: lane 1, prestained molecular-weight marker proteins; lane 2, lipopolysaccharide; lane 3, membrane-associated proteins extracted by incubation of bacterial cells at 60°C for 30 min; and lane 4, 14-kDa fimbrial protein. Numbers on the right indicate the molecular weights. The procedures are as described in Materials and Methods. From Thiagarajan et al. (1996).

hens. Thus, virulence properties of *S.* Enteritidis that determine the dissemination of the organism from the intestines to the ovaries and subsequent contamination of the egg have not been addressed.

Members of the family Enterobacteriaceae, such as *Escherichia coli* and *S.* Enteritidis, express fimbriae on their surface that mediate the attachment of cultured mammalian cells (Mett et al., 1983; Baloda et al., 1988; Aslanzadeh and Paulissen, 1992). The relevance of fimbrial expression in the pathogenesis of *S.* Enteritidis infection in chickens has not been examined so far. In this study, three *S.* Enteritidis PT8 strains that differ in their fimbrial expression were used for experimental infection of adult laying hens. All of the strains used in this study belonged to PT8. They were also similar in their plasmid profiles: strains 9 and 21 carried a 62-kb plasmid, and strain 30 carried a 68-kb plasmid (A.M. Saeed, unpublished data). These strains were compared based on organ invasion, fecal shedding, and ability to elicit serum immune responses in laying hens after oral inoculation.

Comparison between the three PT8 strains (PT9, PT21, and PT30) revealed that the frequency of isolation of *S.* Enteritidis from ceca of hens inoculated with strain 21 was lower than that of the other two groups. A similar trend was observed in fecal shedding of *S.* Enteritidis during the first weeks after inoculation. Taken together, these observations

suggest that strain 21 could not effectively colonize the intestinal tract. This inability could be due to the absence of surface structures that mediate specific, successful attachment. Alternatively, it could also be due to the inability of the organism to survive the intestinal environment of the host. The normal resident microbial flora that competes for nutrients in the intestinal tract might be a contributing factor.

An important consideration in this infectivity trial was isolation of *S.* Enteritidis from the reproductive tract and egg contents after oral inoculation. Of interest was the difference, if any, between the three strains of *S.* Enteritidis in terms of ovarian colonization and laying of contaminated eggs. The results of the study did not reveal a correlation between fimbrial expression and the proportions of hens that were positive for *S.* Enteritidis isolation from the reproductive organs. Similarly, no differences were apparent in terms of laying of contaminated eggs between the three groups of hens. The incidence of contaminated eggs was sporadic and was usually observed in weeks 2 and 3 after inoculation. One possible explanation could be that, following oral inoculation, a small number of organisms may penetrate the intestinal mucous membrane, leading to seeding of various internal organs without successful cecal colonization. However, it is not clear whether such an invasion would occur under natural conditions where the density of the inoculum may not be as high as was used in this study. Persistent, intestinal colonization by *S.* Enteritidis was not found to be a prerequisite for laying of contaminated eggs (Gast and Beard, 1990a). In addition, experimental infection of 300 laying hens with *S.* Enteritidis showed that laying of contaminated eggs was independent of the frequency and duration of positive isolation from the internal organs (Saeed et al., chapter 23 in this book). The fact that *S.* Enteritidis strain 21 used in this study was isolated from the reproductive organs at a similar frequency as the other two strains in the absence of effective cecal colonization supports these observations.

Comparison of hens inoculated with strain 21 showed that they mounted a strong antibody response at the end of week 2. During the following weeks, the antibody titer dropped to a lower level. In contrast, antibody titers of hens inoculated with strains 9 and 30 remained higher at the end of week 3 after inoculation (Table 24.3). The isolation of *S.* Enteritidis from the liver and spleen, which are components of the reticuloendothelial system, was similar, indicating that the immune system might have been primed in all three groups of hens. Since strain 21 was unable to colonize ceca successfully, constant antigenic stimulation from the intestinal tract might not have been present in this group. In contrast, successful cecal colonization in a larger number of hens inoculated with strains 9 and 30 would lead to a strong immune response. At the end of 9 weeks, antibody titers rose again in these two groups but not in the strain-21 group. This seems to suggest that restimulation of the immune system might have occurred in the hens inoculated with *S.* Enteritidis strains 9 and 30 but not in the group inoculated with strain 21. This restimulation could have occurred because of multiplication of the organism in the gut after stress or been due to the decline

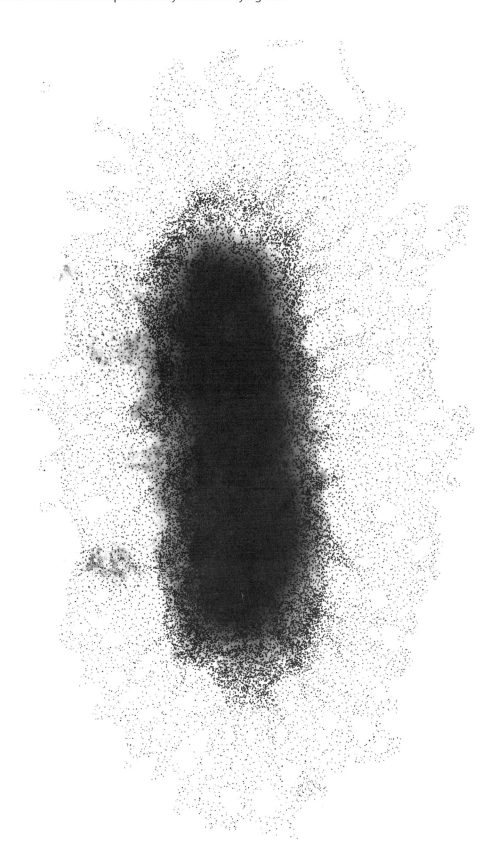

FIGURE 24.3 Transmission electron micrograph (×50,000) shows *Salmonella* Enteritidis phage type 8 (strain 9) immunogold-labeled by using monoclonal antibody as described in Materials and Methods.

of the systemic and local immune responses. This phenomenon during experimental infection of the chickens has been described previously (Lindell et al., 1994).

Immunoblot using antiserum obtained from a single hen revealed that the humoral immune response against *S.* Enteritidis oral infection consisted of antibodies against the LPS, the membrane-associated proteins, and the 14-kDa fimbrial protein expressed by strain 9. Commercial *S.* Enteritidis LPS was used as the antigen in the ELISA described in this study. The results of the immunoblot reiterate the presence of antibodies against LPS. The antiserum used in the immunoblot was collected 9 weeks after oral inoculation of hens. Thus, the humoral immune response elicited by live *S.* Enteritidis organisms administered orally appears to last for a long time. The LPS-specific antibodies were present in the serum of inoculated hens until the end of the infectivity trial. A similar observation was made by Humphrey et al. (1991) in the case of specific pathogen–free (SPF) hens inoculated with *S.* Enteritidis. The outer-membrane proteins including fimbriae may be relevant in immune response against *S.* Enteritidis. Peralta et al. (1994) have reported that immunization of hens with the 14-kDa fimbrial protein results in egg-yolk antibodies against the protein. These antibodies were effective in inhibiting the attachment of *S.* Enteritidis to mouse intestinal epithelial cells (Peralta et al., 1994). The protective role of this fimbrial protein against *S.* Enteritidis infection needs to be examined in chickens.

We cloned the gene that encodes for the fimbrial protein (14 kDa), using a PTX101 vector (Francisco et al., 1992), into an *E. coli*. Expression of this cloned gene resulted in the conversion of the nonattaching *E. coli* into a transformant strain that expressed a similar attachment pattern as *S.* Enteritidis PT9 (donor of a 14-kDa gene) on HEP-2 cells (Rank, 1996).

The results presented in this study indicate a role for fimbriae in the pathogenesis of and immune response to *S.* Enteritidis infection in chickens. No correlation was evident between the expression of particular type of fimbrial protein and ovarian colonization leading to laying of contaminated eggs, suggesting that invasiveness may be mediated by a different set of salmonella virulence attributes. However, fimbrial proteins may be necessary in cecal colonization and subsequent elicitation of a strong immune response. This was suggested by the fact that fimbriae may mediate the attachment of *S.* Enteritidis to the target tissue, such as cecal tonsils (Thorns et al., 1996). The fimbriae may also be relevant in environmental contamination because *S.* Enteritidis isolates endowed with a particular type of fimbriae may be able to colonize the ceca longer, leading to persistent fecal shedding.

REFERENCES

Aslanzadeh, J., and Paulissen, L.J. 1992. Role of type 1 and type 3 fimbriae on the adherence and pathogenesis of *Salmonella enteritidis* in mice. Microbiol. Immunol. 36:351–359.

Baloda, S.B. 1988. Characterization of fibronectin binding to *Salmonella enteritidis* strain 27655R. FEMS Microbiol. Lett. 49:483–488.

Baloda, S.B., Faris, A., and Krovacek, K. 1988. Cell surface properties of enterotoxigenic and cytotoxic *Salmonella enteritidis* and *Salmonella typhimurium*: studies on hemagglutination, cell-surface hydrophobicity, attachment to human intestinal cells and fibronectin binding. Microbiol. Immunol. 32:447–459.

Barrow, P.A. 1991. Experimental infection of chickens with *Salmonella enteritidis*. Avian Pathol. 20:145–153.

Barrow, P.A., and Lovell, M.A. 1991. Experimental infection of egg laying hens with *Salmonella enteritidis* phage type 4. Avian Pathol. 20:335–348.

Bygrave, A.C., and Gallagher, J. 1989. Transmission of *Salmonella enteritidis* in poultry. Vet. Rec. 125:571.

Centers for Disease Control. 1988. Update: *Salmonella enteritidis* infections and grade A shell eggs—United States. MMWR 37:490–496.

Centers for Disease Control. 1990. Update: *Salmonella enteritidis* infections and shell eggs in the United States. MMWR 39:909–912.

Chart, H. 1994. Sodium dodecyl sulfate–polyacrylamide gel electrophoresis for separation and resolution of bacterial components. In: Chart, H., ed. Methods in practical laboratory bacteriology. Boca Raton, FL: CRC, pp. 21–33.

Chart, H., Threlfall, E.J., and Rowe B. 1989. Virulence of *Salmonella enteritidis* phage type 4 is related to the possession of a 38 Mda plasmid. FEMS Microbiol. Lett. 58:299–304.

Chart, H., Threlfall, E.J., and Rowe, B. 1991. Virulence studies of *Salmonella enteritidis* phage types. Lett. Appl. Microbiol. 12:188–191.

Cooper, G.L., Nicholas, R.A., and Bracewell, C.D. 1989. Serological and bacteriological investigations of chickens from flocks naturally infected with *Salmonella enteritidis*. Vet. Rec. 125:567–572.

Cowden, J.M., Chishom, D., O'Mahoney, M., Lynch, D., Mawer, S.L., Spain, G.E., Ward, L., and Rowe, B. 1989a. Two outbreaks of *Salmonella enteritidis* phage type 4 infection associated with the consumption of fresh shell-egg products. Epidemiol. Infect. 103:47–52.

Cowden, J.M., Lynch, D., Joseph, C.A., O'Mahoney, M., Mawer, S.L., Rowe, B., and Bartlett, C.L.R. 1989b. Case-control study of infections with *Salmonella enteritidis* phage type 4 in England. BMJ 299:771–773.

Coyle, E.F., Ribiero, C.D., Howard, A.J., Palmer, S.R., Jones, H.I., Ward, L., and Rowe, B. 1988. *Salmonella enteritidis* phage type 4 infection: association with hens' eggs. Lancet 2:1295–1297.

Duguid, J.P., Anderson, E.S., and Campbell, I. 1966. Fimbriae and adhesive properties in salmonellae. J. Pathol. Bacteriol. 92:107–138.

Edwards, P.R., and Ewing, W.H. 1986. Identification of Enterobacteriaceae, 4th ed. New York: Elsevier Science.

Feutrier, J., Kay, W.W., and Trust, T.J. 1986. Purification and characterization of fimbriae from *Salmonella enteritidis*. J. Bacteriol. 168:221–227.

Finlay, B.B., and Falkow, S. 1989. Common themes in microbial pathogenicity. Microbiol. Rev. 53:210–230.

Francisco, J.A., Eahart, C.F., and Georgiou, G. 1992. Transport and anchoring of β-lactamase to the external surface of *Escherichia coli*. Proc. Natl. Acad. Sci. USA 89:2713–2717.

Gast, R.K., and Beard, C.W. 1990a. Production of *Salmonella enteritidis* contaminated eggs by experimentally infected hens. Avian Dis. 34:438–446.

Gast, R.K., and Beard, C.W. 1990b. Isolation of *Salmonella enteritidis* from internal organs of experimentally infected hens. Avian Dis. 34:991–993.

Gast, R.K., and Beard, C.W. 1991. Evaluation of a chick mortality model for predicting the consequences of *Salmonella enteritidis* infection in laying hens. Poult. Sci. 71:281–287.

Halavatkar, H., and Barrow, P.A. 1993. The role of a 54-kb plasmid in the virulence of strains of *Salmonella enteritidis* of phage type 4 for chickens and mice. J. Med. Microbiol. 38:171–176.

Hedberg, C.W., David, J.J., White, K.E., MacDonald, K.L., and Osterholm, M.T. 1993. Role of egg consumption in sporadic *S. enteritidis* and *S. typhimurium* infection in Minnesota. J. Infect. Dis. 176:107–111.

Hinton, M., Threlfall, E.J., and Rowe, B. 1990a. The invasive potential of *Salmonella enteritidis* phage types for young chickens. Lett. Appl. Microbiol. 10:237–239.

Hinton, M., Threlfall, E.J., and Rowe, B. 1990b. The invasiveness of different strains of *Salmonella enteritidis* phage type 4 for young chickens. FEMS Microbiol. Lett. 70:193–196.

Hopper, S.A., and Mawer, S. 1988. *Salmonella enteritidis* in a commercial layer flock. Vet. Rec. 123:351.

Konrad, H., Smith, B.P., Dilling, G.W., and House, J.K. 1994. Production of *Salmonella* serogroup D(O9)-specific enzyme-linked immunosorbent assay antigen. Am. J. Vet. Res. 55:1647–1651.

Laemmli, U.K. 1970. Cleavage of structural protein during the assembly of the head of bacteriophage T4. Nature 227:680–685.

Lin, F.-Y.C., Morris, J.G., Jr., Trump, D., Tilghman, D., Wood, P.K., Jackman, N., Israel, E., and Libonati, J.P. 1988. Investigation of an outbreak of *Salmonella enteritidis* gastroenteritis associated with consumption of eggs in a restaurant chain in Maryland. Am. J. Epidemiol. 128:839–844.

Lindell, K.A., Saeed, A.M., and McCabe, G.P. 1994. Evaluation of resistance of four strains of commercial laying hens to experimental infection with *Salmonella enteritidis* phage type eight. Poult. Sci. 73:757–762.

Lister, S.A. 1988. *Salmonella enteritidis* infection in broilers and broiler breeders. Vet. Rec. 123:350.

Mett, H., Kloetzlen, L., and Vosbeck, K. 1983. Properties of pili from *Escherichia coli* SS142 that mediate mannose-resistant adhesion to mammalian cells. J. Bacteriol. 153:1038–1044.

Miller, R.G., and Tate, C.R. 1991. Xylose-lysine-tergitol 4: an improved selective agar medium for the isolation of *Salmonella*. Poult. Sci. 70:2429–2432.

Muller, K.H., Collinson, S.K., Trust, T.J., and Kay, W.W. 1991. Type 1 fimbriae of *Salmonella enteritidis*. J. Bacteriol. 173:4765–4772.

Peralta, R.C., Yokoyama, H., Ikemori, Y., Kuroki, M., and Kodoma, Y. 1994. Passive immunisation against experimental salmonellosis in mice by orally administered hen egg-yolk antibodies specific for 14-kD fimbriae of *Salmonella enteritidis*. J. Med. Microbiol. 41:29–35.

Rank, D.L. 1996. Development of a potential genetically-engineered oral subunit vaccine against *Salmonella enteritidis* in poultry (Master thesis). West Lafayette, IN: Purdue University.

SAS Institute, 1989. SAS/STAT® user's guide, version 6, 4th ed., vols. 1 and 2. Cary, NC: SAS Institute.

Shivaprasad, H.L., Timoney, J.F., Morales, S., Lucio, B., and Baker, R.C. 1990. Pathogenesis of *Salmonella enteritidis* infection in laying chickens. I. Studies on egg transmission, clinical signs, fecal shedding, and serologic responses. Avian Dis. 34:548–557.

St. Louis, M.E., Morse, D.L., Potter, M.E., DeMelfi, T.M., Guzewich, J.J., Tauxe, R.V., and Blake, P.A. 1988. The emergence of grade A eggs as a major source of *Salmonella enteritidis* infections: new implications for the control of salmonellosis. JAMA 259:2103–2107.

Thiagarajan, D., Saeed, A.M., and Asem, E.K. 1994. Mechanism of transovarian transmission of *Salmonella enteritidis* in laying hens. Poult. Sci. 73:89–98.

Thorns, C.J., Sojka, M.G., McLaren, I.M., and Dibb-Fuller, M. 1992. Characterization of monoclonal antibodies against a fimbrial structure of *Salmonella enteritidis* and certain other serogroup D salmonellae and their application as serotyping reagents. Res. Vet. Sci. 53:300–308.

Thorns, C.J., Turcitte, C., Gemmell, C.G., and Woodward, M.J. 1996. Studies into the role of the SEF14 fimbrial antigen in the pathogenesis of *Salmonella enteritidis* Microb. Pathog. 20:235–246.

Timoney, J.F., Shivaprasad, H.L., Baker, R.C., and Rowe, B. 1989. Egg transmission after infection of hens with *Salmonella enteritidis* phage type IV. Vet. Rec. 125:600–601.

Towbin, H., Staehelin, T., and Gordon, J. 1984. Electrophoretic transfer of proteins from polyacrylamide gels to nitrocellulose sheets: procedure and applications. Proc. Natl. Acad. Sci. USA 76:4350–4354.

Van Tuinen, E., and Riezman, H. 1987. Immunolocalization of glyceraldehyde-3-phosphate dehydrogenase, hexokinase, and carboxypeptidase Y in yeast cells at the ultrastructural level. J. Histochem. Cytochem. 35:327–333.

Part IV
Prevention and Control

Introduction: *Salmonella enterica* Serovar Enteritidis Current Status and a Recommendation for Its Prevention and Control

J. Mason

In its May 16, 1996, issue, the *New England Journal of Medicine* published a report on "A National Outbreak of *Salmonella* Enteritidis (*S.* Enteritidis) Infections from Ice Cream": the outbreak was estimated to have caused up to 224,000 cases of illness in persons who used a nationally distributed brand of ice cream in the fall of 1994. There has been a slow decline in *S.* Enteritidis outbreaks from a high of 77 in 1989, to 70 in 1990, 68 in 1991, 59 in 1992, 63 in 1993, 44 in 1994, 56 in 1995, and 49 in 1996. Unfortunately, the *S.* Enteritidis case incidence has not shown a similar downward trend and, in fact, is now rising. Some 10,091 cases were recorded in 1994, from a low of some 6500 in 1992, and the total for 1995 was 10,201. *Salmonella* Enteritidis was the leading human *Salmonella* serovar in 1995, with 25% of all *Salmonella* isolates, surpassing *Salmonella* Typhimurium, the usual leader, with 24%.

As many will recall, human *S.* Enteritidis cases in the United States began to rise in the late 1970s, and more sharply in the mid-1980s, particularly in the Northeastern and Middle Atlantic states. This increase turned out to be part of a pandemic, with similar, almost simultaneous increases around the world, and particularly in Great Britain and other European countries. To everyone's surprise, these increases were found to be associated with fresh eggs or egg-containing foods. Evidently some strains of *S.* Enteritidis had become more invasive in chickens, and eggs were being laid already infected with *S.* Enteritidis organisms.

The surge of *S.* Enteritidis cases and outbreaks in humans resulted in an emergency test and slaughter program in Great Britain in 1988, with compensation to the owners of *S.* Enteritidis–positive layer flocks. This program was discontinued a few years later, after millions of pounds had been spent and hundreds of thousands of birds destroyed. A less drastic program was started in the United States in 1990 to trace back from human *S.* Enteritidis outbreaks where eggs were implicated, to the flocks of origin, to test them for *S.* Enteritidis, and to divert the eggs from positive flocks to pasteurization plants. During the 6 years that this program was in operation, until its funds were cut off in 1996, some 334 *S.* Enteritidis outbreaks were reported, some 38 flocks were tested, and some 1.3 billion eggs were diverted to pasteurization.

Although there was some decrease in *S.* Enteritidis cases in 1992 and 1993, and some of this may have been due to the traceback program, it is more likely that control efforts by the egg producers themselves, perhaps stimulated by the fear of tracebacks to their flocks, were responsible. These efforts resulted finally in the formation of a number of organized preventive quality-assurance programs, such as the early one in Maine, started in 1989, followed by a more inclusive one in Pennsylvania in 1992, and, more recently, one in California. In addition, the United Egg Producers, which represents some 80% of the egg industry, is now promoting a national egg-quality-assurance program.

Unfortunately, liquid-egg and spent-hen surveys carried out by Animal and Plant Health Inspection Service and Food Safety Inspection Service in 1995, to compare with similar surveys in 1991, showed that *S.* Enteritidis was still widely distributed in egg-layer flocks, that the rates had not decreased, and that *S.* Enteritidis was even more prevalent in some areas than before. Even more disturbing was the news that phage type 4, an *S.* Enteritidis variant that had not been found previously in poultry in the United States but was the type mainly responsible for the rapid spread and increase in European countries, had been found in California and possibly other states.

In view of the current situation, with an increasing *S. Enteritidis* incidence in humans and evidence of fairly widespread distribution of *S. Enteritidis* in egg-layer flocks, and with no clearly defined federal government program, what should be done by egg producers themselves, by their associations, and by state and federal agencies?

There is now little likelihood that any federal agency will recommend a national program to test all layer flocks for *S. Enteritidis*, with either depopulation of the positive flocks or the diversion of their eggs to "breaker" plants. Such a program would be difficult to organize and carry out, would be very expensive, and would certainly bankrupt the egg industry. In addition, a testing program alone, without any parallel programs to prevent or eliminate *S. Enteritidis* in the flocks, would do little to solve the basic problems that maintain *S. Enteritidis* transmission.

Actually, the original U.S. Department of Agriculture (USDA) *S. Enteritidis* regulation, adopted in 1990 and amended in 1991, is still in effect but is not being enforced, because no funds have been allocated for this purpose by the fiscal year 1996 Congress. A few states that still consider *S. Enteritidis* a problem are trying to set up their own traceback programs. This will be difficult to coordinate without some national oversight, especially if the outbreaks and the suspected source flocks are in different states. Under the previous USDA *S. Enteritidis* Control Program, the epidemiological information was carefully reviewed to provide some assurances that the outbreak was really egg related, and then someone with some experience was detailed to carry out the egg trace in an effort to find a single source flock.

With the deferral of federal funding for the FSIS *S. Enteritidis* program, the FDA announced on July 5, 1996, that it would assume responsibility for the outbreak traceback program, since it continues to hold the regulatory authority for shell eggs involved in interstate commerce. However, the continuation of the outbreak traceback program by the FDA provides no great benefit in regard to *S. Enteritidis* prevention or control. Even if a source flock is found quickly, tested without delay, and, if positive, the eggs diverted to pasteurization plants, there may be little effect on the overall risk of exposure to *S. Enteritidis*. The eggs that would be diverted would more than likely be replaced in the shell-egg market by eggs from flocks that might be equally contaminated with *S. Enteritidis*. Based on the recent spent-hen survey results that up to 45% of the layer flocks in the United States may be positive for *S. Enteritidis*, with some regional differences, it is doubtful whether an outbreak traceback program alone could have much effect in reducing *S. Enteritidis* in layer flocks. So what can be done, short of destructive and costly government testing programs, or ineffective traceback programs, to lower the incidence of *S. Enteritidis* in humans? In addition to the obvious need to improve food-handling practices, what can be done by the producers themselves to lower the level of *S. Enteritidis* in their flocks? Based on the experience over the last 5 years of the Pennsylvania Egg Quality Assurance Program (PEQAP), I would recommend that a voluntary, preventive program, modeled after the

Pennsylvania program, be started and implemented wherever *S. Enteritidis* is considered a problem.

The elements of the Pennsylvania program are summarized below, and additional information can be provided on request. But why should this program be adopted by egg producers, when there is no governmental requirement for them to participate, and especially since *S. Enteritidis* does not actually cause any additional morbidity or mortality in their birds or even lower egg production? Should producers participate in this type of program, at their own expense, if they are not compelled to do so? One obvious benefit from a program of this kind is that it affords producers some protection from liability in case of an outbreak, on the basis of the legal principle that all reasonable and acceptable methods are being used to prevent *S. Enteritidis*. However, another more immediate cost benefit would result from the beneficial effects of the stringent programs of cleaning and disinfection, rodent control, and heightened biosecurity that are required, which should help to prevent or control poultry diseases other than *S. Enteritidis*.

The findings of the Pennsylvania *S. Enteritidis* Pilot Project, which was carried out in 1992 and 1993 and was the forerunner of the PEQAP, demonstrated that *S. Enteritidis* is difficult to eliminate once it is established in a henhouse. Following the PEQAP protocol diligently should reduce *S. Enteritidis* and possibly even eliminate it over time. However, what should be done in the short term to lower the risk of *S. Enteritidis* for egg consumers while *S. Enteritidis* in the birds is being eliminated in the long term? How can this type of program be affordable to producers, if the price of eggs sent to "breaker" plants usually is somewhat less than the price of shell eggs? Currently, some 25%–30% of all eggs produced in the United States are being sent to "breaker" plants. In the PEQAP, the participating producers can use open-ended contracts with pasteurization plants to shift their stocks of eggs around, and generally reserve the eggs from their positive flocks for pasteurization. This satisfies their commitments for "breaker" eggs and, at the same time, gives them the opportunity to provide "safer" table eggs, protect their market, and reduce considerably the risk that their eggs might be involved in an outbreak.

This type of marketing policy obviously favors large producers with many separate houses and premises, and the integrators, who contract to market eggs from many different producers. Although the Pennsylvania program is not readily adaptable to all situations, it does permit the larger producers or marketing groups to gain some commercial advantage by claiming that their eggs are "safer" and are produced under more sanitary conditions. However, these claims must be substantiated by some type of independent monitoring to confirm compliance with the control and testing protocols.

Undoubtedly, many individual producers are now carrying out their own *S. Enteritidis* control programs, which include many of the measures of the Pennsylvania program. At present, there are no nationally recognized standards for an acceptable egg-quality-assurance program. With the withdrawal of the USDA from its leadership role in the *S.* Enteritidis Control Program, it is uncertain that there will be any federal government efforts in this direction in the near future. Currently, the United States Animal Health Association (USAHA) is trying to supply this need and has set up an *S.* Enteritidis Committee, which has formulated recommendations for such standards, which include all "the recognized *S.* Enteritidis prevention and control measures, short of testing for *S.* Enteritidis or diversion of eggs from positive flocks." The committee's proposals have been approved by the USAHA Board of Trustees.

Any well-designed quality-assurance program, with independent monitoring for compliance, should reduce the *S.* Enteritidis burden in layer houses, in time, even if no testing for *S.* Enteritidis is carried out. However, *S.* Enteritidis is difficult to eliminate and, even with the best efforts, success may not be achieved for a number of years. Without some type of testing for *S. enteritidis,* at least in the environment, there would be no objective indication that the measures applied were effective. There would also be no effort to eliminate any infected eggs from the table-egg market until the program did succeed.

Egg producers in the United States are not now required legally to carry out any *S.* Enteritidis prevention or control programs. With the rising incidence of human *S.* Enteritidis cases, however, they should consider establishing their own voluntary programs, preferably modeled after the program now operating successfully in Pennsylvania. An agreement has just been adopted jointly by the Pennsylvania Departments of Agriculture and Health, and the Pennsylvania Poultry Federation, which covers the operation of this program and provides an excellent model for a hazard-analysis critical control point–type egg-quality-assurance program of this kind. Until more suitable national standards are adopted, this agreement can serve as a guide for anyone interested in starting a similar service.

25

Economic Consequences of *Salmonella enterica* Serovar Enteritidis Infection in Humans and the U.S. Egg Industry

R.A. Morales and R.M. McDowell

INTRODUCTION

In the United Kingdom, the economic impact of the 1988 events regarding the risks associated with shell-egg consumption effectively illustrates the influence of consumer food-safety perceptions on the economic health of a food-producing industry. A food scare initiated by a senior U.K. health official's comment linking salmonellosis with eggs immediately resulted in a 60% decline in table-egg consumption. Until recently, egg consumption in the U.K. remained at 25% below prescare consumption levels (Kinderlerer, 1994). Such market impacts are not unique to the egg industry, and analogous food scares have occurred in other food-producing industries. Alar in apples in the United States, bovine spongiform encephalopathy in cattle in Europe, and, most recently, *Pfiesteria* in fish in Maryland have caused precipitous declines in demand for those foods. What is becoming increasingly clear is that food safety is a significant factor for market stability and that consumers are starting to perceive and perhaps even demand safety as a quality attribute of foods. An increasing demand for food safety ultimately affects not just individual consumers or producers but also market supply and demand and industry prices and quantities.

Several factors are propelling the economic analysis of food-safety problems beyond traditional farm-level approaches. Market effects can stem from a variety of sources other than the purely biological aspects of food-

borne pathogens. In the case of *Salmonella enterica* serovar Enteritidis (*S*. Enteritidis), these include but are not limited to media information, political considerations such as regulatory actions, corollary health concerns such as heart disease and cholesterol content in eggs, and cultural values. Although *S*. Enteritidis as an animal pathogen does not result in direct economic losses stemming from morbidity and mortality, nonetheless the biological factors promoting the *S*. Enteritidis pandemic in the 1980s and those presently encouraging the emergence of *S*. Enteritidis phage type 4 (PT4) will engender indirect economic effects. Industry response and regulatory action in response to this public health threat will ultimately determine the economic impacts. Although the term *emerging pathogen* is now part of the epidemiological lexicon, and *S*. Enteritidis is an excellent example of an emerging pathogen, there are unfortunately few studies to guide us toward a comprehensive analysis of the economic impact of this or other emerging foodborne pathogens.

The science of economics plays a critical role in the intelligent management of microbial foodborne hazards. Economics enlightens decision making by monetizing consequences of disease and their control, and providing guidelines for evaluating different animal and public health policy options, their cost effectiveness, and distributional effects among different groups. At a national level, economics has several roles. It aids in setting priorities for mitigation, that is, the hazards that should take priority in resource allocation decisions, both in total and at the margin. It provides guidance for determining the appropriate level of risk reduction. It also helps decision makers to devise policies that most efficiently achieve our desired safety goals (McDowell et al., 1995). Economics plays a number of other roles in the decision process. One vital role is that of "gatekeeper" in helping to prevent inefficient policies from being enacted (Antle, 1996). Another is in assisting food producers in understanding how food safety and public perception affect consumer demand for their products, and ultimately determining the economic health of their industry (Morales, 1997a). Economics also has the prescriptive role of specifying the most economically efficient way to achieve a given level of safety or maximize hazard reduction for a given outlay of resources.

In this chapter, we briefly trace the emergence of the worldwide S. Enteritidis pandemic and describe economic trends and statistics for the poultry industry, which has been the focus of the epidemic. Next, the economic impacts of S. Enteritidis on consumers and producers are addressed. Economic consequences of S. Enteritidis interventions are discussed in the context of alternative industry options for controlling S. Enteritidis. The importance of evaluating the potential effects of S. Enteritidis control programs on supply and demand, and on industry prices and quantities, is discussed. Finally, this chapter addresses the opportunities for marketing food safety as a product-quality attribute.

WORLDWIDE EMERGENCE OF *SALMONELLA* ENTERITIDIS AS A POULTRY PATHOGEN

Salmonella Enteritidis became an increasing problem in many parts of the world in the late 1970s, emerging as a major source of salmonellosis in Europe, North America, and South America by the mid-1980s (Rodrigue et al., 1990). The growth in S. Enteritidis foodborne illness, as indicated by its proportion of all salmonella isolates reported to public health organizations, illustrates both the explosive growth of S. Enteritidis as a human health problem and its considerable geographical variation. Between 1975 and 1987, the proportion of all salmonella isolates represented by S. Enteritidis doubled in the United States, tripled in several European countries, and increased by a factor of 275 in Argentina. The proportion of S. Enteritidis out of all salmonellae increased in 11 of 12 European countries, averaging a 3.3-fold increase (Rodrigue et al., 1990). The S. Enteritidis pandemic continued through the late 1980s, and S. Enteritidis incidence increased in two-thirds of the 35 countries reporting to the World Health Organization (Gomez et al., 1997). England and Wales were particularly affected, with S. Enteritidis comprising 6.3% of all salmonella isolates in 1979, increasing to 33% in 1985 and 57% in 1994 (Henson, 1995). Concurrently, S. Enteritidis PT4 rapidly emerged as the primary S. Enteritidis serovar in England and Wales, accounting for 75% of all S. Enteritidis isolated in 1994.

In the United States, S. Enteritidis comprised 25% of all salmonella isolates by 1995, compared with 5% in 1985 (Gomez et al., 1997). *Salmonella* Enteritidis isolates and the proportion of all salmonella isolates also increased in Europe and South America, and S. Enteritidis PT4 emerged. The spread of S. Enteritidis and S. Enteritidis PT4 geographically became the cause of an increasing number of human cases of salmonellosis and began to exact a considerable toll on public health (both in terms of surveillance costs and in human morbidity and mortality) and on the eggs and broilers as public confidence in the safety of eggs began to decline (Gomez et al., 1997).

For reasons not clearly understood, the emergence of S. Enteritidis in Canada has not been as marked as in the United States, South America, or Europe. By 1991, S. Enteritidis accounted for 12.5% of all salmonella isolates in Canada. A nationwide survey of S. Enteritidis in Canadian poultry flocks found that about 3% of broiler and layer flocks were infected with S. Enteritidis (Poppe, 1994). Similar surveys in the United States showed that nearly half of the egg-laying flocks in some regions were infected with S. Enteritidis (Ebel et al., 1992, 1993). The prevalence of S. Enteritidis–contaminated eggs from infected Canadian flocks was less than 0.06% (Poppe, 1994), about the same rate as reported for most U.S. flocks from which S. Enteritidis–positive eggs were isolated (Mason, 1994). Also, unlike Europe and a growing area of the United States, S. Enteritidis PT4 is rarely found in Canada. The striking differences between Canada and the United States, particularly the northeast regions, suggest that carefully designed and conducted epidemiological studies comparing egg-laying flocks in the two countries might shed considerable light on the explanatory variables that determine prevalence of S. Enteritidis among egg-laying flocks.

The emergence of S. Enteritidis in the 1980s as a significant public health problem and its relationship to the egg industry was manifested as a rise in foodborne outbreaks of S. Enteritidis traced to intact, grade-A shell eggs, a food vehicle formerly not associated with foodborne disease. In addition to foodborne outbreaks, S. Enteritidis isolates from human cases also began increasing both in absolute number as well as in proportion of all salmonella isolates. The increase in human cases and the geographical spread of S. Enteritidis in the United States can be tracked by the relative frequency of S. Enteritidis isolates in all salmonella isolates. In 1977, S. Enteritidis was comparatively insignificant with respect to other salmonella serovars; in only one state did S. Enteritidis represent more than 15% of all salmonella isolates (Fig. 25.1). By 1980, S. Enteritidis accounted for 15%–25% of all salmonella isolates in seven states and exceeded 25% in four states. Over the next decade, S. Enteritidis began emerging across the United States, comprising 1%–25% of all salmonella isolates in 16 states in 1990 and in 22 states in 1994 (Tauxe, 1997). Nationwide surveys of spent laying hens have demonstrated that S. Enteritidis has infected a substantial proportion of the U.S. laying flock in all regions of the country (Ebel et al., 1992, 1993; Hogue et al., 1997).

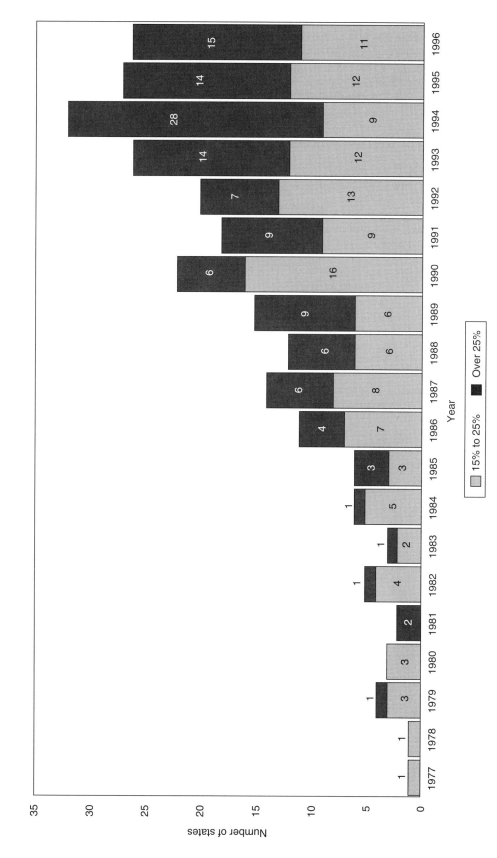

FIGURE 25.1 Total number of states with *Salmonella* Enteritidis constituting over 15% of all salmonella isolates, 1977–96.

The increasing trend was not just relative to all salmonella isolates. The rate of *S.* Enteritidis isolates reported per 100,000 population began increasing in the northeastern United States in the 1970s, doubling between 1975 and 1980 and again between 1980 and 1985, and increasing by 20% between 1985 and 1995. The 1995 rate per 100,000 population in the northeast was five times the rate in 1970 (Table 25.1). This trend was repeated in other regions of the country: rates in the mid-Atlantic region increased six-fold between 1980 and 1985, and isolates quadrupled in the Pacific region between 1985 and 1995. Overall, total isolation rates in the United States increased from one to four per 100,000 between 1970 and 1995.

More recent trends suggest that the number of *S.* Enteritidis outbreaks and associated deaths have decreased, a trend that may in part be attributable to the adoption of the recommendations of the Centers for Disease Control and Prevention (CDC) regarding proper egg handling and preparation as well as increased use of pasteurized egg products in nursing homes and hospitals (Table 25.2). However, while outbreak-related cases have declined, *S.* Enteritidis isolation rates have trended upward since 1985, suggesting that the number of sporadic cases increased. *Salmonella* Enteritidis has emerged from its former position as a minor foodborne pathogen and currently represents about 25% of all salmonella foodborne infections in humans in the United States. Moreover, with the emer-

gence of *S.* Enteritidis PT4 in the western United States, the disease patterns for *S.* Enteritidis in the United States are becoming reminiscent of those in the U.K. *S.* Enteritidis epidemic affecting both layer and broiler industries in that country.

Relatively early in the pandemic, shell eggs were epidemiologically identified as the most frequently associated food vehicle in *S.* Enteritidis outbreaks (St. Louis et al., 1988). In 1990, the U.S. Department of Agriculture (USDA) instituted two new programs to control *S.* Enteritidis in egg-laying operations. First, a voluntary *S.* Enteritidis testing program for breeder flocks was begun to eliminate vertical transmission to laying hens and, subsequently, their environments. Second, a traceback program to identify flocks implicated in human foodborne outbreaks of salmonellosis was initiated. Under this traceback program, if *S.* Enteritidis was detected at the farm of origin of the implicated eggs, then eggs from that flock could not be sold as shell eggs. Producers with *S.* Enteritidis test-positive flocks had two available options. They could depopulate flocks early, clean and disinfect premises, and then restock with *S.* Enteritidis–negative pullets or, alternatively, keep the infected flock but divert eggs for the remaining life of the flock to the breaking-egg market for subsequent sale as pasteurized egg products. During the first 2 years of the USDA traceback program, 19 of 25 laying flocks involved in a traceback were restricted, resulting in the voluntary depopulation of 3.1 million birds and

TABLE 25.1 Incidence of *Salmonella* Enteritidis isolates in the United States per 100,000 population by region, 1970–95.

Year	Region				
	Mid-Atlantic	Northeast	Pacific	Other	U.S. total
1970	1	2	1	1	1
1975	1	2	1	1	1
1980	1	4	1	1	1
1985	6	8	1	1	2
1990	8	9	2	2	3
1995	5	10	4	2	4

TABLE 25.2 *Salmonella* Enteritidis outbreaks, cases, deaths, and isolates, 1985–96

Year	Outbreaks	Cases	Deaths	Isolates	
				Total	Proportion of all salmonellae (%)
1985	26	1159	1	5657	10
1986	47	1444	6	6036	14
1987	53	2511	15	7052	15
1988	42	995	11	7063	16
1989	77	2467	14	8766	20
1990	70	2327	3	8764	21
1991	68	2398	5	7755	19
1992	59	2438	4	6578	19
1993	53	2217	6	8071	22
1994	47	5498	2	9866	26
1995	57	1332	0	10,201	25
1996	51	1461	2	9566	23

the diversion of 1.2 billion eggs (1% of U.S. egg production per year of the traceback program) (Mason and Ebel, 1991).

In 1992, a voluntary cooperative effort (named the *S. Enteritidis* Pilot Project) between federal and state agencies, universities, and the poultry industry in Pennsylvania was initiated to identify on-farm management practices to reduce *S. Enteritidis*. In April 1994, the first of the quality-assurance programs initiated by the egg industry—the Pennsylvania Egg Quality Assurance Program—began as a continuation of the *S. Enteritidis* Pilot Project (White et al., 1997). Since then, several states and industry groups have developed their own egg-quality-assurance programs. Management and control measures used in each of these programs vary widely and may include testing poults, feed, or environment for *S. Enteritidis*; cleaning and disinfecting houses and equipment; controlling rodents and pests; and refrigerating eggs immediately after collection. In October 1995, as private and state-level *S. Enteritidis* quality-assurance programs emerged, Congress deferred federal funding, thus discontinuing all USDA on-farm *S. Enteritidis* programs.

The U.S. egg industry, the focus of the *S. Enteritidis* epidemic, is one of the most highly integrated livestock production systems whose structure has evolved toward fewer but larger firms. Positive productivity trends in both laying-egg and broiler industries reflect the high level of efficiency attained in these food production systems, trends that have been achieved through advances in production technology, genetics, and disease control. In the U.S. laying-egg industry, total egg production has been dramatically increasing despite the shrinking size of our national laying flock. In 1970, a total of 324 million hens produced an average of 218 eggs per hen annually. Today, a national laying flock of 283 million hens produces an average of 256 eggs per hen annually. The U.S. broiler industry likewise is producing heavier birds with better feed efficiencies in a shorter grow-out period. Since the 1970s, average live weight has increased by roughly half a pound per decade, from 3.8 pounds in the mid-1970s to current average live weights of 4.8 pounds, while the grow-out period has shortened by almost 1 week per decade.

Total U.S. egg production is 64 billion eggs annually, generating approximately $4 billion per year in revenues. The United States is a net exporter of eggs, although exports constitute a small share (4%) of total egg production. Approximately 22%–25% of all eggs are broken and further processed and pasteurized, with the remainder sold as shell eggs. The price differential between shell eggs and ungraded, heavy nest-run eggs for breaking ranges from 6 to 14 cents per dozen. The standard discount for breaking eggs increases as egg quality declines.

Processed egg production has doubled since 1980, although various egg products are still produced in similar proportions (approximately 50% processed as whole eggs, 27% as liquid egg whites, 13% as liquid egg yolks, and 10% as dried egg products). Liquid egg products are either sold for immediate consumption or frozen.

U.S. total egg consumption patterns have also been changing dramatically over the past three decades. Annual per capita egg consumption (both shell eggs and egg prod-

ucts) has steadily declined from a peak of 403 in 1945 to 239 currently. Several factors have been postulated to explain these changes in consumption patterns. They include the concern for cholesterol, increased use of convenience foods such as cereals and breakfast bars, less time spent on at-home food preparation, the rise in two-worker households, and the increasing awareness of the link between foodborne salmonellosis and shell-egg consumption. The decline in total egg consumption is also reflected in per capita consumption of shell eggs, which declined from 292 in 1960 to 178 currently. On the other hand, pasteurized egg-product consumption has been steadily increasing to 61 shell-egg equivalents per capita currently, more than double the 1960 levels (29 shell-egg equivalents).

The American Egg Board reports that institutional use of pasteurized egg products has increased from 10 in 1980 to 16 pasteurized eggs per capita in 1992, and a further increase to 28 per capita is projected by the year 2000. The growth in pasteurized egg consumption has been accompanied by an increasing proportion of liquid eggs sold for immediate consumption. Data from 1994 show that 59% (836 million pounds) of liquid egg products were sold for immediate consumption, up from 34% in 1980. Simultaneously, frozen egg products have declined from 53% (330 million pounds) in 1980 to current levels of 31% (430 million pounds in 1994) (Fig. 25.2).

Considering the high degree of integration and larger production volume in this industry, it is easy to see that slight changes in prices and market quantities will affect producer profit margins as well as consumer demand. Stability of supply and demand is critical to the industry's economic future. *Salmonella* Enteritidis can have direct and indirect effects on both the supply and the demand for eggs. Hence, recognizing the economic implications of *S. Enteritidis* and its control is necessary for understanding and resolving this complex infection in animals and humans.

ECONOMIC IMPLICATIONS OF *SALMONELLA* ENTERITIDIS FOR CONSUMERS

Salmonellosis is an acute intestinal infection that is characterized by diarrhea, nausea, abdominal cramping, and fever, often lasting for a week or more. The incidence is highest in infants, but people of all ages are susceptible to the infection. Although most cases resolve without specific treatment, antibiotic treatment can be lifesaving in severe cases (Tauxe, 1996).

In certain high-risk groups such as the very young, the elderly, and immune-compromised individuals (including persons with diabetes, HIV, chronic diseases, and cancer, or persons undergoing immunosuppressive therapy as an adjunct to organ transplant or cancer treatment), infection can spread to the bloodstream, bone marrow, or meningeal lining of the brain, leading to a severe and occasionally fatal illness. The size of this high-risk group is the subject of some dispute, although published estimates suggest that anywhere

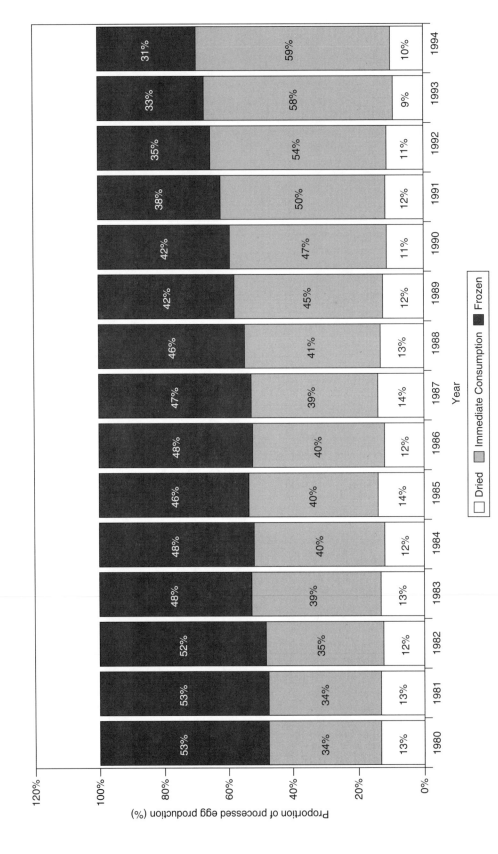

FIGURE 25.2 Processed egg production by product type, 1980–94.

from 10% [Council for Agricultural Science and Technology (CAST), 1994] to 20% (Gerba et al., 1996) of the U.S. population is particularly susceptible to foodborne diseases.

In addition to the acute form of the disease, salmonellosis may be accompanied by long-term sequelae. Cardiac inflation, neural infections, reactive arthritis, splenomegaly, and osteomyelitis are some of the chronic sequelae that have been reported following salmonellosis (D'Aoust, 1989). About 2%–3% of nontyphoid salmonella infection cases develop postinfection complications in the form of recurring joint pain and arthritis (Tauxe, 1996). In persons with a specific genetic susceptibility, up to 20% may exhibit these complications (Edmonds, 1984; Smith et al., 1993).

The economic impacts of human salmonellosis and other foodborne diseases have been estimated and reported for England (Roberts and Sockett, 1994), Canada (Todd, 1989a), and the United States (Cohen et al., 1978; Archer and Kvenberg, 1985; Roberts, 1989; Todd, 1989b; Buzby et al., 1996). In general, economic losses have been computed by estimating the number of cases of specific diseases, taking into account the sources of undercounting common to most foodborne-disease reporting, and multiplying the number of cases by an estimated cost per case. These costs are typically developed for different disease outcomes corresponding to case severity. Most of the U.S. cost estimates for salmonellosis cases are derived primarily from a single investigation of an outbreak of salmonellosis (Cohen et al., 1978).

The most recent evaluation of the economic impacts of salmonella and other foodborne pathogens updated the cost estimates from the Cohen et al. (1978) study, adding a value-of-life component to the estimate and willingness to pay to avoid foodborne illness (Buzby et al., 1996). Economic losses from salmonellosis are calculated for each of four case outcomes (no physician visit, physician visit, hospitalization, and death). This study also reports a relative frequency of occurrence of each of these outcomes. Using the updated estimates from the Buzby et al. (1996) study of economic losses due to salmonellosis and weighting these losses by the relative frequency of each outcome, the weighted economic costs associated with each of four case outcomes were estimated, with the weighted average cost per case (in 1993 dollars) equal to $1018.00 (Table 25.3). Buzby et al. (1996) estimate a range of costs per case from $371 (no physician visit) to $385,000 (death). Note that

these two categories account for 34% and 45%, respectively, of the weighted average cost. The outcomes that required medical intervention followed by patient recovery account for only 20% of the weighted average cost per case. Note further that the weighted average cost per case is about half the value estimated by Archer and Kvenberg (1985).

Estimating the economic losses from *S.* Enteritidis requires an estimate of the number of annual human cases due to *S.* Enteritidis foodborne illness. To represent adequately the increasing trend due to sporadic cases in spite of the decline in outbreaks, the average of *S.* Enteritidis isolates from 1993 to 1995 is used. *Salmonella* Enteritidis isolates averaged 9884 annually in the United States during this 3-year period. Multipliers have been used to account for the underreporting that is common with foodborne illness. Those used by the CDC range from 20 to 100, that is, only one in 20–100 cases is reported to the CDC. Based on their outbreak investigation, Mishu et al. (1994) evaluated this multiplier at 38. Buzby et al. (1996) used a factor of 50 in their economic evaluations. These multipliers are used to estimate the number of cases and corresponding economic losses. Applying this range of multipliers, approximately 200,000 to 1 million *S.* Enteritidis cases are estimated to occur annually (Table 25.4). Multiplying the number of estimated cases by the weighted average cost per case of $1018, and assuming that the average cost of a case of salmonellosis due to *S.* Enteritidis is similar to that of other salmonellosis cases, estimated economic losses due to *S.* Enteritidis foodborne illness ranges from $200 million to $1 billion annually (1993 dollars) for various levels of underreporting.

No single study provides a definitive measure of the true economic losses attributable to *S.* Enteritidis infections in humans. The limitations inherent in many of these cost assessments are considerable. These estimates are based primarily on a single study (Cohen et al., 1978) from one outbreak involving fewer than 300 people. Since that time, changes in population demographics, medical technology and costs, proportion of population covered by health insurance (which influences willingness to incur medical costs), emergence of a potentially more pathogenic strain of salmonella in *S.* Enteritidis PT4, and a host of other factors make extrapolation of the 1976 data to current economic losses less than satisfactory. Since 1976, the number of persons susceptible to foodborne diseases has increased considerably: currently, between one-tenth to one-fifth of the

TABLE 25.3   Average economic losses from a case of salmonellosis weighted by frequency of occurrence and severity of consequences

Case outcome category	Frequency of outcome (weight)[a]	Economic loss ($)[b]	Weighted economic loss ($)	Weighted loss as % of total cost
No physician visit	0.93	371	345.03	33.9
Physician visit	0.05	794	39.70	3.9
Hospitalization	0.0188	9087	170.84	16.8
Death	0.0012	385,355	462.43	45.4
Total	1.0000	—	1018.00	100.00

[a]Buzby et al. (1996).
[b]Economic estimates adapted from Buzby et al. (1996).

TABLE 25.4   Estimated annual human cases and associated economic losses from *Salmonella* Enteritidis foodborne illness

S. Enteritidis isolates	Multiplier	Estimated cases	Weighted average cost per case (1993 dollars)	Estimated economic losses (million $)
9884	20[a]	197,680	$1,018.00[d]	201
9884	38[b]	375,592	$1,018.00	382
9884	50[c]	494,200	$1,018.00	503
9884	100[a]	988,400	$1,018.00	1006

[a]CDC multipliers.
[b]Mishu et al. (1994) multiplier.
[c]Buzby et al. (1996) multiplier.
[d]See Table 25.3 for calculation of weighted average cost per case.

U.S. population is considered susceptible to foodborne pathogens. These individuals typically become ill with lower doses of pathogen (Hennessy et al., 1996), experience more serious health outcomes [see Baker et al. (1997) for a review], and may be at greater risk of dying of an *S.* Enteritidis infection. The size of the susceptible population or high-risk subpopulation may significantly affect the relative frequency of various case outcomes and thus the weighted average cost per case.

Published estimates of the economic losses due to salmonellosis do not include costs for long-term consequences or sequelae to salmonella infections, a potentially large source of underestimation of costs. These long-term effects can include reactive arthritis and Reiter's syndrome. Recent reviews suggest that 2%–3% of people experiencing foodborne illness (including *S.* Enteritidis and *Salmonella* Typhimurium) may develop reactive arthritides (Smith, 1994; Tauxe, 1996; McDowell and McElvaine, 1997). Two recent studies suggest that the frequency of long-term sequelae may be 6–7 times higher than the estimates reported in the literature. Locht and others (1993) followed the outcomes of 108 physicians infected with *S.* Enteritidis from a foodborne outbreak traced to eggs and found that 16% of those with acute illness subsequently suffered some form of reactive arthritis. Smith (1994) cites a foodborne outbreak due to *S.* Typhimurium in which 16.4% of 116 patients developed reactive arthritis and 9.5% developed conjunctivitis. Nearly 40% of those who developed reactive arthritis had symptoms persisting over 1 year. No comprehensive or systematic study of the medical costs, productivity losses, or willingness to pay to avoid reactive arthritis is available in the literature on costs of foodborne illness, so the economic consequences of this aspect of *S.* Enteritidis–related salmonellosis cannot be included in the cost estimates at this time. Since long-term chronic complications are often an important part of an economic evaluation of foodborne disease, the economic losses from *S.* Enteritidis may be significantly underestimated.

Finally, the estimated economic losses are primarily those in the "measured economy," that is, items included in the gross national product. These losses do not include any compensation for pain and suffering associated with acute disease, loss of nonwork time, or consideration of people's willingness to pay to avoid being ill. The work of Harrington and Portney (1987) concluded that direct medical costs and productivity losses may form the lower boundary of the true economic value of losses from disease or accidents. The use of experimental auctions to value reductions in the likelihood of foodborne disease suggests that the value is 2–3 times higher than previously speculated in the published literature (Hayes et al., 1995). This suggests that there are other costs, still unaccounted for in great part, that are not insignificant to the economic evaluation of foodborne illness.

ECONOMIC IMPLICATIONS OF *SALMONELLA* ENTERITIDIS TO PRODUCERS

Salmonella Enteritidis has not been consistently associated with significant morbidity or mortality in commercial egg production, yet several researchers have demonstrated a decline in egg production with experimental *S.* Enteritidis infection. Shivaprasad et al. (1990) demonstrated reduced egg production, depression, anorexia, diarrhea, and slightly increased mortality among hens inoculated with 10^8 cells via oral or intravenous route. Gast and Beard's (1990) research quantified a 10%–30% decline in egg production after the administration of oral doses of 10^9 colony-forming units to 27-week-old to 62-week-old birds. Barrow and Lovell (1991) likewise noted a 10% drop in egg production that persisted over a 4-week period in layers inoculated intravenously with 10^5 *S.* Enteritidis organisms. A survey of farms involved in a traceback (Morales, 1996) showed that the youngest flocks testing positive for *S.* Enteritidis were 35 weeks of age (that is, in the peak of egg production) whereas the oldest test-positive flocks were at the end of their production cycle (70 weeks). If one assumes a prevalence of up to 45% among flocks (Hogue et al., 1997), a decline in egg production in younger hens could affect profitability significantly (Table 25.5).

Farm-level costs for *S.* Enteritidis control in laying flocks can vary by flock size, housing and equipment type and age, environmental conditions, and management practices. Moreover, short-run producer costs of compliance with regulatory protocol can be exceedingly high regardless of whether eggs are diverted or an infected flock is depopulated (Morales, 1995). No indemnities are paid if a producer depopulates, and the income stream from that flock's egg production is

TABLE 25.5 Management practice changes and additional costs for *Salmonella* Enteritidis control

Cost-of-compliance survey question	Range of responses
Number of houses with *S*. Enteritidis(+) status during any one traceback period	1–10 houses
Age of layers at traceback	35–70 weeks
Percent production of the flock at restriction	65%–92%
Age of *S*. Enteritidis(+) flock when sold	68–70 weeks
Number of weeks *S*. Enteritidis(+) flock was in production	48–51 weeks
Downtime in *S*. Enteritidis(+) houses	2–8 weeks
Total number of eggs diverted to breakers	1246.5–487,500 cases
Additional breaker discount for *S*. Enteritidis(+) eggs	Less than $0.05–$0.08 per dozen
Changes in quarterly egg production during the traceback period	Less than 5.5%–15% of normal production
Percent of eggs typically sold to breakers prior to traceback	0%–60%
Percent of eggs sold to breakers during the year after regaining *S*. Enteritidis(−) status	60%–75%
Additional labor hours during *S*. Enteritidis(+) status	
Management/field service personnel	0–29 h per month
Hired labor	0–40 h per month
Paid consultants	3–20 h per month
Additional labor costs during *S*. Enteritidis(+) status	$660–$1000 per month
Additional expenses during *S*. Enteritidis(+) status	
Repairs and maintenance	$0–$300 per month
Animal-health supplies	$10–$400 per month
Miscellaneous supplies	$0–$100 per month
Average feed costs per layer prior to *S*. Enteritidis(+) status	$5.63–$5.96 per layer (52 weeks)
Average feed costs per layer during *S*. Enteritidis(+) status	$5.65–$6.14 per layer (52 weeks)
Cleaning and disinfecting costs (Per house basis)	
Dry-cleaning	$600–$1508
Average pressure-washing	$2500–$4000
Fumigation	$280–$500
Heat-treatment[a]	$1000
Disinfection	$225–$800
Cost of *S*. Enteritidis testing in pullets	$0.003–$0.02 per pullet
Cost of environmental testing in layer houses	$200–$250 per house
S. Enteritidis vaccine costs	$0–$0.16 per bird
Rodent control costs[a]	$60 per month
Fly control[a]	$210 per month
Feed additive costs for *S*. Enteritidis control[a]	$0.005 per lb feed

[a]Only one respondent reported using this method and/or incurring this cost.

lost. If replacement pullets are not immediately available, then producers incur the opportunity cost of idle capital (land, housing, and equipment). If producers opt to retain flocks and divert eggs to the egg-product market for pasteurization, they lose the shell-egg premium from selling eggs for breaking. Moreover, eggs from an identified *S*. Enteritidis–positive flock are further discounted an additional 5–8 cents per dozen eggs. In either case (depopulation or diversion), producers must fulfill existing contracts and may need to purchase shell eggs in the open market to meet contract obligations (Morales, 1996). They also incur the costs of cleaning and disinfecting laying houses, which can range from $2500 to $10,000 per house (Mason and Ebel, 1991). Cleaning and disinfecting procedures generally require an additional 2–4 weeks of downtime between flocks (standard industry practice is 2 weeks), further increasing the opportunity costs of idle capital. Other secondary costs associated with tracebacks include liability claims, increased insurance premiums or canceled coverage, loss of consumer confidence, and, less frequently, recalls and bans.

With the *S*. Enteritidis traceback program in place, producer cooperation in voluntary control programs was understandably less than satisfactory for several reasons. With the possible exception of *S*. Enteritidis PT4, *S*. Enteritidis produces few observable symptoms at the commercial flock level. Thus, the direct losses incurred by producers from *S*. Enteritidis as a disease entity are minimal or not distinct. Furthermore, since salmonellae are ubiquitous in nature with many sources of contamination, complete elimination of *S*. Enteritidis may not be a realistic goal. None of the existing control methods, alone or in combination, seem to guarantee elimination of *S*. Enteritidis from a flock or premises. However, as consumer concerns regarding *S*. Enteritidis mounted, the egg industry proactively developed egg-quality-assurance programs in several states. Instituting egg-quality assurance has successfully stabilized demand for many firms. However, as most producers have been unable to pass the costs on to consumers in the form of a price premium for safer products, there is limited incentive for aggressive control measures from the egg industry.

Other indirect costs and benefits accrue to producers from *S*. Enteritidis control programs. The most significant indirect effects arise from exogenous shifts in consumer demand. The classic example in the egg industry of how consumers' changing risk perceptions affect demand is the decline in shell-egg consumption attributed to increased concern about cholesterol content in foods and the link with coronary heart disease.

Microbiological studies have implicated contaminated poultry and eggs in foodborne salmonellosis for many years, yet the consuming public has only recently become conscious of this risk. This increasing perception of risk associated with the consumption of these foods could change the demand for shell eggs in several ways. If consumers are confident that producers and/or regulators have instituted effective control programs that lower the risk of salmonellosis, then demand for shell eggs could conceivably rise. This means that at any given shell-egg price, the quantity of eggs purchased by consumers would increase. As a result, prices for shell eggs would also increase. If all else remains the same, this means increased revenues for shell-egg producers.

On the other hand, if consumers think that there is an increased risk of salmonellosis from eating shell eggs, they will purchase fewer eggs and producer revenues will fall. The size of the price fall, assuming the supply of eggs remains unchanged, is a measure of the importance that consumers attach to salmonellosis risk. However, a degree of substitutability exists between shell eggs and pasteurized egg products, so a decline in shell-egg consumption due to changing consumer risk perceptions would increase pasteurized egg consumption.

In an attempt to quantify the effect of changing consumer risk perceptions on demand, an econometric analysis of the effect of adverse information on salmonellosis on shell-egg and pasteurized egg consumption was conducted (Morales, 1997a). A salmonella information variable was created using information from popular press releases relating specifically to salmonella in eggs, including reports of egg-associated disease outbreaks caused by salmonella serovars. Adverse information specifically linking salmonellosis to egg consumption was associated with a statistically significant decline in both shell-egg and pasteurized egg consumption (1% and 0.1%, respectively), indicating the negative effect that adverse publicity can have on product demand.

Instituting *S*. Enteritidis control increases production costs, which translates eventually into reduced profits and higher prices. However, the indirect producer benefits from instituting *S*. Enteritidis control programs cannot be discounted. One such benefit is stabilizing product demand and maintaining market share by holding consumer confidence. Another is the ability to limit liability and fulfill the legal requirements for due diligence. Although there have been few successfully litigated cases against producers whose eggs or laying flocks were implicated in human outbreaks of salmonellosis, legal proceedings are costly and time-consuming. Furthermore, although the research in this area is limited, improvements in biosecurity and pathogen control invariably prove beneficial to increasing productivity and decreasing the incidence of other diseases.

Finally, although export markets do not constitute a significant share of the egg industry, assuring market stability is critical to any industry maintaining its competitiveness in international trade. The devastating effects of food-safety-related import restrictions on a large exporting industry was evidenced in the recent Russian ban on U.S. broilers. Food-safety programs are now becoming an increasing requirement among trading countries, and guidelines are being developed within various institutions, such as the Codex Alimentarius Commission, the World Trade Organization, and the Sanitary and Phytosanitary Agreements of the General Agreement on Tariffs and Trade (GATT).

INTERVENTION OPTIONS AND MARKETING OPPORTUNITIES

Opportunities for marketing food safety exist. Altering the safety attributes of products generally offers increased sales, especially if consumers are informed about the improved safety features. Markets for improved safety attributes are affected by at least five considerations: those problems of concern to consumers, consumer preferences among alternative food-safety strategies, size of the potential market for products with improved safety attributes, consumer willingness to pay for improved attributes, and the food-safety regulatory environment.

Consumers can address food-safety concerns in several ways. They can avoid or reduce consumption, adopt safe handling and cooking practices, trust the industry to provide foods with safety characteristics, or delegate accountability for food safety to government regulation. Successful firms will be able to anticipate future regulatory environments that could erode or increase product value. For example, Alar-free apples (once sold at a premium) were no different from other apples after Alar was banned. Firms capturing marketing opportunities will also be able to anticipate consumers' priority concerns rapidly enough for product development and market positioning. These firms recognize that consumer confidence and preferences influence product demand.

The strength of consumer demand for safer products will depend on the sources, the accountability for food-safety problems, and how mitigation strategies reduce the perceived risk of foodborne hazards. Demographic changes suggest that markets for food safety will expand with an aging U.S. population, creating a niche market among high-risk individuals. The key to marketing food safety is identifying either niche markets or sizable enough markets for safety-improved products. Consumers must also be willing to pay for safer foods, and research indicates that consumers are willing to do so for risks that concern them. Safer products also seem less valuable if consumers feel they have to rely on their own means to ensure safety than if they rely on producers or regulators (Roberts et al., 1997).

As with most food-safety problems, the most successful efforts to reduce the public health risk from *S*. Enteritidis in eggs will include control options over many stages of the

TABLE 25.6   Cost estimate of selected input requirements for *Salmonella* Enteritidis control and prevention

Control method	Cost of control (cents per layer per year)
Environmental testing	0.25–0.31
Fumigation	0.4–0.5
Pressure washing	3.5–4
Cleaning and disinfecting	0.5–1.8
Labor and supplies	1.7–2.0
Pullet testing	0.3–2.0
Rodent control	9.0
Total cost per layer	15.65–19.61
Total cost per dozen eggs	0.745–0.981[a]

[a]Assumes 20–21 dozen eggs per layer per year.

farm-to-table continuum, rather than focusing on any one particular strategy. Producers, processors, wholesalers, transporters, retailers, and consumers alike can reduce the risk of *S.* Enteritidis illness from egg consumption.

Although a variety of solutions has been developed and adopted in many countries, the epidemiology of *S.* Enteritidis infection in poultry is still not well understood, and a comprehensive understanding of the factors that determine *S.* Enteritidis infection in poultry operations still eludes researchers (Mason, 1994). The appropriate control strategies and public policies will vary, depending on the industry, epidemiological factors, the efficacy and cost of mitigation strategies, and the current impacts of *S.* Enteritidis on public health.

Intervention strategies can be broadly categorized by their place in the farm-to-table continuum: production and preproduction, processing and distribution, and preparation and consumption. Systems theory suggests, and practical experience has demonstrated, that no single approach is superior. The overwhelming record in the field of pollution control shows that it is almost always more economically efficient to control pollution by adjusting the processes that generate it than by attempting abatement efforts after the process is completed (Knesse and Schultze, 1975). Because systematic epidemiological and economic analysis has been used to evaluate only a few intervention strategies, most information on the viability of specific interventions is based on practical experience and experimentation.

Epidemiological analysis of the routes of *S.* Enteritidis introduction into poultry flocks, both vertically and horizontally, has yielded a number of solutions (Noordhuizen and Frankena, 1994). Monitoring and sampling strategies play a critical role in preventing or identifying infections. Preventing infection by controlling *S.* Enteritidis at the breeder-flock level has been advocated and used in several countries (Edel, 1994; Mason, 1994). At the producer or farm level, the basic practices have evolved into a set of control strategies that constitute most egg-quality-assurance programs: *S.* Enteritidis–free pullets placed in *S.* Enteritidis–free houses, assuring feed and water are free from *S.* Enteritidis, aggressive rodent control, environmental testing to determine status of laying environment, rigorous disinfection to eliminate residual *S.* Enteritidis contamination, and, for some programs, egg testing. At the

processing and distribution stages, refrigerating eggs to prevent *S.* Enteritidis growth during distribution and storage has been advocated by a number of researchers. To date, the economics of refrigeration and different temperature regimens (specific temperatures, and internal versus ambient temperatures) have not been analyzed. Recommendations at the preparation and consumption stage include using pasteurized egg products when egg pooling is required or when feeding susceptible populations, and increased education of food servers and homemakers on proper storage and preparation of shell eggs.

Although a number of researchers have analyzed interventions from an epidemiological standpoint, few have evaluated the efficacy (reduction in the prevalence of *S.* Enteritidis–infected flocks or eggs), costs, and consequent economic efficiency of specific interventions. Thus, although these studies provide a starting point for evaluating risk-reducing interventions, they do not provide any guidance as to their practical value or relative cost-effectiveness.

A simulation model of infection over time in Dutch poultry farms by van de Giessen and others (1994) evaluated hypothetical cumulative infection curves to identify interventions appropriate for specific situations. The authors concluded that most infections in the Netherlands arise not from infected laying stock but from contaminated laying-house environments, suggesting appropriate interventions include environmental testing prior to stocking houses, and cleaning and disinfecting farm premises that are test positive (Table 25.6). Ament and others (1993) used a benefit–cost framework including efficacy estimates, intervention costs, and explicit evaluation of the public health benefits achieved by prospective interventions. In particular, they analyzed a policy of monitoring laying flocks by sampling fecal material to detect *S.* Enteritidis infections and destroyed infected flocks. Their analysis included effectiveness of sampling (probability of detecting infection), cost of sampling and culturing samples, cost of destroying flocks, subsequent reduction in frequency of human disease, and the value of this reduction based on numbers of cases and previously reported costs per cases of salmonellosis. The authors concluded that *S.* Enteritidis screening and subsequently destroying infected flocks was economically justified by savings in human-disease costs. Their model of the Dutch system of egg production also evaluated optimal sampling frequency in which sampling three times over the life of the flock provided the highest net benefits.

A third evaluation of producer-level intervention strategies in the Netherlands (Edel, 1994) addressed effectiveness of specific actions but provided no information on costs, benefits, or impacts on public health. However, it evaluated a commonly recommended intervention of eradicating *S.* Enteritidis in breeder flocks. Their top-down approach of eradicating *S.* Enteritidis from breeder flocks and then maintaining stringent hygiene standards in the rest of the industry apparently has been successful at clearing *S.* Enteritidis from the national flock. Two additional approaches—using competitive exclusion flora to prevent or reduce *S.* Enteritidis colonization of hens' intestinal tracts, and using antibiotics in lieu of destroying infected flocks—were determined to be effective, but the economic efficiency of these interventions was not evaluated.

Simulation modeling was used to evaluate the cost effectiveness of several farm-level interventions in the United States (McDowell, 1995). The analysis evaluated three testing strategies: (a) environmental testing followed by egg testing for positive environmental tests, and diversion of infected eggs; (b) egg testing of all flocks and diverting all eggs from infected flocks to pasteurization; and (c) environmental testing of all flocks, and diverting all eggs from infected flocks to pasteurization.

The model included all sampling and culturing costs, as well as producer losses from diverting eggs to pasteurization, simulating the results for a 180-flock region with a 45% flock prevalence with *S.* Enteritidis. Sampling 100 eggs weekly from all flocks with diversion to pasteurization for all egg-positive flocks reduced the frequency of *S.* Enteritidis–positive eggs released to the shell-egg market from 1.5 million to 138,000 annually, a 90% reduction at a cost of about $33.4 million. Although the use of proxy data for an important model parameter—the sensitivity and specificity of environmental testing as an indicator of egg positivity—limits the usefulness of some model outputs, the analytical framework is useful for modeling specific policy options and accounting for the costs and change in the number of *S.* Enteritidis–positive eggs available for human consumption. If linked to an appropriate model of public health benefits from reduced exposure to *S.* Enteritidis–

positive eggs, models such as this can provide decision makers with valuable information on the economic efficiency and distributional impacts of risk-management policies. The comprehensive risk assessment for shell eggs and egg products in progress at the USDA at the time of this writing will provide for the first time a systematic appraisal of the costs and benefits of specific management options to reduce the risk of foodborne disease from *S.* Enteritidis in eggs (Baker et al., 1997).

Detailed cost–benefit analyses of salmonella reduction strategies in poultry have been conducted in Canada by Curtin (1984, 1986) and by Finn and Mehr (1977) and in Germany [see Todd (1989a,b) for a review of the German study]. Each study relied on a number of assumptions specific to the epidemiology and economics of its country to determine the cost-effectiveness of interventions to reduce poultry-related salmonellosis. All studies were characterized by relatively low numbers of cases (and rates) and low costs per case of human illness; thus, these studies may not be applicable to other countries. Finn and Mehr (1977) examined salmonella eradication from poultry, concluding that the expected costs were 13 times the expected savings from reducing poultry-associated salmonellosis. Curtin's work compared the expected control program costs with the expected savings from disease-related costs, assuming reductions in foodborne disease with the adoption of specific practices. The interventions included a broad range of both low-technology and high-technology approaches to reduce the frequency of contaminated product or increase the frequency of proper storage and food preparation practices. The benefit–cost ratios calculated by Curtin (1984, 1986) range from 0.2 to 16.3 (Table 25.7). The most economically efficient options (those with the highest benefit–cost ratio) were the low-technology options: educating consumers and food-service workers, cleaning crates, and disinfecting carcasses. Some practices common to modern *S.* Enteritidis quality-assurance programs (such as *S.* Enteritidis–free feed and water, and cleaning and disinfecting poultry houses) had benefit–cost ratios of less than 1, indicating that they were not economically feasible. It is interesting to note that the ranking of interventions according to net benefits does not correspond to the ranking by benefit–cost ratio. The latter statistic provides a better measure of economic efficiency.

TABLE 25.7   Net benefits and benefit–cost ratios for salmonella reduction interventions in the Canadian poultry industry

Intervention	Net benefits (million $, base = 1982)	Benefit–cost ratio
Education of food-service workers	12.1	9.7
Chlorine dioxide for carcass decontamination	9.5	16.3
Poultry irradiation	7.1	1.5
Clean crates	4.6	8.3
Homemaker education	3.8	12.0
Clean poultry processing	2.9	7.5
Clean rendering products	0.5	1.5
Clean feed	(1.7)	0.6
Clean barns	(1.9)	0.7
Clean hatcheries and eggs	(2.4)	0.2
Competitive exclusion	(8.5)	0.5

Adapted from Curtin (1984, 1986).

A benefit–cost analysis of the current Swedish program for controlling salmonella infections in the livestock industry to reduce human illness examined the net benefits and the distribution of benefits and costs by determining the effect of discontinuing the existing programs (Engvall and Anderson, 1993). Using official reported cases, published estimates of direct and indirect costs of illness, and the public and private costs for prophylaxis, the number of human cases that would occur without their current program was extrapolated from experiences of other European countries with similar livestock industries. Their results are striking: the human-disease costs and salmonella control costs are nearly identical with and without the control programs by using minimum estimates, but the distribution of costs is reversed. With existing programs, illness and death costs are estimated at SEK 4.8 million, and control costs at SEK 107.5 million, for a total of SEK 112 million annually. Without a control program, the estimated total costs are SEK 117 million annually, with illness and death costs estimated at SEK 115.2 million and control costs at SEK 2 million annually. Assuming a margin of error of 10% in the figures, neither option is preferable to the other on the basis of total costs or on the basis of economic efficiency. Electing to spend money on control and prophylaxis instead of incurring the same costs as a result of direct and indirect costs of illness is a social choice that presumably reflects the values of the country's citizens. Were such analyses more commonly done, decision makers and the public could make better informed choices about national food-safety policies.

Recent attempts to evaluate the usefulness of risk-reducing activities in poultry production in Europe utilize the Delphi technique to assess opinion from a large group of experts. Henson (1995) assembled a group of 45 experts to evaluate the relative usefulness of specific mitigation strategies to reduce nontyphi salmonella in egg and broiler production. Three rounds of data collection and evaluation on seven options produced median and maximum efficacy estimates (that is, percent hazard reduction) ranging from 5% (median estimate for pasteurized eggs) to 80% [maximum values for irradiation, hazard-analysis critical control point (HACCP) implementation, and reducing contamination in feed and stock](Table 25.8).

The conflicting results of the various studies and the incompatibility of some of the research results with the accumulated experience of producers and epidemiologists highlight a feature of the research on disease and control option costs, and

economic feasibility. Most research results are specific to a particular country at a particular time and may not be transferable to other economic or epidemiological settings. Further, all estimates of disease losses must be considered as indicative of the general magnitude of the problem, not as a definitive measurement. Sound epidemiological research and economic analysis will help to generate research results that are more transferable and durable in their temporal significance.

A recent technological advancement that may capture a marketing opportunity for *S.* Enteritidis–free eggs has led to the development of in-shell pasteurization methods designed to kill any *S.* Enteritidis that may be present inside the shell egg. Pasteurization methods may also add to the shelf life of eggs. Several processes are being evaluated that involve heat and hyperpasteurization, a system to force oxygen into the eggs at high pressure. In April 1996, Minneapolis-based Michael Foods began test marketing in-shell pasteurized eggs marked with a stylized "P" for easy identification by shoppers; the eggs were packaged in a clear plastic carton allowing visual inspection. The pasteurized shell eggs were priced between $1.39 and $1.59 per dozen, compared with $1.00 per dozen for untreated eggs in the test-market area. In May 1996, a New Hampshire–based firm, Pasteurized Eggs, L.P., received Food and Drug Administration approval for a new technology that can pasteurize up to 225 cases of eggs per hour at a projected cost of 2 cents per egg.

SAMPLING FOR *SALMONELLA* ENTERITIDIS

Sampling plays a crucial role in *S.* Enteritidis control and quality-assurance programs for testing flock environments for *S.* Enteritidis, detecting *S.* Enteritidis–positive eggs, and estimating the prevalence of infected eggs in infected flocks' output. In all cases, test sensitivity and specificity influence the interpretation of test results. Unfortunately, the relationship between environmental tests, hens' sera or organ tests, and egg tests is not well understood with respect to sensitivity and specificity for egg positivity. Thus, the economics of substituting or combining tests is poorly understood.

Most individual producers, quality-assurance programs, and regulatory agencies are more interested in determining

TABLE 25.8 Delphi estimates of efficacy of risk-mitigation practices to reduce the total incidence of nontyphi salmonella in poultry and eggs

Practice	Estimated hazard reduction			
	Median (%)	Rank	Maximum (%)	Rank
Food irradiation	35	1	80	1
HACCP implementation	25	2	80	1
Reduced contamination of feed and livestock	20	3	80	1
Competitive exclusion	20	3	50	2
Vaccines	20	3	50	2
Cold-egg distribution	10	4	20	4
Pasteurized eggs	5	5	25	3

HACCP, hazard-analysis critical control point. Adapted from Henson (1995).

whether flocks are infected with, than in measuring the prevalence of, *S*. Enteritidis–positive eggs in a flock's output. Our work with regulatory officials and epidemiologists working to reduce the *S*. Enteritidis problem suggests that decision making and policy formulation could be improved if the general principles and economics of discovery sampling for defective (for example, infected) items in populations were more clearly and widely understood. The underlying statistical theory is rarely included in the statistical training of most biological and physical scientists; thus, a brief discussion to illuminate the limitations of such sampling for improving food safety is warranted.

Discovery sampling is a special case of acceptance sampling with one objective: to determine whether the prevalence of "defectives" in a population is greater than or equal to some threshold value, with a user-specified level of statistical assurance that the inference is correct. (Although most sampling plans are designed to detect the presence of defective items in a population, the pejorative is not necessarily implied. These sampling plans can also be used to determine the presence of "exceptional" items that have some categorical attribute that differs from those of the "normal" members of the population.) Sampling procedures based on the hypergeometrical distribution (the model for sampling without replacement) to discover or detect the presence of diseased or otherwise defective members of animal populations were developed during the 1960s (Beal, 1983, 1988) and have been used extensively by the USDA since then. These

procedures have been adapted by animal-health authorities in many other parts of the world (Cannon and Roe, 1982).

Many animal-health and food-safety issues involve hazards with no acceptable tolerance, so we are often interested in determining whether a particular population is *free* of a particular hazard. However, short of conducting a census or using Bayesian methods, the mathematics of sampling precludes sampling to make inferences about sampled populations having zero members with specific characteristics. In discovery sampling, sample size depends on three parameters: the size of the population in question; a minimum or threshold prevalence of defectives; and sample reliability, or probability, that the sample will detect one or more defective items at the specified threshold prevalence.

Positive economics of intensity or scale exist for one of these parameters: the size of the population being sampled. As population increases, threshold prevalence rate, and sample reliability hold constant, sample size becomes asymptotic (Fig. 25.3). For example, sample sizes to detect a 0.1% defect rate in populations of 20,000 or larger are essentially equal (about 1500 for 80% reliability). Thus, larger populations can be sampled at proportionately smaller rates; the converse, unfortunately for smaller producers, is that small populations must be sampled at increasingly higher rates as population size declines.

Unfortunately, positive returns to scale or intensity of discovery sampling stop there. The other parameters that influence sample size—threshold defect rate and sample

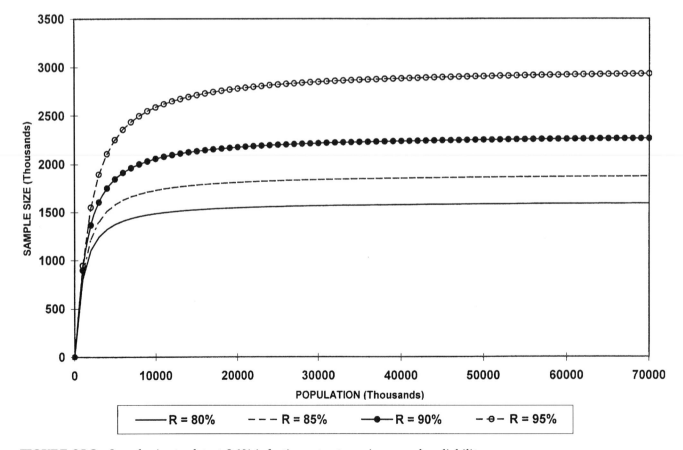

FIGURE 25.3 Sample size to detect 0.1% infection rate at varying sample reliability.

reliability—are enhanced at increasing marginal cost (in terms of sample size) at almost all points in the sampling continuum. The vertical distance between the sample size curves in Figure 25.3 demonstrates this decreasing return to sample reliability for incremental increases in sample size. The specific values for sample sizes (for a population of 70,000) at varying sample reliability levels illustrate this more concretely: for detecting a 0.1% defect rate, increasing sample reliability from 70% to 80% increases sample size by 3317, whereas increasing reliability from 80% to 90% increases sample size by 5243. Thus, the 10% increase in sample reliability increases sample size by 58%. Sample reliability increases with increasing sample size but increases as a decreasing rate (Figs. 25.4, 25.5); each additional increment in sample reliability requires a larger increment in sample size than the previous increment in reliability. The practical significance is that generating information with extremely high reliability comes at the price of very large sample sizes.

Increasing the *resolution* of discovery sampling by decreasing the threshold prevalence level requires constantly increasing sample sizes. The shape of the curves in Figure 25.6 clearly illustrates that sample size increases at an increasing rate as threshold prevalence declines. Examining the curve for reliability = 0.95, decreasing threshold prevalence from 0.01 to 0.001 increases sample size by 2634 (from 297 to 2931). Decreasing threshold prevalence from 0.001 to 0.0001 increases sample size from 2391 to 24,370, a net increase of

21,439. The prevalence values in Figure 25.6 encompass published estimates of prevalence of *S.* Enteritidis–positive eggs in infected flocks in the United States and Canada.

Combining low threshold prevalence rates with high sample reliability generates sample sizes that approach the size of the population. Should such samples be undertaken, the cost of randomizing the sample would often make a census (100% sample) more economical. Unfortunately, this situation frequently characterizes the quality of information desired by public and private decision makers faced with determining the safety of products that may be contaminated with pathogens such as *S.* Enteritidis, *Escherichia coli* O157:H7, or bovine spongiform encephalopathy. In such cases, it is typically not economically feasible to obtain such assurance through sampling. Other technologies or approaches must be developed or adopted to achieve the desired level of safety assurance at a socially acceptable cost.

Computing the sampling costs to detect *S.* Enteritidis–positive eggs in a day's run of 70,000 eggs illustrates the need (a) to develop alternative sampling procedures to detect *S.* Enteritidis–positive eggs at low prevalence, and (b) to understand more fully the relationship between egg positivity and *S.* Enteritidis positivity in less expensive environmental or bird tissue samples. Sampling costs include labor for sample collection, costs of culturing or processing samples, and the value of eggs taken in the sample. The *S.* Enteritidis Pilot Program sampling protocol specified dividing the sample into 20-egg pools cultured for *S.* Enteritidis. At the

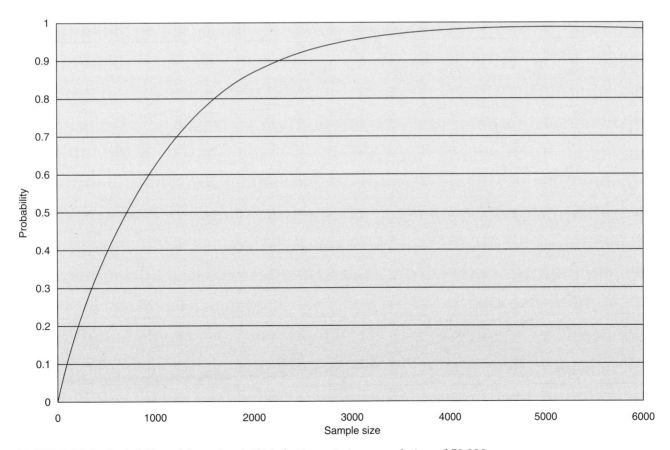

FIGURE 25.4   Probability of detecting 0.1% infection rate in a population of 70,000.

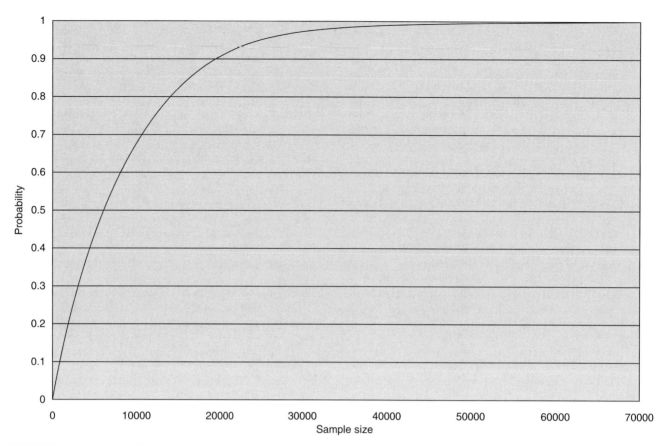

FIGURE 25.5 Probability of detecting 0.01% infection rate in a population of 70,000.

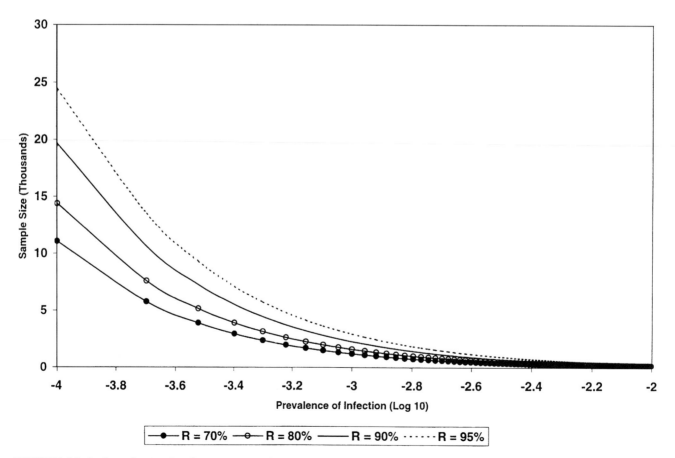

FIGURE 25.6 Sample size for discovery sampling in a population of 70,000.

low prevalences observed in commercial flocks, positive pools represent one positive egg. The culturing cost was approximately $30 per pool. The total costs for discovery sampling to detect contamination rates of 0.1% and 0.01% with 95% confidence by using this protocol and per pool culturing costs are shown in Table 25.9.

Note the total sampling cost for detecting 0.1% egg prevalence exceeds the total gross value of one day's production (70,000 eggs valued at 60 cents per dozen). These clearly prohibitive costs explain, in part, why smaller sample sizes were and are used in various public and private quality-assurance programs. The dramatically increasing costs as threshold contamination rates decrease and/or sample reliability increases make clear that sampling product for rare defective items is not an economically efficient way to meet the important public health goal of identifying and removing contaminated product from the market. This phenomenon applies to other food hazards, such as *E. coli* O157:H7 in hamburger, where the acceptable level of contamination is zero or quite low compared with conventional microbial standards. In these situations, traditional discovery sampling coupled with conventional microbial culturing methods to identify unacceptable product is simply uneconomical. If government and private interests are to assure food safety in a cost-effective manner, other approaches and techniques must be adapted or developed that simultaneously meet our criteria for accuracy and economic viability.

The results of experimental studies of naturally and artificially infected hens suggest that negative sample results (either egg, environment, or bird/tissues) should be evaluated carefully before assuming type-II errors are the only cause for failing to detect infected or defective items. Humphrey's 1994 review (see also chapter 18 in this book) of *S*. Enteritidis contamination in eggs identified several phenomena that can produce sampling anomalies: hens lay *S*. Enteritidis–positive eggs for up to 6 weeks after they cease shedding *S*. Enteritidis in their feces; some *S*. Enteritidis–infected hens produce *S*. Enteritidis–positive eggs but never produce *S*. Enteritidis–positive feces; some hens infected with *S*. Enteritidis PT4 show infection of internal organs with *S*. Enteritidis without intestinal colonization by *S*. Enteritidis; culturing time and egg-handling practices prior to culturing significantly alter the isolation rate of *S*. Enteritidis–positive eggs; the *S*. Enteritidis egg-positivity rate (proportion of eggs laid by *S*. Enteritidis–positive hens that were *S*. Enteritidis–positive) varied from 1% to 20% on a daily basis. Additional evidence of temporal clumping of *S*. Enteritidis–positive eggs comes from outbreak data (Vugia et al., 1993). These factors all provide the possibility of false-negative results when either infected hens or infected eggs are present.

Alternatives to egg sampling exist but have not been systematically analyzed to determine their effectiveness (for example, the sensitivity of various environmental tests), nor has the concordance between various tests or their reliability as indicators of *S*. Enteritidis–positive eggs. The data from spent-hen surveys (Ebel et al., 1992; Hogue et al., 1997) indicate that sampling birds or their immediate environment may be much more economical. Spent-hen surveys show average infection rates (measured by culturing internal organs) of about 2%–5% in infected flocks. Looking for infected birds at 5% prevalence may be much cheaper than looking for infected eggs at 0.01%–0.001% prevalence. Detecting a 5% infection rate (with 95% reliability) in a 70,000-bird flock requires a sample of 58; detecting a 0.1% infection rate takes a sample of 2931.

In addition to sampling alternative objects, alternatives for testing methods may provide more economical approaches to detecting infected flocks. Enzyme-linked immunosorbent assay can be used on eggs or sera and may be an economically viable alternative to traditional *S*. Enteritidis–culturing methods (Barrow, 1994). Further, the test is quite robust from the standpoint of collecting and preserving samples. As yet, the economics of alternative diagnostics have not been analyzed to identify economically efficient alternatives to conventional egg or environmental sampling. Given that the cost of egg sampling to detect a 0.1% egg prevalence with 95% reliability exceeds $4500 for a flock producing 70,000 eggs per day, ample opportunity exists to find less expensive yet equally or more reliable testing methods.

When the concordance between egg positivity and other less expensive (but more equivocal) tests is better understood, their accuracy can be framed in the standard context of diagnostic tests: test sensitivity and specificity. These data, plus information on prevalence of infected flocks, can be combined in the standard Bayesian manner to give producers and epidemiologists the same type of information available to clinicians using a diagnostic test: the positive and negative predictive values of test results (that is, probability of *S*. Enteritidis ± eggs given test ± results). The predictive values and the consequences of various misclassifications will permit more informed, optimal decision making, given specific test results.

TABLE 25.9 Total costs of egg sampling and testing for detecting *Salmonella* Enteritidis infections in laying flocks

Contamination rate (%)	Sample size[a]	Value of eggs[b] ($)	Testing costs[c] ($)	Total costs ($)
1	297	15	446	460
0.1	2310	147	4397	4543
0.01	24,370	1219	36,555	37,774

[a]Sample sizes based on 95% sample reliability (probability of obtaining one or more positive eggs = 0.95, given the true prevalence of *S*. Enteritidis–positive eggs in the population is equal to the stated contamination rate).
[b]Eggs valued at $0.60 per dozen.
[c]Testing costs (calculated for pools of 20 eggs at $30 per pool).

INDUSTRY IMPLICATIONS OF *SALMONELLA* ENTERITIDIS: WHO PAYS FOR FOOD-SAFETY PROGRAMS?

Control programs can be costly. With increasing demands on our scarce resources, efficient resource allocation must become the objective of decision makers involved in instituting disease-control programs. Government costs and farm-level costs can generally be readily determined when evaluating many disease-control programs. However, some potential market responses (specifically, changes in supply and demand, market prices, and quantities) cannot be directly assessed but are nonetheless critical to the long-term success of control programs. Anticipating these market responses and evaluating the potential *distributional* effects of animal-health programs (that is, who bears the costs and who benefits) are necessary to maintaining industry structure and integrity.

Evaluating market price and quantity changes for the egg industry requires considering both shell-egg and egg-product (breaking egg) supply and demand. This is so because of their high degree of substitutability in supply (that is, most eggs can be processed into either shell eggs or breaking eggs) and, to a lesser extent, in demand (for example, restaurants and some institutions use shell eggs and egg products interchangeably). There are several requisites to accomplish this analysis: one is using an economic analytical approach such as multimarket equilibrium welfare analysis, and the other is availability of information on control-program options and their costs (Morales, 1995, 1996). For example, information that could be used to evaluate the market effects of *S.* Enteritidis control programs includes the effectiveness and cost of control options such as certified *S.* Enteritidis–free pullets, in-house testing and monitoring, rodent control, competitive exclusion, strict temperature controls, improved egg-handling practices, and diversion of eggs to the breaking-egg market for pasteurization (Morales, 1995, 1997b).

Table 25.10 illustrates the burden and distribution of costs from a hypothetical *S.* Enteritidis control program that increases production costs by 1 cent per dozen eggs: the net surplus changes (the cost of the program to society) are equivalent whether egg diversion is or is not a policy option ($39 million annually). However, producers could minimize their short-term losses if egg diversion was a program option, particularly if they produced predominantly shell eggs ($21.5 million under a diversion program versus $37.5 million otherwise). Table 25.11 illustrates the distribution of program costs over time for an *S.* Enteritidis control program that increases input costs by 1 cent per dozen eggs but permits recovering a portion of egg production costs by diverting eggs to pasteurization. Over the short term, the burden of program costs falls primarily on shell-egg producers ($41 million annually). In the long run, a larger portion of the program costs will be passed on to consumers in the form of higher prices, and the cost burden will be shared more equally between producers and consumers.

TABLE 25.10   Consumer and producer gains and losses (long run) under a *Salmonella* Enteritidis control program with and without diversion of eggs for pasteurization as a policy option (annual)

	With diversion (million $)	Without diversion (million $)
Consumer surplus		
Shell-egg market	(17.90)	(1.95)
Breaking-egg market	2.24	(0.09)
Total	(15.66)	(2.04)
Producer surplus		
Shell-egg market	(21.50)	(37.45)
Breaking-egg market	(2.24)	0.09
Total	(23.75)	(37.36)
Net surplus change	(39.41)	(39.40)

TABLE 25.11   Short-run and long-run consumer and producer gains and losses under a *Salmonella* enteritidis control program with diversion of eggs for pasteurization (annual)

	Short run (million $)	Long run (million $)
Consumer surplus		
Shell-egg market	(6.67)	(17.90)
Breaking-egg market	4.24	2.24
Total	(2.43)	(15.66)
Producer surplus		
Shell-egg market	(40.62)	(21.50)
Breaking-egg market	(4.25)	(2.24)
Total	(44.87)	(23.75)
Net surplus change	(47.32)	(39.41)

The value of the information gained through this type of analysis is significant because it enables regulatory officials, producers, and consumers to evaluate a variety of options based on an objective evaluation of who pays, who benefits, and by how much. Better information should promote better decisions with fewer unanticipated effects. This is particularly important to industry because disease-control or disease-eradication program effects are likely to show up in firm production costs and profitability. Finally, least-cost programs can be identified and then compared with the benefits attained by reducing the public health risk from foodborne illness due to S. Enteritidis, improving our ability to allocate efficiently those resources devoted to control programs.

SUMMARY AND CONCLUSIONS

The economic consequences of S. Enteritidis to the egg industry are diverse in effect and magnitude. Analyzing these impacts in conjunction with epidemiological methods and risk analysis will provide more complete information for evaluating alternative intervention strategies and policy options. The distinction between the measurement of benefits versus the costs of policy becomes even more critical with food-safety regulation.

REFERENCES

Ament, A.J.H.A., Janner, J., van de Giessen, A., and Notermans, S. 1993. Cost benefit analysis of a screening strategy for *Salmonella* Enteritidis in poultry. Vet. Q. 15:33–37.

Antle, J.M. 1996. Efficient food safety regulation in the food manufacturing sector. Am. J. Agric. Econ. 75:1242–1247.

Archer, D.L., and Kvenberg, J.E. 1985. Incidence and cost of food-borne diarrheal disease in the United States. J. Food Prot. 48:887–894.

Baker, A., Ebel, E.D., Hogue, A.T., McDowell, R.M., Morales, R.A., Schlosser, W., and Whiting, R.A. 1997. Parameter values for a risk assessment of *Salmonella* Enteritidis in shell eggs and egg products. USDA Food Safety and Inspection Service Draft Report, August. Washington, DC: U.S. Department of Agriculture.

Barrow, P.A. 1994. Serological diagnosis of *Salmonella* serotype Enteritidis infections in poultry by ELISA and other tests. Int. J. Food Microbiol. 21:55–68.

Barrow, P.A., and Lovell, M.A. 1991. Experimental infection of egg-laying hens with *Salmonella enteritidis* phage type 4. Avian Pathol. 20:335–348.

Beal, V.C. 1983. Regulatory statistics, vol. 1. Riverdale, MD: Animal and Plant Health Inspection Service, U.S. Department of Agriculture.

Beal, V.C. 1988. Regulatory statistics, vol. 2-B. Riverdale, MD: Animal and Plant Health Inspection Service, U.S. Department of Agriculture.

Buzby, J.C., Roberts, T., Lin, C.-T.J., and McDonald, J.M. 1996. Bacterial foodborne disease: medical costs and productivity losses. Agricultural Economics Report 741. Washington, DC: Food and Consumer Economics Division, Economic Research Service, U.S. Department of Agriculture.

Cannon, R.M., and Roe, R.T. 1982. Livestock disease surveys: a field manual for veterinarians. Canberra: Australian Bureau of Animal Health.

Cohen, M.L., Fontaine, R.E., Pollard, R.A., Von Allmen, S.D., Vernon, T.M., and Gangarosa, E.J. 1978. An assessment of patient-related economic costs in an outbreak of salmonellosis. N. Engl. J. Med. 299:459–460.

Council for Agricultural Science and Technology (CAST). 1994. Foodborne pathogens: risks and consequences. Task Force Report 122. Ames, IA: CAST.

Curtin, L. 1984. Economic study of *Salmonella* food poisoning and control measures in Canada. Working Paper 11-84. Ottawa: Marketing and Economics Branch, Agriculture Canada.

Curtin, L. 1986. Analysis of *Salmonella* food poisoning and control measures in the Canadian poultry industry. In: Proceedings, second world congress of foodborne infections and intoxications. Berlin: Institute of Veterinary Medicine.

D'Aoust, J.Y. 1989. Salmonella. In: Doyle, M.P., ed. Foodborne bacterial pathogens. New York: Marcel Dekker.

Ebel, E.D., David, M.J., and Mason, J. 1992. Occurrence of *Salmonella enteritidis* in the U.S. commercial egg industry: report on a national spent hen survey. Avian Dis. 36:646–654.

Ebel, E.D., Mason, J., Thomas, L.A., Ferris, K.E., Beckman, M.G., Cummins, D.R., Tucker, L.S., Sutherlin, W.D., Glasshoff, R.L., and Smithhisler, N.M. 1993. Occurrence of *Salmonella enteritidis* in unpasteurized liquid egg in the United States. Avian Dis. 37:135–142.

Edel, W. 1994. *Salmonella enteritidis* eradication programme in poultry breeder flocks in the Netherlands. Int. J. Food Microbiol. 21:171–178.

Edmonds, J. 1984. Reactive arthritis. Aust. J. Med. 14:81–88.

Engvall, A., and Anderson, Y. 1993. The economics of Swedish salmonella control: a cost/benefit analysis. Working Paper. Stockholm: Swedish Institute of Infectious Disease Control.

Finn, P.J., and Mehr, B. 1977. A benefit–cost analysis of eradicating *Salmonella* infection in chicken produced in Canada. In: Proceedings, international symposium on salmonella and prospects for control, 8–11 June 1977. Guelph, Canada: University of Guelph.

Gast, R.K., and Beard, C.W. 1990. Production of *Salmonella enteritidis*-contaminated eggs by experimentally infected hens. Avian Dis. 34:438–446.

Gerba, C.P., Rose, J.P., and Haas, C.N. 1996. Sensitive populations: who is at the greatest risk? Int. J. Food Microbiol. 30:113–123.

Gomez, T.M., Molarjemi, Y., Miyagawa, S., Kaferstein, F.K., and Stohr, K. 1997. Foodborne salmonellosis. World Health Stat. Q. 50:81–89.

Harrington, W., and Portney, P.R. 1987. Valuing the benefits of health and safety regulations. J. Urban Econ. 22:101–112.

Hayes, D.J., Shogren, J.F., Shin, S.Y., and Kliebenstein, J.B. 1995. Valuing food safety in experimental auction markets. Am. J. Agric. Econ. 77:40–53.

Hennessy, T.W., Hedberg, C.W., Slutsker, L., White, K.E., Besser-Wiek, J.M., Moen, M.E., Feldman, J., Coleman, W.W., Edmonson, L.M., MacDonald, K.L., Osterholm, M.T., and the Investigation Team. 1996. A national outbreak of *Salmonella* Enteritidis infections from ice cream. N. Engl. J. Med. 334:1281–1286.

Henson, S. 1995. Estimating the incidence of foodborne *Salmonella* and the effectiveness of alternative control measures. In: Proceedings, NE-165 Conference, 6–7 June 1995, Washington, DC. Storrs: Food Marketing Policy Center, Department of Agricultural and Resource Economics, University of Connecticut.

Hogue, A.T., Ebel, E.D., Thomas, L.A., Schlosser, W., Bufano, N., and Ferris K. 1997. Surveys of *Salmonella enteritidis* in unpasteurized liquid egg and spent hens at slaughter. J. Food. Prot. 60:1194–1200.

Humphrey, T.J. 1994. Contamination of egg shells and contents with *Salmonella* Enteritidis: a review. Int. J. Food Microbiol. 21:31–40

Kinderlerer, J.L. 1994. Salmonella in eggs. BNF Nutr. Bull. 19:11–18.

Knesse, A.V., and Schultze, C.L., 1975. Pollution, prices, and public policy. Washington, DC: Brookings Institute.

Locht, H.E., Kihlstrom, E., and Linstrom, F.D. 1993. Reactive arthritis after salmonella among medical doctors: study of an outbreak. Rheumatology 20:845–848.

Mason, J. 1994. *Salmonella enteritidis* control programs in the United States. Int. J. Food Microbiol. 21:155–169.

Mason, J., and Ebel, E.D. 1991. APHIS *Salmonella enteritidis* Control Program. In: Proceedings, symposium on the diagnosis and control of salmonella. San Diego, CA: U.S. Animal Health Association.

McDowell, R.M. 1995. A simulation of the cost and effectiveness of risk mitigation options for reducing *Salmonella enteritidis* in commercial laying flocks. Unpublished staff report. Riverdale, MD: Animal and Plant Health Inspection Service, Risk Analysis Systems Staff, U.S. Department of Agriculture.

McDowell, R.M., Kaplan, S., Ahl, A., and Roberts, T. 1995. Managing risks from foodborne microbial hazards. In: Roberts, T., Jensen, H., and Unnevehr, L., eds. Tracking foodborne pathogens from farm to table: data needs to evaluate control options. USDA ERS Miscellaneous Publication. Washington, DC: U.S. Department of Agriculture.

McDowell, R.M., and McElvaine, M.D. 1997. Long-term sequelae to foodborne disease. In: Ahl, A., and Sutmoller, P., eds. Food safety special issue. Sci. Tech. Rev. OIE 16:337–341.

Mishu, B., Koehler, J., Lee, L.A., Rodrigue, D., Brenner, F.H., Blake, P., and Tauxe, R.V. 1994. Outbreaks of *Salmonella enteritidis* infections in the United States, 1985–1991. J. Infect. Dis. 169:547–552.

Morales, R.A. 1995. Equilibrium welfare analysis of food safety regulation: the case of *Salmonella enteritidis* in eggs (Ph.D. dissertation). Raleigh: Department of Agricultural and Resource Economics, North Carolina State University.

Morales, R.A. 1996. Farm-level costs for control of *Salmonella enteritidis* in laying flocks. In: Caswell, J.A., ed. The economics of reducing health risk from food. Storrs: University of Connecticut Press.

Morales, R.A. 1997a. The effect of media information regarding *Salmonella enteritidis* on the demand for shell eggs and pasteurized egg products. Epidemiol. Sante Anim. 31–32:10.08.1–10.08.3.

Morales, R.A. 1997b. The use of equilibrium welfare analysis for evaluating the industry effects of disease control programs with applications to *Salmonella enteritidis* in eggs. Epidemiol. Sante Anim. 31–32:10.07.1–10.07.3.

Noordhuizen, J.P., and Frankena, K. 1994. *Salmonella enteritidis*: clinical epidemiological approaches for prevention and control of *S. Enteritidis* in poultry production. Int. J. Food Microbiol. 21:131–143.

Poppe, C. 1994. *Salmonella enteritidis* in Canada. Int. J. Food Microbiol. 21:1–5.

Roberts, J.A., and Sockett, P.N. 1994. The socio-economic impact of human *Salmonella enteritidis* infection. Int. J. Food Microbiol. 21:117–129.

Roberts, T. 1989. Human illness costs of foodborne bacteria. Am. J. Agric. Econ. 71:468–474.

Roberts, T., Morales, R.A., Lin, C.-T.J., Caswell, J.A., and Hooker, N.H. 1997. Worldwide opportunities to market food safety. In: Wallace, T., and Schroder, W., eds. Perspectives on food industry/government linkages. Hingham, MA: Kluwer Academic.

Rodrigue, D.C., Tauxe, R.V., and Rowe, B. 1990. International increase in *Salmonella enteritidis*: a new pandemic? Epidemiol. Infect. 105:21–27.

Shivaprasad, H.L., Timoney, J.F., Morales, S., Lucio, B., and Baker, R.C. 1990. Pathogenesis of *Salmonella enteritidis* infection in laying chickens. I. Studies on egg transmission, clinical signs, fecal shedding, and serologic responses. Avian Dis. 34:548–557.

Smith, J.L. 1994. Arthritis and foodborne bacteria. J. Food Prot. 57:935–941.

Smith, J.L., Palumbo, S.A., and Walls, I. 1993. Relationship between foodborne bacterial pathogens and the reactive arthritis. J. Food Saf. 13:209–236.

St. Louis, M.E., Morse, D.L., Potter, M.E., DeMelfi, T.M., Guzewich, J.J., Tauxe, R.V., and Blake, P.A. 1988. The emergence of grade A eggs as a major source of *Salmonella enteritidis* infections: new implications for the control of salmonellosis. JAMA 259:2103–2107.

Tauxe, R.V. 1996. An update on *Salmonella*. Health Environ. Digest 10:1–4.

Tauxe, R.V. 1997. The continuing challenge of *Salmonella* Enteritidis infections in the United States: a public health perspective. Paper presented at the Joint FDA/FSIS shell eggs and egg products risk assessment technical meeting, Arlington, VA, 3 September 1997.

Todd, E.C.D. 1989a. Preliminary estimates of costs of foodborne disease in Canada and costs to reduce salmonellosis. J. Food Prot. 52:586–594.

Todd, E.C.D. 1989b. Preliminary estimates of costs of foodborne disease in the United States. J. Food Prot. 52:595–601.

van de Giessen, A.W., Ament, A.J.H.A., and Notermans, S.H.W. 1994. Intervention strategies for *Salmonella enteritidis* in poultry flocks: a basic approach. Int. J. Food Microbiol. 21:145–154.

Vugia, D.J., Mishu, B., Smith, M., Travis, D.R., Hickman-Brenner, F.W., and Tauxe, R.V. 1993. *Salmonella enteritidis* outbreak in a restaurant chain: the continuing challenges of prevention. Epidemiol. Infect. 110:49–61.

White, P.D., Schlosser, W., Benson, C.E., Maddox, C., and Hogue, A. 1997. Environmental survey by manure drag sampling for *Salmonella enteritidis* in chicken layer houses. J. Food Prot. 60:1189–1193.

26

Control of *Salmonella enterica* Serovar Enteritidis in Sweden

A. Engvall and Y. Anderson

INTRODUCTION

The salmonella control programs in Sweden have gained considerable international interest in recent decades, especially since the pandemic spread of *Salmonella enterica* serovar Enteritidis (*S.* Enteritidis) began (Watson, 1976; Wierup, 1992; Anon., 1994; Bögel, 1994; Wierup et al., 1995b). The present programs involve different parts of the pre-meat-harvesting and post-meat-harvesting industry. The latest changes in the programs have been due to the Swedish accession to the European Union (EU). In addition to programs in the animal sector, control of the spread of salmonellae is based on close cooperation between authorities in the human health, food, and veterinary fields. Sweden thus has a long tradition of controlling salmonellae in food-producing animals but also of surveillance of salmonellae in humans and the follow-up of infected persons. These precautions have led to Sweden having a very low number of indigenous salmonellosis cases, including *S.* Enteritidis, in humans. *Salmonella* Enteritidis has not gained access to the Swedish poultry industry, mainly because of measures taken within the framework of the control programs that have included all salmonella serovars, thereby preventing the introduction of new emerging serovars.

LAWS, REGULATIONS, AND CONTROL PROGRAMS

Since 1874, Sweden has had laws regulating measures to prevent the spread of infectious diseases. Clinical reporting of salmonellosis in humans started in 1875 (Anderson et al., 1994). Since 1946, typhoid fever and, since 1965, paratyphoid fever and salmonellosis have been reported

separately. New legislation introduced in 1968 classified salmonellosis as a serious infectious disease and detailed rules for notification, record keeping, and prophylactic measures were laid down. In the latest legislation (dated 1988), many of these measures are still intact.

According to the Swedish food act of 1971, salmonella-contaminated food is considered unfit for human consumption and will be destroyed. In the veterinary field, the first laws for salmonella control were adopted in 1961. A large salmonella outbreak in 1953–54, involving more than 9000 people and causing the death of more than 90 persons, had demonstrated the need for better control (Lundbeck et al., 1955). The outbreak, which was caused by *Salmonella* Typhimurium, originated in a slaughterhouse in Alvesta in the south of Sweden and spread through contaminated meat products. It is one of the largest salmonella outbreaks ever reported and spurred new legislation in both the human health and the veterinary fields.

In 1983, laws were adopted that, for example, made bacteriological testing of broiler flocks compulsory. In recent years, legislation has been modified, mainly due to the Swedish accession to the EU.

Common principles of the control programs for animals have been reviewed by Wierup (1994), Wierup and Nordblom (1985), and Wierup et al. (1992a, 1995). Those principles were mainly introduced in the salmonellosis act of 1961 and are essentially still intact. They involve, for instance, mandatory notification by veterinary laboratories of all salmonella isolations; confirmation and serotyping of all salmonella isolates from animals, food, and feedstuffs, and phage typing of *Salmonella* serovars Typhimurium and Enteritidis; testing schemes and rules for feed hygiene and biosecurity, especially for poultry; and official investigations of holdings or farms found infected and restrictions put on such establishments until they are considered salmonella free. Additionally, apart from the broiler sector, the government also pays compensation to animal owners for actions taken as a result of regulations.

POULTRY

Structure of the Poultry Industry

Production of poultry is concentrated in the south of Sweden. The broiler production has increased in recent years. In 1960, a total of 3 million broilers were produced, as compared with 60 million in 1996. There are approximately 150 establishments for broiler production producing approximately 3500 flocks for slaughter annually in Sweden. The turkey, duck, and geese industry is very small. There are roughly 10,000 farms holding 6 million laying hens. More than 80% of layers are kept in 300 farms with more than 5000 hens each.

The broiler and layer industries are strictly organized with breeding pyramids, similar to the situation in other countries with a developed poultry industry. All grandparent birds are imported as day-old chicks and quarantined. Practically all parent birds and all production birds are hatched in domestic hatcheries.

CONTROL OF MEAT-PRODUCING POULTRY

In 1970, governmental regulations introducing a voluntary program for controlling salmonellae, primarily in the broiler sector, were instituted (Lindgren, 1973). The program contained important control points (Lindgren et al., 1980; Svedberg, 1983, 1988; Wierup and Nordblom, 1985), such as

- Production stock must originate from parent birds participating in the control program.
- Hatcheries from which birds originate must participate.
- Feed given to birds must be heat treated.
- Biosecurity at the farm level should be strengthened and standardized.
- Rules for bacteriological testing of breeder and production flocks were introduced.
- All flocks are to be supervised by an official veterinarian.

Earlier regulations stipulating the compulsory destruction of all flocks found to be salmonella positive were still in force, and animal owners were economically compensated. All breeding flocks were included, and approximately 90% of all broiler producers joined the program.

In 1984, mandatory bacteriological testing of broiler and other meat-producing poultry flocks was started, while other parts still were voluntary. Economic compensation was also changed. Governmental reimbursements were removed, and producers had to buy insurance to cover the risk. Because insurance companies demanded that producers must join the voluntary program in order to be able to insure a flock, affiliation rates were very high.

In 1992, the regulations were relaxed to allow feeding of broilers with non-heat-treated wheat, if it was handled and stored under hygienic conditions.

In 1994, testing of breeder flocks and hatcheries was made mandatory. Present testing schemes for breeder and production flocks are outlined in Tables 26.1 and 26.2, respectively.

After accession to the EU, programs for poultry (including layer) breeding flocks were defined and adjusted according to Council Directives 90/539/EEC and 92/117/EEC. Programs were also amended in accordance with Commission Decision 95/50 (Anon., 1995) in order to be able to document clearly the salmonella situation at the postharvest stage. At slaughterhouses, poultry neck skins are sampled. The testing schemes introduced are outlined in Tables 26.3 and 26.4.

RESULTS AND FINDINGS

The numbers of notified salmonella-infected flocks of meat-producing poultry in 1968–96 are shown in Figure 26.1.

During 1972–79, a yearly mean of 38,681 birds was investigated within the frame of the program for broilers, turkeys, ducks, and geese, and, altogether, 171, 22, and 10 salmonella-positive flocks were found, respectively. Only in one broiler flock was S. Enteritidis isolated. An investigation in 1975 at the eight largest poultry-processing plants, comprising samples from 3480 broilers, revealed 15 positive samples from one plant, indicating a prevalence of contaminated birds well under 1% (Svedberg, 1988).

An investigation in 1990 (Wahlström et al., 1994) showed that of 2730 broilers sampled, 0.7% were salmonella positive: serovars Livingstone, Infantis, Orion, and Anatum were found.

Results of the control program for breeder and production flocks for 1995–96 are outlined in Table 26.5 (Anon., 1996, 1997). In 1996, S. Enteritidis phage type 4 (PT4) was found in four backyard flocks of geese. Infection was traced to a small hatchery.

CONTROL OF COMMERCIAL LAYERS

The control among layers has been reviewed by Engström and Wierup (1989) and Wierup et al. (1995a). The voluntary program introduced in 1970 also covered layers. Very few producers remained in the program, though, mainly because of high costs, and only one breeding company was affiliated. Because of the increasing awareness of the international S. Enteritidis situation, action was taken in 1988–89. Hatcheries, breeder flocks, and eggs delivered to four plants producing pasteurized egg powder were tested for the presence of salmonellae. Breeding flocks and hatcheries were found to be salmonella free. Of 381 pools of egg yolks and whole eggs investigated, salmonellae were found in 18 (4.7%). The following serovars were found: Typhimurium, Haifa, Mons, and Livingstone.

The results of the study motivated the industry to initiate a testing program for layers, which was introduced in 1991. Each layer flock had to be tested before slaughter. Three samples, each consisting of 30 fresh fecal droppings, were investigated from each flock. In 1991, approximately 5% of flocks were found to be infected; in 1992, 2% were found to be infected; and, in 1993, less than 1% were found to be infected (Wierup et al., 1995a). In 1994, testing of breeder flocks, hatcheries (Table 26.1), and commercial layer flocks was made mandatory.

A modified voluntary control program specially adapted for layers was introduced during 1993–95. This

TABLE 26.1   Sampling scheme for flocks of breeders of layers, broilers, turkeys, ducks, and geese and for hatcheries

Category	Sampling occasion[a]	No. of samples from birds[b]	No. of fecal samples[c]
Flocks			
Elite and grandparents			
Rearing	Day old	All dead birds	Samples from 10 internal linings of the chicken boxes
	1–2, 4, 9–11, and 2 weeks before moving/start of laying	10 dead birds	60
Egg production	Once a month, last sample 2 weeks before slaughter		60
Parents			
Rearing	Day old	10 dead birds	Samples from 10 internal linings of the chicken boxes
	4 and 2 weeks before moving/start of laying	10 dead birds	60
Egg production			
Hatchery capacity >1000[d]	Once a month, last sample 2 weeks before slaughter		60
Hatchery capacity <1000[d]	Every 2 weeks		60
Hatchery			
Capacity >1000[d]	Every 2 weeks from each parent group		One sample of meconium pooled from 250 chicks

[a]Age of birds is in weeks unless otherwise indicated.
[b]The cecum is removed from dead or killed chicks. Ceca from 10 birds are collected to form a pooled sample.
[c]Fresh fecal samples with cecal droppings are collected; 30 fecal samples constitute one pooled sample to be examined at the laboratory.
[d]Chickens per year.

TABLE 26.2   Sampling scheme for poultry flocks for meat production

Meat-producing poultry	Sampling occasion	No. of samples from birds[a]	No. of fecal samples[b]
Broilers	1–2 weeks before slaughter	30	30
Broilers (<500 birds per poultry pen)	1–2 weeks before slaughter	10	60
Turkeys, ducks, and geese	1–2 weeks before slaughter	5	60
Divided slaughter[c]	1–2 weeks before slaughter		90

[a]The cecum is removed from dead or killed chicks. Ceca from 10 birds are collected to form a pooled sample.
[b]Fresh fecal samples with cecal droppings are collected; 30 fecal samples constitute one pooled sample to be examined at the laboratory.
[c]If part of a flock is slaughtered at a later time, only fecal samples are taken, 1–2 weeks before slaughter of that part.

TABLE 26.3   Sampling scheme of poultry at slaughterhouses

Place of sampling	Sample	Sampling	Annual no. of samples
All major slaughterhouses[a]	Neck skin	Daily sampling	≥3000
All minor slaughterhouses[b]	Neck skin	—	60

[a]Annual slaughter of >150,000 poultry per slaughterhouse.
[b]Annual slaughter of <150,000 poultry per slaughterhouse.

TABLE 26.4   Sampling scheme for poultry meat, beef, and pork at cutting plants

Capacity in tons of plant (per week)	Sample	Sampling	Number of samples in 1996	
			Beef/pork	Poultry meat
>100	Meat, scrapings	Daily		
>20 to <100	Meat, scrapings	Weekly	5510	581
>5 to <20	Meat, scrapings	Monthly		
<5	Meat, scrapings	Biannually		

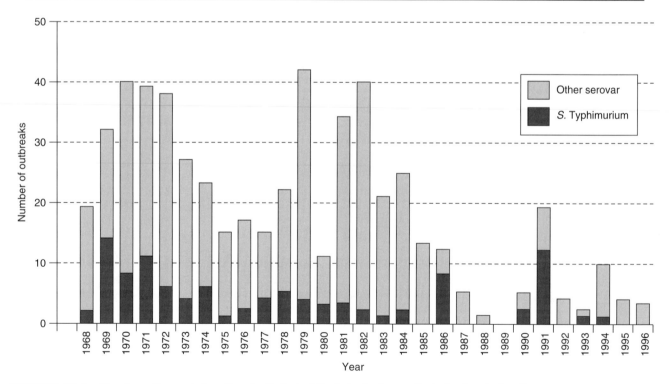

FIGURE 26.1   Number of reported outbreaks (infected flocks) of salmonella infection in broilers.

TABLE 26.5   Findings of salmonella in the Swedish salmonella control program for poultry, 1995–96

Year	Grandparent flocks					Parent flocks					Production flocks					Single animals tested at slaughter (mainly broilers)
	Layers	Broilers	Turkeys	Ducks	Geese	Layers	Broilers	Turkeys	Ducks	Geese	Layers	Broilers	Turkeys	Ducks	Geese	
1995	6/0[1]	7/0	—	—	—	24/0	77/0	17/0	4/0	3/0	2350/10[2]	3727/4[3]	39/1[4]	—	—	2778/2[9]
1996	6/0	11/0	—	—	—	33/0	116/0	?/0	?/0	?/0	800/6[5]	3300/4[6]	62/0	?/1[7]	?/7[8]	3922/2[10]

[1]Number of flocks examined through number of salmonella-positive flocks.
[2]Serovars Livingstone, Infantis, Mbandaka, Cubana, and Enteritidis (one flock).
[3]Serovars Livingstone, Bovis-morbificans, and Infantis.
[4]Serovar Mbandaka.
[5]Serovars Livingstone, Mbandaka, and subspecies 1 (6, 7:d).
[6]Serovars Havana, Livingstone, and Newport.
[7]Serovar Typhimurium.
[8]Serovars Enteritidis (four flocks) and Muenster.
[9]Serovars Livingstone and Infantis (layers).
[10]Serovar Livingstone (layers).

involved, for example, building standards, hygienic standards, biosecurity measures, and mandatory heat treatment of all feed except on-farm-produced grain, handled and stored under hygienic conditions. Affiliation with this program is at present much lower than with the broiler control program. In 1995, testing schemes for layer flocks were slightly modified as outlined in Table 26.6.

RESULTS AND FINDINGS

The total number of flocks found to be infected with *S.* Enteritidis and other salmonella serovars is shown in Figure 26.2. *Salmonella* Enteritidis has never been found in breeder flocks or at hatcheries. Altogether, *S.* Enteritidis has been found in seven layer flocks since 1987 (Wierup et al., 1995a). In five flocks, PT4 has been isolated and, in one flock each, PT1 and PT6.

Measures If Salmonellae Are Isolated

When an infected flock is found, the establishment has always been placed under restrictions and an official investigation performed with the aim of finding sources of infection and clearing the infection from the flocks as quickly as possible.

Infected breeding flocks have always been destroyed, irrespective of the serovar isolated. Before 1982, all infected broiler flocks were destroyed. Beginning in 1982, a new system was introduced, which implied that flocks infected with *S.* Typhimurium were still to be destroyed, but a second investigation was made if other serovars were found. Depending on the prevalence found, different procedures were followed (Engström and Wierup, 1989). Since 1991, all salmonella-infected flocks of meat-producing poultry found have been destroyed, irrespective of serovar, based on decisions by the competent authority.

TABLE 26.6   Sampling scheme for layer flocks (table-egg production)

Laying hens	Sampling occasion[a]	No. of fecal samples[b]
Rearing of pullets[c]	2 weeks before transport to a laying unit	90
Egg production	25–30, 50, and 3–4 weeks before slaughter	90
Egg production (floor production or <1000 birds/poultry pen)	25–30, 50, and 3–4 weeks before slaughter	60

[a]Age of birds is in weeks unless otherwise indicated.
[b]Fresh fecal samples with cecal droppings are collected; 30 fecal samples constitute one pooled sample to be examined at the laboratory.
[c]Flocks comprising more than 200 birds.

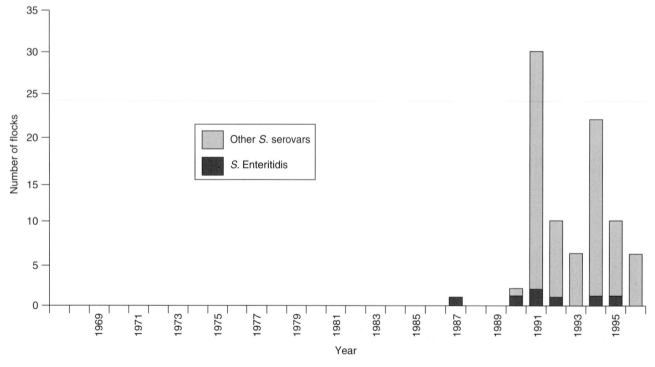

FIGURE 26.2   Number of reported outbreaks (infected flocks) of salmonella infection in layers. From the Swedish Board of Agriculture.

In layers, findings of salmonellae were extremely rare before 1990. In 1990, rules were applied that differentiated *S.* Enteritidis from other serovars. If *S.* Enteritidis was found, the flock was immediately destroyed. If other serovars were isolated, the flock was allowed to produce eggs during its productive period. After accession to the EU, the regulations have been changed. The finding of so-called invasive serovars, according to the Scientific Veterinary Committee Opinion of 10 June 1994 (Gallinarum, Pullorum, Enteritidis, Berta, Typhimurium, Thompson, Infantis), will always lead to the immediate destruction of a flock. The finding of other serovars means that eggs can be delivered only to egg-powder plants for pasteurization and that the flock is eventually destroyed or sanitarily slaughtered.

After the slaughter or destruction of infected poultry flocks, the establishments are cleaned and disinfected under official supervision. Environmental samples are taken to verify the results of cleaning and disinfection. Restrictions are lifted when the holding is considered free of salmonella contamination. In addition, the two consecutive broiler flocks raised in units where salmonellae have been found must be treated with competitive exclusion using Broilact (Pivnick and Nurmi, 1982; Wierup et al., 1988, 1992b).

The cost of the poultry programs has been calculated by Lindgren et al. (1980), Wierup and Nordblom (1985), and Engvall et al. (1994).

CATTLE, SWINE, AND SHEEP

Control Program

In food-producing animals other than poultry, regular testing programs in herds or flocks have not been used. However, basic parts of the program (such as clinical observations in the field, autopsies, compulsory bacteriological examinations of all animals that are sanitarily slaughtered, and compulsory notification of and restrictions imposed on infected farms) prevail also for these species (Wierup, 1994; Wierup et al., 1995a). When Sweden acceded to the EU, a testing scheme for cattle and swine was introduced so that the country had additional guarantees regarding salmonellae when importing live animals and animal products, because the salmonella status in Sweden had to be

documented. The program is detailed in Commission Decision 95/50 (Anon., 1995).

Sheep are not part of a regular testing scheme in herds or at slaughter, but should salmonellae be found, actions are taken. Investigations performed on sanitarily slaughtered swine, sheep, and cattle at normal slaughter in 1975 and 1990–92 showed a salmonella prevalence of less than 1% (Robertsson, 1976; Wahlström et al., 1994). No *S.* Enteritidis isolates were found in cattle, swine, or sheep in 1995–96.

Measures If Salmonellae Are Isolated

If salmonellae are found, the farm of origin is placed under restrictions. Official investigations are conducted, including animal sampling. Animal movements are also restricted. Restrictions are lifted after cleanup and disinfection and when the property is considered salmonella free. Two consecutive whole-herd tests with normal results need to be performed before restrictions are lifted.

Feed Control

The control of feed, including import and production control, has been detailed by Engström and Wierup (1989) and by Häggblom (1994, 1996).

The monitoring of animal feed had already begun in the late 1940s. In 1958, the major feed companies in Sweden formed the Association of Veterinary Feed Control (AVFC). Until 1993, almost all feed for livestock was monitored for salmonellae by the AVFC.

The import of finished feed for cloven-hoofed animals or raw materials containing animal products has to be licensed by authorities and the material examined for salmonellae. Also, imported raw materials of vegetable origin, such as rapeseed meal and soybean meal, are tested for salmonellae before the products can be used by the feed industry. An extensive hygiene and testing program for feed factories has been operational for several years. In 1991, the testing program, which was earlier an end-product control, changed to a hazard-analysis critical control point (HACCP) system. The number of positive samples increased in connection with this change.

Table 26.7 shows the number of samples and salmonella findings in feed raw materials of animal origin intended for

TABLE 26.7   Number of samples taken and findings of salmonella and of *Salmonella* Enteritidis in connection with the import control of feedstuff of animal origin in Sweden, 1963–92

	Time period					
	1963–67	**1968–72**	**1973–77**	**1978–82**	**1983–87**	**1988–92**
No. of samples	42,502	39,480	10,483	6234	12,243	18,930
No. of salmonella isolates	482	356	67	67	238	363
	1%	1%	0.6%	1%	2%	2%
No. of *S.* Enteritidis isolates	0	0	0	0	0	1[a]

[a]Feather meal.

import to Sweden in 1963–92. *Salmonella* Enteritidis was not found in imported or domestically produced feedstuffs in 1995 or 1996 (Anon., 1996, 1997). It is obvious from these results that raw feed materials are not a significant source of *S.* Enteritidis infection in animals.

Import Control of Animals

Until the Swedish accession to the EU, cattle, swine, and sheep intended for import to Sweden were not regularly examined for salmonellae. Very few animals were imported, though. After the accession, cattle and swine not included in the salmonella control programs, including imported animals, are examined for salmonellae before being moved into a controlled herd.

Since the introduction of salmonella control, imported poultry have been quarantined and examined for salmonellae. Importation has mainly been restricted to breeding animals, especially grandparent flocks (Engström and Wierup, 1989). Wierup et al. (1995a) showed that between 1982 and 1992, among 124 imported grandparent flocks, 18 (14.5%) were found to be salmonella positive when examined in quarantine. No *S.* Enteritidis was found. All infected flocks were destroyed. The control of imported poultry is the main reason why *S.* Enteritidis has not gained access to the Swedish poultry-breeding pyramid.

After accession to the EU, Sweden retained the required testing for the presence of salmonellae in commercial poultry flocks due to be imported, provided they had not been included in a control program considered equivalent to the Swedish one. When intended for import from other EU countries, layers may be tested for invasive serovars, and breeder flocks and day-old chicks of production flocks may be tested for all serovars, in accordance with Commission Decisions 95/160 and 95/161.

Import Control of Food

The import control system before the Swedish accession to the EU has been described by Stenson (1994). Essentially non-heat-treated meat and meat products had to be examined before import, except for those from a few countries (such as Norway, Finland, and Iceland) considered to have very good salmonella control programs. Samples were taken according to the number of packages in the consignments. Initially, consignments not contaminated with *S.* Typhimurium or having less than 5% of samples positive for other salmonella serovars were allowed to be imported. This system was changed in 1993. In the new system, enough samples (n = 60) are collected to detect a 5% prevalence of salmonellae, with 90%–99% confidence (the confidence level depends on the size of the imported consignments). If salmonellae are found, the consignment is rejected. After the accession to the EU, the system still applies for import from Third-World countries. The import of table eggs, poultry meat, pork, and beef from EU countries is limited by additional guarantees, whereas other meat and meat products can be imported without testing. Additional guarantees mean that consignments are tested in the establishment of origin before export to Sweden, provided they do not come from an establishment

included in a control program considered equivalent to the Swedish one.

During 1988–92, *S.* Enteritidis was found in 51 consignments of meat intended for export to Sweden from 12 countries (Wierup et al., 1995a).

SALMONELLA FINDINGS IN 1947–92

Statistics regarding findings of salmonellae in animals and feedstuffs have been published regularly (Karlsson et al., 1963; Hurvell et al., 1969; Gunnarsson et al., 1974; Sandstedt et al., 1980; Mårtensson et al., 1984; Eld et al., 1991; Malmqvist et al., 1995). Table 26.8 lists the total number of isolates of salmonella strains and *S.* Enteritidis for 1963–92. Table 26.9 presents numbers, for the same period, of all isolates from animals, where *S.* Enteritidis has been isolated at least once. Findings of *S.* Enteritidis in wild animals during 1947–85 are summarized in Table 26.10 (Borg, 1985).

THE HUMAN SITUATION

The number of cases of human salmonella infection reported by laboratories in Sweden was about 5000 a year between 1986 and 1994, with a decrease in 1995 to 3659 and a small increase in 1996 to 4098. The total incidence was about 50 cases per 100,000 inhabitants. Approximately 50% of the reported cases were caused by *S.* Enteritidis. In the last decade, in about 85% of the reported cases, the infected individuals contracted the infection while abroad (Fig. 26.3). The reported indigenous cases are normally around 400–800 each year, and the indigenous incidence is 8–10 cases per 100,000 inhabitants.

CONTROL OF SALMONELLAE

The National Food Administration is supposed to be notified of any known foodborne disease outbreak in the country by environmental and public health local boards and medical and veterinary officers. Salmonella-infected individuals are reported if they are found to be infected when tested (see the following section: *Definition of a Human Case*).

Reported outbreaks and individual cases of salmonellosis are investigated to identify sources of infection. If food or animals are incriminated or suspected as the sources, extended investigations are conducted. Close cooperation between veterinary, food, and human-health authorities is essential in finding and eliminating the sources. Such cooperation has often proven successful in tracing and controlling indigenous salmonellae, as when a sudden increase in human cases of indigenous *S.* Enteritidis PT4 was observed. The investigation quickly led to an *S.* Enteritidis–infected poultry farm being identified and the flock being destroyed.

TABLE 26.8 Total number of serotyped salmonella isolates and *Salmonella* Enteritidis isolates from animals in Sweden, 1963–92

	Time period					
	1963–67	1968–72	1973–77	1978–82	1983–87	1988–92
No. of salmonella isolates	835	1746	1106	1266	760	602
No. of S. Enteritidis isolates	8	22	9	7	0	9
%	1	1.3	0.8	0.6	0	1.5

TABLE 26.9 Total number of isolates of *Salmonella* Enteritidis and total number of salmonella isolates in Sweden according to animal species, 1963–92

Species	No. of S. Enteritidis isolates	Total no. of isolates
Cattle	21	2681
Swine	5	393
Horse	1	84
Hen and chicken	5	729
Geese and duck	1	59
Wild bird	3	1269
Monkey	1	15
Dog	1	151
Cat	3	52
Seal	1	2
Chinchilla	1	2
Cage bird	2	134
Hedgehog	4	4
Reptile	1	396
Zoo animal	1	12
Mouse and rat	3	10
Total	54	5993

TABLE 26.10 Investigations of wild animals in Sweden, 1947–82

Species	No. of animals investigated	Total no. of salmonella isolates	S. Enteritidis isolates
Fox (*Vulpes vulpes*)	2452	34	4
Hare (serovar *Lepus*)	7864	11	0
Seagull (serovar *Larus*)	892	28	0
Bird of prey	2645	29	1
Crow (serovar *Corvus*)	820	0	0
Various birds	4009	35	2
Passerines	2495	938[a]	—

[a]Only *S.* Typhimurium isolates. Data regarding other serovars are not available.

DEFINITION OF A HUMAN CASE

A human case of salmonella infection is defined as a case where salmonellae have been isolated from fecal or other samples from a person, irrespective of whether clinical symptoms have been noticed. Suspected cases of salmonellae will be confirmed by the laboratory investigation. Normally, all human strains will be serotyped and, for *S.* Enteritidis and *S.* Typhimurium, also phage typed.

A case is defined as indigenous even if the source of infection is imported or the case is secondary to a patient who has contracted the infection abroad. Cases from ferries flying the Swedish flag are also reported as domestic, even if the food is foreign and has not been inspected according to Swedish law. This means that the number of truly domestic cases is even lower than that shown in figures and tables.

A case is defined as infected abroad if the person became sick during the trip abroad or during the first days after returning to Sweden. Suspected foodborne infections on airplanes are also investigated. Certain risk groups are tested when returning from abroad. Such persons found to be infected are defined as cases having contracted the infection abroad, even though clinical symptoms may be absent. For

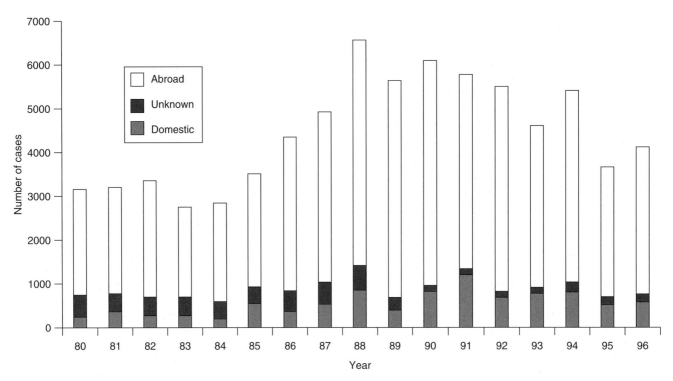

FIGURE 26.3   Number of laboratory-reported cases of salmonella infection in humans: indigenous and infected abroad, 1980–96.

example, until 1 January 1997, it was mandatory for food handlers to submit a feces sample for the investigation of salmonella/shigella after being abroad (outside the Nordic countries) for more than 5 days.

The sampling of risk groups who have been abroad and the willingness to see a family doctor if you suspect a disease from abroad, as well as the attitude of physicians about taking samples from sick persons returning from holidays in foreign countries, are probably important reasons why so many cases coming from abroad are reported.

DIFFERENT SEROVARS

About 130 different serovars are reported in Sweden each year. About 20 are common in Sweden and, generally, the same serovars prevail each year. The number of cases and the two most frequently reported serovars are shown in Figure 26.4. *Salmonella* Typhimurium was the most common serovar at the beginning of 1980. Since 1985, *S.* Enteritidis has predominated. This has mostly been due to the spread of *S.* Enteritidis in eggs and chickens in Europe (Schmidt, 1995).

THE *SALMONELLA* ENTERITIDIS SITUATION BEFORE 1980

After the large salmonella outbreak in 1953, the epidemiological surveillance of communicable diseases was reor-

ganized and the Department of Epidemiology was started at the National Bacteriological Institute, now the Swedish Institute for Infectious Disease Control. In the beginning, the department took great interest in investigating outbreaks on the spot, before the local authorities were organized in a better way.

Between 1953 and 1979, a total of 11 foodborne outbreaks of *S.* Enteritidis were reported, with a total of more than 4500 cases. Infection sources of different types have been involved, such as chickens, farm cattle, cured meats, and provisions, but on several occasions the source of infection has been unknown. During this period, two large foodborne outbreaks were reported:

Outbreak 1

In the latter part of August 1976, people ferrying between Gothenburg in Sweden and Fredrikshamn in Denmark contracted salmonellosis. The ferry staff also fell sick. Among the kitchen staff, 12 of 22 were positive for salmonellae and at least five were carriers. About 8000 people traveled on that ferry on the days concerned, and 7000 meals were served. During the investigation of the outbreak, 150 food samples were taken. Salmonellae were isolated from different food items, both from raw and from prepared food. This showed that the standard of food hygiene had been low, and that cross-contamination was possible. Among other things, the same cutting boards had been used for cutting both raw meat and prepared food (Böttiger et al., 1977).

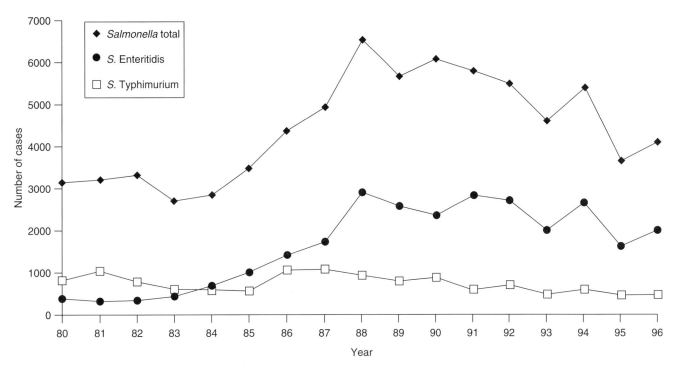

FIGURE 26.4   Number of laboratory-reported cases of salmonella infection and the two most commonly found serovars in humans, 1980–96.

Outbreak 2

In October 1977, a large outbreak caused by *S.* Enteritidis PT4 that occurred in Tensta, a suburb of Stockholm, emanated from a large canteen handling food for 28 schools in that part of Stockholm. The day before the outbreak started, they served fish and remoulade sauce. Mustard dressing also had been served before the outbreak, and mayonnaise was a major ingredient in that, as well. *Salmonella* Enteritidis was isolated from the remoulade sauce, which was prepared from fresh eggs the day before the food was served. About 3000 persons, mostly schoolchildren and their teachers, contracted the disease, and the attack rate was about 30% (Hellström, 1980). Of these persons, 80% were between 7 and 16 years of age, and 25% were asymptomatic carriers. It appeared that 6% of the cases were secondary. Of the sick persons, 80 were hospitalized, but none died.

SALMONELLA ENTERITIDIS IN SWEDEN SINCE 1980

Table 26.11 shows the number of laboratory-reported cases of *S.* Enteritidis divided into indigenous cases and cases infected abroad. It is clear that the number of cases infected abroad closely follows the changes in the total number of reported cases during different years. The total number of *S.* Enteritidis cases has been rather stable since 1988 (2886), except for decreases in 1993 and 1995. There is no good explanation for these changes, but a change in traveling habits may be one explanation, because most cases are con-

tracted abroad. A decrease in *S.* Enteritidis has also been observed in some other European countries during 1993–95 (Fisher, 1997). This decrease may be a result of new control measures being adopted or of more hygienic handling of food, especially raw eggs (Schmidt, 1995).

The number of reported indigenous cases has been low for a long time (normally about 100–200 cases have been reported each year). No increase in indigenous cases of *S.* Enteritidis was seen in Sweden until 1991, when 486 cases were reported (Table 26.11). In 1989, only 3.5% of *S.* Enteritidis cases were indigenous, but the percentage increased during 1991 to 17.2%. This increase was due to several outbreaks of *S.* Enteritidis PT4 originating from a single poultry farm (see below).

OUTBREAKS FROM THE SAME SOURCE

The number of indigenous, reported cases of salmonellae increased during 1991. The increase in outbreaks and also in sporadic indigenous cases was due to the spread of *S.* Enteritidis PT4 in Sweden. Ten outbreaks of *S.* Enteritidis PT4 were reported. In two of the outbreaks, *S.* Enteritidis was also found in the food: in a pyramid cake (made of eggs and baked on a spit) and in an "American type of cheese cake." In the majority of the *S.* Enteritidis PT4 outbreaks, the patients recalled consuming eggs. The majority of the outbreaks and also the sporadic cases occurred in the south of Sweden. Two outbreaks and a few sporadic cases

TABLE 26.11   Number of laboratory-reported *Salmonella* Enteritidis cases: indigenous and infected abroad, 1987–96

Year	Total no. of cases	Indigenous		Infected abroad		Place of infection unknown	
		No.	%	No.	%	No.	%
1987	1712	97	5.7	1466	85.6	149	8.7
1988	2886	132	4.6	2555	88.5	199	6.9
1989	2537	88	3.5	2334	92.0	115	4.5
1990	2321	248	10.7	2041	88.0	32	1.3
1991	2824	486	17.2	2311	81.8	27	1.0
1992	2726	274	10.1	2404	88.2	48	1.7
1993	1973	145	7.3	1795	91.0	33	1.7
1994	2656	154	5.8	2439	91.8	63	2.4
1995	1594	124	7.8	1427	89.5	43	2.7
1996	2003	217	10.8	1736	86.7	50	2.5

occurred in the far north. This geographical distribution was a bit confusing, but the investigation revealed that the eggs in the north were generally produced in the south, since very few poultry farms are situated in the far north. The incriminated eggs were traced to one egg purveyor in the south of Sweden and further on to one suspect farm. Sampling from this farm showed that only 2% of samples (three samples) were positive for *S.* Enteritidis. This indicates how difficult it can be to identify an infected farm.

DISTRIBUTION OF *SALMONELLA* ENTERITIDIS CASES DURING THE YEAR

Most cases infected abroad appear in the summer months, when package tours are common. The increase in the number of cases starts in June and lasts until September or October. There is a delay in the figures because of the notification system. The reporting system is based on the day of report and not on the day of onset of clinical symptoms.

The number of indigenous cases increases slightly in the summer, but there are normally very few. One explanation may be that they are secondary cases that should increase as the number of reported cases infected abroad increases. There are normally no signs of an increased domestic threat of *S.* Enteritidis during any time of the year.

AGE AND SEX DISTRIBUTIONS OF THE CASES

Most cases are reported from persons who are 25–64 years of age, which generally means people traveling abroad. There is no difference in the number of cases, except for a slight increase in the number of women in the 45–64 age group. The domestic cases are very few, and no real difference is obvious in the different age groups. Figure 26.5 outlines the distribution according to age and sex for the year 1996.

OUTBREAKS OF *SALMONELLA* ENTERITIDIS

Though 50% of all salmonella cases reported in Sweden are due to *S.* Enteritidis, that serovar is not predominant among the indigenous cases. Generally, if there is an outbreak with any serovar, that serovar will predominate in that year.

There were only six outbreaks involving *S.* Enteritidis in 1980–89, with a total of 96 cases (Table 26.12). All of the outbreaks were rather small. The types of food involved were béarnaise sauce (two outbreaks) and salad (one outbreak). The source of infection was unknown in three outbreaks. In 1990–96, a total of 17 outbreaks was reported, 10 of them during 1991. Except for the outbreaks during 1991, where eggs were proven or suspected as the original source of infection, the immediate sources of infection were egg sauce, a fish dish, and shellfish; for the rest, the source of infection was unknown.

DIFFERENT PHAGE TYPES OF *SALMONELLA* ENTERITIDIS

Phage typing started in Sweden in 1990. The English phage-typing system is used (Ward et al., 1987). The most commonly found phage types that have been reported are, as in most other countries, *S.* Enteritidis PT4, but PT1, PT6a, and PT8 also are rather frequently reported. Swedish tourists travel particularly to the south of Europe and other countries around the Mediterranean Sea. Especially *S.* Enteritidis is contracted in the south of Europe, and particularly PT4 and PT6a. *Salmonella* Enteritidis PT1 is mostly seen in tourists returning from eastern Europe.

The rather high number of indigenous cases of *S.* Enteritidis PT6a reported in 1992 might be explained by a foodborne outbreak on a ferry. During 1996, indigenous cases of *S.* Enteritidis PT8 suddenly increased: at least 33 persons, mainly children, had contracted *S.* Enteritidis PT8 after contact with turtles. Table 26.13 shows the distribution of *S.* Enteritidis phage types isolated from persons in Sweden.

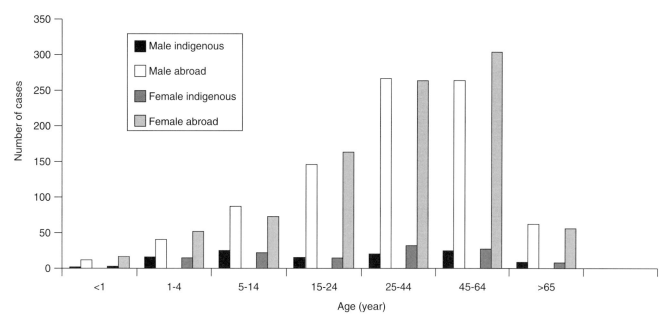

FIGURE 26.5 Total number of laboratory-reported *Salmonella* Enteritidis cases by age and sex: indigenous and infected abroad (including unknown cases), 1996.

TABLE 26.12 Total number of outbreaks in humans caused by salmonella and outbreaks due to *S.* Enteritidis, 1980–96

Year	S. Enteritidis		Other serovars	
	No. of outbreaks	No. of cases	No. of outbreaks	No. of cases
1980	—	—	7	68
1981	—	—	4	152
1982	—	—	7	218
1983	—	—	5	127
1984	—	—	4	114
1985	2	48	8	364
1986	1	16	6	421
1987	1	9	7	184
1988	2	23	8	345
1989	—	—	7	86
1990	2	157	10	440
1991	10	207	15	630
1992	3	118	7	181
1993	1	9	8	313
1994	—	—	2	336
1995	—	—	3	74
1996	1	14	8	73
Total	20	537	75	2662

TABLE 26.13 The most common phage type of *Salmonella* Enteritidis isolated from humans, 1992–96

Year	PT1	PT4	PT6	PT6a	PT8	PT13	PT14	PT21
1992	301 (28)[a]	1460 (56)	204 (22)	283 (91)	166 (26)	13	32 (2)	52 (2)
1993	213 (26)	1146 (61)	92 (4)	152 (14)	90 (22)	52	14 (1)	68 (1)
1994	224 (12)	1349 (75)	119 (4)	534 (16)	103 (16)	19 (4)	36 (11)	39 (2)
1995	135 (9)	840 (39)	63 (12)	248 (12)	91 (25)	9	13 (1)	19
1996	236 (12)	1000 (52)	95 (11)	185 (5)	196 (105)	44	35 (14)	15

[a]Number of domestic cases is in parentheses.

SUMMARY AND CONCLUSIONS

The total number of human S. Enteritidis infections in Sweden has increased in the last 15 years. Less than 15% of all cases are infected in the country, though. The incidence rate of indigenous S. Enteritidis infections in humans is 3–5 cases per 100,000 inhabitants in Sweden. This is a low figure compared with many other countries. Several factors have contributed to this: The salmonella control programs in animals have proven effective in controlling S. Enteritidis. Health authorities have always investigated known cases of salmonellosis in order to identify sources of infection. When such investigations have pointed to the involvement of animals or animal products, close cooperation between human-health and veterinary authorities have been initiated. In this way, tracing of human salmonellosis to domestic sources of infection has been efficient and has enabled rapid action, for example, in infected flocks. The extensive investigations of infected persons also provides an important standard against which the effectiveness of the salmonella control programs in animals can be measured.

Food is very seldom contaminated with S. Enteritidis in Sweden, thanks to stringent import control and the Swedish control programs. *Salmonella* Enteritidis has not been found in Swedish broiler flocks since 1972 and only in seven flocks of layers since 1987. In fact, S. Enteritidis has been more frequently isolated from cattle herds than from poultry flocks in Sweden. Two factors have probably been of great importance in keeping Swedish poultry practically free of S. Enteritidis: (a) the import control of grandparent chickens, which means that imported infected flocks are destroyed, irrespective of serovars found; and (b) the salmonella control programs include all salmonella serovars, thus preventing the proliferation of serovars that later may turn out to be of great significance to human health.

Salmonella enteritidis has, over the years, been isolated from several species of wild animals and birds. The significance of these infected species for the salmonella situation in domestic animals and humans seems to be limited.

In conclusion, because of the measures adopted, Swedish poultry production has so far not been involved in the pandemic spread of S. Enteritidis, and Swedish poultry meat and eggs can be considered practically free of S. Enteritidis. Other significant sources of infection do not seem to exist in Sweden and, as a result, S. Enteritidis does not constitute a significant domestic problem.

REFERENCES

Anderson, Y., de Jong, B., and Böttiger, M. 1994. The public health aspects of salmonellosis: the incidence and epidemiological surveillance at the national level. In: Öjeberg-Bengtsson, S., ed. NVI/WHO international course on salmonella control in animal production and products, Malmö, Sweden, August 21–27, 1993. Uppsala: National Veterinary Institute.

Anonymous. 1994. Control of food borne diseases in humans and animals: strategies and approaches at the animal production level—the Swedish salmonella control programme. WHO report 1994. WHO/Zoon/94.171. Geneva: WHO, pp. 1–73.

Anonymous. 1995. Report to the EEC Commission. 1995. Swedish salmonella control programmes for live animals, eggs and meat. Uppsala: National Veterinary Institute, Swedish Board of Agriculture and National Food Administration, pp. 1–47.

Anonymous. 1996. Report to the EEC Commission in accordance with EEC Directive 92/117: Swedish report to the commission concerning trends and sources of zoonotic infections recorded in Sweden during 1995. Uppsala: National Veterinary Institute, Swedish Board of Agriculture and National Food Administration, pp. 1–42.

Anonymous. 1997. Report to the EEC Commission in accordance with EEC Directive 92/117: Swedish report to the commission concerning trends and sources of zoonotic infections recorded in Sweden during 1996. Uppsala: National Veterinary Institute, Swedish Board of Agriculture and National Food Administration, pp. 1–51.

Bögel, K. 1994. The current international salmonella situation: availability and quality of surveillance data. In: Öjeberg-Bengtsson, S., ed. NVI/WHO international course on salmonella control in animal production and products, Malmö, Sweden, August 21–27, 1993. Uppsala: National Veterinary Institute.

Borg, K. 1985. Spread of infection through wild animals: account of 35 years' study. Sven. Vet. 37:111–128.

Böttiger, M., Hansson, T., and Malmvall, B.-E. 1977. Salmonella i sensommarvärme. Swed. Med. J. 74:3546–3551.

Eld, K., Gunnarsson, A., Holmberg, T., Hurvell, B., and Wierup, M. 1991. Salmonella isolated from animals and feedstuffs in Sweden during 1983–1987. Acta Vet. Scand. 32:261–277.

Engström, B., and Wierup, M. 1989. Salmonella control in poultry in Sweden. In: Report of WHO consultation on epidemiological emergency in poultry and egg salmonellosis, 20–23 March 1989. Geneva: World Health Organization.

Engvall, A., Anderson, Y., and Cerenius, F. 1994. The economics of the Swedish salmonella control: a cost/benefit analysis. In: Öjeberg-Bengtsson, S., ed. NVI/WHO international course on salmonella control in animal production and products, Malmö, Sweden, August 21–27, 1993. Uppsala: National Veterinary Institute.

Fisher, I. 1997. *Salmonella enteritidis* and S. typhimurium in Western Europe in 1993–1995: a surveillance report from Salmnet. Eurosurveillance 1:4–6.

Gunnarsson, A., Hurvell, B., Nordblom, B., Rutqvist, L., and Thal, E. 1974. Salmonella isolated from animals and feedstuffs in Sweden over the period 1968–1972. Nord. Vet. Med. 26:9, 499–517.

Häggblom, P. 1994. Monitoring and control of salmonella in animal feed. In: Öjeberg-Bengtsson, S., ed. NVI/WHO international course on salmonella control in animal production and products, Malmö, Sweden, August 21–27, 1993. Uppsala: National Veterinary Institute.

Häggblom, P. 1996. Control of salmonella in feedingstuffs. In: 47th annual meeting of the EAAP, Lillehammer, Norway, 25–29 August 1996.

Hellström, L. 1980. Food-transmitted S. *enteritidis* epidemic in 28 schools. In: Proceedings of world congress on foodborne infections and intoxications, West Berlin, pp. 1–20 and 397–400.

Hurvell, B., Lagerquist, U., Rutqvist, L., and Thal, E. 1969. Salmonella isolated from animals and feed stuffs in Sweden during 1963–1967. Nord. Vet. Med. 21:289–305.

Karlsson, K.A., Rutqvist, L., and Thal, E. 1963. Salmonella isolated from animals and animal feeds in Sweden during 1958–1962. Nord. Vet. Med. 15:833–850.

Lindgren, N.-O. 1973. Geflügel Salmonellose: ein Program für ihre Bekämpfung in Schweden. In: Fifth international congress of the World Veterinary Poultry Association, Munich, 1973, vol. 1, pp. 691–724.

Lindgren, N.-O., Sandstedt, K., and Nordblom, B. 1980. An evaluation of an avian salmonellosis control programme in Sweden. In: Sixth European Geflugelkonferenz, Hamburg, 8–12 September 1980, vol. 1, pp. 196–205.

Lundbeck, H., Plazikowski, U., and Silverstolpe, L. 1955. The Swedish salmonella outbreaks of 1953. J. Appl. Bacteriol. 18:535–548.

Malmqvist, M., Jacobsson, K.G., Häggblom, P., Cerenius, F., Sjöland, L., and Gunnarsson, A. 1995. Salmonella isolated from animals and feedstuffs in Sweden during 1988–1992. Acta Vet. Scand. 36:21–39.

Mårtensson, L., Holmberg, T., Hurvell, B., Rutqvist, L., Sandstedt, K., and Wierup, M. 1984. Salmonella isolated from animals and feed stuffs in Sweden during 1978–1982. Nord. Veterinaermed. 36:371–393.

Pivnick, H., and Nurmi, E. 1982. The Nurmi concept and its role in the control of salmonella in poultry. In: Davies, R., ed. Developments in food microbiology 1. Barking, UK: Applied Science, pp. 41–70.

Robertsson, J.-Å. 1976. Investigation of the frequency of salmonella infection in animals normally slaughtered in Sweden. Sven. Vet. 28:699–702.

Sandstedt, K., Gunnarsson, A., Hurvell, B., Nordblom, B., Rutqvist, L., and Söderlind, O. 1980. Salmonella isolated from animals and feed stuffs in Sweden during 1973–1977. Nord. Veterinaermed. 32:57–74.

Schmidt, K. 1995. WHO surveillance programme for control of foodborne infections and intoxications in Europe. In: Sixth report 1990–1992. Berlin: Federal Institute for Health Protection of Consumers and Veterinary Medicine (FAO/WHO Collaborating Centre for Research and Training in Food Hygiene).

Stenson, H. 1994. Import control. In: Öjeberg-Bengtsson, S., ed. NVI/WHO international course on salmonella control in animal production and products, Malmö, Sweden, August 21–27, 1993. Uppsala: National Veterinary Institute.

Svedberg, J. 1983. The Swedish salmonella control programme for broiler production: a method to detect infected birds before slaughter. In: Proceedings of the eighth international symposium of the world association of veterinary food hygienists, Dublin, 30th August–4th September 1981, pp. 53–55.

Svedberg, J. 1988. The Swedish salmonella control programme for broiler production: methods to detect infected birds before slaughter—environment and animal health. In: Ekesbo, I., ed. Proceedings of the sixth international congress on animal hygiene, 14–17 June 1988, Skara, Sweden, vol. 1, pp. 270–274.

Wahlström, H., Wierup, M., Olsson, E., and Engvall, A. 1994. Prevalence of salmonella in swine, cattle and broiler carcasses after slaughter in Sweden. In: Öjeberg-Bengtsson, S., ed. NVI/WHO international course on salmonella control in animal production and products, Malmö, Sweden, August 21–27, 1993. Uppsala: National Veterinary Institute.

Ward, L.R., De Sa, J.D.H., and Rowe, B. 1987. A phage-typing scheme for *Salmonella enteritidis*. Epidemiol. Infect. 99:291–294.

Watson, W.A. 1976. Salmonella control in certain European countries. R. Soc. Health J. 96:21–25.

Wierup, M. 1992. Control of salmonella in food producing animals. In: Proceedings of Joint FAO/WHO Food Standards Programme. Codex Coordinating Committee for Europe, 18th session, Stockholm, 11–15 May 1992.

Wierup, M. 1994. Control of salmonella in animal production and products in Sweden. In: Öjeberg-Bengtsson, S., ed. NVI/WHO international course on salmonella control in animal production and products, Malmö, Sweden, August 21–27, 1993. Uppsala: National Veterinary Institute.

Wierup, M., and Nordblom, B. 1985. The salmonella control program in Sweden with special reference to poultry. In: Snoeyenbos, G.H., ed. Proceedings of the international symposium on salmonella, New Orleans, 19–20 July 1984, pp. 94–108.

Wierup, M., Wold-Troell, M., Nurmi, E., and Häkkinen, M. 1988. Epidemiological evaluation of the salmonella controlling effect of a nationwide use of a competitive exclusion culture in poultry. Poult. Sci. 67:1026–1033.

Wierup, M., Engström, B., Engvall, A., and Wahlström, H. 1992a. Control of salmonella in food-producing animals in Sweden. In: CNEVA international symposium for salmonella and salmonellosis, September 15–17, Ploufragan/Saint-Brieuc, France, pp. 386–398.

Wierup, M., Wahlström, H., and Engström, B. 1992b. Experience of a 10-year use of competitive exclusion treatment as part of the salmonella control programme in Sweden. Int. J. Food Microbiol. 15:287–291.

Wierup, M., Engström, B., Engvall, A., and Wahlström, H. 1995a. Control of *Salmonella enteritidis* in Sweden. Int. J. Food Microbiol. 25:219–226.

Weirup, M., Engvall, A., Olsson, E., Engström, B., Häggblom, P. 1995b. Control of salmonella infection in broilers: the Swedish model. Zootec. Int. 18:48–51.

27

Control of *Salmonella enterica* Serovar Enteritidis Under the U.S. National Poultry Improvement Plan

A.R. Rhorer

SALMONELLA PULLORUM

Raising chickens, turkeys, and other types of poultry—whether for profit or pleasure—entails undertaking the serious responsibility of disease prevention. Probably the greatest single factor that limited the early expansion of the U.S. poultry industry was the disease known as *bacillary white diarrhea*, caused by *Salmonella* Pullorum. This disease, later called *pullorum disease*, was rampant in poultry and could cause upward of 80% mortality in baby chicks. Poultrymen recognized the problem but were unable to manage it until the causative organism was discovered by Dr. Leio Rettger in 1899 and a diagnostic blood test was developed by Dr. F.S. Jones in 1913.

Following these two discoveries, individual poultrymen started to test their birds for pullorum disease and eliminate the reactors from the breeding flocks, but the disease was so widespread that a coordinated effort was necessary. A number of states started statewide pullorum testing programs in the early 1920s and, before long, a few breeding flocks were being identified as free of pullorum.

At about this same time, some of the early poultrymen started to exert a conscientious effort to improve the genetic production capabilities of their stock. Even though a thorough understanding of genetics was lacking, considerable improvement was made through trapnesting programs that identified superior individual birds. This would be expanded later to include individual male matting and family selection as tools to improve production potential.

As news of the availability of better stock spread and as better transportation of baby chicks became available, largely through the U.S. mail, breeders became overwhelmed with orders for baby chicks from all over the country. It was then more important than ever that stock be free of pullorum disease and that production efficiencies be improved to even higher levels.

Equally important was terminology. States having pullorum testing programs devised their own criteria and terminology to identify the various levels of freedom from the disease. Those having statewide breeding programs also used sundry terms that meant different things to different people. With the distribution of stock over a wide geographical area, it soon became apparent that nationwide criteria and touchstone terminology for both breeding and disease control programs were necessary for the poultry industry to take advantage of the improvements that were being made.

In the early 1930s, members of the poultry-breeding and poultry-hatching industries, through the International Baby Chick Association (IBCA), started to discern the profit of a national program for the improvement of poultry. It was presumed that such a program would distribute the good points of the individual state breeding and disease control programs and develop standard terminology that would be uniform in all areas of the country.

Naturally, many divergent opinions were voiced as to what areas should be covered by a national program. State poultry extension specialists and administrators of existing state improvement programs were drawn into the discussions. Since the proposed program would dictate some type of federal coordination, the U.S. Department of Agriculture (USDA) became involved. Committees and subcommittees were formed to hammer out details regarding the different sectors of the emerging poultry improvement program.

After a few years, several IBCA conventions, a myriad of committee meetings, and innumerable hours of reflection, the provisions for the first nationwide poultry improvement program were finalized in 1934. This program, which was named the National Poultry Improvement Plan (NPIP), was subsequently adopted by 47 states, which became responsible for the blood testing and subsequent classification for various disease control programs for over 2.3 billion breeding chickens and 200 million breeding turkeys during the next 63 years.

The NPIP is a voluntary cooperative state–federal program in which approximately 99% of the U.S. breeding and hatchery industry participates. The major role of the USDA is one of program coordination and supplying certain laboratory material and services. This accounts for approximately 3% of the total program cost. States, through a Memorandum of Understanding with the U.S. Department of Agriculture, agree to provide personnel necessary to conduct blood tests and related laboratory services, make inspections, keep records, and generally supervise the program. This is estimated to account for 30% of the total cost of the program. The industry members participate through an agreement with their state agency and pay approximately 67% of the total cost. This, of course, varies from state to state.

PROVISIONS OF THE NATIONAL POULTRY IMPROVEMENT PLAN

The provisions governing the NPIP are contained in Title 9, Code of Federal Regulations [chapter 1, Animal and Plant Health Inspection Service (APHIS)]. As needs arise for increased control measures for certain diseases or as new disease-control techniques are developed, these provisions are modified to keep current with the changing requirements of the industry. They are amended through recommendations made at the biennial National Plan Conference by delegates representing the industry within their states. Except during World War II, these were annual conferences until 1950, when they became biennial.

General Conference Committee

An important part of the NPIP provisions provides for the General Conference Committee, which is an official advisory committee to the Secretary of Agriculture. The delegates to the National Plan Conference elect seven members to this committee, one from each of the six regions and one member at large. This committee provides the industry a direct line of communication to the Secretary of Agriculture on matters relating to poultry health.

The duties and functions of the General Conference Committee are as follow:

1) Assist the Department in planning, organizing, and conducting the biennial NPIP Conference.
2) Recommend whether new proposals (i.e., proposals that have been submitted as provided in §147.44) should be considered by the delegates to the NPIP Conference.
3) During the interim between Plan Conferences, represent the cooperating state in:
   a) Advising the Department with respect to the administrative procedures and interpretations of the Plan provisions as contained in 9 Code of Federal Regulations.
   b) Assisting the Department in evaluating comments received from interested persons concerning proposed amendments to the Plan provisions.
   c) Recommending to the Secretary of Agriculture any changes in the provisions of the Plan as may be necessitated by unforeseen conditions when postponement until the next NPIP Conference would seriously impair the operation of the program. Such recommendations shall remain in effect only until confirmed or rejected by the next Plan Conference, or until rescinded by the Committee.
4) Serve as a forum for the study of problems relating to poultry health and as the need arises, to make specific recommendations to the Secretary of Agriculture concerning ways in which the Department may assist the industry in solving these problems.

Programs

At present, programs under the NPIP include control of *Salmonella enterica* serovar Pullorum (*S.* Pullorum), *S.* Gallinarum, *S.* Enteritidis, *Mycoplasma gallisepticum*, *M. synoviae*, *M. meleagridis*, and all potential *Salmonella* pathogens. In addition, recommended and/or required sanitation practices and the testing and laboratory protocol and techniques for the identification and isolation of infected specimens or samples are included in the provisions.

STATES THAT ARE U.S. PULLORUM-TYPHOID CLEAN

In 1968, the NPIP provisions were amended to permit a breeding flock to be qualified as a "U.S. Pullorum-Typhoid Clean" flock based on modified testing requirements if the entire state where the flock is located meets certain requirements. These requirements follow:

1. All hatcheries are in the Plan or equivalent program.
2. All breeding flocks are in the Plan or equivalent program.
3. All imports into the state are "U.S. Pullorum-Typhoid Clean" or equivalent.

4. All pullorum and fowl typhoid isolations are reported.
5. All pullorum and fowl typhoid isolations are investigated to determine source.
6. All flocks infected with pullorum or fowl typhoid are quarantined.
7. All exhibited poultry are blood tested or are from a pullorum typhoid–negative flock.

In 1974, the National Plan provisions were again amended to provide for the recognition of a state as a *U.S. Pullorum-Typhoid Clean State* if it had the above requirements as part of its state animal-health regulations and if it was enforcing them. The interpretation was made that this amendment would be made retroactive to 1968. This would allow for immediate recognition of any state that was implementing these regulations prior to 1974. Thus, nine states were given the status of a U.S. Pullorum-Typhoid Clean State at that time. Since then, a total of 42 states have earned that recognition.

SALMONELLA ENTERITIDIS

The consumption of clean, intact, shell eggs or foods containing eggs became implicated as a major factor in the increased incidence of human salmonellosis in the mid-1980s (St. Louis, et al., 1988; Centers for Disease Control, 1992). Epidemiological investigations into several *S. Enteritidis* outbreaks traced implicated eggs back to infected laying flocks (Telzak et al., 1990; Mishu et al., 1991). The human outbreaks were largely associated with one serovar of *Salmonella: S. Enteritidis*.

Initial reactions to the evidence that associated human illness due to *S. Enteritidis* with the consumption of eggs included substantial disbelief. After implementation of the Egg Products Inspection Act in 1970, uncracked and sanitized eggs had a long history of being considered safe (even if consumed uncooked). A similar involvement of eggs in human *S. Enteritidis* outbreaks in the United Kingdom resulted in a precipitous drop in egg consumption that had devastating economic consequences for the British egg industry. To address the threat to public health posed by contaminated eggs and to protect the economic viability of the egg industry, the NPIP considered a control program for egg-type breeding chickens in an attempt to prevent vertical transmission.

The modifications to the U.S. Sanitation Monitored program for egg-type breeding chickens were considered at the 1988 biennial Plan Conference in Portland, Maine. The new U.S. Sanitation Monitored program for egg-type breeding chickens took effect in July 1989. This voluntary testing program—which was modeled after the Model State Program for the Control of *S. Enteritidis* developed by the Northeastern Conference on Avian Diseases—was intended to be the basis from which the egg-type breeding-hatching industry could conduct a program for the prevention and control of salmonellosis. The program was intended to reduce the incidence of *S. Enteritidis* in hatching eggs and chicks through an effective and practical sanitation program at the breeder farm and in the hatchery.

In response to the alarming number of human outbreaks of *S. Enteritidis*, the USDA APHIS published an interim rule entitled "Poultry Affected by *S. Enteritidis*," 9 Code of Federal Regulations (CFR) Parts 71 and 82. Under 9 CFR 82, egg-type breeding flocks must be classified as U.S. Sanitation Monitored by the NPIP, or meet a state plan determined by the administrator to be equivalent, in order for the hatching eggs and newly hatched chicks from the flocks to be moved interstate. The name of the *S. Enteritidis* control program for egg-type breeding chickens in the NPIP was changed from U.S. Sanitation Monitored to U.S. *S. Enteritidis* Monitored at the biennial Plan Conference in 1994.

The following are the present requirements of the U.S. *S. Enteritidis* Monitored program of the NPIP (Fig. 27.1):

1) A flock and the hatching eggs and chicks produced from it which have met the following requirements as determined by the Official State Agency:
   i) The flock originated from a U.S. *S. Enteritidis* Monitored flock, or meconium from the chick boxes and a sample of chicks that died within 7 days after hatching are examined bacteriologically for salmonella at an authorized laboratory. Cultures from positive samples shall be serotyped.
   ii) All feed fed to the flock shall meet the following requirements:
      A) Pelletized feed shall contain either no animal protein or only animal protein products produced under the Animal Protein Products Industry (APPI) Salmonella Education/Reduction Program. The protein products must have a minimum moisture content of 14.5% and must have been heated throughout to a minimum temperature of 190°F, or above, or to a minimum temperature of 165°F for at least 20 minutes, or to a minimum temperature of 184°F under 70 lbs. pressure during the manufacturing process.
      B) Mash feed shall contain either no animal protein or only animal protein products supplement manufactured in pellet form and crumbled.

■ Monthly environmental samples
■ 300 birds evaluated serologically
■ Positive bird isolates loses status
■ Group-D *Salmonella* shall be serotyped

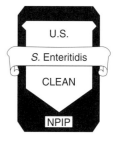

FIGURE 27.1 U.S. *Salmonella* Enteritidis Clean Program for primary meat-type breeding-chicken flocks. NPIP, National Poultry Improvement Plan.

iii) Feed shall be stored and transported in such a manner as to prevent possible contamination;

iv) The flock is maintained in compliance with §§147.21, 147.24(a), and 147.26 of this chapter;

v) Environmental samples shall be collected from the flock and by an Authorized Agent, as described in §147.12 of this chapter, when the flock is 2 to 4 weeks of age. The Authorized Agent shall also collect samples every 30 days after the first sample has been collected. The samples shall be examined bacteriologically for group D salmonella at an authorized laboratory. Cultures from positive samples shall be serotyped.

vi) A federally licensed S. Enteritidis bacterin may be used in multiplier breeding flocks that are negative for S. Enteritidis upon bacteriological examination as described in paragraph (d)(1)(v) of this section, provided that a sample of 350 birds, which will be banded for identification, shall remain unvaccinated until the flock reaches at least 4 months of age. Following negative serological and bacteriological examinations as described in paragraph (d)(1)(vii) of this section, the banded, non-vaccinated birds shall be vaccinated.

vii) Blood samples from 300 non-vaccinated birds as described in paragraph (d)(1)(vi) of this section shall be tested with either pullorum antigen or by a federally licensed S. Enteritidis enzyme-linked immunosorbent assay (ELISA) test when the flock is more than 4 months of age. All birds with positive or inconclusive reactions, up to a maximum of 25 birds, shall be submitted to an authorized laboratory and examined for the presence of group D salmonella, as described in §147.11 of this chapter. Cultures from positive samples shall be serotyped.

viii) Hatching eggs are collected as quickly as possible and are handled as described in §147.25 of this chapter).

ix) Hatching eggs produced by the flock are incubated in a hatchery that is in compliance with the recommendations in §§147.23 and 147.24(b) of this chapter, and sanitized either by a procedure approved by the Official State Agency or fumigated (see §147.25 of this chapter).

2) A flock shall not be eligible for this classification if S. Enteritidis is isolated from a specimen taken from a bird in the flock. Isolation of S. Enteritidis from an environmental or other specimen as described in section (d)(1)(v) of this paragraph will require bacteriological examination for S. Enteritidis in an authorized laboratory, as described in 147.11(a) of this chapter, of a random sample of 60 live birds from a flock of 5,000 birds or more, or 30 live birds from a flock with fewer than 5,000 birds. If only one specimen is found positive for S. Enteritidis, the participant may request bacteriological examination of a second sample, equal in size to the first sample, from the flock. If no S. Enteritidis is recovered from any of the specimens in the second sample, the flock will be eligible for the classification.

3) A flock shall be eligible for this classification if S. Enteritidis is isolated from an environmental sample collected from the flock in accordance with paragraph (d)(v) of this section, provided that testing is conducted in accordance with paragraph (d)(1)(vi) of this section each 30 days and no positive samples are found.

4) In order for a hatchery to sell products of this classification, all products handled shall meet the requirements of the classification.

5) This classification may be revoked by the Official State Agency if the participant fails to follow recommended corrective measures.

During the first 6 years of the NPIP S. Enteritidis control program for egg-type breeding-chicken flocks, 36 were determined to be environmental positive, six were dead-germ positive, and 15 were bird positive (Table 27.1; Figs. 27.2, 27.3) Of those that were found to be S. Enteritidis positive, 40% were phage type 8 (PT8), 16% were PT13, 16% were PT13a, and the rest were various other phage types (Fig. 27.4). The majority of the positive egg-type breeding-chicken flocks were located in Pennsylvania, Indiana, and Ohio (Fig. 27.5). All of the infected flocks were multiplier breeding flocks. There were no primary breeding flocks found positive during the first 6 years of the program.

TABLE 27.1.   Progress made in the control of *Salmonella* Enteritidis in egg-type breeding chickens on farms participating in the National Poultry Improvement Plan

Year	Flocks (no.)	Birds participating	Environment-positive flocks	Dead-germ-positive flocks	Bird-positive flocks
1989	347	3,947,680	—	0	—
1990	351	4,111,680	4	6	3
1991	270	2,717,788	8	—	4
1992	344	3,429,123	10	—	4
1993	288	2,892,630	5	—	2
1994	273	3,255,206	3	—	1
1995	281	3,044,984	3	—	1
1996	293	3,443,623	3	—	—

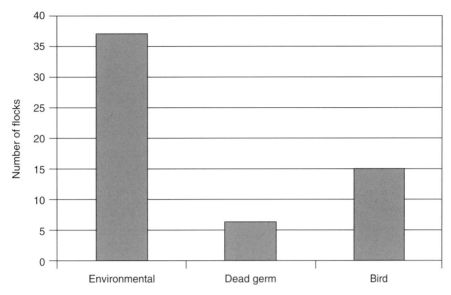

FIGURE 27.2   Number of egg-type chicken-breeding flocks with *Salmonella* Enteritidis isolates (environmental, dead germ, and bird), 1990–96.

- 1990: 11 of 340 flocks positive, 3.1%
- 1991: 8 of 270 flocks positive, 2.9%
- 1995: 2 of 265 flocks positive, 0.7%
- 1996: 4 of 293 flocks positive, 1.3%

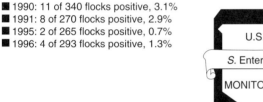

FIGURE 27.3   Progress in the control of *Salmonella* Enteritidis in egg-type breeding chickens. NPIP, National Poultry Improvement Plan.

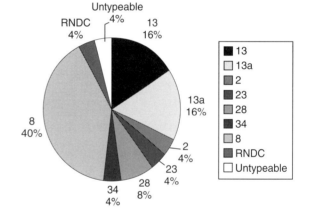

FIGURE 27.4   Phage types of *Salmonella* Enteritidis isolates from egg-type breeding-chicken flocks (environmental, dead germ, and bird), 1990–96. RNDC, reacts but does not conform.

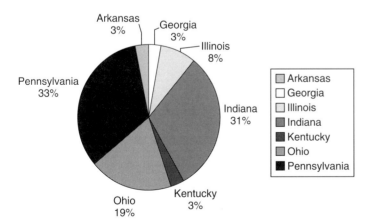

FIGURE 27.5   States with *Salmonella* Enteritidis isolates from egg-type breeding-chicken flocks (environmental, dead germ, and bird), 1990–96.

REFERENCES

Centers for Disease Control. 1992. Outbreak of *Salmonella enteritidis* infection associated with consumption of raw shell eggs, 1991. MMWR 41:369–372.

Mishu, B., Griffin, P.M., Tauxe, R.V., Cameron, D.N., Hutcheson, R.H., and Schaffner, W. 1991. *Salmonella enteritidis* gastroenteritis transmitted by intact chicken eggs. Ann. Intern. Med. 115:190–194.

St. Louis, M.E., Morse, D.L., Potter, M.E., DeMelfi, T.M., Guzegich, J.J., Tauxe, R.V., and Blake, P.A. 1988. The emergence of grade A eggs as a major source of *Salmonella enteritidis* infections: new implication for the control of Salmonellosis. JAMA 259:2103–2107.

Telzak, E.E., Budnick, L.D., Greenburg, M.S.Z., Blum, S., Shayegani, M., Benson, C.E., and Schultz, S. 1990. A nosocomial outbreak of *Salmonella enteritidis* infection due to the consumption of raw eggs. N. Engl. J. Med. 322:394–397.

28

Epidemiology of *Salmonella enterica* Serovar Enteritidis Infection in British Poultry Flocks

S.J. Evans, R.H. Davies, and C. Wray

INTRODUCTION

More than 2300 different salmonella serovars have been described, and they differ widely in their host range and pathogenicity. Infections are common in domestic poultry, and, although many serovars have been identified, one serovar may be predominant for a number of years before being replaced by another. Since 1987, *Salmonella enterica* serovar Enteritidis (*S.* Enteritidis) has been the most frequent serovar isolated from the national poultry flock in Great Britain. This increase was associated with the emergence of phage type 4 (PT4) (Table 28.1).

Salmonella Enteritidis is well adapted to poultry, and infection is not usually associated with clinical disease (Hopper and Mawer, 1988; Humphrey et al., 1989). In 1994, less than a quarter of isolations reported to the Ministry of Agriculture, Fisheries and Food (MAFF) were associated with clinical disease. However, *S.* Enteritidis can cause systemic infection, and morbidity rates ranging from 5% to 20%, with mortality rates of 6%, have been recorded during the first week of life in several chicken flocks (O'Brien, 1988; McIlroy et al., 1989). In affected chicks, the pathological findings include pericarditis, necrotic foci in the liver, and indurated yolk-sac remnants.

TABLE 28.1 *Salmonella* Enteritidis: number of cultures sensitive to all antimicrobials used for testing

Year	PT4	%	All phage types	%	No. of different phage types
1995	473/488	96.9	536/557	96.2	11
1994	556/580	95.9	748/800	93.5	18
1993	1303/1347	96.7	1825/1946	93.8	22
1992	2628/2681	98.0	3380/3656	92.5	21
1991	3093/3195	96.8	3922/4270	91.9	24
1990	2481/2597	95.5	2677/3074	87.1	4
1989	1246/1318	94.5	1625/1815	89.5	24
1988	458/470	97.4	570/585	97.4	13

PT4, phage type 4.

Adult chickens infected naturally with *S.* Enteritidis are usually symptomless carriers of the organism, although it may be isolated from the ovaries and oviduct, liver, spleen, and peritoneum (Hopper and Mawer, 1988; Cooper et al., 1989). Infected breeder and layer flocks usually show no decrease in egg production, although some chickens may become chronic carriers and excrete the organism intermittently (Williams, 1972; Williams and Whittemore, 1976). When chickens come into lay, infection may spread rapidly and many chickens may become infected. The organism has also been isolated from a composite sample of tests from 23-week-old chickens (Bygrave and Gallagher, 1989), but the role of male chickens in the maintenance and spread of infection is not known.

Stresses such as food and water deprivation and intercurrent disease may increase the susceptibility of chickens to *S.* Enteritidis (Arakawa et al., 1992; Holt, 1993; Nakamura et al., 1995) and also enhance the severity (Phillips and Opitz, 1995), increase speed of transmission between chickens (Holt, 1995), or cause recrudescence of infection (Qin et al., 1995). It has been shown that PT4 is more virulent and invasive in poultry than other phage types of *S.* Enteritidis (Hinton et al., 1990a; Barrow, 1991). A gradation has also been found in the ability of strains of PT4 isolated in 1978, 1984, and 1988 to invade chicken livers (Hinton et al., 1990b), suggesting an increase in the virulence of this strain during that period.

Salmonella is a frequent foodborne infection of humans, and contaminated poultry products are a major source of infection (Coyle et al., 1988; Humphrey et al., 1988; Cowden et al., 1989; Roberts and Socket, 1994). Efforts to control salmonellae in domestic poultry are mainly driven by public health implications.

DETECTION

Salmonellae are Gram-negative, nonsporing rods that lack capsules. They grow readily on ordinary media, forming large, thick, grayish-white colonies. The bacteria can be isolated from infected tissues by direct culture, and the ceca are the most likely site for isolation in adult chickens. Population-screening methods must be capable of detecting low-incidence infections of poultry, which are common, and methods have been developed to sample the environment as an indirect indicator of flock infection.

Various isolation methods are in current use and most involve a pre-enrichment step followed by selective enrichment in selenite, tetrathionate, or Rapport-Vassiliadis medium, and incubation at 41°–42°C, and then the use of a selective plating medium, such as MacConkey, deoxycholate citrate, or brilliant green agar (Davies and Wray, 1994b). Colonies suspected of being salmonellae are tested by a slide agglutination test, and further biochemical and serological tests are used to identify the serovar. Further subdivisions for epidemiological purposes can be achieved by phage-typing schemes, plasmid profile analysis and other genetic techniques, biotyping, and antimicrobial sensitivity testing.

A number of serological tests are available for the diagnosis of salmonellae in poultry. The enzyme-linked immunosorbent assay (ELISA) is used in many countries for the identification of *S.* Enteritidis–infected flocks although, because of a lack of specificity, bacteriological confirmation is recommended. Two systems are in current use: indirect ELISA and competitive double-antibody-blocking ELISA, the former being favored for monitoring purposes in Great Britain. Another disadvantage of using diagnosis based on serology is that positive serology does not necessarily mean that the chicken is still infected, and negative serology can be compatible with the early stages of infection prior to the development of an immune response. Interpretation of serological tests is further complicated by vaccination or antibiotic treatment of flocks.

EPIDEMIOLOGY OF INFECTION

Prevalence

Between 1981 and 1986, *S.* Enteritidis accounted for 2.2% of the salmonella incidents recorded from domestic fowl by the MAFF, but the number of reports of this serovar tripled in 1987, and this dramatic increase continued in 1988, by which stage *S.* Enteritidis accounted for 50% of the poultry salmonella reports. The number of incident reports continued to rise and peaked in 1990–91 and then gradually declined during 1992–93, followed by a more marked decline in 1994 (Fig. 28.1). In response to the epidemic, in 1989 the British government introduced a compulsory monitoring scheme for salmonella infection of poultry flocks. This scheme is discussed later, but the increased level of monitoring may have resulted in an increase in the number of reports of salmonellae from poultry and thus complicates the interpretation of trends over time, particularly early in the epidemic. Throughout this epidemic, the predominant strain of *S.* Enteritidis has been PT4, which has been isolated from more than 75% of incidents (MAFF, 1995a). Surveys conducted by the Public Health Laboratory Service of English retail premises suggest that at the peak of the epidemic about 40%–60% of fresh and frozen chickens were contaminated with salmonellae and *S.* Enteritidis PT4 was the most common type found (Public Health Laboratory Service, 1989; Roberts, 1991). Similar surveys of retail eggs suggested that 0.9% were contaminated with salmonellae, again predominantly *S.* Enteritidis PT4 (de Louvois, 1993). However, a survey of retail raw chicken in the winter and spring of 1993–94 showed that the level of salmonella contamination had decreased to 33% of fresh and 41% of frozen chickens sampled, and *S.* Enteritidis PT4 was isolated from 16% of all chickens sampled (HMSO, 1996).

Sources of Infection

VERTICAL TRANSMISSION
The poultry industry is separated into egg and meat production enterprises, each of which has its own breeding-flock

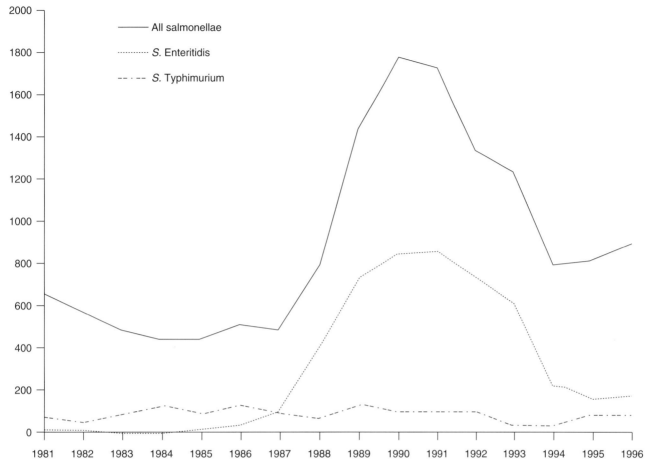

FIGURE 28.1   The number of reports of salmonella serovar cases, 1981–96.

hierarchy. Elite breeder flocks contain the primary genetic stock, whose offspring form the grandparent flocks, which, in turn, produce parent breeder flocks. Breeding and production flocks from both sectors of the British poultry industry have been involved in the *S.* Enteritidis epidemic. The hierarchical structure of the industry and the ability of *S.* Enteritidis to be transmitted vertically to offspring via eggs may partly explain the widespread nature of the epidemic (Lister, 1988; O'Brien, 1988). There have been no confirmed flock infections with *S.* Enteritidis in elite or grandparent breeding flocks since the start of the compulsory monitoring scheme for salmonellae in 1989. However, *S.* Enteritidis PT4 was isolated from the ovules of two hens from a British grandparent flock, type unspecified, which was examined at depletion in 1988 (O'Brien, 1990). Anecdotal evidence from other countries suggests that primary breeding flocks were infected in the late 1980s, because *S.* Enteritidis was isolated in Japan from broiler parent chicks that had been imported from England and from a broiler grandparent flock in the Netherlands that had been hatched from eggs imported from the United Kingdom (Nakamura et al., 1993; Edel, 1994).

When a breeding flock is infected with *S.* Enteritidis, a cycle can be established by which the organism passes via the eggs to the progeny and even to chicks hatched from

eggs laid by infected progeny. This cycle can occur by true ovarian transmission or, as is much more likely to happen, through fecal contamination of the egg surface. As the egg passes through the cloaca, salmonellae in feces attach themselves to the warm, wet shell surface and may be drawn inside as it cools. Surface contamination may also occur in the nest boxes.

Hatcheries can serve as reservoirs of infection, and cross-contamination in the hatchery may dramatically increase the prevalence of salmonella-infected chicks leaving the hatchery compared with the low prevalence of infected eggs entering the hatchery. Bailey et al. (1994) demonstrated that a single salmonella-contaminated egg could substantially contaminate other eggs and chicks in the hatching cabinet.

We carried out a comparative study of salmonella contamination in 11 commercial hatcheries (Davies and Wray, 1994b), which indicated the effective and less effective key cross-contamination hazard points.

Of the egg-sanitization programs, the most intensive was washing eggs with an automatic spray machine on the farm, fogging with a peroxygen compound during transit, and fumigation with formaldehyde upon arrival at the hatchery. This resulted in no detectable salmonella contamination of the egg-storage and egg-handling areas. In contrast, in the hatchery that accepted eggs dipped in a sanitizer on the farm and disinfectant fogging on arrival at the hatchery, 26% of the samples from the egg reception and store were contaminated with salmonellae.

In the setters where the trolleys and protective floor belting could be moved to assist cleaning, the salmonella contamination rate was much lower when compared with setters with fixed tray turners, which did not allow easy removal of shell debris. Among the automatic suction cups for egg transfer, 50%–83% were found to be contaminated, and we found that regular disinfection using a spray during operation could prevent contamination.

Hatching of eggs from an infected flock liberated large quantities of chick dust and fluff, which contained 10^4 cfu salmonellae per gram. Sampling the interiors and air-intake ducts of hatchers showed that the use of continuous formaldehyde fumigation during hatching in addition to a well-sealed dust-trap corridor controlled salmonella contamination and prevented the surface contamination that occurred in poorly run hatcheries.

In the chick-handling area, there is a high potential for cross-contamination, but salmonella contamination can be reduced significantly by good organization, hygiene management, and disinfection practices. Likewise, marked differences were observed between the hatcheries in the efficacy of tray sanitization: salmonellae were not isolated in some, whereas 25% contamination rates were observed in others.

Recent studies in the Netherlands concluded that vertical transmission of *S.* Enteritidis to parent breeders and to commercial laying flocks did not appear to be important, at least in recent years, as infections during the rearing period were rare (van de Giessen et al., 1994; Fris and van den Bos, 1995). A case-control study carried out by the Central Veterinary Laboratory has also shown that vertical transmission was not a source of *S.* Enteritidis PT4 infection for parent breeding chickens infected since 1992 (Evans and Sayers, unpublished data).

FEED CONTAMINATION

Early speculation suggested that contaminated feed was involved in this epidemic, but, although a recognized source of some salmonella serovars (Jones et al., 1989), there is controversy as to the importance of feed in the epidemiology of *S.* Enteritidis infection (HMSO, 1992; Jones and Richardson, 1996). The main reason for this controversy is that there appears to be little correlation between the salmonella serovars isolated from poultry and those found in feed. The incidence of salmonella contamination in feeds, detected by official MAFF testing of animal protein and finished feeds, is generally low, but contamination rates were higher than current levels at the start of the epidemic. In 1989, of home-produced animal protein samples tested by the MAFF, 5% were positive for salmonellae, but only four (7%) of these contained *S.* Enteritidis. Since then, the salmonella contamination rate of home-produced animal protein has gradually decreased to about 2%, although the proportion of isolates found to be *S.* Enteri-

tidis has remained constant. Although salmonellae are isolated more frequently from consignments of imported animal protein, *S.* Enteritidis is rarely found. In recent years, finished poultry-feed samples have also been monitored for salmonellae, but in 1993 and 1994 less than 2.7% of samples tested were positive and less than 2% of these contained *S.* Enteritidis (HMSO, 1992; MAFF, 1995a). However, it has been observed that, due to the heterogeneity of infection in feed (Veldman et al., 1995), the sensitivity of current monitoring procedures is relatively poor (Davies, 1992). The ability of the organisms to multiply from nondetectable numbers during improper feed storage has also been recognized (Davies, 1992). It is also essential that finished feed does not become contaminated in transport or storage before it is consumed by poultry. It has been shown that chicks can be infected with feed containing less than 1 salmonella per gram (Hinton, 1988), but not every serovar or phage type has the same colonization potential, and poultry may become selectively colonized by the more virulent strains in feeds, such as *S.* Enteritidis PT4. Horizontal spread between chickens may further spread feedborne infection.

A second reason for the disputed role of feed as a source of *S.* Enteritidis is the limited epidemiological evidence from field investigations. The levels of *S.* Enteritidis in poultry in Northern Ireland are lower than those in the rest of the United Kingdom, and all breeder feed has been heat treated since early epidemiological investigations revealed that feed was a possible source of *S.* Enteritidis for these flocks (McIlroy et al., 1989). However, heat treatment of breeder feed is only one aspect of the comprehensive control policy adopted by the poultry industry in Northern Ireland. Humphrey and Lanning (1988) found that formic acid treatment of breeder feed significantly reduced the number of salmonella isolations from feed, litter, hatchery waste, and chick box liners, indicating that the feed was a source of salmonellae. Other recent studies have also implicated feed as a source of salmonellae for poultry flocks, although this risk may be associated with serovars other than *S.* Enteritidis (Henken et al., 1992; Jacobs-Reitsma et al., 1994; Angen et al., 1996). More convincingly, the recent case-control study of *S.* Enteritidis PT4 infection of breeding flocks in Great Britain found a significant protective effect of heat-treated poultry feed, indicating that, despite apparently low levels of contamination detected by MAFF monitoring, feed remains an important source of infection (Evans and Sayers, unpublished data).

THE ROLE OF WILDLIFE

Elimination of the persistent contamination of some poultry-breeder units was one of the most difficult problems in the control of *S.* Enteritidis and other salmonella serovars in many poultry flocks in Great Britain and other countries (Baggesen et al., 1992; Brown et al., 1992). Such persistent contamination may be caused by failure of disinfection routines (discussed later) or the presence of wildlife carriers or vectors.

Although *S.* Enteritidis infection in mice in poultry units was reported 15 years previously (Krabisch and Dorn,

1980), the significance of mice as vectors of *S.* Enteritidis in poultry units has only received widespread attention relatively recently (Henzler and Opitz, 1992). Naturally infected mice, captured at depletion in poultry units, where *S.* Enteritidis infection had been confirmed in the chickens, excreted the organism for up to 18 weeks (Davies and Wray, 1995a). Excretion was intermittent, and reactivation of infection occurred during periods of stress. The prevalence of *S.* Enteritidis in individual fecal pellets was usually low [<10 colony-forming units (CFU)], but one pellet contained 10^2–10^3 organisms. Salmonella contamination in the environment may be amplified by mice defecating into feed troughs and on egg-collection belts and may be spread further throughout the house by automated feeding, egg conveyors, and manure-removal equipment.

We detected *S.* Enteritidis–infected mice in a single poultry house for more than 2 years, and, after depopulation, they constitute a reservoir of infection that can infect the next flock. Infected dead mice or droppings were found on 50% of the broiler breeder or layer breeder units that were investigated after cleaning and disinfection. Many areas in poultry units may become infested with rodents, and an intensive and sustained rodent control program is necessary for the control of salmonellae: the program needs to be well planned, flexible, and continuous, and its effectiveness must be monitored (World Health Organization, 1994). Trapping of rodents may also be used to monitor salmonella contamination, because mice remain infected even after environmental contamination becomes difficult to detect by standard sampling techniques.

Salmonella infection has also been detected in many species of wild birds. At hatcheries and poultry-processing units, salmonellae were detected in wild-bird droppings, which may contaminate clean equipment left outside buildings (Davies and Wray, 1994c).

Flies have frequently been shown to be contaminated with salmonellae, and Edel et al. (1973) found that 1.5% of 202 flytraps examined were contaminated with salmonellae. Blowfly larvae (*Lucilia serricata*) have also been shown to be contaminated with salmonellae, and studies have shown that maggots are a potent vehicle of salmonella infection for chickens (Davies and Wray, 1994d). Maggots, which may contain up to 300 CFU of salmonellae, are attractive to chickens, and, when ingested, the cuticle has a protective effect so that the bactericidal effect of gastric acidity, and so on, is bypassed.

It has been suggested that mealworm beetles (*Alphitobius diaperinus*) may also be important in persistence and transmission of salmonella infections in poultry units (Baggesen et al., 1992; Brown et al., 1992). In our studies, 500 live *Alphitobius* beetles were collected before cleansing and disinfection in two poultry units, and although the environmental contamination with salmonellae was high, the organism was not isolated from the beetles. Likewise, we failed to infect the beetles by artificial contamination with salmonellae, although von Geissler and Kösters (1972) found that artificially infected beetles excreted salmonellae for 15 days.

ENVIRONMENTAL CONTAMINATION

Persistent environmental contamination of houses is an important factor in the maintenance of *S.* Enteritidis, and other salmonellae, in poultry flocks (Kradel and Miller, 1991; Baggesen et al., 1992). The effective decontamination of salmonella-infected houses before repopulation is a highly important consideration in a *hazard analysis critical control point* approach for poultry units. A high standard of disinfection is necessary to avoid infection of poultry placed in previously infected houses, because it has been shown experimentally that an infective dose of salmonellae for chickens can be fewer than five cells (Milner and Shaffer, 1952), or 100 cells for adult chickens, following conjunctival inoculation (Humphrey et al., 1992). Intercurrent disease may make the chickens even more susceptible (Arakawa et al., 1992; Holt, 1993; Nakamura et al., 1995). A number of analytical studies have associated salmonella infection with poor hygiene standards at poultry sites (Henzler and Opitz, 1992; Opitz, 1992; Fris and van den Bos, 1995). The tendency toward reinfection on farms is widely recognized, and, in a case-control study of British poultry-breeding flocks, *S.* Enteritidis PT4 infection was associated with a history of salmonellae at the poultry site, highlighting the importance of farm environment in the epidemiology of infection (Evans and Sayers, in press). This was similarly reported by a study of broiler flocks in Denmark (Angen et al., 1996).

Our studies in breeder houses found a threefold higher salmonella isolation rate from nest-box floors and dust on in-house slave feed hoppers than from drinkers, chain feeders, slats, perches, and dust on beams and ventilation ducts. In broiler breeder houses, salmonellae were isolated from egg-sorting tables and 75% of the egg-collecting trolleys that were sampled.

In a study of 16 commercial broiler and layer breeder houses after cleaning and disinfection, the most sensitive sites, in decreasing order, for detection of salmonellae were floor sweepings and nest-box floors, slave feed hoppers, hydrated wall-fabric junctions, and high beams and pipes.

Studies carried out at the Central Veterinary Laboratory and in the field identified many potential problems during disinfection of poultry units naturally contaminated with *S.* Enteritidis (Davies and Wray, 1995b). Variations in the efficacy of commonly used disinfectants were apparent within a disinfectant group. It was possible for salmonella contamination to be amplified during pressure washing or steam cleaning, and, if an effective terminal disinfectant was not used, the high numbers of salmonellae were likely to persist. The efficacy of the disinfection regimen was not directly dependent on the standard of physical cleaning if this was carried out to an adequate standard, because elimination of salmonellae could be achieved even in the presence of substantial quantities of residual organic matter. Regimens involving formaldehyde, either as part of a terminal compound or as a fogging agent, were found to be the most effective. Humans can also act as mechanical carriers of salmonellae on contaminated clothing, footwear, and hands.

Although many sources of salmonella infection for poultry are established and have been discussed, the relative importance of these in the field is not known. It is also thought likely that the major routes of infection may be different for different serovars and flock types, and their relative risk may have changed over time. A summary of the cycle of salmonella infection in poultry is presented in Figure 28.2.

PREVENTION AND CONTROL

There are three major points at which poultry-associated human cases of *S.* Enteritidis infection can be controlled. These are the prevention of infection in live chickens, slaughterhouse interventions to control contamination of carcasses, and education of the public as to the necessity of adequate cooking of chicken meat and eggs and the prevention of cross-contamination of other foods in the kitchen. There are currently no acceptable slaughterhouse interventions that will ensure salmonella-free meat, and consumer food-hygiene education has had only limited success. Therefore, control of the epidemic of *S.* Enteritidis is centered on the eradication of infection in poultry. It is necessary to eliminate infection from both breeding and production flocks, and experience from control schemes in various countries has shown that a *top-down* approach, by first controlling infection in breeding flocks to prevent vertical transmission of infection to progeny, is most successful.

Statutory Aspects of the Control of Salmonellae in Great Britain

In 1989, a new Zoonoses Order replaced and broadened the scope of the previous order that was first enacted in 1975. The main provisions of Zoonoses Order of 1989 are the requirement to report the results of tests that identify the presence of salmonellae, the provision of a culture to the MAFF, the taking of live chickens and other samples for diagnostic purposes, the imposition of movement restrictions and isolation requirements, as well as a requirement for the cleaning and disinfection of premises and vehicles. The order also applies the provision of the Animal Health Act of 1981 (HMSO, 1981) with regard to the compulsory slaughter of salmonella-infected poultry flocks and compensation.

To combat *S.* Enteritidis infection in poultry, the Poultry Laying Flocks (Registration and Testing) Order (HMSO, 1989a) and Poultry Breeding Flocks and Hatcheries (Registration and Testing) Order (HMSO, 1989b) were enacted in 1989. These orders required the testing of poultry for salmonellae on a regular basis. The purposes of these two orders were to prevent transmission of salmonellae to humans through eggs and to reduce vertical transmission of salmonellae so that chickens for commercial rearing did not take infection onto premises. These two orders were revoked in 1993 with the implementation of the Poultry Breeding Flocks and Hatcheries Order (HMSO, 1993), which brought salmonella-control measures in poultry into line with European Union Directive 92/117/EEC (Anon., 1993). This order requires the regular monitoring of breeding flocks and hatcheries for *S.* Enteri-

tidis and *Salmonella* Typhimurium by a prescribed program using methods laid down in the order. If either *S.* Enteritidis or *S.* Typhimurium is isolated from any chickens in a flock, Directive 92/117/EEC requires that all chickens in the affected poultry house be slaughtered and the owner compensated. The directive also makes provision for alternatives, such as antibiotic treatment, but, to date, most flock owners have opted for slaughter.

Since 1993, there has been no statutory requirement to monitor turkeys, ducks, geese, or the commercial generations of domestic fowl. In addition, flock owners have been encouraged to adopt good management practices for the control of salmonellae by following voluntary Codes of Practice that have been developed by the MAFF in collaboration with the poultry industry and the veterinary profession (MAFF, 1993, 1995b).

Feedstuffs have always been a potential source of salmonellae for poultry, and the Processed Animal Protein Order of 1989 (HMSO, 1989c) requires those who process animal protein to be registered with the MAFF and to test each day's consignment for salmonellae in an authorized laboratory. If salmonellae are isolated, the processor is required to ensure that no contaminated material is incorporated into animal feedstuffs. As part of its package of control measures, the MAFF, in cooperation with the feedstuff industry, introduced a number of voluntary Codes of Practice for the production, storage, handling, and transport of animal feedstuff (MAFF, 1995c–g). Heat treatment and chemical treatment of feed to control salmonella contamination are known to be effective, provided adequate temperatures or adequate levels of chemicals are used (Jones and Richardson, 1996). A recent government report strongly recommended the effective heat treatment of all poultry feeds (HMSO, 1996).

The Processed Animal Protein Order of 1989 also prohibits the landing in Great Britain of any processed animal protein or of any product containing processed animal protein except under the authority of a license. The conditions imposed in the import license reflect the likely contamination status of imported materials. In the case of some countries, these conditions may require detention of every imported consignment at the port of landing until negative salmonella test results have been obtained.

There is now evidence that these measures to eradicate infection in the British poultry industry have had some success. Primary breeder flocks are free of infection, and there is a declining trend in reports from parent breeding flocks (Figs. 28.3, 28.4). However, eradication is still likely to be some time in the future. Therefore, attention has also been directed at interventions to protect chickens from infection. The most feasible are competitive exclusion, antibiotic treatment, and vaccination. Competitive exclusion refers to the colonization control in live chickens by the establishment of protective populations of intestinal bacteria (Nurmi and Rantala, 1973). Despite success under experimental conditions, it has shown mixed results in the field in its ability to protect against salmonella infection (Goren et al., 1988; Mead, 1991; Mulder and Bolder, 1991). In general, protection is superior with undefined

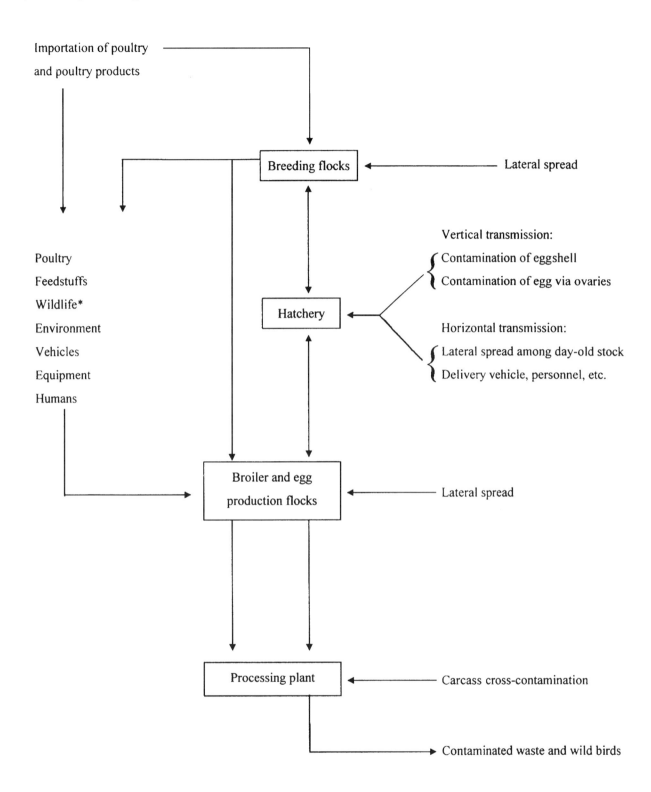

*Wildlife includes vermin, wild birds, and insects

FIGURE 28.2   Cycle of salmonella infection.

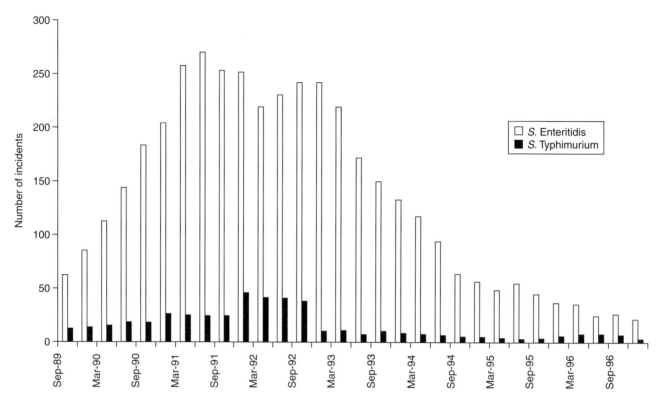

FIGURE 28.3 Number of reported salmonella incidents in British broiler breeding flocks in 12-month periods, 1989–96. From the Ministry of Agriculture, Fisheries and Food (MAFF).

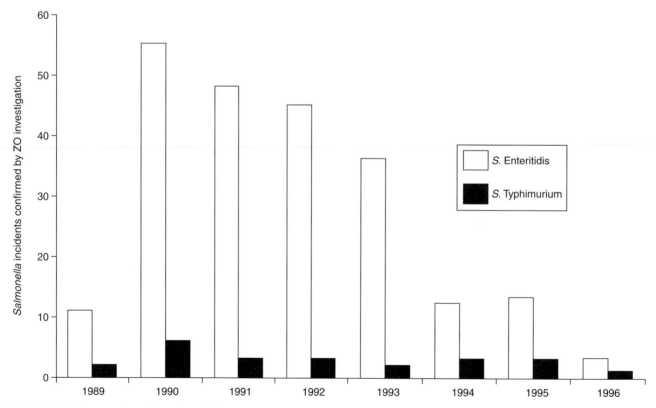

FIGURE 28.4 Number of confirmed [by Zoonoses Order (ZO) investigation] incidents of *Salmonella* in British broiler breeding flocks, 1989–96.

cultures that contain a broad range of bacteria (Stavric et al., 1991). There is also a risk of spreading pathogens to recipient chickens. The use of antibiotic treatment is controversial because of the risk of selection of resistant strains of bacteria (particularly if quinolone drugs are used). Recent trials in British breeder flocks infected with *S. Enteritidis* have shown that a combination of antibiotic treatment and competitive exclusion reduced the prevalence of infection but was not successful in totally eliminating the organism (HMSO, 1996). Control by vaccination is still in the development stages, although an inactivated vaccine has been available in recent years in the United Kingdom and has been used in breeding flocks. One disadvantage to vaccination is the interference with the results of serological monitoring of flocks for infection. All three methods of intervention are likely to be most successful when used as part of a comprehensive salmonella-control program.

REFERENCES

Angen, O., Skov, M.N., Chriel, M., Agger, J.F., and Bisgaard, M. 1996. A retrospective study on *Salmonella* infection in Danish broiler flocks. Prev. Vet. Med. 26:223–237.

Anonymous. 1993. Council Directive 92/117/EEC of 17 December 1992 concerning measures for protection against specified zoonoses and specified zoonotic agents in animals and products of animal origin in order to prevent outbreaks of foodborne infections and intoxications. Off. J. Eur. Community 62:38–48.

Arakawa, A., Fukaton, T., Baba, E., McDougald, L.R., Bailey, J.S., and Blankenship, L.C. 1992. Influence of coccidiosis on colonisation in broiler chickens under floor pen conditions. Poult. Sci. 71:59–63.

Baggesen, D.L., Olsen, L.E., and Bisgaard, M. 1992. Plasmid profiles and phage types of *Salmonella typhimurium* isolated from successive flocks of chickens on three poultry stock farms. Avian Pathol. 21:568–579.

Bailey, J.S., Cox, N.A., and Berrang, M.E. 1994. Hatchery acquired salmonellae in broiler chicks. Poult. Sci. 73:1153–1157.

Barrow, P.A. 1991. Experimental infection of chickens with *Salmonella enteritidis*. Avian Pathol. 20:145–153.

Brown, D.J., Olsen, J.E., and Bisgaard, M. 1992. *Salmonella enteritidis* infection, cross-infection and persistence within the environment of a broiler parent stock unit in Denmark. Zentralbl. Bakteriol. 277:129–138.

Bygrave, A.C., and Gallagher, J. 1989. Transmission of *Salmonella enteritidis* in poultry. Vet. Rec. 124:333.

Cooper, G.L., Nicholas, R.A., and Bracewell, C.D. 1989. Serological and bacteriological investigations of chickens from flocks naturally infected with *Salmonella enteritidis*. Vet. Rec. 125:567–572.

Cowden, J.M., Lynch, D., Joseph, C.A., O'Mahony, M., Mawser, S.L., Spain, G.E., Ward, L., and Rowe, B. 1989. Case control study of infections with *Salmonella enteritidis* phage type 4 in England. BMJ 299:771–773.

Coyle, E.F., Palmer, S.P., Ribeiro, C.D., Jones, H.I., Howard, A.J., and Ward, L. 1988. *Salmonella enteritidis* phage type 4 infection: association with hens' eggs. Lancet 2:1295–1297.

Davies, R.H. 1992. Salmonella: the feedstuffs connection. In: Thrusfield, M.V., ed. Proceedings of the Society of Veterinary Epidemiology and Preventive Medicine, Edinburgh, pp. 47–59.

Davies, R.H., and Wray, C. 1994a. An approach to reduction of *Salmonella* infection in broiler chicken flocks through intensive sampling and identification of cross-contamination hazards in commercial hatcheries. Int. J. Food Microbiol. 24:147–160.

Davies, R.H., and Wray, C. 1994b. Evaluation of a rapid cultural method for identification of salmonellas in naturally contaminated veterinary samples. J. Appl. Bacteriol. 77:237–241.

Davies, R.H., and Wray, C. 1994c. *Salmonella* pollution in poultry units and associated enterprises. In: Dewi, I.A.P., Axford, R.F.F., Maria, I.F.M., and Umed, H., eds. Pollution in livestock systems. Oxon, UK: CAB, pp. 137–166.

Davies, R.H., and Wray, C. 1994d. Use of larvae of *Lucilia serricata* in colonisation and invasion studies of *Salmonella enteritidis* infection in poultry. In: Pusztail, A., Hinton, M.H., and Mulder, R.W.A.W., eds. Flair 6.10: the attachment of bacteria to the gut. Het Spelderholt: COVP-DLO, pp. 117–123.

Davies, R.H., and Wray, C. 1995a. Mice as carriers of *Salmonella enteritidis* on persistently infected poultry units. Vet. Rec. 137:337–341.

Davies, R.H., and Wray, C. 1995b. Observations on disinfection regimes used on *Salmonella enteritidis* infected poultry units. Poult. Sci. 74:638–647.

de Louvois, J. 1993. *Salmonella* contamination of eggs: a potential source of human salmonellosis. PHLS Microbiol. Digest 10:159–163.

Edel, W. 1994. *Salmonella enteritidis* eradication programme in poultry breeder flocks in the Netherlands. Int. J. Food Microbiol. 21:171–178.

Edel, W., van Schothorst, M., Guinee, P.A.M., and Kampelmacher, E.H. 1973. Mechanisms and prevention of salmonella infections in animals. In: Hobbs, B.C., and Christian, J.H.B., eds. The microbiological safety of food. London: Academic, pp. 247–256.

Fris, C., and van den Bos, J. 1995. A retrospective case control study of risk factors associated with *Salmonella enteritidis* infections on Dutch broiler breeder farms. Avian Pathol. 24:255–272.

Goren, E., de Jong, W.A., Doornenbal, P., Bolder, N.M., Molder, R.W.A.W., and Jansen, A. 1988. Reduction of salmonella infection of broilers by spray application of intestinal microflora: a longitudinal study. Vet. Q. 10:249–255.

Henken, A.M., Frankena, K., Geolema, J.O., Graat, E.A.M., and Noordhuizen, J.P.T.M. 1992. Multivariate epidemiological approach to salmonellosis in broiler breeder flocks. Poult. Sci. 71:838–843.

Henzler, D.J., and Opitz, H.M. 1992. The role of mice in the epizootiology of *Salmonella enteritidis* infection on chicken layer farms. Avian Dis. 36:625–631.

Hinton, M. 1988. *Salmonella* infection in chicks following the consumption of artificially contaminated feed. Epidemiol. Infect. 100:247–256.

Hinton, M., Threlfall, E.J., and Rowe, B. 1990a. The invasive potential of *Salmonella enteritidis* phage types for young chickens. Lett. Appl. Microbiol. 10:237–239.

Hinton, M.H., Threlfall, E.J., and Rowe, B. 1990b. The invasiveness of different strains of *Salmonella enteritidis* phage type 4 for young chickens. FEMS Microbiol. Lett. 70:193–196.

HMSO. 1981. The animal health act 1981. Statutory Instrument 1975 No. 1030.

HMSO. 1989a. The poultry laying flocks (registration and testing) order 1989. Statutory Instrument 1989 No. 1964.

HMSO. 1989b. The poultry breeding flocks and hatcheries (registration and testing) order 1989. Statutory Instrument 1989 No. 1963.

HMSO. 1989c. The processed animal protein order 1989. Statutory Instrument 1989 No. 661.

HMSO. 1992. The report of the expert group on animal feedingstuffs. Lamming, E., chairman.

HMSO. 1993. The poultry breeding flocks and hatcheries order 1993. Statutory Instrument 1993 No. 1898.

HMSO. 1996. Report on poultry meat. Advisory Committee on the Microbiological Safety of Food.

Holt, P.S. 1993. Effect of induced molting on the susceptibility of white leghorn hens to a *Salmonella enteritidis* infection. Avian Dis. 37:412–417.

Holt, P.S. 1995. Horizontal transmission of *Salmonella enteritidis* in molted and unmolted laying chickens. Avian Dis. 39:239–249.

Hopper, S.A., and Mawer, S.L. 1988. *Salmonella enteritidis* in a commercial layer flock. Vet. Rec. 123:351.

Humphrey, T.J., and Lanning, D.G. 1988. The vertical transmission of *Salmonella* and formic acid treatment of chicken feed. Epidemiol. Infect. 100:43–49.

Humphrey, T.J., Mead, G.C., and Rowe, B. 1988. Poultry meat as a source of human salmonellosis in England and Wales. Epidemiol. Infect. 100:175–184.

Humphrey, T.J., Baskerville, A., Chart, H., and Rowe, B. 1989. Infection of egg-laying hens with *Salmonella enteritidis* PT4 by oral inoculation. Vet. Rec. 125:531–532.

Humphrey, T.J., Baskerville, A., Chart, H., Rowe, B., and Whitehead, A. 1992. Infection of laying hens with *Salmonella enteritidis* PT4 by conjunctival challenge. Vet. Rec. 131:386–388.

Jacobs-Reitsma, W.F., Bolder, N.M., and Molder, R.W.A.W. 1994. Cecal carriage of *Campylobacter* and *Salmonella* in Dutch broiler flocks at slaughter: a one year study. Poult. Sci. 73:1260–1266.

Jones, F.T., and Richardson, K.E. 1996. Fallacies exist in current understanding of *Salmonella*. Feedstuffs 68:22–25.

Jones, F.T., Axtell, R.C., Rives, D.V., Scheideler, S.E., Tarver, F.R., Walker, R.L., and Wineland, M.L. 1989. *Salmonella* contamination sources in modern broiler production and processing systems. In: Proceedings of the 10th annual meeting of the Southern Poultry Science Society, p. 23.

Krabisch, P., and Dorn, P. 1980. Zur epidemiologischen Bedeuntung von Lebendvektoren bei Verbreitung von Salmo-

nellen in der Geflugelmast. Berl. Muench. Tierarztl. Wochenschr. 92:232–235.

Kradel, D.C., and Miller, W.L. 1991. *Salmonella enteritidis* observations on field related problems. In: Proceedings 40th western poultry disease conference, Acapulco, Mexico, pp. 146–150.

Lister, S.A. 1988. *Salmonella enteritidis* infection in broilers and broiler breeders. Vet. Rec. 123:350.

McIlroy, S.G., McCracken, R.M., Neill, S.D., and O'Brien, J.J. 1989. Control, prevention and eradication of *Salmonella enteritidis* infection in broiler and broiler breeder flocks. Vet. Rec. 125:545–548.

Mead, G.C. 1991. Developments in competitive exclusion to control *Salmonella* carriage in poultry. In: Blankenship, L.C., ed. Colonization of human bacterial enteropathogens in poultry. San Diego, CA: Academic, pp. 91–104.

Milner, K.C., and Shaffer, M.F. 1952. Bacteriologic studies of experimental *Salmonella* infections in chickens. J. Infect. Dis. 90:81–85.

Ministry of Agriculture, Fisheries and Food (MAFF). 1993. Code of Practice for the prevention and control of *Salmonella* in breeding flocks and hatcheries. London: MAFF.

Ministry of Agriculture, Fisheries and Food (MAFF). 1995a. *Salmonella* in animal and poultry production 1994. London: MAFF.

Ministry of Agriculture, Fisheries and Food (MAFF). 1995b. Code of Practice for the prevention and control of *Salmonella* in commercial egg laying flocks. London: MAFF.

Ministry of Agriculture, Fisheries and Food (MAFF). 1995c. Code of Practice for the control of *Salmonella* during the storage, handling and transport of raw materials intended for incorporation into, or direct use as, animal feedingstuffs. London: MAFF, 1989; revised May 1995.

Ministry of Agriculture, Fisheries and Food (MAFF). 1995d. Code of Practice for the control of *Salmonella* in the animal by-products rendering industry. London: MAFF, 1989; revised May 1995.

Ministry of Agriculture, Fisheries and Food (MAFF). 1995e. Code of Practice for the control of *Salmonella* for the UK fish meal industry. London: MAFF, 1989; revised May 1995.

Ministry of Agriculture, Fisheries and Food (MAFF). 1995f. Code of Practice for the control of *Salmonella* in the production of final feed for livestock in premises producing less than 10,000 tonnes per annum. London: MAFF, 1989; revised May 1995.

Ministry of Agriculture, Fisheries and Food (MAFF). 1995g. Code of Practice for the control of *Salmonella* in the production of final feed for livestock in premises producing over 10,000 tonnes per annum. London: MAFF, 1989; revised May 1995.

Ministry of Agriculture, Fisheries and Food (MAFF). 1996. *Salmonella* in livestock production 1995. London: MAFF.

Mulder, R.A.W., and Bolder, N.M. 1991. Experience with competitive exclusion in the Netherlands. In: Blankenship, L.C., ed. Colonization of human bacterial enteropathogens in poultry. San Diego, CA: Academic, pp. 77–90.

Nakamura, M., Nagamine, N., Norimatsu, M., Suzuki, S., Ohishi, K., Kijima, M., Tamura, Y., and Sato, S. 1993. The ability of *Salmonella enteritidis* isolated from chicks imported from England to cause transovarian infection. J. Vet. Med. Sci. 55:135–136.

Nakamura, M., Nagamine, N., Takahashi, T., Norimatsu, M., Suzuki, S., and Sato, S. 1995. Intratracheal infection of chickens with *Salmonella enteritidis* and the effect of feed and water deprivation. Avian Dis. 39:853–858.

Nurmi, E., and Rantala, M. 1973. New aspects of *Salmonella* infections in broiler production. Nature 241:210–211.

O'Brien, J.D.P. 1988. *Salmonella enteritidis* infection in broiler chickens. Vet. Rec. 122:214.

O'Brien, J.D.P. 1990. Aspects of *Salmonella* enteritidis control in poultry. World Poult. Sci. J. 46:119–124.

Opitz, H.M. 1992. Progress being made in *Salmonella enteritidis* reduction on the farm. Poult. Digest March:16–22.

Phillips, R.A., and Opitz H.M. 1995. Pathogenicity and persistence of *Salmonella enteritidis* and egg contamination in normal and infectious bursar disease virus–infected leghorn chicks. Avian Dis. 39:778–787.

Public Health Laboratory Service (PHLS). 1989. Memorandum of evidence to the Agriculture Committee enquiry on *Salmonella* in eggs. PHLS Microbiol. Digest 6:1–10.

Qin, Z.R., Arakawa, A., Baba, E., Fukata, T., Miyamoto, T., Sasai, K., and Withanage G.S.K. 1995. *Eimeria tenella* infection induces recrudescence of previous *Salmonella enteritidis* infection in chickens. Poult. Sci. 74:1786–1792.

Reynolds, D.J., Davies, R.H., Richards, M., and Wray, C. 1997. Evaluation of combined antibiotic and competitive exclusion in broiler breeder flocks infected with *Salmonella enterica* serovar Enteritidis. Avian Pathol. 26:83–92.

Roberts, D. 1991. *Salmonella* in chilled and frozen chicken. Lancet 337:984–985.

Roberts, J.A., and Sockett, P.N. 1994. The socio-economic impact of human *Salmonella enteritidis* infection. Int. J. Food Microbiol. 21:117–129.

Stavric, S., Gleeson, T.M., and Blanchfield, B. 1991. Efficacy of undefined and defined bacterial treatment in competitive exclusion of *Salmonella* from chicks. In: Blankenship, L.C., ed. Colonization of human bacterial enteropathogens in poultry. San Diego, CA: Academic, pp. 323–330.

van de Giessen, A.W., Ament, A.J.H.A., and Notermans, S.H.W. 1994. Intervention strategies for *Salmonella enteritidis* in poultry flocks: a basic approach. Int. J. Food Microbiol. 21:145–154.

Veldman, A., Vahl, H.A., Borggreve, G.J., and Fuller, D.C. 1995. A survey of the incidence of *Salmonella* species and Enterobacteriaceae in poultry feeds and feed components. Vet. Rec. 136:169–172.

von Geissler, H., and Kösters, J. 1972. Die hygienishche Bedeuntung des Getreideschimmelkafers (*Alphitobius diaperinus* panz) in der Geflugelmast. Dtsch. Tierartzl. Wochenschr. 79:177–181.

Williams, J.E. 1972. Observations on *Salmonella thompson as* a poultry pathogen. Avian Pathol. 1:69–73.

Williams, J.E., and Whittemore, A.D. 1976. Comparison of six methods of detecting *Salmonella* typhimurium infection in chickens. Avian Dis. 20:728–734.

World Health Organization (WHO). 1994. Guidelines on cleaning, disinfection and vector control in *Salmonella* infected poultry flocks. Geneva: WHO.

29

Occurrence of *Salmonella enterica* Serovar Enteritidis in Poultry and Other Animals in the United States, 1989–96

K.E. Ferris

IDENTIFICATION AND CHARACTERIZATION

Salmonella enterica serovar Enteritidis (*S.* Enteritidis) is identified by serotyping a bacterial isolate that has been confirmed biochemically to be salmonella. The cell wall (somatic or O) and flagellar (H) antigens are identified by agglutination reactions by using antisera produced in rabbits against specific salmonella antigens. A blood-agar-base (BAB) slant for O antigens and a tube of trypticase soy with tryptose (TST) broth for H antigens are inoculated and incubated at 37°C for 18–24 h. A suspension of cells (from the BAB slant) in physiological saline is used in a slide agglutination test to determine the somatic antigens. The somatic antigen of *S.* Enteritidis is group D1 (1, 9, 12). Physiological saline with 0.6% formalin is added to the TST broth and allowed to stand for at least 1 h. This antigen is used in a tube agglutination test to determine the flagellar antigens. *Salmonella* Enteritidis will agglutinate in g complex and single factor m antisera, but will be negative in factors f, s, t, p, q, and u. The Kauffman-White typing scheme for *S.* Enteritidis also lists a phase-2 antigen 1,7 in brackets, which indicates the antigen may not be expressed by all isolates. *Salmonella* Enteritidis is usually monophasic with the antigenic formula 1,9,12: g,m:- (Ewing, 1986).

Isolates that have been identified as *S.* Enteritidis can be further classified by phage type. The salmonella-serotyping laboratory of the National Veterinary Services Laboratories (NVSL) began phage typing *S.* Enteritidis isolates in 1990. As *S.* Enteritidis became the most common serovar isolated from people with salmonellosis in Great Britain, isolations of this serovar were increasing in the United States. Phage type 4 (PT4) was the predominant strain found in Great Britain, but this phage type had been found in fewer human isolates in the United States. Phage typing of animal isolates of *S.* Enteritidis was begun in order to assist in epidemiological investigations of human outbreaks and to try to prevent the introduction of *S.* Enteritidis PT4 into animal populations in the United States. Phage-typing data have been collected by the NVSL since 1990 and have not previously been presented.

At the NVSL, the set of 10 phages isolated in Great Britain is used (Ward et al., 1987). The pattern of lysis produced by these phages determines the phage type (Table 29.1). An isolate is transferred to a tube of nutrient broth and incubated until growth is visible. A nutrient-agar plate is dried in a 37°C incubator for 2 h and then flooded with the nutrient broth, with the excess liquid removed. A drop of each of the phages at the routine test dilution is then applied to the plate, and the plate is incubated at 35°C. The areas and degrees of lysis are recorded after 18–24 h of incubation, and the phage type is determined (Ward et al., 1987).

TABLE 29.1 Reactions of the *Salmonella* Enteritidis–type strains

PT	Phage									
	1	2	3	4	5	6	7	8	9	10
3	OL	–	–	–	–	–	–	OL	–	OL
4	–	SCL	CL	OL	CL	SCL	CL	SCL	OL	OL
8	–	–	SCL	OL	CL	SCL	SCL	SCL	OL	OL
13	–	–	–	OL	–	SCL	–	–	OL	–
13a	–	–	–	SCL	–	SCL	–	SCL	OL	SCL
14b	–	–	–	–	–	OL	–	–	+	–
23	–	–	–	OL	–	–	–	–	OL	–
28	–	–	++	SCL	SCL	OL	+	SCL	OL	OL
34	–	–	–	–	–	–	–	OL	–	OL

PT, phage type; –, no reaction; +, 1–40 plaques; ++, 41–80 plaques; SCL, semiconfluent lysis; CL, confluent lysis; OL, confluent opaque lysis.

SOURCES AND PHAGE TYPES OF *SALMONELLA* ENTERITIDIS

Salmonella Enteritidis was the most common serovar identified from animals and related sources in 1991–94 (Ferris and Miller, 1991, 1992; Ferris and Thomas, 1993–95). In 1995 and 1996, it was the second most common serovar, although it was still the most frequently isolated salmonella from chickens in both years (Ferris and Thomas, 1995; Ferris and Miller, 1996). The first year in which a significant increase in isolation of *S.* Enteritidis was noted was 1990 (Ferris and Miller, 1990). The number of isolates increased from 488 (13th most common serovar) in 1989 (Ferris and Miller, 1989) to 1499 (third most common serovar) in 1990. This increase was partially due to a large number of isolates submitted from research projects and *S.* Enteritidis Task Force investigation isolates. Isolates from 1989 and 1990 are grouped together in the 1990 phage-type data presented here because all of the 1989 isolates were phage typed in 1990.

The NVSL is dependent on the laboratories submitting isolates for accurate information about the origin of the isolates. Many chicken isolates were identified only as "avian" or "environmental." This is most important when interpreting Figure 29.1 (*S.* Enteritidis by source). The number of submissions from environmental sources correlates with the number from chickens until 1994–96, when those identified only as "environmental" declined as more submissions were identified with the animal species of origin. Those identified only as "avian" declined rapidly after 1990. If the isolates from chickens and environmental sources are added together (Fig. 29.2), the picture of salmonella activity in the United States for the years 1989–96 is easier to visualize. It should be emphasized that many isolates were from research studies, surveys, and tracebacks from human outbreaks. The number of isolates from rodents peaked in 1993 at 1508 as the relationship between rodents and infected chickens was studied.

Salmonella Enteritidis is not a host-adapted serovar, but the number of isolates from sources other than chickens remained fairly constant from 1989 to 1996. There was a slight increase in isolations from cattle, peaking in 1993

(Fig. 29.3), but it is interesting that the number of isolates from turkeys decreased from the 1989–90 level and remained low throughout the period described.

Not all *S.* Enteritidis isolates submitted to the NVSL were phage typed. Figure 29.4 shows the number that were phage typed, as well as the total number of isolates identified from 1989–90 to 1996. At least one isolate was phage typed from each sample or submission.

The phage-typing results are presented in Figures 29.5 and 29.6. PT8 was the most common phage type identified from 1989–90 until 1995, when PT13a was identified more frequently. In 1991, of the isolates phage typed, 39% were PT8. In 1996, only 23% were PT8, and PT13a increased from 20% of the total in 1991 to 27% in 1996. PT28 remained fairly constant throughout this time, and it now accounts for 18% of the *S.* Enteritidis phage types, compared with 9.5% in 1991. The numbers of PT3 and PT34 have remained relatively low throughout the years. PT14b was identified 388 times in 1989–90 but decreased to 110 in 1991 and was not identified in 1996. PT13 was identified more than 100 times each year from 1991 to 1993 but only 21 times in 1996. PT4 increased from eight in 1993 to 167 in 1994. There were 71 isolates of PT4 identified in 1995 and 61 in 1996 (6% of the total).

Although *S.* Enteritidis was isolated from animals throughout the United States, the majority of isolates each year came from states that had flocks involved in traceback investigations. In 1989–90, isolates were received from 38 states and the District of Columbia, but 73% of the isolates were from Pennsylvania (1672), Maryland (342), New Jersey (322), and Maine (227). Isolates from 36 states and the District of Columbia were identified as *S.* Enteritidis in 1991, but 87% were from five states: Indiana (2139), Pennsylvania (926), New Jersey (772), Maryland (426), Maine (241), and Georgia (134). In 1992, there were 80.5% from Pennsylvania and Maryland and, in 1993, there were 85% from Pennsylvania and Indiana. In 1994, of the isolates received, 85% were from Pennsylvania, Indiana, and California, and 83% of the PT4 isolates were from California. In 1995 and 1996, isolates were received from 31 and 30 states, respectively, and for a large number (854 in 1995 and 591 in 1996) a state of origin was not listed.

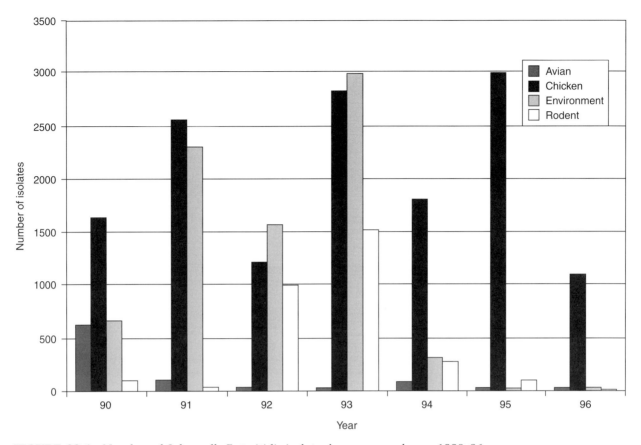

FIGURE 29.1   Number of *Salmonella* Enteritidis isolates by source and year, 1990–96.

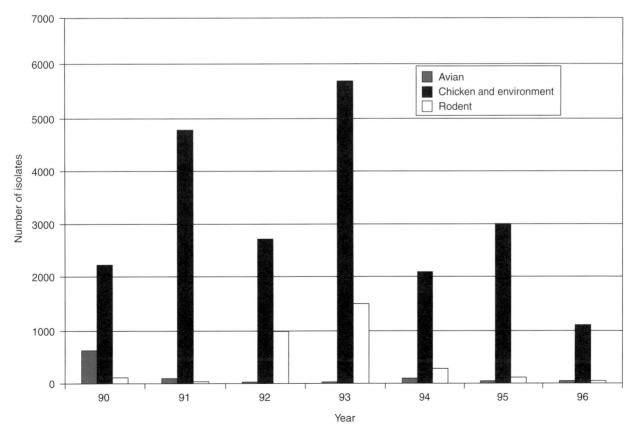

FIGURE 29.2   Number of *Salmonella* Enteritidis isolates by source and year, 1990–96.

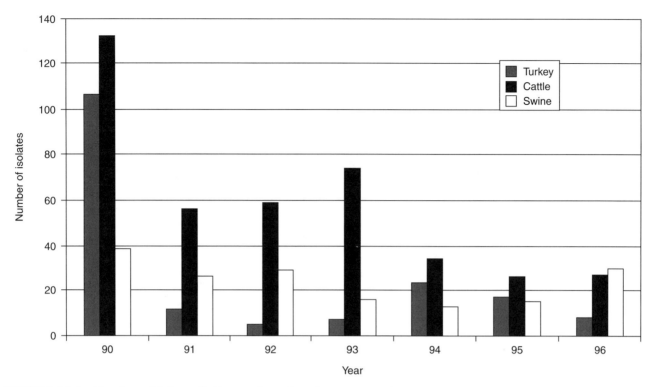

FIGURE 29.3   Number of *Salmonella* Enteritidis isolates by source and year, 1990–96.

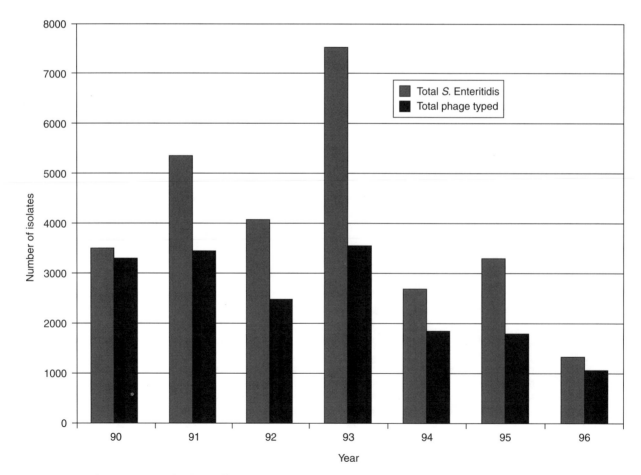

FIGURE 29.4   Phage typing of *Salmonella* Enteritidis, 1990–96.

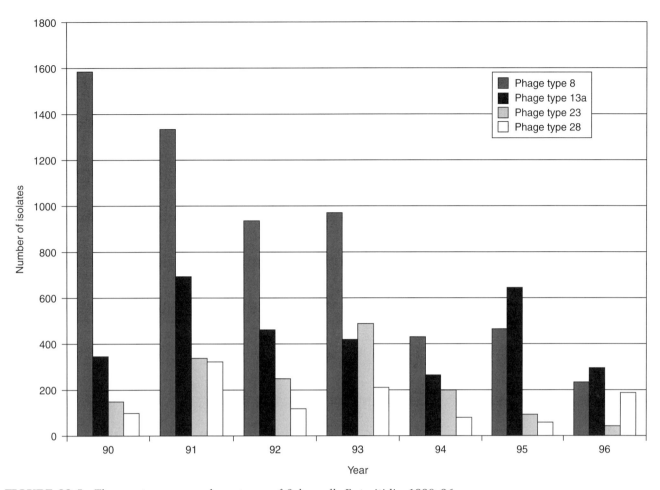

FIGURE 29.5   The most common phage types of *Salmonella* Enteritidis, 1990–96.

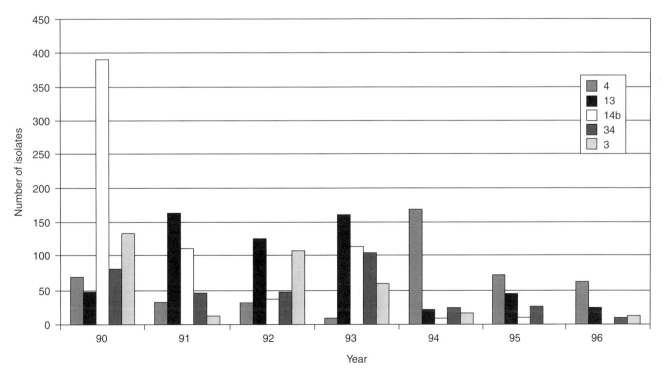

FIGURE 29.6   The less common phage types of *Salmonella* Enteritidis, 1990–96.

Throughout the years, the majority of isolates from cattle and swine were from cases of clinical disease (primary or secondary infection). From 1989–90 to 1995, an average of 86% of the isolates from cattle were from clinical disease. In 1996, there were 52% identified as "surveillance/monitor" or "other." Of the swine isolates, 87% were from clinical disease from 1989–90 to 1994. In 1995, the clinical isolates were 47% of the total, and 63% were monitor samples in 1996. An average of 70.5% of the isolates from chickens were environmental, monitor samples, "other," or research from 1989–90 to 1993. In 1994, this percentage rose to 85%, and it was 97% in 1995 and 1996.

There was no apparent association between phage type and clinical role. Interpreting the data is difficult because many submitters did not indicate a clinical role. In 1989–90, there was no information on clinical role for 33% of the submissions. This percentage was even higher in 1991–93, with 65% in 1991 and 1992, and 69% in 1993, lacking information on the clinical role. In 1994, of the submissions, 34% did not list the clinical role, but only 2% and 1.5% of the isolates in 1995 and 1996, respectively, were submitted without this information.

REFERENCES

Ewing, W.H. 1986. Edwards and Ewing's identification of Enterobacteriaceae, 4th ed. New York: Elsevier Science.

Ferris, K.E., and Miller, D.A. 1989. Salmonella serotypes from animals and related sources reported during July 1988–June 1989. Proc. U.S. Anim. Health Assoc. 93:521–538.

Ferris, K.E., and Miller, D.A. 1990. Salmonella serotypes from animals and related sources reported during July 1989–June 1990. Proc. U.S. Anim. Health Assoc. 94:463–478.

Ferris, K.E., and Miller, D.A. 1991. Salmonella serotypes from animals and related sources reported during July 1990–June 1991. Proc. U.S. Anim. Health Assoc. 95:440–454.

Ferris, K.E., and Miller, D.A. 1992. Salmonella serotypes from animals and related sources reported during July 1991–June 1992. Proc. U.S. Anim. Health Assoc. 96:492–504.

Ferris, K.E., and Miller, D.A. 1996. Salmonella serotypes from animals and related sources reported during July 1995–June 1996. Proc. U.S. Anim. Health Assoc. 100:505–526

Ferris, K.E., and Thomas, L.A. 1993. Salmonella serotypes from animals and related sources reported during July 1992–June 1993. Proc. U.S. Anim. Health Assoc. 97:524–539.

Ferris, K.E., and Thomas, L.A. 1994. Salmonella serotypes from animals and related sources reported during July 1993–June 1994. Proc. U.S. Anim. Health Assoc. 98:443–461.

Ferris, K.E., and Thomas, L.A. 1995. Salmonella serotypes from animals and related sources reported during July 1994–June 1995. Proc. U.S. Anim. Health Assoc. 99:510–524.

Ward, L.R., De Sa, J.D.H., and Rowe, B. 1987. A phage-typing scheme for Salmonella enteritidis. Epidemiol. Infect. 99:291–294.

30

Role of Rodents in the Epidemiology of *Salmonella enterica* Serovar Enteritidis and Other Salmonella Serovars in Poultry Farms

D.J. Henzler and H.M. Opitz

INTRODUCTION

The emergence of *Salmonella enterica* serovar Enteritidis (*S.* Enteritidis) as a cause of foodborne salmonellosis, regionally in the mid-Atlantic and northeastern United States, and as a worldwide pandemic has concerned both veterinary and human public health professionals (St. Louis et al., 1988; Rodrigue et al., 1990). Epidemiological evidence strongly supports the role of commensal rodents in the on-farm contamination of poultry feed and environments with salmonellae, and specifically *S.* Enteritidis, and is highly suggestive of direct infectious spread to chickens (Krabisch and Dorn, 1980; Henzler and Opitz, 1992; Davies and Wray, 1995; Kinde et al., 1996a,b). Specific subtypes of *S.* Enteritidis isolated from mice are capable of undergoing spontaneous swarm migration on selective agar and have a very high O-antigen–core ratio, both features of increased invasiveness and pathogenicity (Guard-Petter et al., 1997).

Producers are typically unaware of the high numbers of house mice (*Mus musculus*) living in poultry houses. Mouse populations are easily underestimated because of their chiefly nocturnal activities and the acceptance of "a few mice" as normal in commercial poultry buildings. Ample shelter, food, and water in poultry dwellings, and

the previous lack of practical methods for quantifying rodents, have contributed to high rodent densities within poultry houses. Furthermore, rodent damage to poultry houses, through gnawing and nest building, create "infectious pockets" within the confines of walls and attics of facilities, providing a source of exposure to salmonella-clean rodents entering these areas. These sites are not easily sanitized and escape traditional cleaning and disinfection methods.

SALMONELLA SEROVARS ASSOCIATED WITH COMMENSAL RODENTS

Commensal rodents are commonly associated with human dwellings and human activities, such as intensive poultry and livestock production. Commensal rodents are not native to the United States. These rodents—the house mouse (*M. musculus*), Norway rat (*Rattus norvegicus*), and roof rat (*Rattus rattus*)—established themselves in the United States and other places they were not native by traveling on ships that early settlers used in transportation from their native homelands of Europe.

Salmonellae have been isolated from commensal rodents in urban, rural, and agricultural habitats worldwide (Savage and Read, 1913; Robinson and Daniel, 1968; Taylor 1968; Goyal and Singh, 1970; McKiel et al., 1970; Sato et al., 1970; Jones and Twigg, 1976; Singh et al., 1980; Henzler and Opitz, 1992; Davies and Wray, 1995; Guard-Petter et al., 1997). *Salmonella* Enteritidis and *S.* Typhimurium are the most frequent serovars associated with these rodents, particularly in poultry houses (Sato et al., 1970; Singh et al., 1980; Henzler and Opitz, 1992; Davies and Wray, 1995; Kinde et al., 1996a,b; Guard-Petter et al., 1997; D.J. Henzler, unpublished data).

Salmonella Enteritidis (*Bacillus enteritidis*, Gaertner organisms) has been associated with rats (presumably Norway rats) since as early as 1913 (Savage and Read, 1913). Of 41 rats, five (12.2%) had *B. enteritidis* isolated from the spleen, and two of these rats also had the bacterium isolated from the liver. Norway rats were implicated in the transmission of *S.* Enteritidis and *S.* Newington on a farm associated with broilers and vertically infected carrier chickens in Japan. Rats were thought to be the source of introduction of the flock to *S.* Newington. *Salmonella* Enteritidis was isolated from one of 14 and from five of 37 rats from a farm where *S.* Enteritidis was also isolated from chicks over a several-year period (Sato et al., 1970). *Salmonella* Anatum and *S.* Stanley were isolated from rats on a poultry farm in a country where *S.* Anatum is one of the most common serovars for salmonellosis in humans, animals, and birds (Goyal and Singh, 1970). *Salmonella* Enteritidis was one of five serovars isolated from 254 rats and one of two serovars isolated from 109 house mice trapped from dairy and poultry premises, feed stores, and around residential buildings in India (Singh et al., 1980). In New Zealand, of 42 Norway rats cultured for salmonellae, 15 were positive with *S.* Typhimurium and *S.* Bovis-morbificans. These rats were trapped on three sheep farms where *S.* Bovis-morbificans was an enzootic subtype. These rats were believed to have been contaminated by feeding on sheep carcasses or by the environment (Robinson and Daniel, 1968).

A survey of Norway rats (*Rattus norvegicus*) and roof rats (*Rattus rattus*) was done over two separate periods constituting a total of 6 years of study during spring and summer months (McKiel et al., 1970). In total, 16 areas from four Canadian provinces had rats sampled. In total, 39 of 601 rats examined were positive for salmonellae. The salmonella status of the rats was determined by obtaining 1 g of fecal material from a section of the small intestine. Seven of the 601 rats captured were *R. rattus* and the remainder were *R. norvegicus*. Four subtypes of salmonellae were identified as follows: *S.* Enteritidis, *S.* Typhimurium, *S.* Montevideo, *S.* Derby. *Salmonella* Enteritidis accounted for 24 and *S.* Typhimurium for 12 of the 39 salmonella isolates. Within two of the 16 areas, *S.* Enteritidis had an incidence of 19% and 33% of the *R. norvegicus* sampled. In the region that had a 19% incidence, a large number of the rats were captured on a garbage dump. One of two feral cats also sampled at the dump was *S.* Enteritidis positive.

A study in England involved collection and culture of 1269 mammals from both indoor dwellings and the countryside (Jones and Twigg, 1976). Eight of 364 house mice (*M. musculus*) were positive for salmonellae. These mice were collected from livestock-research buildings. Seven mice had *S.* Dublin and were believed to have acquired the infection from experimentally infected cattle that had the same serovar. One mouse had *S.* Typhimurium, which was not a subtype known to be present in any of the cattle. The authors noted that an additional 28 house mice were captured in buildings housing experimentally infected cattle but were not easily infected by salmonellae. The absence of collection of salmonellae from wild free-living populations of mammals other than house mice led the authors to suggest wild mammals are not a significant source of salmonellae in domestic livestock.

Salmonella Enteritidis, *S.* Heidelberg, *S.* Hadar, *S.* Typhimurium, *S.* Anatum, *S.* Mbandaka, *S.* Cerro, and *S.* Schwarzengrund were isolated from 713 house mice (*M. musculus*) and two Norway rats (*R. norvegicus*) collected individually from 46 poultry houses in Maine (Henzler and Opitz, 1992). Poultry houses included in that study housed commercial pullets, laying hens, and broiler breeders. *Salmonella* Enteritidis represented 69% of all salmonella serovars isolated from rodents. *Salmonella* Heidelberg was the second most common serovar cultured from mice, at a frequency of 13.6%. *Salmonella* Typhimurium was isolated from 2.5% of the rodents.

In a 2-year study in Pennsylvania, 621 mouse spleens during the first year and 526 mouse spleens during the second year were cultured for salmonella isolation. *Salmonella* Enteritidis was the most frequent serotype isolated during the 2-year survey, comprising 25.0% and 17.9% of the spleens, respectively. *Salmonella* Typhimurium was isolated from mouse spleens at a much lower frequency of 1.45% and 1.1% during the first and second years of the study, respectively (Guard-Petter et al., 1997).

BIOLOGY OF COMMENSAL RODENTS

Rodents reproduce rapidly in chicken houses, where food, water, and shelter are readily available (Table 30.1). A few mice entering a poultry house can proliferate to high numbers (10,000 or more) during the life of a single flock (D.J. Henzler, unpublished data). Rodents consume feed, destroy insulating and building materials, and undermine building structures through tunneling and nesting. A single mouse consumes two-tenths ounce of chicken feed daily, whereas 2000 mice consume 25 pounds of feed each day. Similarly, Laurie (1945) determined that an adult mouse eats 3.0 g of corn a day and 2000 mice would eat approximately 6 kg.

A study of 1781 wild house mice from two heavy wild populations in confined buildings demonstrated that the natural home range of the mice averaged 12 feet. Of the house mouse movements, 90% were less than 30 feet and

TABLE 30.1   Reproductive and feeding characteristics of the house mouse (*Mus musculus*) and the Norway rat (*Rattus norvegicus*)

Characteristics	House mouse	Norway rat
Home range	9–30 feet usually (up to 150 feet in some houses)	20–300 feet
Longevity	12–15 months	12–15 months
Sexual maturity	45 days	90 days
Litters per year	5–11	4–12
Young per litter	3–11	8–10
Daily feeding sites	Many	Usually 2

70% of the mouse travels were no greater than 10 feet. The greatest distance traveled by a single mouse was no more than 140 feet (Young et al., 1950). The study also demonstrated that the density of mouse populations had little impact on distances moved in the normal home range of mice.

Goodrich examined biological data from 8207 house mice (*M. musculus*) living in four separate wild populations (Laurie, 1945). The average litter size was determined to be 5.83 ± 0.31 mice (range, 2–13 mice). This does not include litters from communal nesting sites, where numbers are considerably higher. Mice harbored in corn ricks (bins) had higher pregnancy levels than did those living in cold meat-storage facilities and were lighter. This increased reproductive performance was speculated to be due to the warmer environments afforded by the corn ricks compared with cold storage. Limited disturbance from predators and humans, and a constant and more complete and unlimited food supply, enabled corn-rick mice to have the highest pregnancy among all four groups studied. No seasonal differences were noted in pregnancy rates among the four groups as is typically noted in noncommensal rodents living in areas predominantly outside of buildings. Annual litter production was determined to be 10.22 ± 0.57 litters for the corn-rick mice. These figures were much higher than those for the other three populations of mice measured, and close to the theoretical maximum number of litters (that is, 13–14) per pregnant female per year.

Several natural populations of house mice were observed under experimental settings that provided ample harborage areas and water, but where feed was restricted in one mouse population (Strecker and Emlen, 1953). The mouse population with feed restriction underwent steady increases in population size until food was restricted, at which time the reproductive performance in female mice was markedly reduced and the data suggested decreasing reproduction in male mice. Litter size of mice was not significantly different at any time in the growing period, including the population peak density, until food was limited.

A study was undertaken on grain-storage areas (ricks) to assess house mouse and Norway rat populations in England during the harvesting seasons from 1939 to 1941 (Venables and Leslie, 1942). Mice were noted to be able to do without a direct supply of water for long periods. Rats were observed drinking rain and dew, and occasionally seen eating green shoots from nearby barley crops. A total

of 85 Norway rat nests were examined with an average of 7.31 young rats per nest (range, 3–13 rats). Another examination of 64 rat nests yielded an average of 6.7 rats per nest. This study noted the existence of both rat and mouse populations in the same ricks, and the longer the grain set before threshing the greater was the increase in rodent populations. Comparison of female rats from ricks and female rats from nonrick areas showed that rick rats had pregnancies of 25%–28% compared with only 3% for rats in the nonrick areas. The chi-squared test showed significant differences in the percent of pregnancies between the populations. These differences were noted for the winter seasons. There were no significant differences in the number of pregnancies between rick rats and nonrick (rural countryside) rats during other seasons. Rick rats were thought to be the source of the rural rats. Additionally, the greater number of female rick-rat pregnancies in the winter months was probably due to the good shelter and the constant abundance of readily available food. House mouse populations multiplied possibly to 3 and 0.5 times within 6 months.

TRANSMISSION AND SHEDDING OF SALMONELLAE AMONG RODENTS

Bartram et al. (1940) infected laboratory rats (presumably white hybrid species of *R. norvegicus*) with various concentrations of a strain of *S.* Enteritidis. In rats dosed with 100 *S.* Enteritidis by stomach tube, the organism was shed in feces intermittently to day 51 after infection. Previously infected rats that had not shed *S.* Enteritidis in feces for 45 days were reinfected by a small dose of bacteria, and *S.* Enteritidis was shed the next day by five of six rats. Excretion of the organism was irregular following this, and most rats discontinued shedding *S.* Enteritidis on day 9, although one rat excreted the bacteria up to day 34. In another experiment, horizontal infection of four rats resulted through exposure to feces of a single rat infected with 100 *S.* Enteritidis organisms. These studies concluded overall that rats infected with *S.* Enteritidis can become carriers and that most rats cease to pass the bacteria by day 15 after infection, although some rats continue to shed

S. Enteritidis for 7 weeks. The authors cite investigations by four independent scientists that the incidence of *S.* Enteritidis infection in wild rats was similar at a range of 11%–13%. In rat feces infected orally with a pathogenic *S.* Enteritidis strain, the bacterium survived for 148 days at room temperature. Horizontal transfer of *S.* Enteritidis occurred through seven separate rat colonies by oral inoculation of a single rat with 100 bacterial cells of an invasive *S.* Enteritidis strain. Similar work with mice was done with horizontal transfer of *S.* Enteritidis infection through three colonies of mice (Welch et al., 1941).

Laboratory rats at age 4 days, 20 days, and 100 days were given doses of *S.* Typhimurium, *S.* Dublin, and *S.* Oranienburg to assess the effect of salmonella strains, dose, and age on the shed of salmonella in feces (Kempelmacher et al., 1969). Salmonellae were given orally through a plastic tube or by direct consumption of the bacterium on minced meat after a 24-h fast. At doses of 5×10^8, most 4-day-old rats died rapidly. With the 20-day-old rats, fecal excretion of salmonellae over 40 days was 100%, except for *S.* Dublin. The shed of salmonellae by 100-day-old rats was less consistent, but a portion of the rats continued to shed salmonellae for up to 40 days. Lower doses of these three strains of salmonellae resulted in less persistent shed of salmonellae in feces. Older rats shed salmonellae less often in feces and, at a 10^2 dose, none of the 100-day-old rats excreted salmonellae in feces, nor could salmonellae be isolated from the intestine or other organs sampled. *Salmonella* Typhimurium was more virulent and was the most persistent of the strains.

The significance of vertical transmission of *S.* Enteritidis in rodent populations is unclear; although some researchers suggest its occurrence in mice, others state that it is unlikely to occur in rats (Davies and Wray, 1995; Henzler et al., 1997b). Mice were fed contaminated feed pellets containing about 10^5 and 10^3 colony-forming units (CFU) per mouse of an *S.* Enteritidis phage type 4 (PT4) isolated from a wild mouse trapped on a poultry farm (Davies and Wray, 1995). One of the mouse groups ceased excreting *S.* Enteritidis at week 15 after feeding and was reinoculated with about 10^5 CFU *S.* Enteritidis; 3 weeks later, the mice stopped fecally excreting the organism. In a group of mice receiving 10^5 organisms, excretion of salmonellae continued for up to 8 months. The higher dose of 10^5 bacteria resulted in longer excretions of *S.* Enteritidis than did a dose of 10^3 bacteria. These studies determined that the excretion of *S.* Enteritidis from the mice was intermittent. Droppings from a group of these mice were added to feed, water in a bell-drinker, or litter that housed 5-week-old chickens, which subsequently became infected with *S.* Enteritidis, as determined by the greater than 10^5 salmonellae isolated per gram of feces.

Salmonella Enteritidis PT4 was confirmed in chickens on two poultry farms, and droppings from two groups of naturally infected mice trapped on these farms were cultured for *S.* Enteritidis (Davies and Wray, 1995). The number of salmonellae isolated per 100 droppings was low (0–10^3), but mice shed *S.* Enteritidis for 7 and 19 weeks. Shedding of *S.* Enteritidis by mice increased in both groups of mice after disturbances or changes in their environment.

In Great Britain, mouse droppings were collected after poultry units were cleaned and disinfected, and although most droppings contained only 1–10 *S.* Enteritidis bacteria, some droppings contained 10^3–10^4 (Davies and Wray, 1995). This is consistent with earlier studies in Maine, where droppings from naturally infected house mice (*M. musculus*), trapped in poultry flocks, contained 2.3×10^5 and 2.5×10^3 *S.* Enteritidis (Henzler and Opitz, 1992). Similarly, the mice in Great Britain produced 111 droppings per day (Davies and Wray, 1995), and Henzler and Opitz (1992) recorded an average of 100 fecal droppings from mice per day.

GENETIC AND NATURAL RESISTANCE

Hormaeche (1979) measured the invasiveness of salmonellae in laboratory mice directly by noting increases in the number of bacterial organisms in the liver and spleen of mice injected with a standard dose of organisms, or indirectly by determining the time of death after dosing. Genetic variation in the resistance to *S.* Enteritidis by laboratory mice was noted with Balb/c mice being more susceptible to intravenous inoculation of this bacterium than were other strains tested. *Salmonella* Enteritidis was the cause of a serious outbreak of clinical disease in a laboratory colony of Balb/c mice known to be susceptible to this subtype of *Salmonella* (Casebolt and Shoeb, 1988). A total of 1200 mice were killed or died as a direct result of *S.* Enteritidis infection. In one group, 80% of the mice died within a week. Clinical signs noted were weight loss, hunched appearance, increased respiratory rate, rough hair coat, and conjunctivitis. Gross pathological lesions included moderate spleen enlargement, and depressed foci on the liver surface and spleen. *Salmonella* Enteritidis was cultured from the liver, gallbladder, and ceca of the mice.

Paratyphoid salmonellae have varying abilities to infect many warm-blooded animals, including rodents and poultry, as well as humans. Prior to the 1950s, rodenticides consisting of live cultures of *S.* Enteritidis var. *danysz* and var. *jena* were used in continental Europe as methods of commensal rodent control (Savage and Read, 1913; Taylor, 1956). Live cultures of these bacterial strains were readily available commercially (in Ratin and in Ratin bread) and applied to "runs" of rodents in bakeries, slaughterhouses, and other establishments where commensal rodents thrived and where the potential for food poisoning existed. The cultures, often referred to as a "virus," were placed on bread. The rodents ingested the bait, developed gastroenteritis, and usually died. Some rodents, though, survived the "virus," recovered, and then shed the *S.* Enteritidis in their droppings, thus contaminating food, which resulted in human food poisoning. *Salmonella* Enteritidis was the second most common type of salmonella food poisoning in 1951, 1952, and 1953 in England. Rodenticide preparations including *S.* Enteritidis var. *danysz* and var. *jena* were implicated in the epidemiology of infection from commensal rodents to humans. The use of *S.* Enteritidis was then banned in the United States and subsequently diminished in Europe.

SIGNIFICANCE IN *SALMONELLA* ENTERITIDIS

Association with Environmental Isolations

Kinde et al. (1996a) cultured isolates for *S.* Enteritidis from a stream that was entirely composed of sewage effluent from a human municipal plant and was suspected to be the only source of water for rodents and feral animals during the summer months. The creek passed within 200 feet of a chicken ranch that was infected with *S.* Enteritidis. Feral animals in the area and on the chicken farm, including mice, were infected with *S.* Enteritidis. The authors strongly suggest that the water may have been the source for contamination of rodents on this farm, which could have contaminated chicken feed bins through the fecal–oral route.

Environmental culture results from samples of the manure and egg-handling equipment among 84 layer flocks in Pennsylvania were compared with mice populations as determined by rodent indexing (RI) (Henzler et al., 1995, 1997a). Flocks with a high RI as compared with a low RI were 4.2 times more likely to have manure samples positive for *S.* Enteritidis. Flocks with a high RI were 4.4 times more likely to have *S.* Enteritidis–positive egg-handling equipment than were flocks with a low RI.

A vector study of salmonellae in broiler operations in Germany revealed that mice were the most frequently infected live vectors, followed by beetles and flies. *Salmonella* Typhimurium and *S.* Enteritidis were the two most frequently isolated serovars (Krabisch and Dorn, 1980). Mice infected with *S.* Enteritidis were often associated with *S.* Enteritidis-contaminated environments. Where mice were positive for *S.* Enteritidis and the environment negative, may be due to lack of sensitivity of the environmental test. Alternatively, mice may remain infected from a previous flock environment that was *S.* Enteritidis positive (Henzler and Opitz, 1992; Guard-Petter et al., 1997).

A comprehensive study of rodents on poultry farms in Maine by Henzler and Opitz (1992) in 46 poultry houses on 10 premises found rodents, particularly the house mouse (*M. musculus*), especially susceptible to *S.* Enteritidis infections over any other salmonella serovars. Mice were infected with *S.* Enteritidis only on farms where *S.* Enteritidis could also be isolated from drag swabs of the manure, poultry-house walkway floors, and hand swabs of the egg belts. In total, 2103 environmental samples, 713 mice, and two rats were tested for salmonellae, and *S.* Enteritidis was isolated from 16.2% of the mice and 5.1% of the environmental samples. On *S.* Enteritidis–contaminated premises, *S.* Enteritidis was cultured from 7.5% of the environmental samples and 24.0% of the rodents. This accounted for 18.0% of the salmonella isolations from environmental samples and 75.3% of all salmonella isolations from mice.

Overall, 168 rodents (23.5%) were positive for salmonellae of the 715 cultured. The rate of *S.* Enteritidis infection in mice on *S.* Enteritidis–contaminated farms ranged from 4.8% to 71.4%, with an average of 24.0%.

Association with Chickens and Eggs

Chicken tissues, eggs, feral animals, and rodents were cultured from a ranch infected with *S.* Enteritidis PT4 (Robinson and Daniel, 1968). Of the 48 mice captured in these houses, six were infected with *S.* Enteritidis and one was infected with *S.* Heidelberg. *Salmonella* Enteritidis was isolated from mice in four of six houses where mice were captured. The range of mice infected with *S.* Enteritidis was 4% to 37.5% in the four houses. Overall, 12.5% of the mice were infected with *S.* Enteritidis.

Chickens housed on dirt and littered floors produced eggs with a higher prevalence of *S.* Enteritidis (14.9–19.1 eggs per 10,000) from two of five flocks infected with *S.* Enteritidis than did chickens on the same ranch housed in cages. Rodents had easy access to the feed bins with the floor-housed chickens, and the feed bins were contaminated with their droppings (Kinde et al., 1996a). Only two mice were cultured in these houses, and *S.* Enteritidis was not isolated from either. Another flock that produced *S.* Enteritidis–positive eggs had *S.* Enteritidis isolated from 37.5% of the mice cultured.

Moderate and high house mice (*M. musculus*) populations as measured by RI in 60 commercial layer flocks in Pennsylvania were not a significant factor for the production of *S.* Enteritidis–contaminated eggs (Henzler et al., 1998). Mouse densities were measured independently of the *S.* Enteritidis status of the mice, and the exposure history of the layers as pullets was unknown. The microbiological flora of the intestinal tract of immature poultry is not well established, and exposure to *S.* Enteritidis, at an early age, may result in a chronically infected bird. Laying hens exposed to mice droppings contaminated with *S.* Enteritidis may likely become infected with *S.* Enteritidis, or such an exposure could exacerbate a previous infection. Alternatively, exposure to *S.* Enteritidis as a chick or pullet may result in subsequent shedding of the bacterium by a laying hen and the production of infected eggs as layers. This could occur either irrespective of, or without exposure to, the presence of *S.* Enteritidis–infected house mice in the layer house.

In total, 621 and 526 mouse spleens were culture positive for *S.* Enteritidis, representing 25.0% and 17.9% from a 2-year study in Pennsylvania in 1992–94. Nine houses where mice were cultured for *S.* Enteritidis produced *S.* Enteritidis–contaminated eggs, and the spleens of four of these mice were also infected (Guard-Petter et al., 1997).

MOLECULAR CHARACTERISTICS OF MOUSE ISOLATES

Epidemiological linkage and significance of *S.* Enteritidis in rodents and chickens can be further supported by molecular characterization of isolates. Identical *S.* Enteritidis phage types were identified from chickens, environmental samples, and mice (Henzler and Opitz, 1992; Kinde et al., 1996a). As part of an epidemiological investigation of the first isolation of *S.* Enteritidis PT4 in the United States in a commercial egg-layer flock, 17 isolates of *S.* Enteritidis were obtained from chickens, eggs, feral animals, and rodents and from effluent from municipal creek water located within 200 feet of the chicken ranch. Plasmid profiles of several isolates from mouse livers, chicken livers, and a chicken egg were identical. Restriction endonuclease plasmid analysis of chicken livers, a mouse liver, and the chicken egg demonstrated identical migration patterns (Kinde et al., 1996b). Isolates from environmental samples, chickens, mice, rats, eggs, and cat feces revealed that all isolates possessed two plasmids of identical size (40.3 and 3.0 MDa). Subtyping of PT14b, using an alternative phage-typing scheme, indicated that isolates from mice and other sources predominantly belonged to the same subtype (Singer et al., 1992). Restriction endonuclease cleavage produced an identical pattern from chicken, environmental, and mice isolates (Singer et al., 1992; Kinde et al., 1996a). No differences in outer-membrane protein profiles between isolates were detected, regardless of plasmid profile, phage type, or source (Singer et al., 1992). Plasmid profile or phage type is not necessarily an indication of the virulence and invasiveness of *S.* Enteritidis in mice or chickens (Halavatkar and Barrow, 1993; Poppe et al., 1993; Guard-Petter et al., 1997). Other researchers suggest that the presence of the large serovar-specific plasmid is essential for virulence expression of *S.* Enteritidis (Helmuth et al., 1985; Nakamura et al., 1985; Montenegro et al., 1991; Suzuki et al., 1992).

Phage types identified from isolates of *S.* Enteritidis from mice were the same as those isolated from the environment (117 mouse and 180 environmental isolates) (Henzler and Opitz, 1992). In chicken flocks on single-house premises, only one phage type of *S.* Enteritidis was isolated from the environment and mice. On multiple-house in-line-layer complexes, multiple phage types were isolated. PT13a and PT14b were the most frequent in environmental and mouse samples.

Other phage types isolated included PT2, PT23, and untypeable. Over nearly a 2-year period of this study, only PT13a was isolated in a single replacement flock on a multiple-house complex, suggesting that the spread of *S.* Enteritidis from mice may be limited. This is supported by the limited home range of the house mouse given ample food, harborage, and possibly water (Young et al., 1950). All of these requirements are present in poultry houses.

Analysis of the *S.* Enteritidis in mouse populations from Pennsylvania layer farms indicated that an emergence of the *S.* Enteritidis population was associated with a great increase in recovery of the bacterium from mice spleens. In total, 19 of 249 *S.* Enteritidis isolations from mice spleens underwent spontaneous swarm migration on 2% brilliant green agar. Six of these isolates were further characterized and yielded an exceptionally high O-antigen–core ratio. Earlier studies demonstrated that avirulent *S.* Enteritidis isolates were associated with an O-antigen–core ratio of 1,

producing chiefly low-molecular-weight lipopolysaccharide (LPS). Previous studies demonstrated that only high-molecular-weight LPS isolates were capable of swarm migration across inhibition agar (Guard-Petter et al., 1996). The ability of bacteria to show swarming migration has been linked to pathogenicity (Allison et al., 1994). Numerous studies have demonstrated the theory that the composition of the LPS is a sensitive indicator of *S.* Enteritidis invasiveness in organs and contaminated chicken eggs (Petter, 1993; Allison et al., 1994; Humphrey et al., 1996). This study supports another tool for investigating the epidemiology of *S.* Enteritidis in mice on farms through the examination of mice spleens, in particular the characterization of the LPS structures and the ability of the isolates to exhibit spontaneous swarming, and contamination of eggs.

PROGRESSION AND PERSISTENCE OF *SALMONELLA* ENTERITIDIS IN MOUSE POPULATIONS

In a study in Pennsylvania, 21 commercial egg-laying houses (some with replacement flocks) had intensive investigations of mouse spleens to evaluate pathogenicity of *S.* Enteritidis. One house (house 5301) that had pullets introduced from vertically infected breeder chicks had a progressive and persistent *S.* Enteritidis infection among the mice. Rodent control was not maintained in this house (RI = 3) and, during the second year of the survey, the percent of mice that were positive for *S.* Enteritidis increased from 16.1% to 47.6% (Guard-Petter et al., 1997). Ineffective control of rodents can result in maintenance of invasive *S.* Enteritidis in mice populations on chicken farms for years (Guard-Petter et al., 1997).

In total, 85 houses in Pennsylvania were evaluated for *S.* Enteritidis in the environment from culture results obtained from drag-swab samples of the manure and hand swabs of the egg belts as part of the *S.* Enteritidis Pilot Project (1992–94). Mice were infected with *S.* Enteritidis in 43 (78%) of 55 *S.* Enteritidis–positive houses, whereas mice were infected with *S.* Enteritidis in six (20%) of 30 *S.* Enteritidis–negative houses. The odds ratio for this association of *S.* Enteritidis in the environment and mice is 14.3 (95% confidence limits of 4.3–50.9). In a previous study in Pennsylvania, mice infected with *S.* Enteritidis were found in *S.* Enteritidis–negative houses (Henzler and Opitz, 1992). It is likely that these mice were exposed to *S.* Enteritidis from the environment of previously housed chickens that may have shed *S.* Enteritidis. Mice are more sensitive indicators of *S.* Enteritidis than are environmental samples; mice were 3.2 times more likely to yield *S.* Enteritidis than were environmental samples from chicken houses contaminated with *S.* Enteritidis (Henzler and Opitz, 1992). Obtaining an adequate sample of mice is important, and some determination of the mouse population through RI is recommended. Where mice are present in moderate or high populations, obtaining a sample of 30 mice for culture of *S.* Enteritidis would indicate whether at least 10% of the mouse population is infected with the bacterium.

MONITORING RODENT POPULATIONS

A variety of methods are available for monitoring rodent populations, but few are practical and adaptable to intensive agriculture poultry production. Traditional methods for estimating rodent populations include direct visual observation, mark and recapture, scoring or counting of rodent tracks from marked tiles, and direct observation of physical signs (for example, rodent droppings, fresh gnawings, and smudge marks). Traditional methods are discussed next, followed by a practical method for quantitation of mice numbers in poultry houses to establish an RI (Henzler, 1993; Guard-Petter et al., 1997; Henzler et al., 1998).

Direct methods for the census of animal populations require marking of the animals and further identification in records for observing these animals in the future (Kaukeinen, 1979). In the case of commensal rodents, these methods often include capturing individual rodents and marking them uniquely with an identifier, such as a toe clip or ear clip. These types of studies are typically done to determine travel patterns, feeding areas, and the effectiveness of rodenticide programs. These methods are very labor-intensive, requiring extensive trapping. Recapture of previously caught rodents can result in their being trap shy, whereas, in other cases, rodents may want to return to a trap for shelter or food. Each of these situations can bias the actual count of rodents. Visual observation and recording of commensal rodents have been done by infrared cameras and by walking through chicken houses at night (Kaukeinen, 1979). These methods are very helpful as a crude estimate of the rodent activity in a house but are limited to only visualizing populations in a portion of the house and for only a component time. In a commercial chicken house, which can be as large as 530 × 60 × 40 feet, directly counting the entire population would be virtually impossible.

Other counting methods known as indirect census of the population include monitoring the amount of consumption of a rodenticide or a commonly eaten food (chicken feed in a poultry house), recording of tracks, and mechanical counting of rodents (Kaukeinen, 1979). Provided census periods are of equal length, the total numbers of bodies counted, food or rodenticide consumption, or tracks noted before or after a treatment can be directly compared.

Mechanical counters are equipped with a photocell and transmit infrared light that does not disturb rodents. The Actimeter system uses a sensing unit as a motion detector, and it detects natural infrared radiation emitted from warm-blooded animals. Rats can be recorded at distances of 2 feet from these counters. Rodents must pass close to the counter to be recorded, and the same rodent can be recorded several times by passing back and forth in front of the counter. This compromises the interpretation of results. These methods are helpful particularly if counters, bait stations, and nontoxic tracking powders (flour) are used, and spaced intervals are required to observe all or most of the rodent population. One method for recording rodent tracks included taking vinyl floor tiles cut into 3 × 6-inch sections, coating them with a mixture of 75% isopropyl alcohol and 25% powdered marking chalk (red or blue), allowing these to air dry, and subsequently recording the animal tracks. This method has been used particularly with Norway rats. Tracks on tiles are then classified as follows: 0 tracks, 1–5 tracks, 6–10 tracks, 10–20 tracks, and more than 20 tracks (Kaukeinen, 1979). They can be specifically located to study a portion of the rodent population in any given area or place. Visual observation and counts of the commensal rodents are difficult because of the primarily nocturnal habits of rodents. Although house mice are curious and can be seen during daylight, their feeding activities are chiefly nocturnal. Rats are generally observed only during daylight hours when their population levels are moderate to high (Kaukeinen, 1979).

An indirect method of censusing Norway rat populations from 14 farms in England was developed using 100 × 200-mm vinyl tracking plates painted with lampblack suspended in methyl alcohol (Quy et al., 1993). Plates were located either in a grid format in areas where rat activity was noted or in places where no visible runs were present, or they were set along walls and in narrow gaps or between vegetation where rats would likely travel. Two indices for recording rat activity were noted: these were based on the presence or absence of tracks on plates (track index score) or the number of footprints noted on a plate. The results of the latter method were scored as follows: 0 = no prints, 1 = 1%–25% of the plate covered with prints, 2 = 26%–95% covered, and 3 = 96%–100% covered. The authors believe this visual assessment is easy and more rapid than counting prints. Plates were scored for 4 consecutive days and averaged. Comparisons were then used after trapping rats as an indicator of the effectiveness of rat reduction. This was combined with measuring consumption of food offered after trapping to estimate the remaining rat population. It is suggested that these methods are helpful as an estimate of population size where trapping methods are not practical. Note that in this study in southern England, fall trapping (September) is affected by immigration of new animals into trap sites with the harvest of field grains.

A study that compared three methods of estimating the number of rats (*R. norvegicus*) in rural garbage dumps included mark and recapture, monitoring of bait consumption, and visual night counts (Taylor et al., 1981). Visual night counts were especially useful in comparison to mark-and-recapture methods, because of the ability to visualize captured rats by their dyed fur. Visual counts were done just after sunset and up to 4 h after dark with the aid of a light. The observer walked quietly and systematically covered all areas of the garbage dump. In total, five nights of visual counts were used for comparison. The visual counts estimated the rat populations to be 3–4 times higher than populations estimated with the mark-and-recapture technique. Monitoring by consumption of bait and visual counts were usually 1.3–7.0 times higher than mark and recapture and were considered more reliable. Central to all population estimates of small mammals using mark-and-recapture techniques is that all animals have the same probability of being caught and recaught. In this study, recapturing animals did not occur at random, and hence population estimates of rats were biased with this technique.

House mice travel well-defined paths along walls or edges in both vertical and horizontal planes, and move out from these areas to feed in limited places, such as feed bins or similar areas. The limited home range of house mice, combined with very little tendency toward territoriality, means that measurements of population densities by using linear units is highly effective (Young et al., 1950).

A practical and efficient method for estimating house mouse (*M. musculus*) populations in poultry houses that has been developed is the RI (Henzler, 1993; Guard-Petter et al., 1997; Henzler et al., 1998; D.J. Henzler, unpublished data). This method encompasses the niche and natural travel patterns of house mice. The RI is a two-step process combining a visual walk-through survey of the poultry house for fresh rodent signs (for example, droppings, insulation pulled out of the walls, and rodent pathways) while using the Pennsylvania Egg Quality Assurance Program Rodent Evaluation Form as a guide, and setting 12 Tin Cat multiple-catch galvanized steel traps. Placed in the traps is 0.5 ounce of chicken feed, and the traps are set in the areas most likely to catch mice (that is, along cage walkways and against walls). The traps, which remain in the house for 7 days, are checked twice within the 7 days, and any trap that did not catch a mouse at the first check is moved a minimum of 15 feet. Traps that caught a mouse are placed back in the same location. At the end of 7 days, the traps are checked a second time. The captured mice are killed, and the total count of mice captured in the 7 days is recorded. The following formula is used to assign an RI:

$$RI = \frac{(\text{number of mice caught in all traps}/\text{number of functioning traps}) \times 12}{\text{number of days traps are set}} \times 7$$

This formula adjusts for periods of time that traps are set that are longer or shorter than 7 days and where more than 12 traps may have been used, and standardizes all mouse catches to a 1-week period using 12 Tin Cat traps. The RIs are grouped as follows: 0–10 mice = 1 (low density), 11–25 mice = 2 (moderate density), and 26 or more mice = 3 (high density).

D.J. Henzler (unpublished data) determined RIs for a total of 51 flocks in Pennsylvania as part of the *S. Enteritidis* Pilot Project in 1992–94. Comparisons were made for three RIs for each flock, with the period between indexes assessed in individual flocks averaging weeks. A total of 29 flocks was considered "first" flocks because RIs were estimated initially in these flocks, followed by RIs determined

TABLE 30.2   Comparison of three rodent indexes determined on 29 "first" flocks in Pennsylvania

No. of flocks	Rodent index	%
11	Maintain (1)	37.9
0	Maintain (2)	0.0
5	Maintain (3)	17.2
8	Increase	27.6
5	Decrease	17.2

TABLE 30.3   Comparison of three rodent indexes determined on 22 "replacement" flocks in Pennsylvania

No. of flocks	Rodent index	%
14	Maintain (1)	63.6
0	Maintain (2)	0.0
2	Maintain (3)	9.1
4	Increase	18.2
2	Decrease	9.1

in 22 replacement flocks (22 flocks replacing "first" flocks in 29 houses). In "first"-flock RI determinations, 11 (37.9%) flocks maintained an RI of 1, and two flocks maintained an RI of 3 (17.2%) (Table 30.2). There were 2.2 times as many flocks maintaining low mice densities as compared with flocks with high mice densities. On determinations of RI in "replacement" flocks, 14 flocks (63.6%) maintained an RI of 1, and two (9.1%) maintained an RI of 3 (9.1%) (Table 30.3). There were 7.0 times as many flocks maintaining low mice densities as compared with flocks with high mice densities. The average time between determination of RIs in "first" flocks and "replacement" flocks was 15.42 weeks and 13.32 weeks, respectively. Rodent-control practices were being extensively developed and information disseminated to the poultry industry during this time. It is likely this effect is partially noted in the increasing proportions of flocks that maintained low rodent populations as determined in "replacement" flocks.

REFERENCES

Allison, C., Emody, L., Coleman, N., and Huges, C. 1994. The role of swarm cell differentiation and multicellular migration in the uropathogenicity of *Proteus mirabilis*. J. Infect. Dis. 169:1155–1158.

Bartram, M.T., Welch, H., and Ostrolenk, M. 1940. Incidence of members of the salmonella group in rats. J. Infect. Dis. 67:222–227.

Casebolt, D.B., and Schoeb, T.R. 1988. An outbreak in mice of salmonellosis caused by *Salmonella enteritidis* serotype Enteritidis. Lab. Anim. Sci. 38:190–192.

Davies, R.H., and Wray, C. 1995. Mice as carriers of *Salmonella enteritidis* on persistently infected poultry units. Vet. Rec. 137:337–341.

Goyal, S.M., and Singh, I.P. 1970. Probable sources of salmonellae on a poultry farm. Br. Vet. J. 126:180–184.

Guard-Petter, J., Keller, L.H., Rahman, M.M., Carlson, R.W., and Silvers, S. 1996. A novel relationship between O-antigen variation, matrix formation, and invasiveness of *Salmonella enteritidis*. Epidemiol. Infect. 117:219–231.

Guard-Petter, J., Henzler, D.J., Rahman, M., and Carlson, R.W. 1997. On-farm monitoring of mouse-invasive *Salmonella enterica* serovar Enteritidis and a model for its association with the production of contaminated eggs. Appl. Environ. Microbiol. 63:1588–1593.

Halavatkar, H., and Barrow, P.A. 1993. The role of a 54-kb plasmid in the virulence of strains of *S. enteritidis* of phage type 4 for chickens and mice. J. Med. Microbiol. 38:171–176.

Helmuth, R., Stephan, R., Bunge, C., Hoog, B., Steinbeck, A., and Bulling, E. 1985. Epidemiology of virulence-associated plasmids and outer membrane patterns within seven common salmonella serotypes. Infect. Immun. 48:175–182.

Henzler, D.J. 1993. Determining the number of mice on farms is a difficult task. Poult. Times 40(6) (15 March).

Henzler, D.J., and Opitz, H.M. 1992. The role of mice in the epizootiology of *Salmonella enteritidis* infection on chicken layer farms. Avian Dis. 36:625–631.

Henzler, D.J., Sischo, W.M., Opitz, H.M., Schlosser, W.D., and Hurd, S.H. 1995. Mice populations and their association with *Salmonella enteritidis* contamination on chicken layer farms [Abstract]. In: Proceedings of the 132nd annual meeting of the American Veterinary Medical Association, July, p. 129.

Henzler, D.J., Kradel, D.C., and Sischo, W.M. 1998. Management and environmental risk factors for *Salmonella enteritidis* contamination of eggs. Am. J. Vet. Res. 59(7):824–829.

Hormaeche, C.E. 1979. Genetics of natural resistance to salmonella in mice. Immunology 37:319–327.

Humphrey, T.J., Rawkins, A., McAlpine, K., Lever, S., Guard-Petter, J., and Cox, J.M. 1996. Isolates of *Salmonella enteritidis* PT4 with enhanced heat and acid tolerance are more virulent in mice and more invasive in chickens. Epidemiol. Infect. 117:79–88.

Jones, P.W., and Twigg, G.I. 1976. Salmonellosis in wild animals. J. Hyg. Camb. 77:51–54.

Kaukeinen, D.E. 1979. Field methods for census taking of commensal rodents in rodenticide evaluations. In: Beck, J.R., ed. Vertebrate pest control and management materials. ASTM STP 680. Philadelphia: American Society for Testing Materials, pp. 68–83.

Kempelmacher, E.H., Guinee, P.A.M., and van Noorle Jansen, L.M. 1969. Artificial salmonella infections in rats. Zentralbl. Vetinarmed. [B] 16:173–182.

Kinde, H., Read, R.H., Ardans, A., Breitmeyer, R.E., Willoughby, D., Little, H.E., Kerr, D., Gireesh, R., and Nagarja, K.V. 1996a. Sewage effluent: likely source of *Salmonella enteritidis*, phage type 4 infection in a commercial chicken layer flock in Southern California. Avian Dis. 40:672–676.

Kinde, H., Read, D.H., Chin, R.P., Bickford, A.A., Walker, R.L., Ardans, A., Brietmeyer, R.E., Willoughby, D., Little, H.E., Kerr, D., and Gardner, I.A. 1996b. *Salmonella enteritidis*, phage type 4 infection in a commercial layer flock in Southern California: bacteriologic and epidemiologic findings. Avian Dis. 40:665–671.

Krabisch, P., and Dorn, P. 1980. Zur epidemiologischen Bedeutung von Lebendvektoren bei der Verbreitung von Salmonellen in der Geflugelmast. Berl. Muench. Tierarztl. Wochenschr. 93:232–235.

Laurie, E.M.O. 1945. The reproduction of the house-mouse (*Mus musculus*) living in different environments. Proc. R. Soc. Lond. [B] 133:248–281.

McKiel, J.A., Rappay, D.E., Cousineau, J.G., Hall, R.R., and McKenna, H.E. 1970. Domestic rats as carriers of leptospires and salmonellae in Eastern Canada. Can. J. Public Health 61:336–340.

Montenegro, M.A., Morelli, G., and Helmuth, R. 1991. Heteroduplex analysis of salmonella virulence plasmids and their prevalence in isolates of defined sources. Microb. Pathog. 11:391–397.

Nakamura, M., Sato, S., Ohya, T., Suzuki, S., and Ikeda, S. 1985. Possible relationship of a 36-megadalton *S. enteritidis* plasmid to virulence in mice. Infect. Immun. 47:831–833.

Petter, J.G. 1993. Detection of two smooth colony phenotypes in a *Salmonella enteritidis* isolate which vary in their ability to contaminate eggs. Appl. Environ. Microbiol. 59:2884–2890.

Poppe, C., Demczuk, W., McFadden, K., and Johnson, R.P. 1993. Virulence of *S. enteritidis* phage types 4, 8, and 13 and other *Salmonella* sp. for day old chicks, hens and mice. Can. J. Vet. Res. 57:281–287.

Quy, R.J., Cowan, D.P., and Swinney, T. 1993. Tracking as an activity index to measure gross changes in Norway rat populations. Wildl. Soc. Bull. 21:122–127.

Robinson, R.A., and Daniel, M.J. 1968. The significance of salmonella isolations from wild birds and rats in New Zealand. N.Z. Vet. J. 16:53–55.

Rodrigue, D.C., Tauxe, R.V., and Rowe, B. 1990. International increase in *Salmonella enteritidis*: a new pandemic? Epidemiol. Infect. 105:21–27.

Sato, G., Miyamae, T., and Miura, S. 1970. A long-term epizootiological study of chicken salmonellosis on a farm with reference to elimination of paratyphoid infection by cloacal swab culture test. Jpn. J. Vet. Res. 18:47–62.

Savage, W.G., and Read, W.J. 1913. Gaertner group bacilli in rats and mice. J. Hyg. 13:343–352.

Singer, J.T., Opitz, H.M., Gershman, M., Hall, M.M., Muniz, I.G., and Rao, S.V. 1992. Molecular characterization of *S. enteritidis* isolates from Maine poultry and poultry farm environments. Avian Dis. 36:324–333.

Singh, S.P., Sethi, M.S., and Sharma, V.D. 1980. The occurrence of salmonellae in rodent, shrew, cockroach and ant. Int. J. Zoonoses 7:58–61.

St. Louis, M.E., Morse, D.L., Potter, M.E., DeMelfi, T.M., Guzewich, J.J., Tauxe, R.V., and Blake, P.A. 1988. The emergence of grade A eggs as a major source of *Salmonella enteritidis* infections. JAMA 259:2103–2107.

Strecker, R.L., and Emlen, J.T., Jr. 1953. Regulatory mechanisms in house-mouse populations: the effect of a limited food supply on a confined population. Ecology 34:375–385.

Suzuki, S., Ohishi, K., Takahashi, T., Tamura, Y., Maramatsu, M., Nakamura, M., and Sato, S. 1992. The role of 36 megadalton plasmid of *S. enteritidis* for the pathogenesis in mice. J. Vet. Med. Sci. 54:845–850.

Taylor, J. 1956. Bacterial rodenticides and infection with *Salmonella enteritidis*. Lancet 1:630–633.

Taylor, J. 1968. Salmonella in wild animals. Symp. Zool. Soc. Lond. 24:53–73.

Taylor, K.D., Quy, R.J., and Gurnell, J. 1981. Comparison of three methods for estimating the numbers of common rats (*Rattus norvegicus*). Mammalia 45:403–413.

Venables, L.S.V., and Leslie, P.H. 1942. The rat and mouse populations of corn ricks. J. Anim. Ecol. 11:44–68.

Welch, H., Ostrolenk, M., and Bartram, M.T. 1941. Role of rats in the spread of food poisoning bacteria of the salmonella group. Am. J. Public Health 31:332–340.

Young, H., Strecker, R.L., and Emlen, J.T., Jr. 1950. Localization of activity in two indoor populations of house mice, *Mus musculus*. J. Mammal. 31:403–410.

31

Prevalence of *Salmonella enterica* Serovar Enteritidis in Unpasteurized Liquid Eggs and Aged Laying Hens at Slaughter: Implications on Epidemiology and Control of the Disease

E.D. Ebel, A.T. Hogue, and W.D. Schlosser

INTRODUCTION

In the late 1980s, researchers showed that human cases of *Salmonella enterica* serovar Enteritidis (*S.* Enteritidis) were increasing in the United States and elsewhere (St. Louis et al., 1988; Cowden et al., 1989; Cowden, 1990). Epidemiological investigations linked many *S.* Enteritidis outbreaks to the consumption of fresh grade-A eggs; from 1985 through 1991, eggs were the implicated vehicles in 82% of human *S.* Enteritidis outbreaks where a food vehicle was identified (Mishu et al., 1994).

In the United States, data on *S.* Enteritidis outbreaks in humans do not indicate a discernible trend in recent years. Human outbreaks of *S.* Enteritidis declined from 70 in 1990 to 44 in 1994. A total of 56 outbreaks was reported in 1995 and 49 in 1996 (Altekruse and Swerdlow, 1996). However, outbreaks are crude indicators of the occurrence of human infection with *S.* Enteritidis. Therefore, reported sporadic cases should also be considered when evaluating trends (Anon., 1992). That these cases are important was demonstrated in a Minnesota case-control study of spo-radic cases of *S.* Enteritidis, where an association with raw/undercooked eggs was found (Hedberg et al., 1993).

In 1991, surveys of unpasteurized liquid egg and aged laying hens were completed to estimate the occurrence and distribution of *S.* Enteritidis in the U.S. commercial egg industry (Ebel et al., 1993). These survey techniques were adopted because of the highly sensitive nature of the *S.* Enteritidis problem in the United States. Given the existence of a regulatory program, with potential economic losses for implicated producers, the U.S. commercial egg industry was reticent to allow on-farm sampling. In contrast to this U.S. situation, Canadian researchers were able to select egg-production houses randomly across Canada from a list of registered producers and then collect environmental samples in these houses to estimate the prevalence of *S.* Enteritidis directly (Poppe et al., 1991).

The 1991 liquid-egg and aged-laying-hen surveys established baseline measures and were intended for comparison with human disease incidence data provided by public health authorities. Survey results were reported by regions (Fig. 31.1). The surveys were repeated in 1995 for comparison

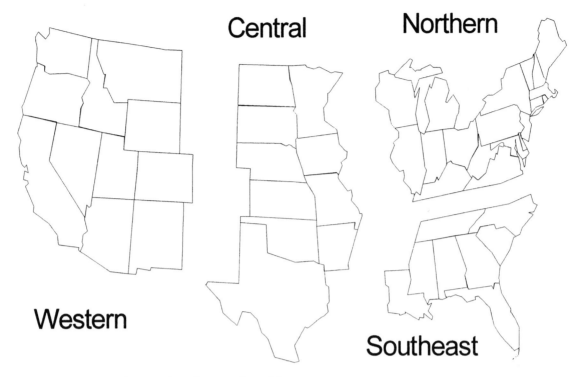

FIGURE 31.1 Regions used in the liquid-egg and aged-hen surveys.

with the baseline data (Hogue et al., 1997). Such a comparison presented an opportunity to evaluate progress of industry initiatives and the effectiveness of the federal *S.* Enteritidis regulation in reducing the occurrence of *S.* Enteritidis in U.S. egg production flocks (Mason, 1994).

METHODS

Unpasteurized Liquid-Egg Surveys

Methodological support for this survey technique came from U.S. Department of Agriculture (USDA)–Agriculture Marketing Service surveys conducted in the years prior to 1991. These surveys demonstrated recovery of *S.* Enteritidis from liquid-egg samples before pasteurization. Although the information from these surveys was valuable, differences in protocol (for example, varying types of liquid egg sampled from different numbers of plants each year) and the limited length of the surveys (typically 5 weeks) made seasonal trends and geographical differences in *S.* Enteritidis occurrence difficult to interpret.

The 1991 and 1995 liquid-egg surveys were designed to follow the same protocol (Ebel et al., 1992, 1993; Hogue et al., 1997), and 20 plants for egg products were selected to cover the four regions (Fig. 31.1); 16 egg-processing plants participated in both surveys. In the 1995 survey, substitutions were made for four plants because one was receiving eggs from flocks outside of its region, two went out of business, and one was not processing during the survey period. In each case, the substituted plant was located in the same

state as the original. Six plants were located in the Northern Region, five each were located in the Central and Western Regions, and four were located in the Southeastern Region. Except for one state in the Western Region, no state had more than one participating plant

For the 1991 survey, sampling was conducted between 11 February 1991 and 7 February 1992. In 1995, sampling was conducted between 31 October 1994 and 28 October 1995. USDA Food Safety and Inspection Service (formerly Agriculture Marketing Service) inspectors in the participating processing plants were instructed to collect 4–6 ounces of unpasteurized liquid whole egg from tanks containing egg products typically produced from flocks within that plant's region. Samples were collected once a week from each plant and may have contained eggs from a single or multiple flocks. Samples were refrigerated and mailed by overnight delivery to National Veterinary Services Laboratories (NVSL) in Ames, Iowa.

For each sample collected, information on the type of eggs was noted by the collector. Eggs brought to egg-processing plants tend to fit into three general categories: graded, restricted, and nest run. Graded eggs are washed and candled before transport to the breaker. Restricted eggs are defined as cracked (checked), dirty, incubator reject, inedible, leaker, or loss eggs. Restricted eggs do not meet the quality standards of consumer grade-AA or grade-A eggs. Nest-run eggs are collected at the farm and then shipped to the processing plant, without having been washed, sized, or candled for quality. Depending on the flock that produced these eggs, egg-handling techniques, and other factors, the quality of nest-run eggs may vary from excellent to poor.

Upon arrival at the breaking plant, eggs are routinely washed and sanitized before breaking. Usually, the eggs are conveyed to a machine that cracks the shell (using a thin knife), allowing the contents to drop into a cup for inspection by a machine operator. Some plants separate egg whites and yolks after inspection and before the liquid product flows via a pipeline system through a filter and cooling system to a holding tank. In the holding tank, the temperature of the product is maintained at 45°F, in accordance with USDA requirements, before it is pasteurized using a plate heat-exchanger system similar to that used in the dairy industry (Anon., 1991).

Culture, serotyping, and phage typing for the 1991 and 1995 surveys were performed by the NVSL using the same protocol. The NVSL reported samples as negative, positive for S. Enteritidis, negative for S. Enteritidis but positive for other salmonellae, or positive for both S. Enteritidis and other salmonellae.

Aged-Laying-Hen Surveys

Methodological support for this survey technique came from Kingston (1981), who showed that intestinal salmonella colonization was correlated with positive environmental sampling results. In addition, research prior to the 1991 survey demonstrated the utility of culturing salmonellae from aged layers' ceca and ovaries (Barnhardt et al., 1991; Dreesen et al., 1992; Waltman et al., 1992).

Both surveys were similarly designed (Ebel et al., 1993; Hogue et al., 1997). For the 1991 survey, the 10 largest slaughter plants—which were responsible for 85% of all aged laying hens (light fowl) annually slaughtered in the United States—were asked to participate. Two plants refused, citing concerns about confidentiality, and one plant was unable to participate because it was not operating. Therefore, seven slaughter plants were enrolled. These were distributed as follows: Northern Region (three plants), Southeastern Region (two plants), and Central Region (two plants). None of the participating plants actually resided in the Western Region.

For the 1995 survey, eight aged-laying-hen slaughter plants were enrolled. These were distributed as follows: Northern Region (three plants), Southeastern Region (two plants), Central Region (one plant), and Western Region (two plants). Five of these plants had also participated in the 1991 survey. One slaughter plant each that had participated in the 1991 survey in the Central and Southeastern Regions no longer slaughtered aged hens in 1995. Therefore, one large Southeastern Region plant was selected to replace these two plants.

The 1991 and 1995 surveys were conducted between April and June 1991 and between July and September 1995, respectively. Samples were collected in each slaughter plant on a twice-weekly schedule by Animal and Plant Health Inspection Services (APHIS) field personnel (except in one 1995 plant where Food Safety Inspection Service personnel collected the samples).

To detect intestinal colonization of birds in a poultry house at 1% prevalence or greater (with 95% confidence),

ceca from each of 300 hens were collected from each unique flock of aged hens presented for slaughter. For these surveys, a *flock* is defined as birds presented for slaughter that originated from the same premises on the same day. These birds typically originate from one poultry house on a premise because houses are usually depopulated and birds sent to slaughter at the same time. The median number of birds per farm is 20,000, and the mean is 280,000, for flocks larger than 10,000 birds (Anon., 1992). The number of birds per farm probably overestimates the number of birds per flock because a farm may contain more than one flock, but these numbers provide an approximation of the number of birds per flock presented for slaughter.

Five ceca samples were pooled in sterile plastic bags, for a total of 60 pooled samples per flock. Sampling was proportioned equally across the total number of trucks from each flock, and across the entire truckload of birds. Collectors wore disposable gloves and changed these after each pool was collected. Flocks were identified by their region of origin, and samples were refrigerated and submitted for immediate culture.

Laboratory support for each plant was contracted with state or university laboratories based on S. Enteritidis–culturing experience and proximity to the plants. Four laboratories participated in both surveys. The total number of pooled samples, the number of salmonella-positive pools, and the number of S. Enteritidis–positive pools were reported for each flock sampled.

Human Disease Surveillance

To compare with commercial egg-industry survey data, 1991 and 1995 S. Enteritidis isolate data reported to the Centers for Disease Control and Prevention from state public health officials were tabulated on a per-capita basis for each region (Altekruse and Swerdlow, 1996).

Estimates of national flock prevalence for each year were completed by modeling each regional estimate as a beta $(s + 1, n - s + 1)$ distribution—where s is the number of positive flocks and n is the number of flocks sampled in each region (Vose, 1996)—and then weighting the regional prevalence by the proportion of U.S. flocks in the region. According to the 1992 U.S. Agriculture Census, the Northern, Southeastern, Central, and Western regions account for 27%, 33%, 26%, and 13% of the egg-laying flocks in the United States, respectively. Using the spreadsheet software Microsoft Excel (Microsoft Corporation, Redmond, WA) and the add-in program @RISK (Palisade Corporation, Newfield, NY), we simulated the national prevalence distribution.

RESULTS

Unpasteurized Liquid-Egg Surveys

PREVALENCE FINDINGS

In 1991, a total of 531 (53%) of 1003 samples of unpasteurized liquid egg was salmonella positive. In 1995, a total of

451 (48%) of 937 samples was salmonella positive (Table 31.1). In both surveys, the Central and Southeastern Regions' proportion of salmonella-positive samples were above, while Western Region results were below, the national averages. For the Northern Region, these results were below and above average in 1991 and 1995, respectively.

In 1991, of the 1003 samples collected, 132 (13%) were *S.* Enteritidis positive. This proportion was slightly more in 1995, when 179 (19%) of 937 samples were *S.* Enteritidis positive. Comparing 1991 and 1995 results, the Northern Region had a higher proportion of *S.* Enteritidis–positive samples than did other regions in both years (Fig. 31.2). The proportion of positive samples doubled, from 20% in 1991 to 40% in 1995, in the Northern Region. The Western Region also had an increase in the proportion of *S.*

Enteritidis–positive samples from 6% in 1991 to 12% in 1995. Only the Central Region showed a decline from 16% to 10% between the two surveys. Southeastern Region results were essentially unchanged in these two surveys.

Detection of *S.* Enteritidis was dependent on other salmonella serovars in the 1991 or 1995 surveys. Analysis of the unpasteurized 1991 liquid-egg results suggested that the likelihood of recovering *S.* Enteritidis from a sample is reduced if other salmonellae are present in the sample. When other salmonella serovars were not detected, the proportion of liquid-egg samples positive for *S.* Enteritidis was 147 (23%) of 630. When other salmonella serovars were detected, the proportion of samples positive for *S.* Enteritidis was 12 (3%) of 418. Similarly, in the 1995 liquid-egg survey, when other salmonella serovars were not detected,

TABLE 31.1 Salmonella samples in unpasteurized liquid-egg samples by regions in 1991 and 1995 surveys

| Region | Year | Number of samples | | | | |
		Tested	Salm. +	(%)	*S.* Enteritidis +	(%)
North	1991	301	131	(44)	59	(20)
	1995	267	146	(55)	106	(40)
Southeast	1991	194	131	(68)	19	(10)
	1995	191	92	(48)	20	(11)
Central	1991	258	197	(76)	40	(16)
	1995	241	131	(55)	24	(10)
West	1991	250	72	(29)	14	(6)
	1995	238	82	(35)	29	(12)
Total	1991	1003	531	(53)	132	(13)
	1995	937	451	(48)	179	(19)

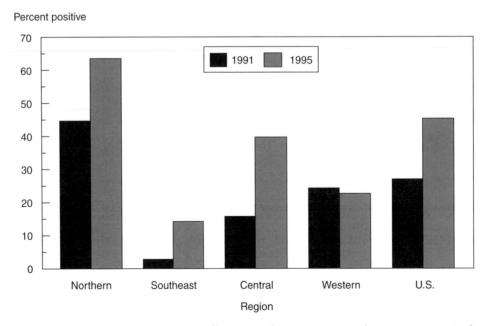

FIGURE 31.2 Percent of *Salmonella* Enteritidis–positive samples in unpasteurized liquid-egg surveys, 1990 and 1995.

the proportion of unpasteurized liquid-egg samples positive for *S.* Enteritidis was 139 (22%) of 623. When other salmonella serovars were detected, the proportion of samples positive for *S.* Enteritidis was 40 (13%) of 314.

The proportions of liquid-egg samples positive for *S.* Enteritidis or other salmonellae were not dramatically different for the different types of eggs sampled (that is, nest run, graded, and restricted) in either the 1991 or 1995 liquid-egg surveys (Table 31.2). Nevertheless, nest-run eggs were the most frequently *S.* Enteritidis–positive

samples in both years. The most common sample in 1991 was a combination of nest-run, graded, and restricted eggs, whereas nest-run eggs were most commonly sampled in 1995. In the 1991 survey, sample collectors did not record egg-type information for the first 6 months.

PHAGE-TYPE OCCURRENCE
A pronounced shift was seen in the dominant *S.* Enteritidis phage type in unpasteurized liquid egg from phage type 8 (PT8) in 1991 to PT13a in 1995 (Fig. 31.3). In 1991, PT8

TABLE 31.2   Frequency of salmonellae in unpasteurized liquid-egg samples by type of eggs sampled in 1991[a] and 1995

Egg type	Year	Total Samples	No. salmonella positive (%)	No *S.* Enteritidis positive (%)
Nest run	1991	121	48 (40)	19 (16)
	1995	373	106 (28)	86 (23)
Graded	1991	2	0 (0)	0 (0)
	1995	4	0 (0)	0 (0)
Restricted	1991	56	23 (41)	3 (5)
	1995	165	61 (37)	22 (13)
Combined nest run and graded	1991	12	4 (33)	1 (8)
	1995	119	38 (32)	21 (18)
Combined nest run, graded,	1991	278	169 (61)	38 (14)
and restricted	1995	267	108 (40)	48 (18)

[a]Egg-type information was collected for approximately one-half of the 1991 survey.

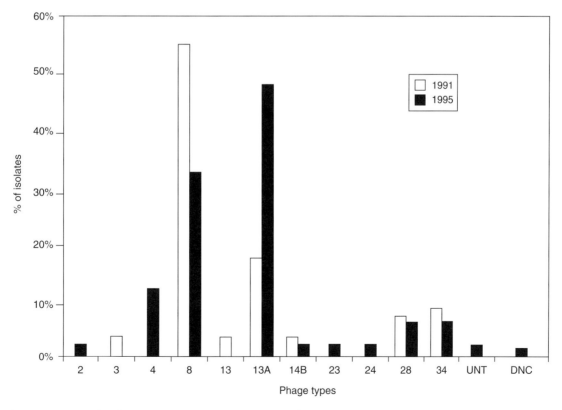

FIGURE 31.3   Percent of *Salmonella* Enteritidis phage types found in unpasteurized liquid-egg samples, 1991 and 1995.

TABLE 31.3　Salmonella prevalence in aged laying hens sampled by region at slaughter, 1991 and 1995

APHIS[a] region	Year	Number of pooled samples[b]					Number of flocks[c]				
		Tested	Salm. +	(%)	S. Enteritidis +	(%)	Tested	Salm. +	(%)	S. Enteritidis +	(%)
North	1991	10,329	2546	(25)	502	(5)	181	147	(81)	81	(45)
	1995	7603	3156	(42)	654	(9)	129	128	(99)	82	(64)
Southeast	1991	3624	1190	(33)	4	(0)	62	60	(97)	2	(3)
	1995	1722	1013	(59)	19	(1)	30	29	(97)	5	(17)
Central	1991	8288	1459	(18)	92	(1)	142	123	(87)	23	(16)
	1995	5316	2371	(45)	203	(4)	90	90	(100)	36	(40)
West	1991	1188	385	(32)	9	(1)	21	21	(100)	5	(24)
	1995	3320	666	(20)	41	(1)	56	51	(91)	13	(23)
Total	1991	23,429	5580	(24)	607	(3)	406	351	(86)	111	(27)
	1995	17,961	7206	(40)	917	(5)	305	298	(98)	136	(45)

[a]APHIS, Animal and Plant Health Inspection Service.
[b]Five ceca were pooled per sample.
[c]The flock was defined as positive if one or more of 60 pooled samples (five ceca per pool) was positive.

represented 55% and PT13a represented 9% of all *S.* Enteritidis isolates. In 1995, PT13a represented 35% of *S.* Enteritidis isolates, whereas PT8 accounted for 27%. On a regional basis, PT8 was most common in the Northern and Central Regions in 1991, whereas PT13a was most common in these regions in 1995. In the Southeastern and Western Regions, PT13 was dominant in 1991. However, PT4 was the most frequent Western Region isolate in 1995 (Fig. 31.3).

Salmonella Enteritidis PT4 was not isolated from unpasteurized liquid-egg samples collected in 1991 but emerged as a major phage type in 1995. PT4 was detected in 21 (12%) of the liquid-egg samples collected throughout the United States in 1995. All but one PT4 isolate came from two of the five plants in the Western Region. The remaining PT4 isolate was detected in the Southeastern Region.

Aged-Laying-Hen Surveys

PREVALENCE FINDINGS

A total of 24,429 pooled samples were collected from 406 flocks in 1991, whereas 17,961 pooled samples were collected from 305 flocks in the 1995 aged-laying-hen survey (Table 31.3). In both surveys, a high proportion (that is, 86%–98%) of all flocks sampled had at least one salmonella-positive pool detected. Overall, 5580 (24%) and 7206 (40%) of pooled samples collected were salmonella positive in 1991 and 1995, respectively. Regionally, the Southeastern Region consistently had the highest sample prevalence of salmonellae in both surveys.

Of the flocks sampled, 111 (27%) and 136 (45%) had at least one *S.* Enteritidis–positive pooled sample detected in 1991 and 1995, respectively. In both years, the majority of positive flocks had just 1–5 (2%–8%) of the 60 pooled samples culture positive for *S.* Enteritidis. Flock prevalence of *S.* Enteritidis was highest in the Northern Region and lowest in the Southeastern Region for both surveys. Between 1991

and 1995, flock prevalence increased in the Northern, Southeastern, and Central Regions, while remaining about the same in the Western Region. Regional patterns for sample prevalence of *S.* Enteritidis were similar to flock prevalence. Overall, 607 (3%) and 917 (5%) of pooled samples were *S.* Enteritidis positive in 1991 and 1995, respectively.

The mean national prevalence in 1991 was 22% (Fig. 31.4). This prevalence can also be represented by a probability distribution with 90% of the values between 18% (5th percentile) and 25% (95th percentile). The mean national prevalence increased to 37% in 1995 with 95% of the values lying between 32% (5th percentile) and 42% (95th percentile).

PHAGE-TYPE OCCURRENCE

There was a slight shift in phage-type distribution between the 1991 and 1995 aged-hen surveys, with PT13a occurring slightly more frequently than PT8 in the 1995 survey (Fig. 31.5). This shift was not as dramatic as that seen in the unpasteurized liquid-egg survey. Together, *S.* Enteritidis PT8 and PT13a made up more than 50% of the isolates recovered from these pooled samples for both the 1991 and the 1995 surveys.

In the 1995 survey, *S.* Enteritidis PT4 was detected in 32 samples and five flocks (2%) in the aged-hen survey. All PT4 positives came from a single slaughter plant in the Western Region.

Human Disease Surveillance

Overall rates of *S.* Enteritidis isolates reported from human cases increased from 3.1 to 3.9 per 100,000 from 1991 to 1995 in the United States. Human *S.* Enteritidis isolation rates increased nearly three times the 1991 rate in the Western Region in 1995. In 1995, the rate of *S.* Enteritidis isolations in the Western Region nearly reached that of the Northern Region. The rate also increased in the Central

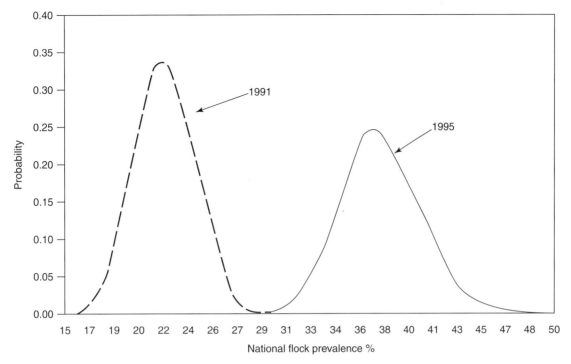

FIGURE 31.4   Probability distribution of the prevalence of *Salmonella* Enteritidis in aged hens processed during 1991 and 1995 surveys, weighted by the proportions of U.S. regional laying-hen flocks.

Percent of isolates

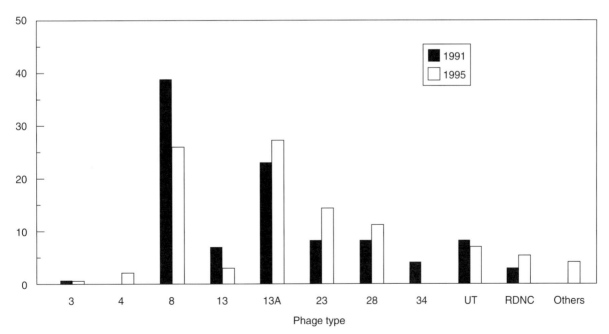

FIGURE 31.5   Percent of *Salmonella* Enteritidis phage types found in aged-hen surveys, 1991 and 1995. UT, untypeable; RDNC, reacts but does not conform; others include PT2 (1%), PT22 (2%), and PT24 (1%).

and Northern Regions and declined slightly in the South-eastern Region.

Temporal Patterns and Survey Relations

A seasonal pattern with a peak in the summer months was seen in a 3-month moving average for salmonella isolation from the 1991 and 1995 unpasteurized liquid-egg surveys. Monthly salmonella prevalence is nearly the same for both years during the peak months of April through October, with some divergence of the curves during the other months.

Data from the 1991 and 1995 aged-hen and liquid-egg surveys suggest a corresponding seasonality in the two datasets. The slope of the data collected from April to June in the 1991 survey appears roughly parallel to the 3-month moving average of liquid-egg data. The aged-laying-hen data collected from July to September in 1995 peak in August as do the data for liquid eggs.

DISCUSSION

Liquid-Egg Survey Implications

Although samples of liquid egg were cultured in 1991 and 1995, these survey results do not enable estimation of the frequency of internal egg contamination with S. Enteritidis. Instead, these results probably reflect environmental and eggshell contamination levels at the time of sampling, in addition to some contribution from internally contaminated eggs. Because other salmonella serovars are not thought to contaminate eggs internally, it seems highly probable that contamination of the egg contents with these serovars originated from eggshells and/or the environment. Similarly, samples positive for both S. Enteritidis and other salmonellae could also be explained by eggshell or environmental contamination. However, an explanation for samples found to contain only S. Enteritidis is less certain.

It is remarkable that we can recover S. Enteritidis from a 10-ml liquid-egg sample collected from bulk tanks containing an average of 10,000 lbs of egg material (as measured in the 1991 survey). This average quantity is equivalent to approximately 90,000 large shell eggs. The average frequency of internally contaminated S. Enteritidis–positive eggs from known-positive flocks is reportedly 2.5 per 10,000 eggs produced (Schlosser et al., 1994), a frequency that predicts 22.5 S. Enteritidis–positive eggs in every 90,000. Furthermore, it is estimated that most internally positive eggs contain 20 or fewer S. Enteritidis organisms per egg (Humphrey et al., 1991). Using these assumptions, a contaminated bulk tank of liquid egg might comprise 450 S. Enteritidis organisms, for a ratio of 1 S. Enteritidis organism per 9354 ml of liquid egg. Because liquid egg is stored in refrigerated tanks designed to inhibit salmonella growth, S. Enteritidis organisms probably are not amplified after egg breaking. For the 10-ml sample size used in the liquid-egg surveys, these assumptions suggest that the likelihood of selecting

a sample containing a single S. Enteritidis organism (contributed by internally contaminated eggs) is nearly one in 1000. Consequently, these assumptions imply that internally contaminated eggs are not responsible for most of the S. Enteritidis–positive samples cultured in the liquid-egg surveys.

Given the high proportion of salmonella-positive samples and flocks in the aged-hen surveys, eggshell contamination with salmonellae is probably a frequent occurrence. Washing, sanitizing, and drying table eggs before placing them in cartons or cases is considered effective in eliminating salmonellae from the surface of shell eggs. Even after routine washing and sanitizing, however, cracked and checked eggs sent to processing plants can harbor salmonellae in shell crevices. Also, salmonellae are more likely to invade thin or checked shells than the typical grade-AA or grade-A shell eggs. Such an explanation is consistent with the relatively frequent isolation of salmonellae from restricted eggs sampled in 1991 and 1995.

Nest-run eggs sampled in 1991 and 1995 were also frequently salmonella positive, yet by definition their shell defects are less prevalent than restricted eggs. More research is required to explain this finding. One possible explanation is that breaker eggs are usually cracked within a few seconds of sanitizing, a time that may be insufficient to kill salmonellae in the breaker plant environment. Another possible explanation is that the surfaces of egg-breaking machinery in contact with contaminated liquid egg may also support replication of salmonella organisms, although this machinery is routinely cleaned at least every 4 h by regulation (Anon., 1991b). Nevertheless, the liquid egg produced during the breaking process is quickly chilled to less than 45°F, so it seems unlikely that much amplification of any salmonella organisms occurs while the liquid is stored prior to pasteurization.

Implications of the Aged-Hen Surveys

The results of the 1991 and 1995 aged-laying-hen surveys are expected to correlate with the prevalence of S. Enteritidis–positive environments in the U.S. commercial layer industry. However, positive environment or cecal sampling results may overestimate the proportion of flocks whose hens produce infected eggs. For example, in the USDA's regulatory program, environmentally positive flocks were retested for evidence of internal organ infection to determine whether eggs were likely contaminated with S. Enteritidis. In the *Salmonella* Enteritidis Pilot Project, eggs were cultured. In both of these programs, about 50% of environmentally positive flocks were found to be organ or egg positive (Mason and Ebel, 1991; Schlosser et al., 1994).

Although these aged-hen survey results are internally consistent for evaluating prevalence trends, they may also overestimate the proportion of environmentally positive flocks. Sensitivity for detecting S. Enteritidis in these aged-hen surveys may be much higher than environmental sampling. A sample size of 300 hen ceca is expected to find at least one positive cecum if the prevalence in the house is more than 1%. Such a sample size is below the level that

Kingston used (that is, 50 ceca per poultry house) to demonstrate the correlation between cecal colonization and environmental swabbing (Kingston, 1981). Therefore, it seems likely that some flocks classified as negative by environmental testing may, in fact, be positive when 300 aged hens are sampled. Such a conclusion is supported by the typically low numbers of pooled samples found positive in the *S*. Enteritidis–positive flocks of the aged-hen surveys. Low numbers of positive samples per flock are especially important given that sampling of aged hens typically followed a stressful transport from farm to slaughter plant. Such a situation likely increases the effective rate of contact and susceptibility of these hosts to *S*. Enteritidis organisms, thereby possibly increasing the prevalence of *S*. Enteritidis–colonized hens in the population to a level at, or above, the detection threshold for our sample size.

In comparison with a Canadian survey (Poppe et al., 1991), the aged-hen surveys suggest a greater prevalence of salmonellae and *S*. Enteritidis in U.S. egg-layer flocks. The Canadian survey found salmonella contamination of 53% of flocks tested, while *S*. Enteritidis was found in 3% of these flocks. Such results may be consistent with the lower occurrence of *S*. Enteritidis infections in humans in Canada, where *S*. Typhimurium is more commonly isolated from human cases than is *S*. Enteritidis (Poppe, 1994).

Implications of Liquid-Egg, Aged-Hen, and Human Data Comparisons

The liquid-egg and aged-hen survey results suggest there was no decline in *S*. Enteritidis occurrence in the commercial egg industry between 1991 and 1995. Levels of salmonellae are higher in summer months, and this seasonal effect may have inflated the 1995 *S*. Enteritidis aged-hen prevalence in comparison to 1991. Nevertheless, levels of *S*. Enteritidis in liquid-egg, aged-hen, and sporadic human isolate data at the national level all increased in frequency between 1991 and 1995. Of human cases cultured, *S*. Enteritidis was the most commonly reported salmonella serovar in the United States in 1995, accounting for 26% of salmonella isolates reported. In 1991, *S*. Enteritidis accounted for 19% of reported human salmonella isolates (Altekruse and Swerdlow, 1996).

The seasonal pattern noted in these surveys matches that seen in a seroprevalence study of poultry. During a 3-year period, researchers in Georgia evaluated the prevalence of pullorum/typhoid test-positive poultry that were sampled for routine regulatory purposes (Waltman and Horne, 1993). Those results showed that the highest seroreactor frequencies occurred between July and September. These poultry results also parallel the seasonal incidence of human outbreaks in the United States. The increased likelihood of human foodborne illnesses in the summer months is thought to be associated with changes in human behavior (for instance, more picnics), as well as generally higher ambient temperatures. These factors increase the likelihood and consequence of mishandling potentially hazardous foods. That a similar pattern is seen in the commercial egg industry suggests the possibility that similar factors are operating within poultry populations (for example, hot weather leads to increased transmission or amplification of salmonellae among layers). Alternatively, increased human outbreaks in the summer months might be a direct result of increased poultry salmonella prevalence caused by, as yet, unexplained factors.

Regional comparisons of the 1995 liquid-egg and aged-hen survey results support some association between the occurrence of *S*. Enteritidis in flocks and liquid egg. Given the differences in egg and aged-hen marketing practices, this finding is remarkable. Such a correlation supports the efficiency of liquid-egg sampling for monitoring *S*. Enteritidis trends in the commercial egg industry. A simple comparison of the numbers of samples collected in the aged-hen survey (for example, 17,961 in 1995) versus the liquid-egg survey (for example, 937 in 1995), together with the longer time period considered in the liquid-egg survey, demonstrates the cost-effectiveness of the sampling of liquid egg. However, sampling of liquid egg is potentially biased by producers preferentially diverting eggs from *S*. Enteritidis–positive flocks to pasteurization plants. Therefore, risk to public health may theoretically decline while liquid-egg results suggest an increase in *S*. Enteritidis occurrence.

Human isolation rates for *S*. Enteritidis by region do not appear to be correlated with aged-hen and unpasteurized liquid-egg data. The most discrepant results exist for the Northern and Western Regions. In the Northern Region, both liquid-egg and aged-hen results indicate a sharply increased *S*. Enteritidis prevalence between 1991 and 1995, whereas human data suggest a slight increase. In the Western Region, liquid-egg and human data show *S*. Enteritidis prevalence increasing between 1991 and 1995, while aged-hen results are essentially unchanged.

One possible explanation for these regional discrepancies is that unpasteurized liquid-egg and aged-layer results are independent of sporadic human isolates. *Salmonella* Enteritidis has been isolated from a wide variety of animal species (Ferris and Thomas, 1995). Thus, sources other than eggs, including humans, may be responsible for human illness (Kinde et al., 1996a,b). On the other hand, eggs are the vehicles implicated in 30% of all human outbreaks that occurred between 1985 and 1991 and in 82% of outbreaks where a food vehicle was identified (Mishu et al., 1994).

A second explanation for the discrepancies is that although liquid-egg, aged-hen, and sporadic human isolate data are not usually independent, marketing practices have skewed the survey results. Some producers may preferentially send positive eggs to pasteurization plants and turn over positive flocks more frequently than negative flocks. This likely occurred in the Northeast, where producers participating in quality-assurance programs divert eggs from *S*. Enteritidis–positive flocks to pasteurization, and may account for the sharply increased occurrence of *S*. Enteritidis in liquid egg and in aged hen flocks, while sporadic human isolates in the region increased only slightly. The increased use of pasteurized egg products and education of food handlers may also reduce human illness independent of producer efforts.

A third explanation for the discrepancies may be that the power of these survey methods is inadequate to demonstrate the association among *S*. Enteritidis in unpasteurized liquid egg, aged hens, and sporadic human isolates. It is estimated that reported salmonella isolates represent 1%–5% of the total salmonella infections (Chalker and Blazer, 1988). This level of detection may be inadequate to demonstrate an association.

Laboratory Implications

Experience with the liquid-egg surveys suggests the need to adjust laboratory methods as the number of salmonella colonies on an agar plate increases. As required in the protocols, three (aged hen) to five (liquid egg) colonies showing typical salmonella reactions on brilliant green novobiocin or xylose-lysine-tergitol 4 agar were selected for testing with group-D antiserum. *Salmonella* Enteritidis was isolated at a higher rate from liquid-egg samples when other salmonella serovars were not concomitantly recovered from the samples. Also, direct enrichment of samples by using a single enrichment medium likely underestimates the levels of contamination. The addition of delayed secondary enrichment to culturing protocols may increase recovery of *S*. Enteritidis (Waltman et al., 1992; Waltman and Horne, 1993).

Phage-Type Implications

The predominance of *S*. Enteritidis PT13a in both 1995 surveys is noteworthy. In the 1991 surveys, PT8 was the predominant phage type of *S*. Enteritidis recovered. This shift in phage type may have occurred due to continuing reintroduction of new *S*. Enteritidis strains into commercial laying flocks. This hypothesis suggests that *S*. Enteritidis is still spreading in the egg industry because some route of introduction into flocks is not adequately controlled. Replacement pullets, feed, rodents, and humans are all possible sources of *S*. Enteritidis introduction into flocks. Alternatively, it is possible that PT13a is better adapted to the ecology in poultry houses and has competitively replaced PT8 since 1991. It is also possible that other strains of *S*. Enteritidis can be transformed into PT13a and that these results simply demonstrate the plasticity of phage typing (Frost et al., 1989).

The emergence of PT4 in the United States presents an opportunity to track the spread of a unique *S*. Enteritidis. It also presents a challenge to protect the commercial egg industry and the public's health. *Salmonella* Enteritidis PT4 was detected in the commercial egg industry in the western states and appears to be a significant source of *S*. Enteritidis in human-associated illness. A study of sporadic human isolates in California showed that 24 (95%) of 26 randomly selected *S*. Enteritidis–case isolates were PT4 (Passaro et al., 1996). Except for one liquid-egg sample, all *S*. Enteritidis PT4 detected in the 1995 liquid-egg and aged-hen surveys came from Western Region samples. In Great Britain and other parts of the world, *S*. Enteritidis PT4 is predominant in the egg industry and is the leading type associated with human illness (Humphrey, 1990; Rodrigue et al., 1990).

Implications for Control

There are difficulties interpreting and comparing these survey results, but there is no disputing the need for perseverance in controlling *S*. Enteritidis in the U.S. commercial egg industry. These survey findings do not support a conclusion that *S*. Enteritidis infection has declined in the U.S. layer industry or in the human population between 1991 and 1995. Instead, they suggest the need for increased involvement of the egg industry and government in preventing or controlling *S*. Enteritidis contamination of flocks.

Successes of past efforts to control *S*. Enteritidis in egg production have been mixed. Some producers in Pennsylvania implemented an on-farm quality-assurance program that demonstrated a reduction in flocks infected with *S*. Enteritidis (White et al., 1997). The program did not eliminate *S*. Enteritidis from all participating flocks, and the effect of this program was not evident at the regional or national level, but it may serve as a prototype for the egg industry. Also, the USDA, until October 1995, enforced the regulation that identified and tested flocks implicated in human *S*. Enteritidis outbreaks, but this regulation apparently did not reduce the level of *S*. Enteritidis in aged hens or liquid-egg samples nationwide. Funding for the USDA regulation was discontinued by Congress in October 1995. As a result, the U.S. Food and Drug Administration took over enforcement of the regulation, using the protocol outlined in a 1993 USDA proposed rule (Anon., 1993).

REFERENCES

Altekruse, S.F., and Swerdlow, D.L. 1996. The changing epidemiology of food borne diseases. Am. J. Med. Sci. 344:23–29.

Anonymous. 1991. Regulations governing the inspection of eggs and egg products. Fed. Reg. 7 CFR part 59.

Anonymous. 1992. Census of agriculture. Washington, DC: U.S. Government Printing Office; U.S. Department of Commerce, Economics and Statistics Administration, Bureau of the Census.

Anonymous. 1993. Chicken disease caused by *Salmonella enteritidis*. Fed. Reg. 58:146.

Barnhardt, H.M., Dreesen, D.W., Bastien, R., and Pancorbo, O.C. 1991. Prevalence of *Salmonella enteritidis* and other serovars in ovaries of layer hens at time of slaughter. J. Food Prot. 54:488–491.

Chalker, R.B., and Blazer, M.J. 1988. A review of human salmonellosis, part 3: magnitude of *Salmonella* infection in the United States. Rev. Infect. Dis. 10:111–118.

Cowden, J.M. 1990. Salmonellosis and eggs: public health, food poisoning, and food hygiene. Curr. Opin. Infect. Dis. 3:246–249.

Cowden, J.M., Lynch, D., Joseph, C.A., et al. 1989. Case-control study of infections with *Salmonella enteritidis* phage type 4 in England. BMJ 299:771–773.

Dreesen, D.W., Barnhart, H.M., Burke, J.L., et al. 1992. Frequency of *Salmonella enteritidis* and other salmonellae in the ceca of spent hens at time of slaughter. Avian Dis. 36:247–250.

Ebel, E.D., David, M.J., and Mason, J. 1992. Occurrence of *Salmonella enteritidis* in the U.S. commercial egg industry: report on a national spent hen survey. Avian Dis. 36:646–654.

Ebel, E.D., Mason, J., Thomas, L.A., et al. 1993. Occurrence of *Salmonella enteritidis* in unpasteurized liquid egg in the United States. Avian Dis. 37:135–142.

Ferris, K.E., and Thomas, L.A. 1995. *Salmonella* serotypes from animals and related sources reported during July 1994–June 1995. Proc. 99th Annu. Meet. U.S. Anim. Health Assoc. 99:510–524.

Frost, J.A., Ward, L.R., and Rowe, B. 1989. Acquisition of a drug resistance plasmid converts *Salmonella enteritidis* phage type 4 to phage type 24. Epidemiol. Infect. 103:234–248.

Hedberg, C.W., David, J.J., White, K.E., et al. 1993. Role of egg consumption in sporadic *Salmonella enteritidis* and *S. typhimurium* infection in Minnesota. J. Infect. Dis. 167:107–111.

Hogue, A.T., Ebel, E.D., Thomas, L.A., et al. 1997. Surveys of *Salmonella enteritidis* in unpasteurized liquid egg and spent hens at slaughter. J. Food Prot. 60:1194–1200.

Humphrey, T.J. 1990. Public health implications of the infection of egg-laying hens with *Salmonella enteritidis* phage type 4. World Poult. Sci. J. 46:5–13.

Humphrey, T.J., Whitehead, A., Gawler, A.H.L., et al. 1991. Numbers of *Salmonella enteritidis* in the contents of naturally contaminated hens' eggs. Epidemiol. Infect. 106:489–496.

Kinde, H., Read, D., Ardans, A., et al. 1996a. Likely source of *Salmonella enteritidis,* phage type 4 infection in a commercial chicken layer flock in southern California. Avian Dis. 40:672–676.

Kinde, H., Read, D., Chin, R., et al. 1996b. *Salmonella enteritidis,* phage type 4 infection in a commercial layer flock in Southern California: bacteriologic and epidemiologic findings. Avian Dis. 40:665–671.

Kingston, D.J. 1981. A comparison of culturing drag swabs and litter for identification of infection with *Salmonella* spp. in commercial chicken flocks. Avian Dis. 25:513–516.

Mason, J. 1994. *Salmonella enteritidis* control programs in the United States. Int. J. Food Microbiol. 21:115–169.

Mason, J., and Ebel, E.D. 1991. The APHIS *Salmonella enteritidis* control program. Animal Health Insight USDA-APHIS, NAHMS (November).

Mishu, B., Koehler, J., Lee, L.A., et al. 1994. Outbreaks of *Salmonella enteritidis* infections in the United States, 1985–1991. J. Infect. Dis. 169:547–552.

Passaro, D.J., Reporter, R., Mascola, L., et al. 1996. Epidemic *Salmonella enteritidis* (SE) infection in Los Angeles County, California: the predominance of phage type 4. West. J. Med. 165:126–130.

Poppe, C. 1994. *Salmonella enteritidis* in Canada. Int. J. Food Microbiol. 212:1–5.

Poppe, C., Irwin, R.J., Forsberg, C.M., et al. 1991. The prevalence of *Salmonella enteritidis* and other *Salmonella* spp. among Canadian registered commercial layer flocks. Epidemiol. Infect. 106:259–270.

Rodrigue, D.C., Tauxe, R., and Rowe, B. 1990. International increase in *Salmonella enteritidis:* a new pandemic? Epidemiol. Infect. 105:21–27.

Schlosser, W.D., Henzler, D.J., Mason, J., and Kradel, D.C. 1994. The *Salmonella enteritidis* pilot project and the Pennsylvania egg quality assurance programs. Proc. 98th Annu. Meet. U.S. Anim. Health Assoc. 98:425–430.

St. Louis, M.E., Morse, D.L., Potter, M.E., et al. 1988. The emergence of grade A eggs as a major source of *Salmonella enteritidis* infections: new implication for control of salmonellosis. JAMA 259:2103–2107.

Vose, D. 1996. Quantitative risk analysis: a guide to Monte Carlo simulation modelling. New York: John Wiley and Sons.

Waltman, W.D., and Horne, A.M. 1993. Isolation of *Salmonella* from chickens reacting in the pullorum-typhoid agglutination test. Avian Dis. 37:805–810.

Waltman, W.D., Horne, A.M., Pirkle, C., and Johnson, D.C. 1992. Prevalence of *Salmonella enteritidis* in spent hens. Avian Dis. 36:251–255.

White, P.L., Schlosser, W., Benson, C.E., et al. 1997. Environmental survey by manure drag sampling for *Salmonella enteritidis* in chicken layer houses. J. Food Prot. 60:1189–1193.

32

The *Salmonella enterica* Serovar Enteritidis Pilot Project

W.D. Schlosser, D.J. Henzler, J. Mason, D. Kradel, L. Shipman, S. Trock, S.H. Hurd, A.T. Hogue, W. Sischo, and E.D. Ebel

INTRODUCTION

Background

In November 1991, a small subcommittee of the *Salmonella enterica* serovar Enteritidis (*S.* Enteritidis) Working Group was formed to organize the *S.* Enteritidis Pilot Project (SEPP) in Pennsylvania. The project was established in Lancaster, Pennsylvania, in April 1992. The project's stated objectives were to develop effective and efficient monitoring procedures for *S.* Enteritidis infection in laying-hen flocks, with the ultimate goal of preventing *S.* Enteritidis from contaminating eggs.

Organization

The SEPP was a voluntary, cooperative effort among the egg industry in Pennsylvania, the Pennsylvania Department of Agriculture, Pennsylvania State University, the University of Pennsylvania, and the United States Department of Agriculture (USDA). An Oversight Committee was established to represent the groups involved. This committee was instrumental in organizing the program and developing conditions for participation and operational protocols. Egg producers provided the flocks to be studied and some assistance in collecting specimens.

Project operations started on 14 April 1992. Flocks were added gradually. Participating flocks were self-selected by producers. The selection may have been biased, with a greater tendency to include known *S.* Enteritidis–positive flocks. As of 31 January 1994, a total of 134 flocks had been, or were being, monitored. These flocks came from 76 different houses, which represented 20%–25% of the total houses in Pennsylvania. There were 38 single houses and 13 farms with multiple houses. There were 53 houses that housed a second flock after the first flock had left. Five of these houses housed a third flock after the second flock had left. Therefore, 58 of the 134 flocks were replacement flocks in previously tested houses. Flocks were accepted into the project at different ages. Some flocks were molted, but most were not. Owners of approximately 50% of the flocks volunteering for the study had positive egg-machinery or manure drag swabs. Most flocks were transferred to a voluntary quality-assurance program in February 1994. The following information, except where noted, is based on data collected from April 1992 through January 1994.

Laboratory Services

The Pennsylvania Department of Agriculture and the two universities provided laboratory services and technical guidance. The USDA Animal and Plant Health Inspection Service–Veterinary Services served as the coordinating agency, provided technical support, and provided additional laboratory services through the National Veterinary Services Laboratories (NVSL).

STUDY METHODS

Owners of flocks entered in the SEPP agreed to adhere to the following testing schedule: an early environmental test when the flock was 26–34 weeks old, a midcycle environmental test when the flock was 35–56 weeks old, and a late environmental test for flocks that were 57 weeks or older until the time the flock was molted. Flocks that were molted were tested again. Additional environmental samples were taken when the house had been cleaned and disinfected after the flock had been depopulated.

Environmental tests consisted of swabs of the manure pit and egg machinery. If any environmental test was positive, the producer submitted 1000 eggs for bacteriological culture every other week until 4000 eggs had been cultured. If any egg pool was positive, the producer diverted eggs from that flock to pasteurization or hard cooking. To resume sale of table eggs, the producer submitted 1000 eggs every other week until 4000 consecutive eggs were culture negative for S. Enteritidis. Flocks with S. Enteritidis–negative environmental samples were considered a low risk for producing S. Enteritidis–positive eggs, and no eggs were cultured from these flocks.

Additionally, swabs from walkways, fans, utility rooms, and egg-processing rooms were collected. The culture results from these swabs were not used to determine flock restrictions. Rather, they were used to assess the value of using other types of samples to determine the environmental status of the house. They were also used to monitor biosecurity and to evaluate cleaning and disinfecting methods.

Rodent density was measured at the time of each environmental test in most houses. This consisted of a visual evaluation and placement of multiple catch-repeating mousetraps. Farm rodent-control procedures were rated by SEPP personnel. Feed was not specifically evaluated as a risk factor for S. Enteritidis because of the difficulty of collecting adequate samples from complete feeds with the necessary frequency to get adequate representation of the large feed tonnages used.

On-Farm Environmental Sampling

Manure pit samples were obtained using two, 4 × 4-inch, 8- or 12-ply gauze sponges that were moistened with canned evaporated skim milk and attached to a pole by a string (Mallinson et al., 1989). Using this apparatus, the gauze sponges were dragged the full length of the manure piles beneath each cage bank. When manure pit areas were inaccessible (less than 5% of the time), samples were taken by hand swabbing areas of the manure drop boards or scrapers.

Egg-machinery samples were obtained by hand swabbing with 4 × 4-inch, 8- or 12-ply gauze sponges moistened with canned evaporated skim milk. At least 50% of the egg deescalators and approximately a 12-foot section of each egg belt at the front of the house were swabbed at each visit.

Transport and Culture of Environmental Samples

All environmental samples for bacteriological examination contained two sponges per sample and were placed in 18-ounce Whirlpack bags. These samples were transported from the farm in coolers with ice packs and transferred to a refrigerator on arrival at the SEPP laboratory. Samples were subsequently shipped to one of the four cooperating diagnostic laboratories.

Culture of Mouse Tissues

Mice collected were cultured according to a previously published protocol (Henzler and Opitz, 1992). The spleen, liver, and all portions of the gastrointestinal tract distal to the esophagus were included in the tissue pools. Tissues from five mice were pooled, except when fewer than five mice were available for culture.

On-Farm Egg Collection

The eggs for culturing were collected systematically, with an equal number of eggs obtained from each cage tier in the house. Project personnel collected unwashed eggs by hand, walking along each row with a pushcart and placing eggs collected on new fiber flats. Visibly dirty eggs and undersized eggs were not included. After collection, eggs were either broken out and contents placed into plastic bags at the SEPP laboratory or transported directly to cooperating laboratories for break-out of egg contents and subsequent culture.

Egg Handling and Culture of Eggs

Prior to breaking the eggs to remove their contents, material adherent to the eggshell was removed by hand, and eggshells were disinfected. The disinfectants used were either iodine or hydrogen peroxide–acetic acid–based sprays. The iodine disinfectant consisted of 3 parts 70% ethyl or isopropyl alcohol to 1 part 10% Lugol's iodine. The hydrogen peroxide–acetic acid sprays were commercial preparations to which a red vegetable dye was added so the disinfectant could be seen on the shell. After the eggs were dried, they were cracked on the lip of a laboratory beaker that had been treated with 70% ethyl alcohol. Eggs were cracked in pools of 10 and placed into sterile 42-ounce plastic bags. Latex gloves were worn to break eggs and changed between each egg pool. The contents of each bag were thoroughly mixed by hand. After mixing, the egg pool was incubated at 25°C for 48 h. Then, 1 ml of sample was transferred to 10 ml of Hajna tetrathionate enrichment broth, which was incubated at 37°C for 24 h. Following this incubation, 0.1 ml of the broth was transferred to a xylose-lysine-deoxycholate (XLD) agar plate and a brilliant green agar plate, and the plates were incubated for 24 h at 37°C. After incubation, three representative salmonella-suspect colonies were selected from the two plates and stabbed into triple-sugar iron and lysine iron agar slants. All presumptive salmonella isolates were sent to the NVSL for serotyping and phage typing. These culture methods apply to egg collections from April 1992 to September 1992.

In September 1992, the time of incubation of the initial egg-pool mixture was extended from 48 h to 72–96 h at

25°C. In January 1993, the protocol was again revised to increase the egg pool from 10 to 20 eggs, which were placed into sterile, 1-gallon freezer plastic bags or quart-sized rigid plastic containers with lids. The egg pools were mixed with a disinfected fork or a sterile wooden stick and incubated for 72–96 h at 25°C. After incubation, instead of an enrichment step, a sterile swab was inserted into the pool mixture, and a short streak of inoculum was applied directly to media plates containing brilliant green agar and XLD agar. An inoculating loop was used to streak the plates from the swabbed area. All plates were incubated according to the original protocol. Heavily contaminated cultures were subcultured to xylose-lysine-tergitol 4 agar or brilliant green agar supplemented with novobiocin. Serotyping and further characterizations were carried out according to the original protocol.

FINDINGS

The Presence of *Salmonella* Enteritidis in the Environment of Layer Houses

1. *Older flocks were more likely to have positive environments than were younger flocks.*

Figure 32.1 shows the prevalence of S. Enteritidis–positive manure-drag swabs by age of flock.

2. *There was no seasonal difference in the percentage of environmental positive tests.*

Figure 32.2 shows the prevalence of S. Enteritidis–positive manure-drag swabs by month of test.

3. *Repeated environmental testing of a house did not give consistent results. Sampling the manure gave* *more consistent results than sampling the egg machinery, though egg-machinery samples were more likely to give positive results.*

One of the difficulties with carrying out studies of S. Enteritidis in egg-layer flocks was selecting the test or tests to be used for determining which flocks were positive. The Northeast Conference on Avian Diseases recommended in 1988 that the environment of layer houses, particularly the manure pits and the egg machinery, be sampled by swabbing. It was assumed that if S. Enteritidis was found in the manure or on the egg machinery, there was a high probability that the birds in the flock were infected. Environmental testing was adopted as a screening device: if it was positive, the eggs were tested; if the environment was negative, no further tests were conducted. Therefore, we were unable to determine the sensitivity of environmental testing for detecting S. Enteritidis in eggs.

The project conducted a study to evaluate the consistency of test results by collecting eight sets of environmental samples from the same flock within 2 days. Ten flocks participated in the study. All houses were deep-pit houses. One pair of technicians collected all samples from the flocks, and a single laboratory processed all samples. The study was conducted from 25 October 1993 to 26 January 1994. Although the study spanned 3 months, once sampling was begun in a house it was completed in 24–36 h.

The collector pair would collect four complete sets of egg-machinery samples. The pair then collected manure samples. Each collector would sample all banks of manure, resulting in two complete sets of manure samples. Upon completion of this sampling, the pair would repeat the manure sampling, collecting a total of four sets of manure samples per house per visit. The collector pair would meet at the same layer house the following day and repeat the

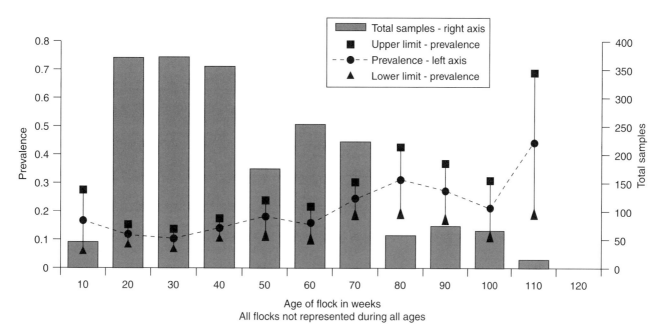

FIGURE 32.1   Prevalence of manure-drag swabs that were positive for *Salmonella* Enteritidis by age of flocks.

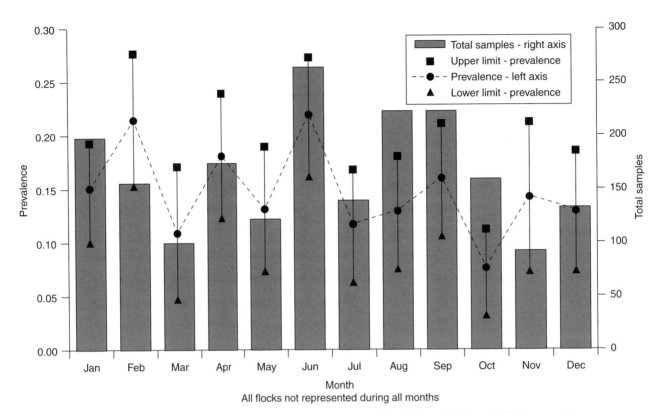

FIGURE 32.2 Prevalence of manure-drag swabs that were positive for *Salmonella* Enteritidis by months.

sample collection. Throughout the study, although collector 2 varied among four individuals, collector 1 remained the same.

All group-D isolates were forwarded to the NVSL for serotyping. Results from the laboratory cultures were compared among the two most closely associated temporal sample collections (that is, sample 1 from collector 1 was compared with sample 1 from collector 2). Concordant and discordant pairs were noted. Concordant pairs were defined as having the same laboratory results between the two collectors, either both positive or both negative for *S.* Enteritidis. Discordant pairs were noted when one collector sample was reported as positive for *S.* Enteritidis and the other collector sample was reported as negative. Five of the houses were negative for *S.* Enteritidis in all samples. The remaining five houses had *S.* Enteritidis recovered from some samples.

Manure sampling yielded more consistent test results than did egg-machinery sampling. Concordant pairs were identified 87.5% of the time during manure sampling, whereas egg-machinery sampling yielded concordant pairs 70% of the time. Although manure sampling appeared to be more consistent among collectors, there was a higher likelihood of isolating *S.* Enteritidis from egg-machinery samples than from the manure samples.

Table 32.1 shows that egg-machinery sampling was more likely to detect *S.* Enteritidis if it was present at lower levels in a layer house. Houses A–C were more lightly contaminated, and all had a higher recovery rate from the egg

machinery than from the manure sampling. In the case of house A, if only manure sampling was conducted this house would be incorrectly labeled as negative for *S.* Enteritidis, because the only positive samples were from the egg machinery.

The Presence of *Salmonella* Enteritidis in Eggs

1. *Of the flocks with S. Enteritidis–positive environments, 50% produced at least one positive egg during the course of testing. Positive eggs were not consistently detected in flocks that had positive environments. The prevalence of S. Enteritidis–positive eggs in the flocks that had positive environments was 2.75 per 10,000, with a range of 0–35 per 10,000. 10% of the isolations from eggs were salmonella other than S. Enteritidis.*

Figure 32.3 shows the prevalences of *S.* Enteritidis–positive eggs in flocks housed in *S.* Enteritidis–positive environments in the SEPP.

The contents of the great majority of eggs tested (more than 99.9%) were free of bacteria. Although eggs were pooled in groups of 10 or 20, it was assumed that when an egg pool was positive for *S.* Enteritidis, a single egg was positive. A total of 647,000 eggs was cultured through 31 January 1994. There were 178 eggs positive for *S.* Enteritidis. The proportion of *S.* Enteritidis–positive eggs was

TABLE 32.1   Summary of layer houses with *Salmonella* Enteritidis–positive samples after eight repeated collections

House	No. positives per no. manure collections	No. positives per no. egg-machinery collections
A	0/8	4/8
B	2/8	3/8
C	1/8	2/8
D	7/8	6/8
E	7/8	5/8

The remaining five houses were negative for all samples (eight per house).

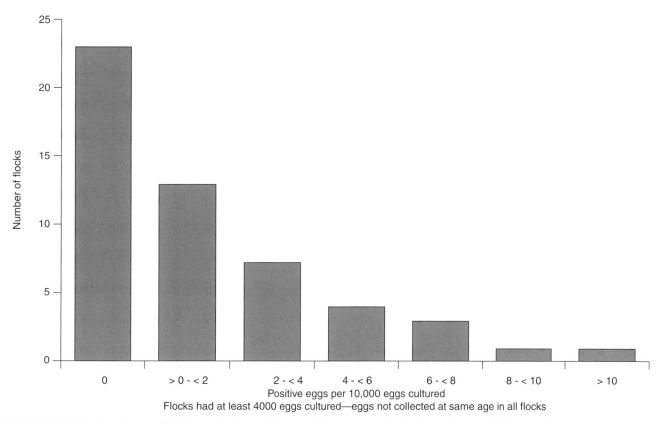

FIGURE 32.3   Prevalence of *Salmonella* Enteritidis–positive eggs in flocks housed in an *S.* Enteritidis-positive environment in the *Salmonella* Enteritidis Pilot Project.

0.000275 or 2.75 per 10,000 eggs from flocks with *S.* Enteritidis–positive environments.

A total of 20 eggs from 11 flocks was positive for salmonellae other than *S.* Enteritidis. This represented a proportion of 0.000031 or 0.31 eggs per 10,000 eggs from flocks with *S.* Enteritidis–contaminated environments. The frequency of egg contamination with non–*S.* Enteritidis isolates was approximately a log base 10 lower than *S.* Enteritidis. Seven serovars were specifically identified as *Salmonella* Typhimurium, Tennessee, Agona, Montevideo, Kentucky, Cerro, and Dublin. Serovars could not be determined for seven other isolates. *Salmonella* Montevideo occurred most frequently, with five isolates, and *S.* Cerro and *S.* Kentucky each with two isolates. All other isolates occurred only once.

2. *Egg-machinery and manure-drag swabs together are better predictors of the potential of a flock to produce positive eggs than is either sample type alone.*

Data from the project were analyzed to determine whether flock environmental status was an accurate predictor of future production of *S.* Enteritidis–positive eggs. Flocks included in the analysis met all of the following criteria: the first environmental sampling in the flock included both egg-machinery and manure-drag swabs; at least 4000 eggs were collected from the flock in the 90 days following the environmental sampling; the flock had not been vaccinated with an *S.* Enteritidis bacterin.

A total of 53 flocks met this criteria. Table 32.2 compares the different types of environmental sampling with the subsequent egg-culture results.

TABLE 32.2 Positive predictive values of environmental samples for *Salmonella* Enteritidis–positive egg pools

Type of environmental sampling	Result of environmental sampling	At least one positive egg pool	No. positive egg pools	Total	Positive predictive value[a]
Egg-machinery swabs	At least one egg-machinery swab positive	10	17	27	37%
	All egg-machinery swabs negative	0	6	6	—
Manure-drag swabs	At least one manure-drag swab positive	9	12	21	43%
	All manure-drag swabs negative	1	11	12	—
Egg-machinery swabs *or* manure-drag swabs	At least one egg-machinery or manure-drag swab positive	10	22	32	31%
	All egg-machinery and manure-drag swabs negative	0	1	1	—
Egg-machinery swabs *and* manure-drag swabs	At least one egg-machinery swab and at least one manure-drag swab positive	9	7	16	56%
	Either all egg-machinery swabs negative or all manure-drag swabs negative	1	16	17	—

[a]Positive predictive value: the probability that a positive egg culture will follow a positive environmental result.

Positive egg-machinery swabs and manure-drag swabs taken individually were both relatively poor predictors of the potential of a flock to produce a detectable level of *S.* Enteritidis–positive eggs. Positive egg-machinery swabs combined with positive manure-drag swabs taken at the same time provided the best predictor of future S. Enteritidis–positive eggs.

3. *Older flocks had a higher proportion of S. Enteritidis-positive eggs than did younger flocks.*

Figure 32.4 shows the prevalence of S. Enteritidis–positive eggs per 10,000 eggs by age of flock.

4. *There was no seasonal difference in the prevalence of* S. *Enteritidis–positive eggs.*

Figure 32.5 shows the prevalence of S. Enteritidis–positive eggs per 10,000 eggs by month of test.

5. *Blood-spot eggs from a flock were more likely to be* S. *Enteritidis positive.*

Blood-spot eggs occur when a blood vessel ruptures during formation of the egg. Blood-spot eggs are discarded during processing for aesthetic reasons. A study was conducted to determine the incidence of S. Enteritidis in blood-spot eggs.

Producers were asked to donate voluntarily all blood-spot eggs from flocks in which eggs were being sampled. SEPP personnel collected blood-spot eggs weekly at the egg processor.

For analysis, all blood-spot egg collections were matched with the nearest ($\pm$ 30 days) regular egg collection. The proportion of positive eggs was compared between blood-spot eggs and regular eggs. Statistical significance was compared using a simple difference-between-proportions test. The proportions were also compared separately for S. Enteritidis–vaccinated and nonvaccinated flocks. Every positive pool of eggs was assumed to contain one contaminated egg.

There were 370 paired collections from 28 flocks, for a total of 54,700 blood-spot eggs collected and 189,000 regular eggs. Only 14 positive blood-spot egg pools were found; 27 positive regular egg pools were detected. The overall proportion of positive blood-spot eggs was almost twice the positive regular egg proportion: 2.56 per 10,000, and 1.43 per 10,000 respectively. This difference was statistically significant ($p < 0.05$).

Blood-spot egg collection appears to be more sensitive, based on the likelihood of blood-spot egg positivity. Nevertheless, the collection of blood-spot eggs may not be feasible for all flocks because only 12 of 28 flocks collected had more than 1000 blood-spot eggs. The average flock (80,000 birds) should produce 150 blood-spot eggs per week and contribute 1000 in 6–7 weeks. The collection of blood-spot eggs depends on the processor's cooperation. It is logistically difficult for some processors to isolate and store blood-spot eggs from individual flocks.

6. *Soiled eggs that had been immersion washed on the farm had a higher prevalence of* S. *Enteritidis contamination.*

In modern, automated egg-layer houses, with 30,000–120,000 birds, some fecal soilage of eggs is unavoidable. During processing, eggs are washed by automatic washers.

Producers occasionally immersion wash soiled eggs that do not come clean in the automatic washer. Some producers immersion wash excessively soiled eggs before the eggs are sent through the automatic washer. Immersion washing entails placing a basket of dirty eggs in a machine with detergent and water heated to about 43°C. The solution is agitated around the eggs for 3–5 min. Water used to wash the eggs that is not changed between washes becomes dirty after several baskets. Warming feces-contaminated eggs followed by cooling facilitates migration of bacteria through the shell and egg membranes into the egg (Forsythe et al., 1953). Immersion-washed eggs were a small proportion of the total flock production (estimated at 0.75%) but may pose a higher risk of salmonellosis to consumers. The project conducted a study to determine whether dirty eggs washed by immersion had a higher prevalence of salmonellae.

Nine flocks were included in this study. Producers were asked to participate if their flock environment was positive for S. Enteritidis and they had a history of immersion washing dirty eggs. The producers washed eggs in the usual manner and set aside up to 1000 immersion-washed eggs each week. The study lasted from August 1993 through June 1994, with flocks entering and leaving the study at different times.

The egg samples were sent to one of two laboratories: Pennsylvania State University or the University of Pennsylvania–New Bolton Center. All of the eggs were pooled and cultured in groups of 20, and we assumed that only a single egg accounted for each positive egg pool. Serotyping of salmonellae isolates was done at the NVSL.

The overall prevalence of S. Enteritidis–positive eggs was 2.2 per 10,000 among the immersion-washed eggs versus 1.4 per 10,000 among the other eggs sampled from the same flocks. The prevalence of salmonellae other than S. Enteritidis was 0.5 per 10,000 among the immersion-washed eggs versus 0.2 per 10,000 among other eggs from the same flocks. The difference was not statistically significant when tested using the Mantel-Haenzel chi-squared test and controlling for flock variation.

There may truly be no difference in salmonellae prevalence between eggs that are immersion washed and those that are not. The sample size in this study, however, was too small to confirm the observed difference.

Management Factors and *Salmonella* Enteritidis

1. *Approximately 50% of* S. *Enteritidis–positive houses that were cleaned and disinfected were culture negative on environmental sampling; 28% of negative houses were culture positive on environmental sampling following the cleaning and disinfecting (C&D).*

Cleaning and disinfecting between flocks is routinely used as a means of reducing disease transmission in poultry houses. All layer houses in the SEPP were cleaned and disinfected between flocks when the houses were empty. The procedure generally consisted of (a) dry cleaning, (b) wet cleaning (soaking, washing, rinsing), (c) disinfection, and, in some cases, (d) formaldehyde fumigation.

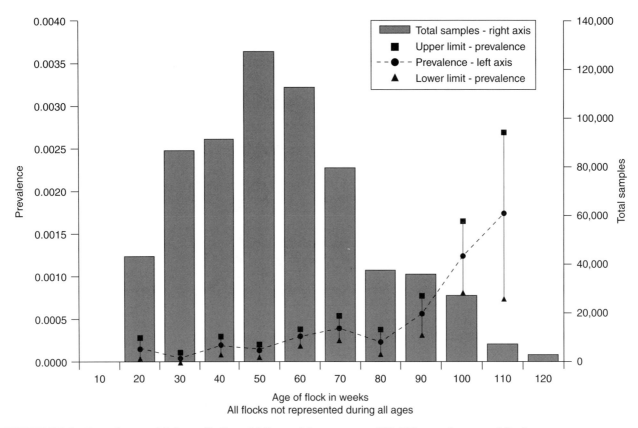

FIGURE 32.4   Prevalence of *Salmonella* Enteritidis–positive eggs per 100,000 eggs by age of flocks.

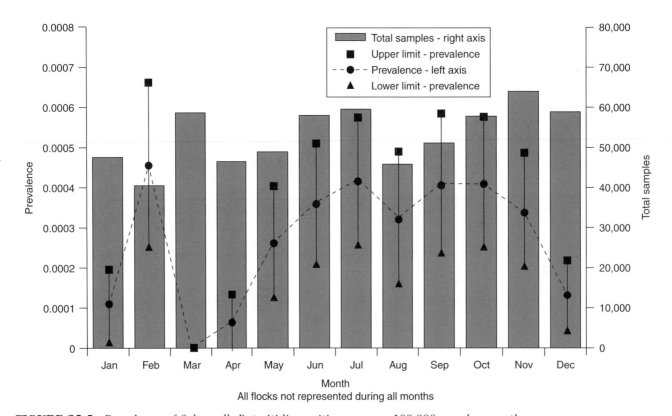

FIGURE 32.5   Prevalence of *Salmonella* Enteritidis–positive eggs per 100,000 eggs by months.

The type of C&D, quality of C&D, and the length of time required to perform C&D varied. Following the C&D of a house but before placement of birds, project personnel collected environmental samples in the house. The types of samples varied but usually included egg-handling equipment, manure area, walkways, fans, and utility rooms. In some cases, personnel collected samples after different stages of the C&D. The number of post-C&D collections varied from 0 to 3. The stage of C&D at which sampling was done was inconsistent. Samples were considered positive or negative based on the presence or absence of *S.* Enteritidis. No attempt was made to quantify the numbers of organisms. Table 32.3 uses only the last post-C&D collection in a house.

A goodness of fit applied to the first row of Table 32.3 determined the likely effectiveness of the C&D procedure in reducing *S.* Enteritidis in a house to below detectable levels to be about 50%.

Of 34 environmentally positive houses that had been cleaned and disinfected, 16 converted to negative status after the procedure. Overall, houses showed a 50% reduction in *S.* Enteritidis–positive samples after C&D.

Table 32.4 compares the proportion of positive samples taken in the 60-day period before C&D to the proportion of positive samples taken on the last post-C&D test before housing the new flock.

Chi squares for comparison of proportions were 1.57 ($p = 0.21$) for egg-handling equipment, 15.3 ($p < 0.01$) for manure pits, 2.3 ($p = 0.13$) for walkways, and 1.31 ($p = 0.25$) for all other environmental samples. The chi square for comparison of proportions for all environmental samples was 17.7 ($p < 0.01$).

When all samples except manure pit samples were counted, 46 (18%) of 250 were positive before C&D and 34 (12%) of 292 samples were positive after C&D. The chi square for comparison of proportions was 4.89 ($p = 0.03$).

Since houses were required to be cleaned and disinfected as a condition of program participation, it is impossible to compare the reductions in contamination that occurred with what would have occurred without C&D.

2. *Molting increases the prevalence of positive eggs in flocks in the immediate postmolt period.*

Data on molting were gathered from 1 May 1992 to 1 May 1994. A total of 31 flocks was molted. Not all molted flocks had eggs gathered during the premolt and postmolt periods. Collections are summarized below for all molted flocks that had eggs collected within 20 weeks before or after molt (Table 32.5).

The proportion of positive eggs in the 0–5 postmolt period was significantly higher ($p < 0.01$) than any of the other periods except for the 20–16 premolt period ($p < 0.1$). This is consistent with the findings of Holt and Porter (1993), who demonstrated that molting is a risk factor for hens being infected with and shedding *S.* Enteritidis.

3. *Data from two complexes (19 flocks) suggest that vaccine may lower the risk of a flock producing contaminated eggs, though an insufficient number of complexes were studied to draw a definite conclusion.*

Some producers administer an *S.* Enteritidis bacterin in their pullet flocks in an effort to ameliorate the effect of *S.* Enteritidis. Data were collected for those flocks in complexes in which *S.* Enteritidis bacterin was used. This was compared with flocks in complexes in which *S.* Enteritidis bacterin was not used.

Two complexes containing a total of nine houses administered an *S.* Enteritidis bacterin to their flocks. As the initial flocks were removed and replaced with new layer birds, the replacement flocks were also administered an *S.* Enteritidis bacterin. The time of administration and number of doses of bacterin were not consistent. A total of 19 flocks in the two complexes were administered bacterin. No single-unit houses elected to use a bacterin. There were eight complexes containing a total of 25 houses with 51 flocks that did not use bacterin.

There was a 12% overall prevalence (84 of 708) of positive egg-machinery and manure-drag swabs in vaccinated flocks. Among the unvaccinated flocks, the prevalence was 16% (200 of 1288). The overall prevalence of *S.* Enteritidis–positive eggs in the vaccinated flocks was 0.37 per 10,000. This compares with 1.50 per 10,000 among the unvaccinated flocks.

It should be noted that the two complexes that used an *S.* Enteritidis bacterin also instituted additional *S.* Enteritidis control measures, such as intensive rodent control. It

TABLE 32.3 *Salmonella* Enteritidis isolation from environmental sampling after cleaning and disinfecting (C&D) but before placement of new flock, compared with environmental sampling results of previous flock

Environmental status of first flock	Environmental status after C&D		
	Positive	Negative	Total
Positive	18	16	34
Negative	2	5	7
Total	20	21	41

This table includes houses that had two flocks and at least one post-C&D environmental collection between the flocks. Houses were considered environmentally positive during the first flock if any sample from any collection during the specified time period was positive. The C&D results represent the last post-C&D collection that was performed.

TABLE 32.4 Isolation of *Salmonella* Enteritidis from environmental samples taken during different times for houses participating in the pilot project: results from 23 houses

Location of samples	Samples collected up to 60 days before C&D			Samples collected at the last post-C&D test before housing new flock		
	Total samples	Total positive samples	% Positive	Total samples	Total positive samples	% Positive
Egg machinery	149	23	15	126	13	10
Manure pits	132	37	28	103	8	8
Walkways	34	14	41	44	11	25
All other environmental samples	67	9	13	122	10	8
Total environmental samples	382	83	22	395	42	11

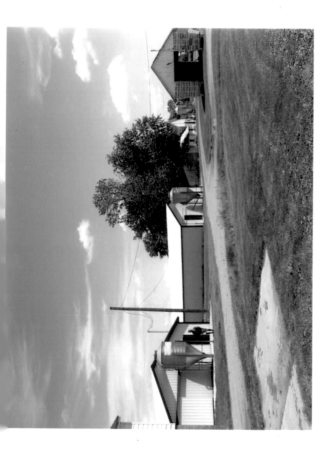

TABLE 32.5 Prevalence of positive eggs for *Salmonella* Enteritidis by 5-week intervals before and after molting in flocks that underwent a molt

Status of flock[a]	No. flocks tested	No. eggs tested	No. positive pools	% Positive eggs
20–16 Premolt	3	7,000	4	0.0571
15–11 Premolt	9	16,000	1	0.0063
10–6 Premolt	12	23,000	4	0.0174
5–0 Premolt	12	21,000	5	0.0238
0–5 Postmolt	6	9,000	13	0.1444
6–10 Postmolt	8	19,000	5	0.0263
11–15 Postmolt	9	18,000	2	0.0125
16–20 Postmolt	10	28,000	11	0.0393

[a]Number of weeks before or after molt.

was not possible to separate other management interventions from the use of the bacterin. It is therefore possible that these other control measures affected the outcome of the study.

4. *Positive chick papers were found in four of 190 collections. Positive pullet environmental swabs were found in six of 79 collections.*

Although participating houses were not required to have chicks or pullets tested, when submitted, samples were tested. Chicks were tested by swabbing every tenth chick paper, and the pullet houses were sampled by drag swabs of the environment.

There were 1404 individual chick-paper swabs from 190 deliveries of chicks. Nine (0.6%) of 1404 samples were positive for *S.* Enteritidis. There were 421 of 1404 samples positive for other salmonella serovars. Four (2.1%) of the 190 deliveries of chicks were positive for *S.* Enteritidis. There were 624 environmental samples collected from 79 pullet flocks (69 houses). These samples were collected on 96 separate visits to the pullet houses. Six (7.6%) of 79 flocks were positive, and 15 (2.4%) of 624 samples were positive.

5. *Eggs, rodents, and the environment often yielded the same phage types within a house.*

Many analyses in this report relied on the relationship between environmental, rodent, or egg isolations of *S.* Enteritidis. Phage typing of these isolates helps determine whether environmental, rodent, and egg isolates are related. *Salmonella* Enteritidis isolates from the SEPP were routinely phage typed by the NVSL.

The most common phage types isolated from the environment and mice were phage type 8 (PT8) and PT23 (Fig. 32.6). The most common phage types isolated from eggs were PT8, untypeable, and PT13a. Flocks usually had the same phage types in the environment as in mice or eggs. This suggests that *S.* Enteritidis infection and transmission in a henhouse exists as an ecological unit, with interdependent connection between the hosts (chickens), the environment, and a possible reservoir (mice).

Progress in Controlling *Salmonella* Enteritidis

1. *Participating houses showed a decrease in the percentage of positive samples in the second flock housed during the SEPP.*

Results of culturing egg-machinery swabs and manure-drag swabs were compared in houses from the first flocks participating in the project to the replacement flocks in the same houses. Tables 32.6 and 32.7 show the results of this comparison.

2. *Producers have continued efforts to control S. Enteritidis in layer flocks.*

Pennsylvania egg producers initiated the Pennsylvania Egg Quality Assurance Program in February 1994, using many of the same control procedures and testing protocols developed in the SEPP. The USDA transferred financial responsibility for this program to producers and Pennsylvania in June 1996. As of January 1997, approximately 85% of the Pennsylvania egg-laying population was enrolled in this voluntary program.

ACKNOWLEDGMENTS

The *Salmonella* Enteritidis Pilot Project required cooperative efforts of many individuals, such as Marlin Henninger, Robert Archer, Mark Nesselrodt, Belvin Markey, Shirley Pflieger, and Patricia White of the SEPP; Carol Maddox and Patty Dunn of Pennsylvania State University; Robert Eckroade and Charles Benson of the University of Pennsylvania; Max Van Buskirk and Tim Secott of the Pennsylvania Department of Agriculture; Lee Ann Thomas of the USDA National Veterinary Services Laboratories; Richard Gast of the USDA Agricultural Research Service; Thomas Gomez of the USDA Animal and Plant Health Inspection Services; John Schwartz of the USDA Cooperative Extension Service; and John Hoffman of the Pennsylvania Poultry Federation.

Despite the efforts of these and other individuals, this project could not have been realized without the cooperation

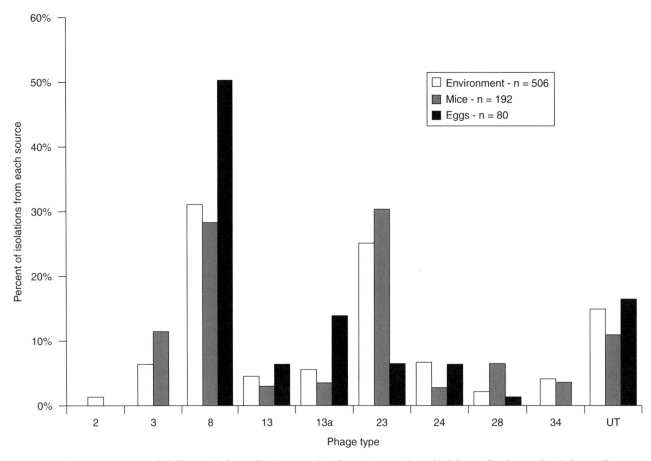

FIGURE 32.6   Frequency of different *Salmonella* Enteritidis phage types identified from flocks in the *Salmonella* Enteritidis Pilot Project. Environmental samples included egg machinery, manure, fans, and walkways. UT, untypeable.

TABLE 32.6   Comparison of egg-machinery swabs in first and second flocks in same house for isolation of *Salmonella* Enteritidis

	First flock			Second flock		
Age in weeks	Samples	No. positive	% Positive	Samples	No. positive	% Positive
20	170	36	21.2	87	16	18.4
30	177	26	14.7	223	34	15.2
40	152	36	23.7	183	10	5.5
50	204	48	23.5	34	7	20.6
60	183	15	8.2	70	9	12.9
70	203	35	17.2	14	2	14.3
Total	1089	196	18.0	611	78	12.8
Age adjusted			18.0			14.1

TABLE 32.7   Comparison of *Salmonella* Enteritidis from manure-drag swabs in first and second flocks in same house

Age in weeks	First flock			Second flock		
	Samples	No. positive	% Positive	Samples	No. positive	% Positive
20	106	19	17.9	216	12	5.6
30	112	9	8.0	209	18	8.6
40	94	26	27.7	189	8	4.2
50	116	25	21.6	34	6	17.6
60	119	17	14.3	64	11	17.2
70	133	36	27.1	14	1	7.1
Total	680	132	19.4	726	56	7.7
Age adjusted			18.5			9.0

and assistance of dozens of Pennsylvania egg producers who opened their flocks and records and invested their time and money in this project.

REFERENCES

Forsythe, R.H., Ayres, J.C., and Radlo, J.L. 1953. Factors affecting the microbial population of shell eggs. Food Technol. 7:49–56.

Henzler, D.J., and Opitz, H.M. 1992. The role of mice in the epizootology of *Salmonella enteritidis* infection on chicken layer farms. Avian Dis. 36:625–631.

Holt, P.S., and Porter, R.E. 1993. Effect of induced molting on the recurrence of a previous *Salmonella enteritidis* infection. Poult. Sci. 72:2069–2078.

Mallinson, E.T., Tate, C.R., Miller, R.G., Bennet, B., and Russek-Cohen, E. 1989. Monitoring poultry farms for *Salmonella* by drag-swab sampling and antigen capture immunoassay. Avian Dis. 33:684–690.

33

Impact of Induced Molting on Immunity and *Salmonella enterica* Serovar Enteritidis Infection in Laying Hens

P.S. Holt

INTRODUCTION

The past 50 years have witnessed a dramatic growth in the commercial egg industry. Currently, an estimated 240 million laying hens in the United States produce close to 60 billion eggs annually. Per-capita egg consumption, while lower than 10–20 years ago, still remains high (Cunningham, 1995; Looper, 1996). To meet the needs of a growing consumer population, industry implemented modern technological innovations such as the development of high-producing genetic stocks of chickens, institution of intensive growing practices, the production of better feeds to increase production efficiency, management of disease through vaccination and biosecurity, and the mechanization of the collecting, packaging, and shipping of product to generate and process eggs faster and more efficiently.

One production topic receiving increased attention over the years was methods to extend the effective egg-laying life of a flock. As a laying flock ages, its ability to lay eggs decreases (Cunningham, 1960; Etches, 1990), and the decline reaches a point where it is no longer economically feasible to keep the flock in lay. At this time, the producer must decide whether to retire the flock and bring a new flock into production, or recycle the current flock to achieve a second, or even third, lay from the hens. Economics guide producers in the recycling decision—factors such as current high egg prices, available cash to bring on a new flock, and the cost to bring a new flock into production versus the cost of

recycling the old flock all play a role. Further, the growing problem of disposal of the spent flock also enters into the equation, because of the growing reluctance of processors to deal with the low meat yields and brittle bones of these hens (Anon., 1993). Because of such factors, flock recycling became a major economic tool for the layer industry. In 1987, an estimated 60% of laying flocks nationally and 90% in California were recycled annually (Bell, 1987), and the popularity of the procedure appears to be increasing.

EFFECT OF MANAGEMENT PRACTICE

A fact that enhanced the popularity of flock recycling, commonly known as induced molting, was that most early studies showed that molting effects on the bird were primarily positive. Compared with their unmolted counterparts, molted birds had increased productivity (Noles, 1966; Lee, 1982; Zimmerman et al., 1987), better feed-to-weight gain ratios (Noles, 1966; Lee, 1982), and less mortality (Lee, 1982). The procedures therefore appeared to have a beneficial effect on laying hens by providing a rest period after an intensive laying cycle (Lee, 1982). This method also synchronized hens for a second laying cycle, which helped maximize efficiency of the operation.

In their text on commercial chicken production, North and Bell (1990) noted that "the best programs must be able to get a flock out of production rapidly and uniformly, experience relatively low mortality, be simple to follow, be inexpensive, and postmolt egg production and egg quality must be only slightly poorer than first-cycle results." There are many methods to molt a bird (Whitehead and Shannon, 1974; Berry and Brake, 1987; Sekimoto et al., 1987; Breeding et al., 1992), but feed removal, combined with reduced photoperiod, remains the method of choice (Bell, 1987; Brake, 1993, 1994). Feed removal can occur on alternate days, with the birds receiving a restricted diet on intervening days, or the birds can remain off feed for extended periods. Alternate-day feed removal can be less stressful on the hens but requires increased work hours to perform the feeding and extends by several weeks the time necessary to bring the hens back into lay (North and Bell, 1990). Extended feed removal remains a favored molting procedure because of the relatively short time needed to return the birds to full lay. Two popular molting regimens, the California and the North Carolina programs, recommend complete feed removal for 10–14 days, coupled with reduction in photoperiod from 16 to 8 h. Targeted weight losses range from 25% (North and Bell, 1990) to 30% (Baker et al., 1983), which is important to get the fat off the reproductive system (North and Bell, 1990; Brake, 1993). Increased body-weight loss correlates with increased postmolt egg production and egg quality (Baker et al., 1983). The flocks require 9–10 weeks before resuming optimum egg lay, which is generally 80%–90% of the maximum lay achieved during the initial cycle.

PHYSIOLOGICAL EFFECTS OF MOLTING

Physiological effects of induced molting include a decline in body weight and size reduction of ovaries, oviduct, and liver (Brake and Thaxton, 1979b) compared with an elevated serum packed blood cell volume and hemoglobin levels (Brake and Thaxton, 1979a; Brake et al., 1982). Spleen weights remain largely unaffected, but the thymus actually exhibits a recrudescence and repopulation (Brake et al., 1981). The ovaries are the targeted organs in this procedure, and the large ovarian follicles are resorbed (Etches et al., 1984; Williams et al., 1985), leaving mainly small follicles. Such a restructuring results in a reproductive tract resembling that of a pre-lay pullet and prepares the hen for an upcoming laying cycle (Brake and Thaxton, 1979b). During the molt, plasma levels of corticosterone and thyroid hormones increase (Brake et al., 1979; Etches et al., 1984) while plasma gonadotropins and sexual steroids decrease (Etches et al., 1984). Increases in plasma corticosterone appear to initiate the reproductive effects, since ovarian regression was observed in hens administered this hormone (Etches et al., 1984; Williams et al., 1985).

Although feed removal provides the benefit of extending the effective egg-laying life of the flock, it may also cause untoward effects on the birds' immune system. Deficient diets have been shown to diminish both humoral immunity (Ben-Nathan et al., 1977, 1981; Gross and Newberne, 1980) and

cell-mediated immunity (Chandra, 1974, 1990; DePasquale-Jardieu and Fraker, 1979) in mammals and birds. An altered immune response was also observed in birds subjected to induced molting through feed withdrawal. Humoral immunity to either sheep red blood cells or *Brucella abortus* antigen remained largely unaffected. However, cell-mediated immunity, as indicated by delayed-type hypersensitivity, graft-versus-host response, and concanavalin-A blastogenesis, was significantly depressed (Holt, 1992b). Total peripheral blood lymphocyte numbers were significantly decreased in molted birds (Holt, 1992b), and a flow-cytometric examination of the lymphocyte subsets showed that the CD4+ T cells, the helper T-cell subset, was significantly decreased in these birds (Holt, 1992a). The B cells and CD8+ T cells were less affected. T-cell function in mammals was similarly shown to be diminished in individuals subjected to deficient diets (DePasquale-Jardieu and Fraker, 1979; Chandra, 1990) and to a variety of other stress situations (Dorian et al., 1982; Glaser et al., 1985b; Kiecolt-Glaser and Glaser, 1988). Elevated levels of serum corticosterone were detected during times of stress, suggesting a possible role for this hormone in the depressed cell-mediated immunity (DePasquale-Jardieu and Fraker, 1979). A similar elevation in this stress hormone was noted in hens subjected to feed removal (Brake et al., 1979; Etches et al., 1984), which may be responsible for observed effects on immunity during an induced molt.

EFFECT OF MOLTING ON IMMUNITY

With the observation that cell-mediated immunity was depressed in birds subjected to feed withdrawal came the inevitable question as to the relevance of such an effect. An intact immune system functions as an important defense against invasion by the multitude of pathogenic microorganisms residing in the environment. Each arm of the immune response protects against different types of pathogens, and a breach of this defense enables these microorganisms to establish a better foothold within the host. Cell-mediated immunity primarily protects against infections caused by intracellular pathogens. Such pathogens can be viruses, bacteria, or parasites and can infect a range of organ sites (Sher and Coffman, 1992; Kaufmann, 1993; Kagi et al., 1996). Protection is mediated by effector T cells and by a battery of hormone messages called lymphokines, which regulate the intensity of the immune response and define which effector cells will play a role in the protection (Lillehoj, 1987; Sher and Coffman, 1992; Kaufmann, 1993). Breaching this immunity can dramatically alter its ability to protect the host against infection.

The discovery that the immune system in molted hens was compromised therefore prompted an investigation into the effect of the procedure on the progression of an infection. *Salmonella enterica* serovar Enteritidis (*S.* Enteritidis) was the organism chosen for the studies, because *S.* Enteritidis is primarily a layer-industry problem (Centers for Disease Control, 1990, 1992, 1996; Gast, 1994; St. Louis et al., 1988), molting is primarily a layer-industry procedure (Bell, 1987), and cell-mediated immunity is important in protecting against a salmonella infection (Collins, 1974; Killar and Eisenstein, 1983). The organism therefore appeared to be the most appropriate choice for the study, directly addressing potential industry problems.

Salmonellae enjoy widespread occurrence in nature and can be recovered from a variety of sources, including feed (Zecha et al., 1977; Cox et al., 1983), insects (Kopanic et al., 1994), rodents (Henzler and Opitz, 1992), litter (Smyser et al., 1966), and other members of the flock (Lahellec and Colin, 1985). These reservoirs serve as ready sources of salmonellae for potentially immunocompromised birds such as may be found during flock recycling. Indeed, hens exposed to an exogenous source of *S.* Enteritidis concomitantly during molt induction exhibited a much more severe infection as compared with their unmolted counterparts. The intestinal shed rate was higher in these birds (Holt and Porter, 1992a,b; Holt et al., 1995), and this is shown in Figure 33.1A. These hens also shed more organisms (Holt and Porter, 1992a,b; Holt, 1993; Holt et al., 1994, 1995) and exhibited significantly more intestinal inflammation, primarily in the colon and cecum, due to the infection (Holt and Porter, 1992b; Porter and Holt, 1993; Holt et al., 1995; Macri et al., 1997). This last point is particularly germane since, except for infections in very young chicks and certain isolated cases in adult birds, *S.* Enteritidis infection in chickens causes little morbidity in the host. However, infection occurring during the molt changes the host-parasite interaction between the *S.* Enteritidis and the hen, resulting in a severe infection more closely resembling a disease state. Tumor necrosis factor, an inflammatory cytokine

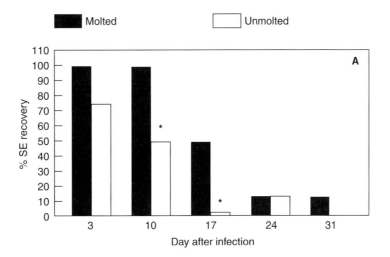

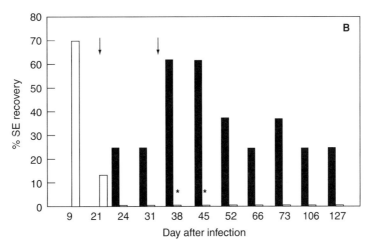

FIGURE 33.1 Intestinal shed rate of *Salmonella* Enteritidis (SE) in molted and unmolted hens infected concurrently with molt (**A**) or 21 days prior to molt (**B**). *Asterisks* indicate significant difference from controls (p < 0.05). *Arrows* indicate the period when feed was removed. From Holt and Porter (1992b) (**A**) and Holt and Porter (1993) (**B**).

previously shown to be responsible for early intestinal pathology in mice infected with *Salmonella* Typhimurium (Arnold et al., 1993), was similarly found to be elevated in molted infected hens (Arnold and Holt, 1996). The potential problems associated with the presence of *S.* Enteritidis in the flock environment therefore become exacerbated when birds are exposed to a stress situation such as feed removal. Even short-term feed removal can increase *S.* Enteritidis shedding by hens (Holt and Porter, 1993; Nakamura et al., 1994a,b), which could affect the eventual flock *S.* Enteritidis status.

Just as molting could affect the progression of a primary *S.* Enteritidis infection in hens, it could also affect an infection already present in the birds. Birds can readily become infected with salmonellae in the hatchery, and these individuals can remain infected for long periods (Bhatia and McNabb, 1980; Cox et al., 1990; Bailey et al., 1994; Cason et al., 1994). Nakamura et al. (1993) showed that a certain percentage of day-old chicks infected with *S.* Enteritidis would remain persistently infected as they matured and went into lay. *Salmonella* Enteritidis can be isolated from the environment of a certain percentage of flocks during their life span (van de Giessen et al., 1994), and 3% of cecal contents from retired laying hens were found to contain the organism (Ebel et al., 1992). Stress situations can reactivate a previous infection (Soave, 1964; Gaskell and Povey, 1977; Rigby and Petit, 1980; Adam, 1982; Glaser et al., 1985a; Hughes et al., 1989), and feed withdrawal to induce a molt can also cause the recurrence of a previous *S.* Enteritidis infection. As was observed with hens molted concurrently with *S.* Enteritidis challenge, recrudescence of infection was found significantly more often in molted birds, and these birds shed significantly more *S.* Enteritidis (Fig. 33.1B) and more readily transmitted the organism to previously uninfected, but contact-exposed, hens (Holt and Porter, 1993). The molted hens also produced more eggs contaminated with the organism. These results indicated that molting can significantly affect an *S.* Enteritidis infection at different times in the infection cycle.

The exacerbation of infection and ready transmission of the organism to previously uninfected hens indicated that the molted hens may be more susceptible to infection by *S.* Enteritidis. Previous studies in mammals provided evidence that fasting could alter the susceptibility of the host to infection by a variety of pathogens (Freter, 1955; Formal et al., 1958; Miller and Bohnhoff, 1962). Similarly, feed removal to induce a molt in hens dramatically increased their susceptibility to *S.* Enteritidis infection. While 10^3–10^4 *S.* Enteritidis were necessary to infect 50% of a test group of unmolted hens, fewer than 10 organisms were required for infection of molted hens (Holt, 1993; Holt et al., 1994). The molted hens were acutely susceptible to *S.* Enteritidis infection, which could put them at risk for any *S.* Enteritidis found in the environment. Special attention therefore needs to be paid to reducing *S.* Enteritidis exposure during this period of high susceptibility to infection.

EFFECT ON TRANSMISSION OF *SALMONELLA* ENTERITIDIS

As was alluded to above, *S.* Enteritidis can originate from a variety of sources, and birds undergoing feed withdrawal and exposed to this organism can become readily infected. What threat do these birds pose to other members of the flock? Nakamura et al. (1993) showed that short-term feed removal could increase horizontal transmission to nearby hens, and Holt and Porter (1992a) found that induced molting increased the horizontal transmission of *S.* Enteritidis to birds in adjacent cages. Holt (1995) further showed that horizontal transmission of *S.* Enteritidis readily occurred down a row of previously uninfected molted hens such that 85%–100% of these birds became infected by day 10 after challenge compared with 10%–30% of unmolted birds (Fig. 33.2). Similar, but less dramatic, effects were observed in birds challenged with a very low

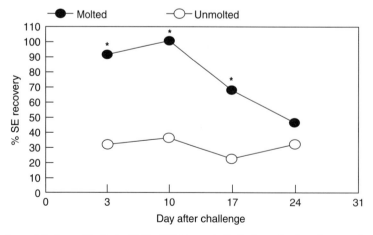

FIGURE 33.2 Transmission of *Salmonella* Enteritidis (SE) to uninfected molted and unmolted hens at various times after challenge. *Asterisks* indicate significantly different from controls (p < 0.05). From Holt (1995).

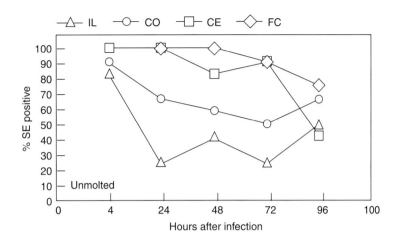

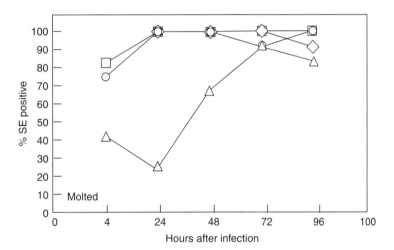

FIGURE 33.3   Recovery of *Salmonella* Enteritidis (SE) from ileum (IL), colon (CO), cecum (CE), and feces (FC) at various times after infection in unmolted and molted hens. From Holt et al. (1995).

dose of *S.* Enteritidis. Several factors appeared to play a role in this rapid transmission, including the amplification of the challenge organism within the intestinal tract of the birds and the subsequent release of large numbers of *S.* Enteritidis into an environment containing highly susceptible birds. Recent work has shown that *S.* Enteritidis can be transmitted to birds in cages a distance away from the infected birds, indicating that airborne transmission of the organism can also occur (Holt et al., 1997). Feed removal therefore has the potential to expand a minor *S.* Enteritidis situation affecting a small number of birds into a major problem within a production facility.

Following ingestion of *S.* Enteritidis, the organism colonizes the gastrointestinal tract of the hen before disseminating to multiple organ sites (Gast and Beard, 1993; Gast, 1994). A hierarchy of intestinal locales is established with regard to colonization. As with other salmonellae, the cecum is the preferred site for colonization by *S.* Enteri-

tidis, followed by the colon and, to a lesser extent, the ileum (Fanelli et al., 1971; Turnbull and Snoeyenbos, 1974; Holt et al., 1995). Feed withdrawal changes this hierarchy so that the infection becomes more evenly distributed along the intestinal tract, including the ileum (Holt et al., 1995) (Fig. 33.3). This alteration occurs rapidly, within 72 h, indicating that factors besides immunodepression may play a part in this scheme. The indigenous bacterial flora was previously shown to be important in modulating the course of salmonella infections in birds, apparently through the production of volatile fatty acids in the intestine (Corrier et al., 1994). The possibility therefore existed that, with the absence of feed, the protective intestinal flora might be modified, with a subsequent alteration in the volatile fatty acid production. However, studies showed that intestinal pH in molted hens did not differ from their fed counterparts (Holt et al., 1994; Corrier et al., 1997) and that the bacterial contents from intestines of molted hens provided competitive exclusion protection against *S.* Enteritidis infection in chicks comparable to intestinal contents from fed hens. While not ruling out the role of intestinal flora changes in the observed alteration in the intestinal colonization patterns in molted birds, these results indicate that other causes also need to be explored.

The realization that a very important economic tool of the layer industry exacerbated an *S.* Enteritidis infection in hens prompted research into methods to ameliorate the situation, either through alternate methods of inducing a molt or through intervention schemes. A low-energy, low-calcium diet, shown previously to cause an egg-lay pause in hens (Rolon et al., 1993), was compared with feed removal as to their relative effects on *S.* Enteritidis infection. Although the *S.* Enteritidis shed rate did not differ between molt groups, birds on the molt diet shed less *S.* Enteritidis, were less susceptible to an infection by this pathogen, and exhibited less intestinal inflammation, compared with fasted birds (Holt et al., 1994). *Salmonella* Enteritidis problems were less pronounced in birds on the molt diet, indicating that such diets may allow producers to recycle their aging hens without the radical exacerbation of an *S.* Enteritidis problem observed during feed removal. Other molt diets (Breeding et al., 1992) may improve the situation further and should be investigated. The use of probiotics currently enjoys widespread popularity within the broiler industry as a method for reducing intestinal colonization of chicks with paratyphoid salmonellae (Blankenship et al., 1993; Corrier et al., 1994). Experimental data documented the efficacy of competitive exclusion as an intervention scheme for broiler and layer chicks, which prompted experiments to test the utility of competitive exclusion as a similar intervention strategy against *S.* Enteritidis in hens during a molt. Studies to date have not demonstrated any protection in molting hens receiving competitive exclusion cultures. However, the administration of lactose in the drinking water during the molt did reduce the cecal carriage and extraintestinal dissemination of an *S.* Enteritidis challenge (Corrier et al., 1997), indicating that some intervention schemes can modify the observed exacerbation of *S.* Enteritidis infection during a molt.

The information provided in this review reflects data from experimental procedures, and caution should be exercised before extrapolating the results derived from the laboratory to on-farm experience. Actual results from the field ultimately will tell the story, and some studies do provide insight into possible effects of molting on commercial flocks. Swayne et al. (1992) observed that intestinal spirochete infections were more severe in molted hens, indicating that, similar to what was observed for *S.* Enteritidis, molting upset the equilibrium normally attained between the host and that parasite. Perhaps more telling is the study conducted by the *S.* Enteritidis Pilot Project in Pennsylvania (U.S. Department of Agriculture, 1995), which showed that the production of eggs contaminated with *S.* Enteritidis increased during molt. These data prompted the authors to categorize molting as a risk factor for *S.* Enteritidis. This information and possibly some of the previ-

ously described experimental data resulted in the implementation of flock monitoring for *S.* Enteritidis problems during the molt as a part of an egg-quality-assurance program (Pennsylvania Poultry Federation, 1994). It remains to be ascertained just what role, if any, molting plays in the current epidemic of eggborne outbreaks of human *S.* Enteritidis infections occurring in this country, and this can only be determined through in-depth surveillance.

REFERENCES

Adam, E. 1982. Herpes simplex virus infections. In: Glaser, R., and Gotlieb-Stematsky, T., eds. Human herpesvirus infections. New York: Marcel Dekker, pp. 1–55.

Anonymous. 1993. Who wants our spent fowl? Poult. Digest 52(12):62.

Arnold, J.W., and Holt, P.S. 1996. Cytotoxicity in chicken alimentary secretions as measured by a derivative of the tumor necrosis factor assay. Poult. Sci. 75:329–334.

Arnold, J.W., Niesel, D.W., Annable, C.R., Hess, C.B., Asuncion, M., Cho, Y.J., Peterson, J.W., and Klimpel, G.R. 1993. Tumor necrosis factor-alpha mediates the early pathology in *Salmonella* infection of the gastrointestinal tract. Microb. Pathog. 14:217–227.

Bailey, J.S., Cox, N.A., and Berrang, M.E. 1994. Hatchery-acquired salmonellae in broiler chicks. Poult. Sci. 73:1153–1157.

Baker, M., Brake, J., and McDaniel, G.R. 1983. The relationship between body weight loss during an induced molt and postmolt egg production, egg weight, and shell quality in caged layers. Poult. Sci. 62:409–413.

Bell, D. 1987. Is molting still a viable replacement alternative? Poult. Trib. 93:32–35.

Ben-Nathan, B., Heller, E.D., and Perek, M. 1977. The effect of starvation on antibody production of chicks. Poult. Sci. 56:1468–1471.

Ben-Nathan, B., Drabkin, N., and Heller, D. 1981. The effect of starvation on the immune response of chickens. Avian Dis. 25:214–217.

Berry, W.D., and Brake, J. 1987. Postmolt performance of laying hens molted by high dietary zinc, low dietary sodium, and fasting: egg production and eggshell quality. Poult. Sci. 66:218–226.

Bhatia, T.R.S., and McNabb, G.D. 1980. Dissemination of *Salmonella* in broiler chicken operations. Avian Dis. 24:616–624.

Blankenship, L.E., Bailey, J.S., Cox, N.A., Stern, N.J., Brewer, R., and Williams, O. 1993. Two-step mucosal competitive exclusion flora treatment to diminish salmonellae in commercial broiler chickens. Poult. Sci. 72:1667–1672.

Brake, J. 1993. Recent advances in induced molting. Poult. Sci. 72:929–931.

Brake, J. 1994. Feed removal remains predominant method of molt induction. Poult. Times 42:6 and 9.

Brake, J., and Thaxton, P. 1979a. Physiological changes in caged layers during a forced molt. 1. Body temperature and selected blood constituents. Poult. Sci. 58:699–706.

Brake, J., and Thaxton, P. 1979b. Physiological changes in caged layers during a forced molt. 2. Gross changes in organs. Poult. Sci. 58:707–716.

Brake, J., Thaxton, P., and Benton, E.H. 1979. Physiological changes in caged layers during a forced molt. 3. Plasma thyroxine, plasma triiodothyronine, adrenal cholesterol, and total adrenal steroids. Poult. Sci. 58:1345–1350.

Brake, J., Morgan, G.W., and Thaxton, P. 1981. Recrudescence of the thymus and repopulation of lymphocytes during an artificially induced molt in the domestic chicken: proposed model system. Dev. Comp. Immunol. 5:105–112.

Brake, J., Baker, M., Morgan, G.W., and Thaxton, P. 1982. Physiological changes in caged layers during a forced molt. 4. Leucocytes and packed cell volume. Poult. Sci. 61:790–795.

Breeding, S.W., Brake, J., Garlich, J.D., and Johnson, A.L. 1992. Molt induced by dietary zinc in a low-calcium diet. Poult. Sci. 71:168–180.

Cason, J.A., Bailey, J.S., and Cox, N.A. 1994. Transmission of *Salmonella typhimurium* during hatching of broiler chicks. Avian Dis. 38:583–588.

Centers for Disease Control. 1990. Update: *Salmonella enteritidis* infections and shell eggs—United States, 1990. MMWR 39:909–912.

Centers for Disease Control. 1992. Outbreak of *Salmonella enteritidis* infection associated with consumption of raw shell eggs, 1991. MMWR 41:369–372.

Centers for Disease Control. 1996. Outbreaks of *Salmonella* serotype Enteritidis infection associated with consumption of raw shell eggs—United States, 1994–1995. MMWR 45:737–742.

Chandra, R.K. 1974. Rosette-forming T lymphocytes and cell-mediated immunity in malnutrition. BMJ 3:608–609.

Chandra, R.K. 1990. Cellular and molecular basis of nutrition-immunity interactions. Adv. Exp. Med. Biol. 282:13–18.

Collins, F.M. 1974. Vaccines and cell-mediated immunity. Bacteriol. Rev. 38:371–402.

Corrier, D.E., Hollister, A.G., Nisbet, D.J., Scanlan, C.M., Beier, R.C., and DeLoach, J.R. 1994. Effect of dietary lactose on cecal pH, bacteriostatic volatile fatty acids, and *Salmonella typhimurium* colonization of broiler chicks. Avian Dis. 34:617–625.

Corrier, D.E., Nisbet, D.J., Hargis, B.M., Holt, P.S., and DeLoach, J.R. 1997. Provision of lactose to molting hens enhances resistance to *Salmonella enteritidis* colonization. J. Food Prot. 60:10–15.

Cox, N.A., Bailey, J.S., Thomson, J.E., and Juven, B.J. 1983. *Salmonella* and other Enterobacteriaceae found in commercial poultry feed. Poult. Sci. 62:2169–2175.

Cox, N.A., Bailey, J.S., Mauldin, J.M., and Blankenship, L.C. 1990. Presence and impact of *Salmonella* contamination in commercial broiler hatcheries. Poult. Sci. 69:1606–1609.

Cunningham, D.L. 1995. The poultry industry in the United States and Georgia: a situation and outlook statement. Athens: University of Georgia Poultry Extension Service, pp. 7–12.

Cunningham, F.E., Cotterill, O.J., and Funk, E.M. 1960. The effect of season and age of birds. 1. On egg size, quality, and yield. Poult. Sci. 39:289–299.

DePasquale-Jardieu, P., and Fraker, P.J. 1979. The role of corticosterone in the loss in immune function in the zinc-deficient A/J mouse. J. Nutr. 109:1847–1855.

Dorian, B., Garfinkel, P., Brown, G., Shore, A., Gladman, D., and Keystone, E. 1982. Aberrations in lymphocyte subpopulations and function during psychological stress. Clin. Exp. Immunol. 50:132–138.

Ebel, E.D., David, M.J., and Mason, J. 1992. Occurrence of *Salmonella enteritidis* in the U.S. commercial egg industry: report on a national spent hen survey. Avian Dis. 36:646–654.

Etches, R.J. 1990. The ovulatory cycle of the hen. Crit. Rev. Poult. Biol. 2:293–318.

Etches, R.J., Williams, J.B., and Rzasa, J. 1984. Effects of corticosterone and dietary changes in the hen on ovarian function, plasma LH and steroids and the response to exogenous LH-RH. J. Reprod. Fertil. 70:121–130.

Fanelli, M.J., Sadler, W.W., Franti, C.E., and Brownell, J.R. 1971. Localization of salmonellae within the intestinal tract of chickens. Avian Dis. 15:366–375.

Formal, S.B., Dammin, G.J., LeBrec, E.H., and Schneider, H. 1958. Experimental *Shigella* infections: characteristics of a fatal infection produced in guinea pigs. J. Bacteriol. 75:604–610.

Freter, R. 1955. The fatal enteric cholera infection of the guinea pig, achieved by inhibition of normal enteric flora. J. Infect. Dis. 97:57–65.

Gaskell, R.M., and Povey, R.C. 1977. Experimental induction of feline viral rhinotracheitis re-excretion in FVR-recovered cats. Vet. Rec. 100:128–133.

Gast, R.K. 1994. Understanding *Salmonella enteritidis* in laying chickens: the contributions of experimental infections. Int. J. Food Microbiol. 21:107–116.

Gast, R.K., and Beard, C.W. 1993. Research to understand and control *Salmonella enteritidis* in chickens and eggs. Poult. Sci. 72:1157–1163.

Giessen, A.W. van de, Ament, A.J.H.A., and Notermans, S.H.W. 1994. Intervention strategies for *Salmonella enteritidis* in poultry flocks: a basic approach. Int. J. Food Microbiol. 21:145–154.

Glaser, R., Kiecolt-Glaser, J.K., Speicher, C.E., and Holliday, J.E. 1985a. Stress, loneliness, and changes in herpesvirus latency. J. Behav. Med. 8:249–260.

Glaser, R., Kiecolt-Glaser, J.K., Stout, J.C., Tarr, K.L., Speicher, C.E., and Holliday, J.E. 1985b. Stress-related impairments in cellular immunity. Psychiatr. Res. 16:233–239.

Gross, R.L., and Newberne, P.M. 1980. Role of nutrition in immunologic function. Physiol. Rev. 60:188–206.

Henzler, D.J., and Opitz, H.M. 1992. The role of mice in the epizootiology of *Salmonella enteritidis* infection on chicken layer farms. Avian Dis. 36:625–631.

Holt, P.S. 1992a. Effect of induced molting on B cell and CT4 and CT8 T cell numbers in spleens and peripheral blood of white leghorn hens. Poult. Sci. 71:2027–2034.

Holt, P.S. 1992b. Effects of induced moulting on immune responses of hens. Br. Poult. Sci. 33:165–175.

Holt, P.S. 1993. Effect of induced molting on the susceptibility of white leghorn hens to a *Salmonella enteritidis* infection. Avian Dis. 37:412–417.

Holt, P.S. 1995. Horizontal transmission of *Salmonella enteritidis* in molted and unmolted laying chickens. Avian Dis. 39:239–249.

Holt, P.S., and Porter, R.E., Jr. 1992a. Effect of induced molting on the course of infection and transmission of *Salmonella enteritidis* in white leghorn hens of different ages. Poult. Sci. 71:1842–1848.

Holt, P.S., and Porter, R.E., Jr. 1992b. Microbiological and histopathological effects of an induced molt fasting procedure on a *Salmonella enteritidis* infection in chickens. Avian Dis. 36:610–618.

Holt, P.S., and Porter, R.E., Jr. 1993. Effect of induced molting on the recurrence of a previous *Salmonella enteritidis* infection. Poult. Sci. 72:2069–2078.

Holt, P.S., Buhr, R.J., Cunningham, D.L., and Porter, R.E., Jr. 1994. Effect of two different molting procedures on a *Salmonella enteritidis* infection. Poult. Sci. 73:1267–1275.

Holt, P.S., Macri, N.P., and Porter, R.E., Jr. 1995. Microbiological analysis of the early *Salmonella enteritidis* infection in molted and unmolted hens. Avian Dis. 39:55–63.

Holt, P.S., Mitchell, B.W., and Gast, R.K. 1998. Airborne horizontal transmission of *Salmonella enteritidis* in molted laying chickens. Avian Dis. 42:45–52.

Hughes, C.S., Gaskell, R.M., Jones, R.C., Bradbury, J.M., and Jordan, F.T.W. 1989. Effects of certain stress factors on the re-excretion of infectious laryngotracheitis virus from latently infected carrier birds. Res. Vet. Sci. 46:274–276.

Kagi, D., Ledermann, B., Burki, J., Zinkernagel, R.M., and Hengartner, H. 1996. Molecular mechanisms of lymphocyte-mediated cytotoxicity and their role in immunological protection and pathogenesis in vivo. Annu. Rev. Immunol. 14:207–232.

Kaufmann, S.H.E. 1993. Immunity to intracellular bacteria. Annu. Rev. Immunol. 11:129–163.

Kiecolt-Glaser, J.K., and Glaser, R. 1988. Psychological influences on immunity: making sense of the relationship between stressful life events and health. In: Chrousos, G.P., Louriaux, D.L., and Gold, P.W., eds. Mechanisms of physical and emotional stress. New York: Plenum, pp. 237–247.

Killar, L., and Eisenstein, T.K. 1983. Strain dependent variation of delayed-type hypersensitivity in *Salmonella typhimurium* infected mice. Adv. Exp. Med. Biol. 162:297–302.

Kopanic, R.J., Jr., Sheldon, B.W., and Wright, C.G. 1994. Cockroaches as vectors of *Salmonella*: laboratory and field trials. J. Food Prot. 57:125–132.

Lahellec, C., and Colin, P. 1985. Relationship between serotypes of salmonellae from hatcheries and rearing farms and those from processed poultry carcasses. Br. Poult. Sci. 26:179–186.

Lee, K. 1982. Effects of forced molt period on postmolt performance of leghorn hens. Poult. Sci. 61:1594–1598.

Lillehoj, H.S. 1987. Effects of immunosuppression on avian coccidiosis: cyclosporin A but not hormonal bursectomy abrogates host protective immunity. Infect. Immun. 55:1616–1621.

Looper, K. 1996. Egg marketing in the United States. Egg Ind. 101:10–15.

Macri, N.P., Porter, R.E., Jr., and Holt, P.S. 1997. The effects of induced molting on the severity of acute intestinal infection caused by *Salmonella enteritidis*. Avian Dis. 41:117–124.

Miller, C.P., and Bohnhoff, M. 1962. A study of experimental *Salmonella* infection in the mouse. J. Infect. Dis. 111:107–116.

Nakamura, M., Nagamine, N., Suzuki, T., Norimatsu, M., Oishi, K., Kijima, M., Tamura, Y., and Sato, S. 1993. Long term shedding of *Salmonella* Enteritidis in chickens which received a contact exposure within 24 hrs of hatching. J. Vet. Med. Sci. 55:649–653.

Nakamura, M., Nagamine, N., Takahashi, T., Suzuki, S., Kijima, M., Tamura, Y., and Sato, S. 1994a. Horizontal transmission of *Salmonella enteritidis* and effect of stress on shedding in laying hens. Avian Dis. 38:282–288.

Nakamura, M., Nagamine, N., Takahashi, T., Suzuki, S., and Sato, S. 1994b. Evaluation of the efficacy of a bacterin against *Salmonella enteritidis* infection and the effect of stress after vaccination. Avian Dis. 38:717–724.

Noles, R.K. 1966. Subsequent production and egg quality of forced molted hens. Poult. Sci. 45:50–57.

North, M.O., and Bell, D.D. 1990. Commercial chicken production manual, 4th ed. New York: Van Nostrand Reinhold, pp. 433–452.

Pennsylvania Poultry Federation (PPF). 1994. Pennsylvania egg quality assurance program. Harrisburg: PPF.

Porter, R.E., Jr., and Holt, P.S. 1993. Effect of induced molting on the severity of intestinal lesions caused by *Salmonella enteritidis* in chickens. Avian Dis. 37:1009–1016.

Rigby, C.E., and Petit, J.R. 1980. Changes in the *Salmonella* status of broiler chickens subjected to simulated shipping conditions. Can. J. Comp. Med. 44:374–381.

Rolon, A., Buhr, R.J., and Cunningham, D.L. 1993. Twenty-four-hour feed withdrawal and limited feeding as alternative methods for induction of molt in laying hens. Poult. Sci. 72:776–785.

Sekimoto, K., Imai, K., Suzuki, M., and Takikawa, H. 1987. Thyroxine-induced molting and gonadal function of laying hens. Poult. Sci. 66:752–756.

Sher, A., and Coffman, R.L. 1992. Regulation of immunity to parasites by T cells and T cell-derived cytokines. Annu. Rev. Immunol. 10:385–409.

Smyser, C.F., Adinarayanan, N., van Roekel, H., and Snoeyenbos, G.H. 1966. Field and laboratory observations on *Salmonella heidelberg* infections in three chicken breeding flocks. Avian Dis. 10:314–329.

Soave, O.A. 1964. Reactivation of rabies virus in a guinea pig due to the stress of crowding. Am. J. Vet. Res. 25:268–269.

St. Louis, M.E., Morse, D.L., Potter, M.E., DeMelfi, T.M., Guzewich, J.J., Tauxe, R.V., and Blake, P.A. 1988. The emergence of grade A eggs as a major source of *Salmonella enteritidis* infections: new implication for the control of salmonellosis. JAMA 259:2103–2107.

Swayne, D.E., Bermudez, A.J., Sagartz, J.E., Eaton, K.A., Monfort, J.D., Stoutenburg, J.W., and Hayes, J.R. 1992. Association of cecal spirochetes with pasty vents and dirty eggshells in layers. Avian Dis. 36:776–781.

Turnbull, P.C.B., and Snoeyenbos, G.H. 1974. Experimental salmonellosis in the chicken. 1. Fate and host response in alimentary canal, liver, and spleen. Avian Dis. 18:153–177.

U.S. Department of Agriculture. 1995. Effect of molting on the prevalence of SE in layer flocks: *Salmonella enteritidis* Pilot Project progress report. Hyattsville, MD: USDA/APHIS, pp. 66–68.

Whitehead, C.C., and Shannon, D.W.F. 1974. The control of egg production using a low-sodium diet. Br. Poult. Sci. 15:429–434.

Williams, J.B., Etches, R.J., and Rzasa, J. 1985. Induction of a pause in laying by corticosterone infusion or by dietary alterations: effects on the reproductive system, food consumption, and body weight. Br. Poult. Sci. 26:25–34.

Zecha, B.C., McCapes, R.H., Dungan, W.M., Holte, R.J., Worcester, W.W., and Williams, J.E. 1977. The Dillon Beach Project: a five year epidemiological study of naturally occurring *Salmonella* infection in turkeys and their environment. Avian Dis. 21:141–159.

Zimmerman, N.G., Andrews, D.K., and McGinnis, J. 1987. Comparison of several induced molting methods on subsequent performance of single comb white leghorn hens. Poult. Sci. 66:408–417.

34

Transmission of *Salmonella enterica* Serovar Enteritidis and Effect of Stress on Shedding in Laying Hens

M. Nakamura

INTRODUCTION

A recent increase in the incidence of *Salmonella enterica* serovar Enteritidis (*S.* Enteritidis) in poultry flocks has been observed in the United States, the United Kingdom, and other countries. Infection with *S.* Enteritidis has been ascribed to transovarian transmission (Gast and Beard, 1990a; Shivaprasad et al., 1990; Nakamura et al., 1993), as well as to oral transmission. Horizontal transmission under normal conditions (Gast and Beard, 1990b) and fasting conditions (Holt and Porter, 1992) has also been reported. Heat and cold stress, short-term withdrawal of feed and water, and induced molting have been reported to be associated with an increase in salmonella isolation from flocks (Jones, 1992; Holt, 1993; Nakamura et al., 1995, 1997).

This chapter analyzes the horizontal transmission of *S.* Enteritidis, including airborne transmission, as well as the effect that short-term stress, which may occur in daily handling, may have on the shedding of *S.* Enteritidis by laying hens.

TRANSMISSION OF *SALMONELLA* ENTERITIDIS IN LAYING HENS

According to Nagaraja et al. (1991), transmission of salmonellae in chickens was thought to be possible through

the following: direct ovarian transmission, eggshell contamination, incubator, hatchery, brooder and environment, poultry feed, other animal sources and humans, and direct spread among adult and young chickens. Among these, direct ovarian transmission, eggshell contamination, and direct spread among adult and young chickens are most important in *S.* Enteritidis transmission among laying hens.

Direct Ovarian Transmission

This has been reviewed by Humphrey (1994). Although cells of *S.* Enteritidis present on eggshells might contaminate egg contents by migration through the shell and associated membrane, it would appear that contamination of the contents of intact eggs is more the result of infection of reproductive tissues. Investigation with naturally contaminated eggs (Mawer et al., 1989; Humphrey et al., 1989b, 1991b) found no association between shell and content contamination. Studies with artificially infected birds have also shown no relationship between the presence of salmonellae on eggshells and the contamination of egg contents (Gast and Beard, 1990a; Humphrey et al., 1991a). During experimental infections of laying hens with *S.* Enteritidis, organisms were isolated from the ovaries and from egg yolk (Shivaprasad et al., 1990; Barrow and Lovell, 1991). The possibility of contamination of yolk in vivo either through a hematogenous spread or colonization of peritoneum by the organism has been reported (Timoney et al.,

1989; Shivaprasad et al., 1990). Thiagarajan et al. (1994) reported that *S.* Enteritidis could be isolated from the membranes of the preovulatory follicles during the first few weeks of infection after oral inoculation of layer birds. They isolated *S.* Enteritidis from the follicular membrane but not from the yolk in 10 of 16 infected birds. Based on this, they suggested that the organism interacts with a cellular component of these follicles. Gast and Beard (1990a,b, 1992) reported that *S.* Enteritidis could be isolated from egg-yolk membranes but not from the yolk of eggs laid by experimentally infected hens. It is conceivable that during transovarian transmission, *S.* Enteritidis remains attached to the egg-yolk membranes and could most frequently be isolated from this part of the egg (Thiagarajan et al., 1994). Thiagarajan et al. (1994) suggested that contamination of the laid egg can occur after the ovulation process and pointed out that the possibility of bacteria reaching the egg through the oviduct cannot be ruled out. Their results suggested that *S.* Enteritidis can colonize the preovulatory follicles by interacting with the ovarian granulosa cells and that adhesive proteins may be involved in this process (Thiagarajan et al., 1996).

The observed prevalence of eggs with salmonella-positive contents can be variable. The prevalence of *S.* Enteritidis in eggs originating from naturally infected laying hens, summarized by Humphrey (1994), was 0.1%–1.0%. However, he pointed out the impact of different laboratory techniques used for the isolation of *S.* Enteritidis. The *Salmonella* Enteritidis Pilot Project (Anon., 1995), which began in April 1992, carried out large-scale surveys. Among 738,000 nest-run eggs, 191 were positive for *S.* Enteritidis. The rate of *S.* Enteritidis–positive eggs was found to be 0.0275%, or 2.75 eggs per 10,000 eggs laid by hens in environmentally positive houses. On the other hand, it is also becoming clear that eggs with salmonella-positive contents can be clustered. This was first observed during outbreak investigation (Humphrey et al., 1989b) and again during studies with naturally infected hens caged individually (Humphrey et al., 1989a). The authors also reported that some stimulus might be causing different hens to lay contaminated eggs at or around the same time. It would seem that, when fresh, contaminated eggs contain only low numbers of *S.* Enteritidis. In a study using naturally contaminated, intact eggs with shells free of fecal contamination, all content-positive eggs examined within 3 weeks of lay contained fewer than 20 cells of *S.* Enteritidis (Humphrey, 1994).

Eggshell Contamination

According to Humphrey (1994), eggshells can become contaminated with salmonellae either as a result of infection of the oviduct or by fecal contamination, and the latter route would seem to be more important with salmonellae other than *S.* Enteritidis. Gast and Beard (1990a) reported that there was a correlation between feces positivity in hens artificially infected with *S.* Enteritidis phage type 13a (PT13a) and eggshell contamination. Humphrey et al. (1991a) found that eggshells were salmonella positive in

the absence of fecal carriage and pointed out that infection of reproductive tissues may be more important with *S.* Enteritidis PT4. Infected birds laid eggs with contaminated shells over 6 weeks after intestinal carriage had ceased. Eggs with contaminated shells were also laid by five birds whose feces were salmonella negative throughout the course of the study. From these results, Humphrey (1994) pointed out the possibility that the shell gland or another part of the oviduct may be a site of infection.

Direct Spread Among Adult and Young Chickens

Contamination of eggshell and egg contents with *S.* Enteritidis would seem to be important as a potential source of human infection. However, direct spread among chickens may be more important in the poultry farms. The oral route of infection may be important in commercial flocks, and experimental investigations have concentrated on infecting birds orally and studying the effects of such factors as organism dose and bird age on the period of bacteria excretion and their distribution in tissues (Humphrey et al., 1989b, 1991a; Timoney et al., 1989; Gast and Beard, 1990b). Baskerville et al. (1992) pointed out, however, that infection may be readily spread by airborne droplets or by dust particles carrying *S.* Enteritidis and that information on the effects of airborne infection with *S.* Enteritidis on laying hens was not available, although Clemmer et al. (1960) had studied experimental airborne salmonellosis in chicks. Therefore, Baskerville et al. investigated the potential of airborne *S.* Enteritidis PT4 to infect laying hens and demonstrated that the exposure of hens to aerosols of *S.* Enteritidis produced a generalized infection and prolonged fecal excretion, even after a low dose. *Salmonella* Enteritidis was present for a similar period in a wide range of alimentary-tract tissues and in the ovary and oviduct. Detailed information on the effects of airborne infection, however, was lacking, because they used only nine hens.

Therefore, the authors (Nakamura et al., 1995) attempted to obtain more information about the distribution of *S.* Enteritidis, which belongs to the same phage type (PT4), in chickens after intratracheal inoculation. Seven-week-old specific pathogen-free (SPF) chickens were inoculated intratracheally with 10^2, 10^5, or 10^8 cells and orally with 10^5 cells. *Salmonella* Enteritidis caused bacteremia within 6 h after intratracheal inoculation, and the organism was isolated from upper-respiratory tissues. At 1 day after inoculation, *S.* Enteritidis was isolated from the upper-respiratory organs, as well as from the liver and spleen. Afterward, almost all organs were positive for the isolation of *S.* Enteritidis. At 14 days after inoculation, the organism was still present in tissues of birds inoculated with 10^8 cells. *Salmonella* Enteritidis was isolated mainly from tissues of the peritoneal cavity, including the reproductive organs, in chickens inoculated with 10^8 cells. The organism was also isolated immediately after challenge from the duodenum and cecum, and was then continuously isolated from the duodenum until 7 days after inoculation and from the cecum until the end of the experiment

(48 days after inoculation). The distribution of *S.* Enteritidis in the alimentary tract was similar to that in orally infected chickens.

It may be most important to understand the pathogenicity of infection with *S.* Enteritidis in chickens. Numerous studies that have been conducted in an attempt to understand the mechanism of transmission of *S.* Enteritidis have provided a substantially better understanding of the *S.* Enteritidis problem in chickens (Holt and Peter, 1992; Holt, 1993). Many questions remain to be answered, however, including those related to horizontal transmission. Holt (1995) reported experiments to determine how readily *S.* Enteritidis can be transmitted from one hen to a group of uninfected hens, which is important for understanding the mechanism of horizontal transmission. He focused on the effect of molting on horizontal transmission and discussed several possible mechanisms of transmission, as described later in this chapter. Recently, the authors (Nakamura et al., 1997) focused on transmission of *S.* Enteritidis with airborne infection among chickens.

Horizontal transmission of *S.* Enteritidis and the effect of airflow on spread were examined in 80 five-week-old chickens divided into five groups (Nakamura et al., 1997); 16 chickens in each group were placed in four wire-floored cages in a row separated by wire, as illustrated in Figure 34.1. The water and feed systems were not shared between cages. In experiment 1, three groups (A–C) of 16 chickens were used. Groups A and B had feed and water withdrawn for 2 days before inoculation and on days 27 and 28 after inoculation. One of four chickens placed in a cage at the downwind end of the row, as illustrated in Figure 34.2, was inoculated orally with 10^9 cells of *S.* Enteritidis HY-1 Rif (Nakamura et al., 1994a).

As shown in Figure 34.3, in group-A chickens on day 1, *S.* Enteritidis was being shed by four hens in the cage where the originally inoculated chicken was placed (hereafter this cage is referred to as the original cage in each group), demonstrating that horizontal transmission occurred rapidly within this cage. However, drinking water and feed were not contaminated. *Salmonella* Enteritidis was not being shed by chickens in the cages adjacent and two and three cages away from the original cage, demonstrating that *S.* Enteritidis did not spread to chickens in other cages. On the other hand, in group-B chickens on day 1, not only

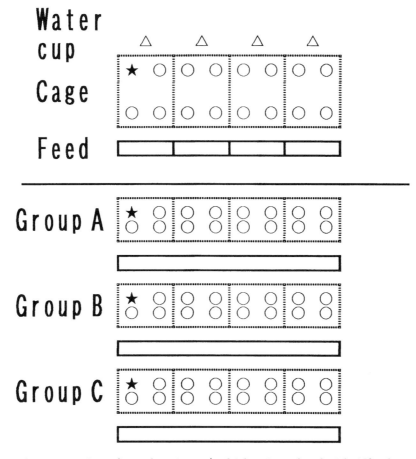

FIGURE 34.1   Schematic presentation of cage locations: ★, chicken inoculated with 10^9 colony-forming units (CFU) of *Salmonella* Enteritidis; ○, uninfected chicken. From Nakamura et al. (1997).

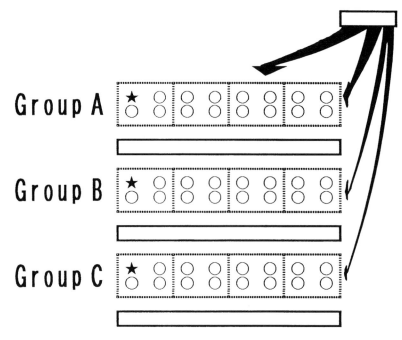

FIGURE 34.2   The airflow by ventilation. From Nakamura et al. (1997).

chickens in the original cage but also three chickens in an adjacent cage and two cages away from the original cage shed *S.* Enteritidis, demonstrating that horizontal transmission rapidly occurred between the chickens in this row by day 1. This horizontal transmission did not occur through feed and water, because *S.* Enteritidis was never detected in the feed and water. In group-C chickens on day 1, two chickens that cohabited with the originally inoculated chicken, and one chicken in the adjacent cage, shed *S.* Enteritidis without contamination of feed and water.

On day 2, horizontal transmission in group-A chickens was still limited to chickens within the original cage, although the feed in the adjacent cage was contaminated with *S.* Enteritidis. In group B, however, *S.* Enteritidis was being shed by all chickens in the adjacent cage and two cages away from the original cage and by one chicken three cages away from the original cage, demonstrating rapid horizontal transmission of *S.* Enteritidis in this row. In group-C chickens, transmission occurred in one chicken three cages away from the original cage, and the feed in all cages was contaminated with *S.* Enteritidis.

After day 3, in group A, most of the chickens that shed *S.* Enteritidis were limited to those within the original cage throughout the experiment (Figs. 34.3, 34.4). In group B, however, not only chickens in the original cage but also chickens in the other three cages shed *S.* Enteritidis and, on days 6 and 7, almost all chickens raised in the four cages in this row shed *S.* Enteritidis. In group C, more than half of the cecal droppings were positive from chickens in the other three cages. These findings show that shedding patterns of *S.* Enteritidis were different between groups A and B. We hypothesized that the difference between these two groups might be a result of the direction of airflow

(Fig. 34.2). The airflow was greater in group A. On the other hand, the airflow in group B was markedly less.

Therefore, experiment 2 was conducted under the same conditions as experiment 1, except that the originally infected chicken was placed in the cage at the upstream side of the airflow in the same row in order to change the airflow direction. Feed and water were withdrawn for 2 days prior to infection, the same as in experiment 1, for 1 day after day 13 of inoculation, and for 2 days after day 21 of inoculation. As shown in Figure 34.5, almost the same shedding pattern as in the group-B chickens of experiment 1 was observed in group D of experiment 2, at least until 12 days after inoculation, suggesting that the direction of the airflow played an important role in the horizontal transmission of *S.* Enteritidis among the chickens. However, rapid transmission occurred also in group-E chickens, where the airflow was much more gentle than in group D.

The effect of contaminated feed and water on the horizontal transmission of *S.* Enteritidis was also examined. Contamination of feed and water did not precede the appearance of cecal droppings positive for *S.* Enteritidis in most cases (Figs. 34.3, 34.4). Moreover, from days 33 to 36 in group B and from days 9 to 15 in group C, *S.* Enteritidis was not isolated from feed and water, although cecal droppings were positive for *S.* Enteritidis during these periods.

Holt (1995) described three possible mechanisms in horizontal transmission: contaminated water supplies, contaminated feathers, and aerosols containing *S.* Enteritidis. First, water can be contaminated with *S.* Enteritidis. Lahellec et al. (1985) reported that drinkers had the highest incidence of salmonella contamination in broiler flocks. In our previous report, contaminated water played an important role in the horizontal transmission of *S.* Enteritidis when contaminated

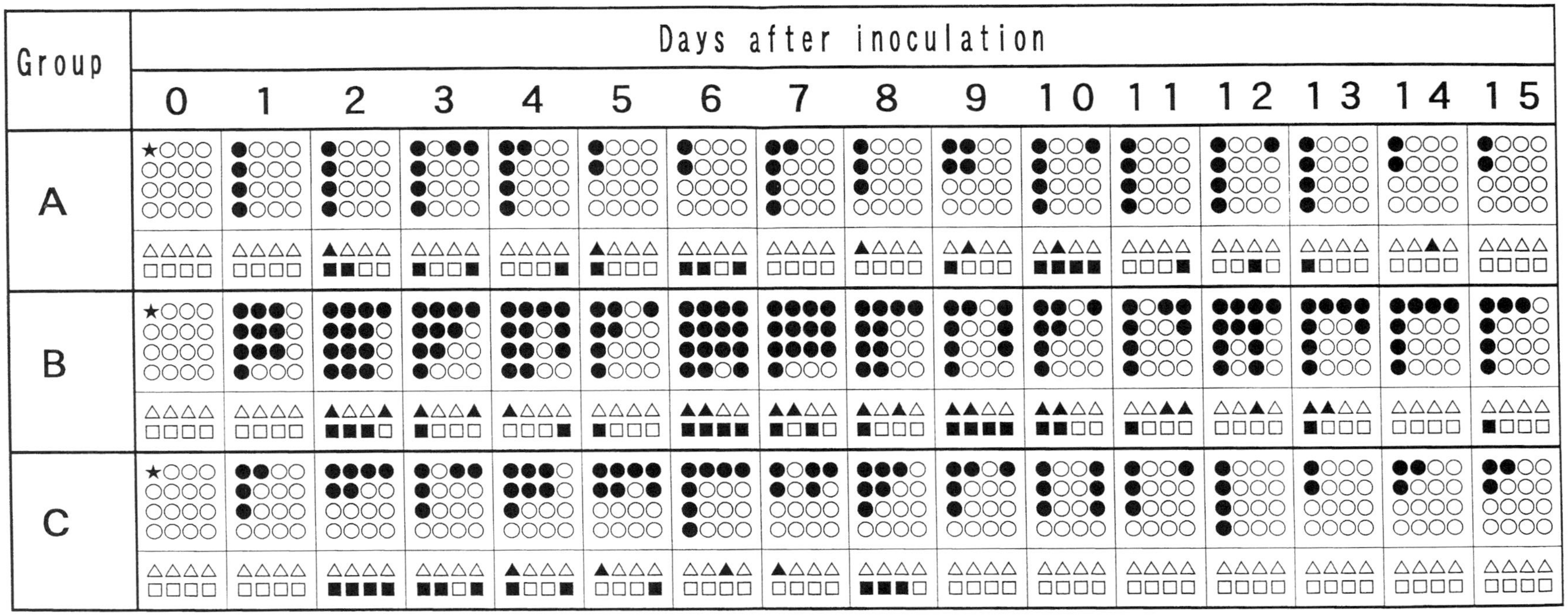

FIGURE 34.3 The horizontal transmission of *Salmonella* Enteritidis in chickens in experiment 1: ★, 10^9 CFU-inoculated chicken; ●, positive cecal dropping; ○, negative cecal dropping; ▲, positive water; △, negative water; ■, positive feed; □, negative feed; groups A and B, withdrawal of food and water for 2 days before inoculation. From Nakamura et al. (1997).

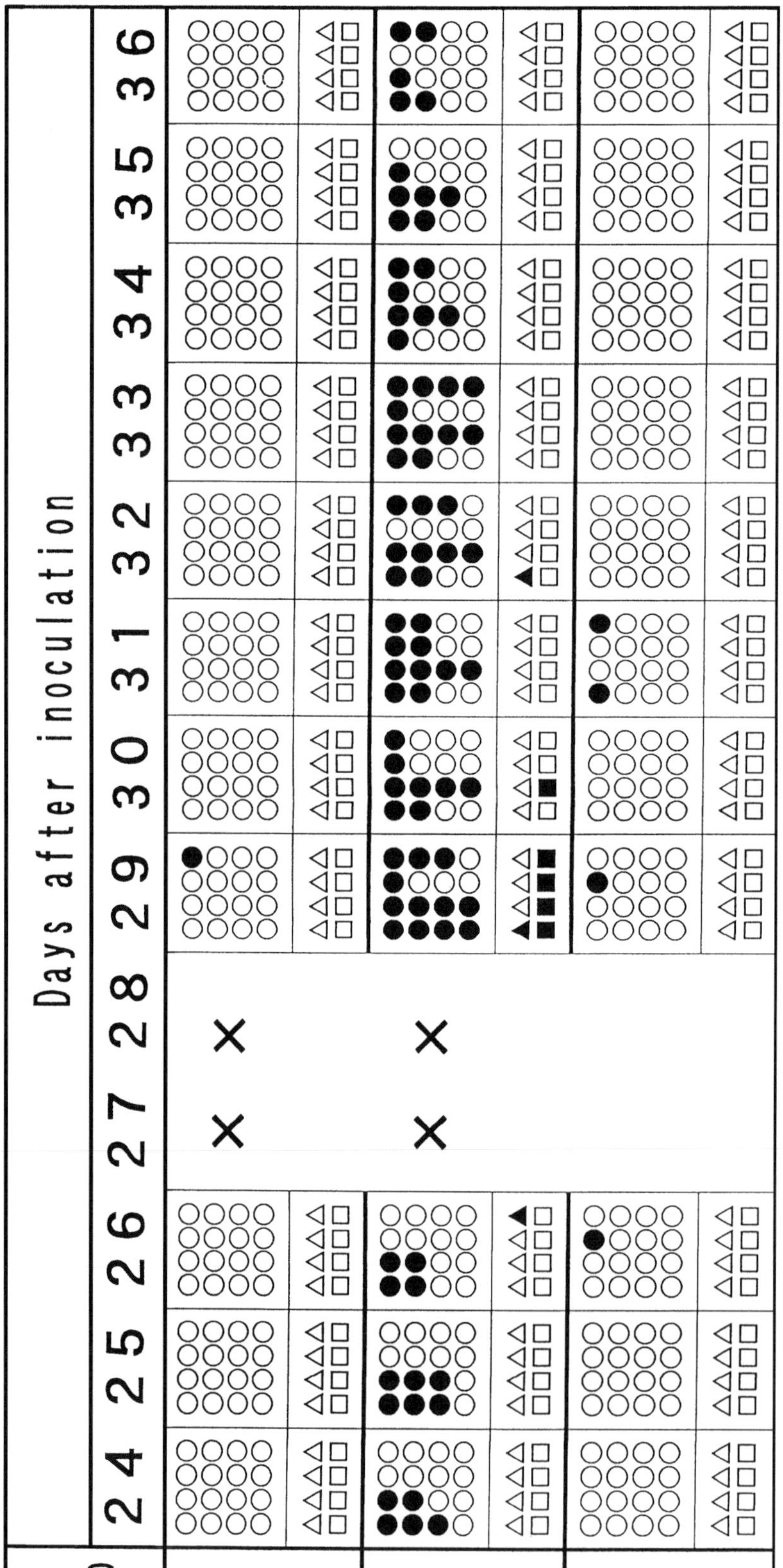

FIGURE 34.4 The effect of withdrawal of food and water on shedding of *Salmonella* Enteritidis by chickens: ★, 10^9 CFU-inoculated chicken; ●, positive cecal dropping; ○, negative cecal dropping; ▲, positive water; △, negative water; ■, positive feed; □, negative feed; groups A and B, withdrawal of food and water for 2 days before inoculation. From Nakamura et al. (1997).

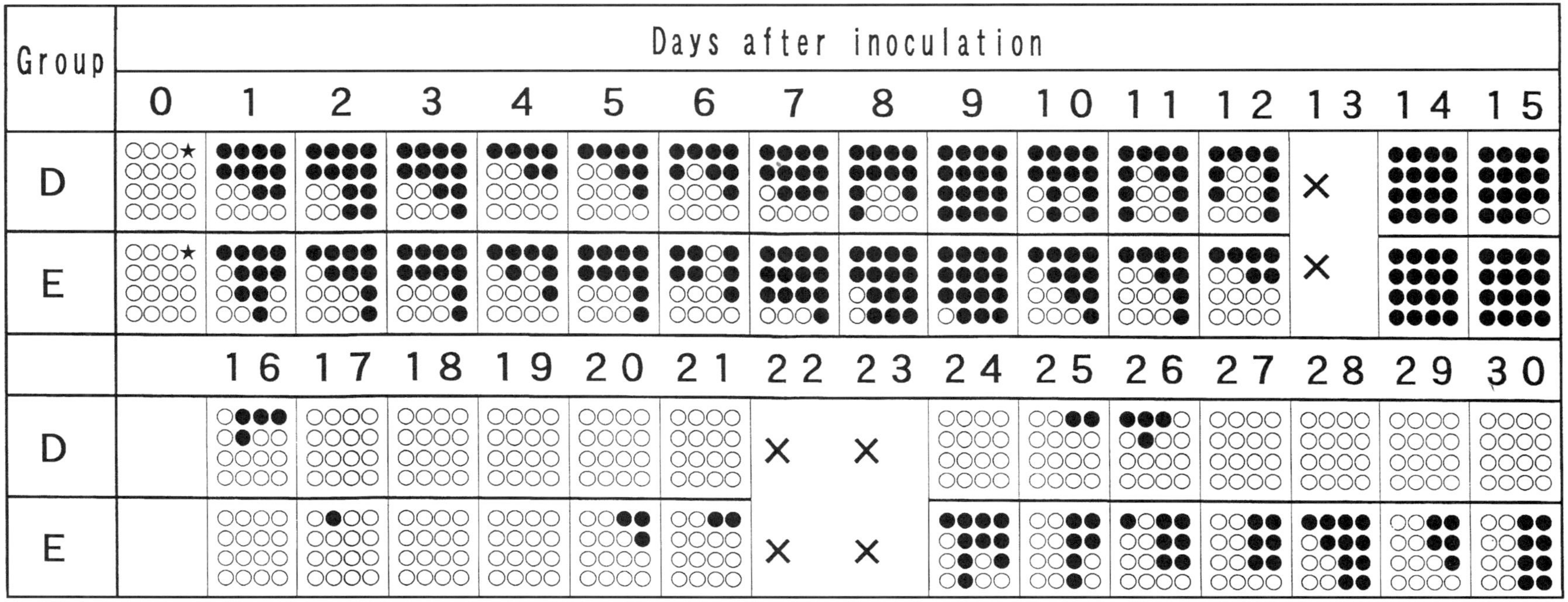

FIGURE 34.5 The horizontal transmission of *Salmonella* Enteritidis in chickens in experiment 2: ★, 10^9 CFU-inoculated chicken; ●, positive cecal dropping; ○, negative cecal dropping; groups D and E, withdrawal of food and water for 2 days before inoculation. From Nakamura et al. (1997).

water was shared among chickens (Nakamura et al., 1994a). In the study described here, however, contamination of water never preceded the appearance of positive cecal droppings. Moreover, *S.* Enteritidis was not isolated from water during a certain period, although cecal droppings of chickens were positive at that time. These findings suggested that, in the present study, *S.* Enteritidis was not transmitted from contaminated water to chickens, but from infected chickens to water. Although contaminated feed has also been implicated (Lahellec et al., 1985), it did not play as important a role in the spread of *S.* Enteritidis among chickens in this study as did contaminated water. Second, feathers can become contaminated with salmonellae and remain contaminated for long periods (Bailey et al., 1990). In the study described here, it was not easy to pluck feathers from chickens in adjacent cages, because the cages were separated with wires. However, contaminated feathers might have played a role in the transmission of *S.* Enteritidis.

The third possible mechanism of transmission could be aerosols containing *S.* Enteritidis. Baskerville et al. (1992) showed that low numbers of *S.* Enteritidis administered by aerosol could cause a disseminated infection. Similar results have been described by Clemmer et al. (1960). Holt (1995) also reported that molted hens can shed high levels of intestinal *S.* Enteritidis, and this may result in large numbers of aerosolized *S.* Enteritidis released into the environment. Humphrey et al. (1992) and the authors (Nakamura et al., 1995) described conjunctival and intratracheal challenge, respectively, and assumed that generalized infection was caused by the potential ability of this organism to invade blood vessels directly. Based on these findings, the author considered that the rapid dissemination among chickens in this study might be caused by airborne droplets or dust particles carrying *S.* Enteritidis. These particles float in the air, and their movement can be affected by the direction of the airflow. By moving the inoculated chickens into the cage with upstream airflow in experiment 2, particles carrying *S.* Enteritidis could float with the airflow. This treatment resulted in rapid dissemination of *S.* Enteritidis in group D. However, rapid transmission also occurred in group-E chickens, where the airflow was much slower than that in group D (Fig. 34.2). Almost the same pattern of transmission was also observed in group C of experiment 1. In both cases, the direction of the airflow was not involved, because the shedding patterns of *S.* Enteritidis were almost the same. It was likely that particles floating in the air could have been inhaled by the chickens within cages in the same row even though the airflow was very weak, because the movement of the chickens themselves caused air movement.

From these findings, the author assumes that the horizontal transmission of *S.* Enteritidis might be caused by airborne infection as a result of aerosol particles carrying the organisms, and the rapidity of spread might be affected by the airflow. However, the present study did not provide enough data to draw conclusions about how individual chickens became infected. Many questions remain to be answered.

EFFECT OF STRESS ON SHEDDING OF *SALMONELLA* ENTERITIDIS BY LAYING HENS

There have been a number of reports on the influence of stress on the shedding of salmonellae. These stresses include social stress, heat and cold, short-term deprivation of feed or water, and induced molting.

Since Jones (1992) reported the effect of stress (including heat stress, exposure to diseases, and management problems) on salmonella isolation rate, some investigators have focused on the effect of stress on the shedding of *S.* Enteritidis.

Social Stress

Social stress has been found to modify the response of chickens to infectious diseases. Social stress was produced in chickens by moving chickens into cages with other chickens (Gross and Siegel, 1965). This daily moving of the visitors into groups of strangers caused social stress for all of the birds, because a new social structure had to be established each day. At the end of the 2-week social-stress period, the stressed birds were more resistant to pathogenic strains of *Escherichia coli* inoculated via air sac than were unstressed controls.

On the other hand, Weinack et al. (1985) reported that only a single replicate group in one of four trials showed a slight increase in the isolation rate of *S.* Typhimurium following stress, which consisted of interchanging contact between two replicate groups for a 2-week period at 3- to 4-day intervals starting at 2 weeks of age.

In our previous study (Nakamura et al., 1994a), 7-month-old SPF chickens were inoculated with *S.* Enteritidis, and, at 20 days after inoculation, 30-day-old SPF chickens were introduced in the same room and raised there for 2 days. This introduction of young chickens into the same rearing room caused a drastic increase in the *S.* Enteritidis recovery rate (from 33% to 94%), although only for 2 days. In Japan, several groups of hens of different ages are raised simultaneously in the same house in order to provide eggs constantly throughout the year. The introduction of a different flock of replacement chickens may be a cause of stress for egg-laying hens, as described here.

Heat and Cold Stress

There have been many reports on the ways in which heat or cold stress affect the shedding of salmonellae (Thaxton et al., 1971, 1974; Soerjadi-Liem et al., 1979; Weinack et al., 1985). Thaxton et al. (1971) reported that when day-old broiler chicks were kept at ambient temperatures of 21°C, 24°C, or 29°C, and 12 h later were challenged with a salmonella serovar, there was a 70% mortality in the challenged birds kept at 21°C, whereas the mortality at 24°C was only 28% and at 29°C it was 0. No mortality was recorded in the unchallenged birds kept at these three temperatures. In a later report, Thaxton et al. (1974) also suggested that the susceptibility of young chickens to the establishment of salmonellae was dependent on body temperature, a normal body temperature being essential if the chickens are to resist establishment of salmonellae in the intestinal tract.

Soerjadi-Liem et al. (1979) reported that day-old chickens kept in a cold environment (18°–22°C) were more susceptible to low and moderate challenges of *S*. Typhimurium than were chickens similarly challenged and kept in a warm environment (32°–36°C). Cold stress at 10°C for 24 h when applied to 12-day-old chickens effectively increased the number of birds shedding organisms. Those authors also reported that similar cold stress on 20-day-old chickens resulted in a less dramatic increase in the number of birds shedding organisms and that, of the 60 birds previously challenged with *S*. Typhimurium and then subjected to cold stress, 16 recommenced shedding and seven with no previous history of shedding began to shed organisms.

Weinack et al. (1985) reported that, using the day-old chicks treated with diluted fecal chicken intestinal microflora, the two stressed groups—one held at 43°C for 2.5 h and the other at 16°C for the same time—had 37% and 45% *S*. Typhimurium recovery rates, respectively, whereas the treated unstressed group had a recovery rate of 20%. However, most groups stressed at 2 weeks of age or older showed a slight or no increase in *S*. Typhimurium isolation rate.

The work of others (Sadler et al., 1969; Rigby and Pettit, 1979; Snoeyenbos et al., 1985) showed that temperature extremes had little effect on the shedding of *S*. Typhimurium in chickens 4–9 weeks of age. However, it was indicated that heat stress reduced the birds' ability to respond immunologically (Ferket and Qureshi, 1992).

Moreover, Jones (1992) showed that exposure to peak temperatures of greater than 90°F was associated with an increase in salmonella isolations from the flock. Therefore, heat stress may have reduced the potential of chickens to respond immunologically, allowing an infection to ensue.

Short-Term Deprivation of Feed and Water

In our previous report (Nakamura et al., 1994a), the effects of short-term deprivation of feed and water on shedding of *S*. Enteritidis were examined in 7-month-old laying hens. At 30 days after *S*. Enteritidis inoculation, feed and water were withdrawn for 2 days, which resulted in an increase in the shedding rate (from about 25% for several days before removal to about 60% for 4 days after removal).

In our experiment described previously in this chapter (Nakamura et al., 1995), the effects of feed and water deprivation on the tissue distribution of bacteria were investigated in intratracheally inoculated chickens. In experiment A, it was shown that the intratracheally inoculated organisms entered the bloodstream immediately after inoculation and produced generalized infection. In experiment B, the effects of feed and water withdrawal on the tissue distribution of bacteria were examined. Three experiments (B-1, B-2, and B-3) were designed as shown in Figure 34.6. Each experiment consisted of three or four groups, with 10 birds in each group. In experiment B-1, suspensions containing 10^5 colony-forming units (CFU)/0.1 ml were inoculated intratracheally, and feed and water were withdrawn for 2 days after inoculation and 2 days before isolation (group A), or 2 days before isolation (group B). Feed and water were

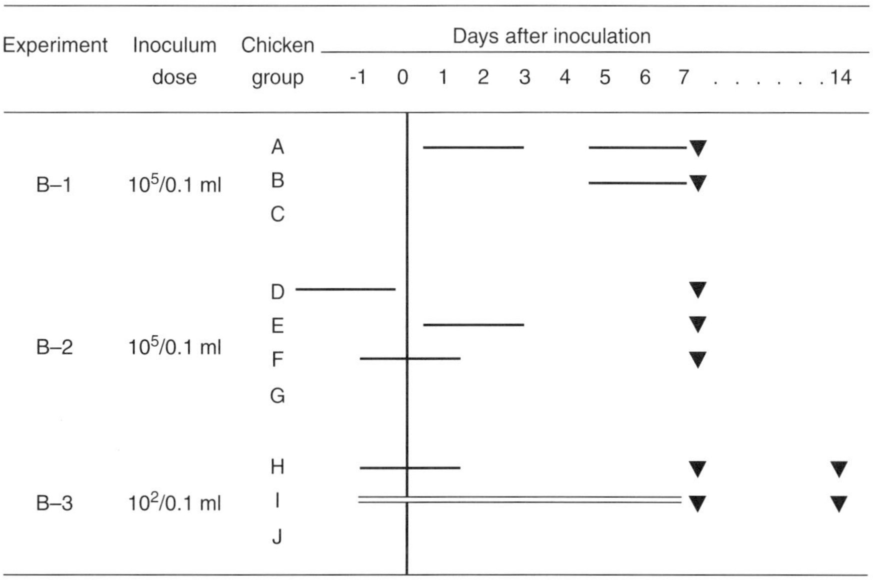

FIGURE 34.6   The period of withdrawal of food and water in experiment B: —, withdrawal of food and water; =, withdrawal of food; ▼, isolation. From Nakamura et al. (1995).

not withdrawn from group C. In experiment B-2, the same dose was inoculated intratracheally. Withdrawal of feed and water for 2 days before (group D) or 2 days after inoculation (group E), and inoculation during 2 days of feed and water withdrawal (group F), were conducted in order to determine the most effective time for withdrawal of feed and water. Feed and water were not withdrawn from group G. In experiment B-3, suspensions containing 10^2 CFU/0.1 ml were inoculated intratracheally. Feed and water were withdrawn for 1 day before and 1 day after inoculation (group H) or for 6 days after inoculation (group I). Feed and water were not withdrawn from group J. Bacteriological examination of tissues was performed 1 or 2 weeks after inoculation.

In experiment B-1, withdrawal of feed and water for 2 days showed a marked effect on the isolation rate of S. Enteritidis in pericardium, trachea, lung, and liver compared with that in group C without the withdrawal (Table 34.1). Moreover, there was a significant difference between groups A and B in the isolation rate of S. Enteritidis from

lung and liver, suggesting that the additional withdrawal of feed and water for 2 days just after inoculation had a marked effect.

The most effective time for the influence of feed and water withdrawal was investigated in experiment B-2. As shown in Table 34.2, two days of withdrawal just before inoculation (group D) had a slight influence on the isolation rate of S. Enteritidis compared with that in group G without withdrawal. Group-E chickens (2 days of withdrawal just after inoculation) and group-F chickens (inoculation during 2 days of withdrawal) were affected significantly.

Horizontal transmission had occurred in the past among chickens raised in the same experimental room as the present one without direct physical contact between birds, and 10^1–10^2 CFU/g of S. Enteritidis organisms were found in the dust collected from the filter of this room. These results showed that horizontal transmission without physical contact occurred with a small number of organisms. Therefore, we changed the inoculum dose from

TABLE 34.1 **Effect of withdrawal of water and feed on the tissue distribution of *Salmonella* Enteritidis in chickens inoculated intratracheally in experiment B-1[a]**

Tissue	No. of positive samples in 10 chickens[b]		
	Group A	Group B	Group C
Pericardium	5[a]	5[a]	0[b]
Trachea	9[a]	6[a]	1[b]
Lung	10[a]	5[b]	4[b]
Liver	10[a]	1[b]	0[b]
Spleen	4[a]	1[a]	4[a]
Gallbladder	0[a]	0[a]	0[a]
Peritoneum	0[a]	1[a]	1[a]
Pancreas	1[a]	0[a]	0[a]
Kidney	0[a]	0[a]	1[a]
Ovary	0[a]	0[a]	1[a]
Duodenum	6[a]	6[a]	3[a]
Cecum	9[a]	7[a]	6[a]
Blood	2[a]	0[a]	0[a]

[a]Period of withdrawal and the isolation of S. Enteritidis is shown in Figure 34.2.
[b]Values within rows followed by different lowercase superscripts differ significantly (p < 0.05).
From Nakamura et al. (1995).

TABLE 34.2 **Effect of withdrawal of water and feed on the tissue distribution of *Salmonella* Enteritidis in chickens inoculated intratracheally in experiment B-2[a]**

Tissue	No. of positive samples in 10 chickens[b]			
	Group D	Group E	Group F	Group G
Pericardium	2[a]	0[a]	3[a]	4[a]
Trachea	6[a]	4[a]	4[a]	4[a]
Lung	8[a]	6[a,b]	9[a]	3[b]
Liver	4[a,b]	8[a]	7[a,b]	3[b]
Spleen	6[a,b]	9[a]	10[a]	2[b]
Cecum	4[b]	9[a]	10[a]	4[b]

[a]Period of withdrawal and the isolation of S. Enteritidis is shown in Figure 34.2.
[b]Values within rows followed by different lowercase superscripts differ significantly (p < 0.05).
From Nakamura et al. (1995).

10^5 CFU/0.1 ml to 10^2 CFU/0.1 ml for experiment B-3. The influence of feed and water withdrawal for 1 day before and 1 day after inoculation and 6 days after inoculation was investigated. As shown in Table 34.3, even with a small inoculum dose, chickens were affected severely, especially group-I chickens with 6 days of feed withdrawal. All group-I chickens still excreted S. Enteritidis 2 weeks after inoculation. The distribution of S. Enteritidis organisms was almost the same as that in chickens inoculated orally with 10^5 CFU/1 ml, demonstrating that severe generalized infection occurred in chickens affected by stress even when a small dose was inoculated intratracheally.

The tissue distribution of S. Enteritidis in intratracheally inoculated chickens was drastically influenced by the withdrawal of feed and water. Based on the results in experiment B-2 (Table 34.2), the effect was not marked when withdrawal was for 2 days before inoculation (group D). On the other hand, the effect of deprivation of feed and water in groups E and F was marked. These results suggest that chickens might become habituated to the stress status by the end of the 2-day period of withdrawal. Recent studies of stress, particularly in relation to induced molting, have focused on the increase in hormone secretion and subsequent changes in the cellular immune responses (Holt, 1992). Deprivation of feed for 48 h markedly increased the corticosteroid concentration in the plasma of 7- to 8-week-old chickens (Freeman et al., 1981; Harvey and Klandorf, 1983). Deprivation of both feed and water might produce a more severe effect in chickens (Nakamura et al., 1994a,b, 1995). Stress had a significant effect on cell-mediated immunity and resulted in a decrease in the number of CD4 T-lymphocytes (Holt, 1992). Although the mechanism of this decrease has not been elucidated, it is assumed that such stress may increase the susceptibility of chickens to salmonella infection and subsequently result in severe generalized infection and in an increase in the shedding rate of S. Enteritidis.

In our recent experiments (Nakamura et al., 1997), the effects of withdrawal of feed and water for 2 days on the shedding of S. Enteritidis were also examined. As shown in

Figure 34.4, the effect of withdrawal of feed and water was marked in group B, where 75% of chickens (12 of 16) shed S. Enteritidis after treatment (on day 29), although only 25% (four of 16) shed before the treatment (on day 26). On the contrary, the effect on chickens in groups A and C, where almost all cecal droppings were negative for S. Enteritidis before treatment (on day 26), was negligible. The viable counts of cecal droppings had increased after withdrawal of feed and water in group B (data not shown). Moreover, as shown in Figure 34.5, after withdrawal of feed and water on days 22 and 23, the number of chickens that excreted S. Enteritidis increased rapidly in group E compared with that in group D. These findings suggest that the effect of withdrawal of feed and water might depend on the infectious status of the chickens just before treatment. Thus, deprivation of feed and water for a short time might aid in the detection of an infection with S. Enteritidis in chickens in which feces or cecal droppings were negative. This procedure might be useful in the isolation of S. Enteritidis in field surveys.

Finally, it should be pointed out from our experiment that not only withdrawal of feed and water but also withdrawal of water under heat stress increased shedding of S. Enteritidis in vaccinated hens, as well as in unvaccinated control hens (Nakamura et al., 1994b).

CONCLUSION

The horizontal transmission of S. Enteritidis might be caused by airborne infection as a result of aerosol particles carrying the organism, and the rapidity of spread might be affected by the airflow, although the oral route of infection may be important in flocks. Short-term stress—including social stress, heat and cold, and deprivation of feed or water—that may occur in daily handling can be associated with an increase in the S. Enteritidis isolation rate. Such stress also increases the shedding of S. Enteritidis in vaccinated hens as well as unvaccinated hens. It has also been

TABLE 34.3   Effect of withdrawal of water and feed on the tissue distribution of *Salmonella* Enteritidis in chickens inoculated intratracheally in experiment B-3[a]

| Tissue | No. of positive samples in 10 chickens[b] | | | | | |
| | 1 Week | | | 2 Weeks | | |
	H	I	J	H	I	J
Pericardium	2[a]	7[b]	1[a]	0[a]	0[a]	0[a]
Trachea	0[a]	4[a]	1[a]	0[a]	0[a]	0[a]
Lung	5[a]	9[a,b]	1[a]	3[a]	2[a]	3[a]
Liver	3[a]	9[b]	0[a]	0[a]	3[a]	0[a]
Spleen	4[a]	10[b]	1[a]	0[a]	2[a]	0[a]
Cecum	6[a]	10[a]	1[b]	6[a]	10[a]	1[b]

[a]Period of withdrawal and the isolation of S. Enteritidis is shown in Figure 34.2.
[b]Values within rows followed by different lowercase superscripts differ significantly (p < 0.05).
From Nakamura et al. (1995).

suggested that certain factors may cause different hens to lay contaminated eggs at or around the same time. The author hypothesizes that clustering of contaminated eggs may be caused by the effect of stress described here.

REFERENCES

Anonymous. 1995. *Salmonella* Enteritidis Pilot Project progress report. Washington, DC: United States Department of Agriculture, pp. 52–54.

Bailey, J.S., Cox, N.A., and Blankenship, L.C. 1990. Persistence and spread of external *Salmonella* contamination during broiler production. Poult. Sci. 69(Suppl.):s154.

Barrow, P.A., and Lovell, M.A. 1991. Experimental infection of egg laying hens with *Salmonella enteritidis* phage type 4. Avian Pathol. 20:335–348.

Baskerville, A., Humphrey, T.J., Fitzgeorgel, R.B., Cook, R.W., Chart, H., Rowe, B., and Whitehead, A. 1992. Airborne infection of laying hens with *Salmonella enteritidis* phage type 4. Vet. Rec. 130:395–398.

Clemmer, D.J., Hickey, J.L.S., Bridges, J.F., Schliessmann, D.J., and Shaffer, M.F. 1960. Bacteriological studies of experimental air-borne salmonellosis in chicks. J. Infect. Dis. 106:197–210.

Ferket, P.R., and Qureshi, M.A. 1992. Performance and immunity of heat-stressed broilers fed vitamin and electrolyte-supplemented drinking water. Poult. Sci. 71:88–97.

Freeman, M.B., Manning, A.C.C., and Flack, I.H. 1981. The effect of restricted feeding on adrenal cortical activity in the immature domestic fowl. Br. Poult. Sci. 22:295–303.

Gast, R.K., and Beard, C.W. 1990a. Production of *Salmonella enteritidis* contaminated eggs by experimentally infected hens. Avian Dis. 34:438–446.

Gast, R.K., and Beard, C.W. 1990b. Isolation of *Salmonella enteritidis* from internal organs of experimentally infected hens. Avian Dis. 34:991–993.

Gast, R.K., and Beard, C.W. 1992. Detection and enumeration of *Salmonella enteritidis* in fresh land stored eggs laid by experimentally infected hens. J. Food Prot. 55:152–156.

Gross, W.E.B., and Siegel, H.S. 1965. The effect of social stress on resistance to infection with *Escherichia coli* or *Mycoplasma gallisepticum*. Poult. Sci. 44:988–1001.

Harvey, S., and Klandorf, H. 1983. Reduced adrenocortical function and increased thyroid function in fasted and refed chickens. J. Endocrinol. 98:129–135.

Holt, P.S. 1992. Effect of induced molting on B cell and CT4 and CT8 T cell numbers in spleens and peripheral blood of white leghorn hens. Poult. Sci. 71:2027–2034.

Holt, P.S. 1993. Effect of induced molting on the susceptibility of white leghorn hens to a *Salmonella enteritidis* infection. Avian Dis. 37:412–417.

Holt, P.S. 1995. Horizontal transmission of *Salmonella enteritidis* in molted and unmolted laying chickens. Avian Dis. 39:239–249.

Holt, P.S., and Porter, R.E., Jr. 1992. Effect of induced molting on the course of infection and transmission of *Salmonella enteritidis* in white leghorn hens of different ages. Poult. Sci. 71:1842–1848.

Humphrey, T.J. 1994. Contamination of egg shell and contents with *Salmonella enteritidis:* a review. Int. J. Food Microbiol. 21:31–40.

Humphrey, T.J., Baskerville, A., Mawer, S.L., Rowe, B., and Hopper, S. 1989a. *Salmonella enteritidis* PT4 from contents of intact eggs: a study involving naturally infected hens. Epidemiol. Infect. 103:415–423.

Humphrey, T.J., Cruickshank, J.G., and Rowe, B. 1989b. *Salmonella enteritidis* PT4 and hens eggs. Lancet 1:281.

Humphrey, T.J., Chart, H., Baskerville, A., and Rowe, B. 1991a. The influence of age on the response of SPF hens to infection with *Salmonella enteritidis* PT4. Epidemiol. Infect. 106:33–43.

Humphrey, T.J., Whitehead, A., Gawler, A.H.L., Henly, A., and Rowe, B. 1991b. Numbers of *Salmonella enteritidis* in the contents of naturally contaminated hens eggs. Epidemiol. Infect. 106:489–496.

Humphrey, T.J., Baskerville, A., Chart, H., Rowe, B., and Whitehead, A. 1992. Infection of laying hens with *Salmonella enteritidis* PT4 by conjunctival challenge. Vet. Rec. 131:386–388.

Jones, F.T. 1992. Breeder flock study shows *Salmonella*-causing factors. Feedstuff 64:22–23.

Lahellec, C., Colin, P., Bennejean, G., Paquin, J., Guillerm, A., and Debois, J.C. 1985. Influence of resident *Salmonella* on contamination of broiler flocks. Br. Poult. Sci. 26:179–186.

Mawer, S.L., Spain, G.E., and Rowe, B. 1989. *S. enteritidis* PT4 and hens eggs. Lancet 1:280–281.

Nagaraja, K.V., Pomeroy, B.S., and Williams, J.E. 1991. Paratyphoid infection. In: Calnek, B.W., Barnes, H.J., Beard, C.W., Reid, W.M., and Yolder, H.W., Jr., eds. Diseases of poultry, 9th ed. Ames: Iowa State University Press, pp. 99–130.

Nakamura, M., Nagamine, N., Norimatsu, M., Suzuki, S., Oishi, K., Kijima, M., Tamura, Y., and Sato, S. 1993. The ability of *Salmonella enteritidis* isolated from chicks imported from England to cause transovarian infection. J. Vet. Med. Sci. 55:135–136.

Nakamura, M., Nagamine, N., Takahashi, T., Suzuki, S., Kijima, M., Tamura, Y., and Sato, S. 1994a. Horizontal transmission of *Salmonella enteritidis* and the effect of stress on shedding in laying hens. Avian Dis. 38:282–288.

Nakamura, M., Nagamine, N., Takahashi, T., Suzuki, S., and Sato, S. 1994b. Evaluation of the efficacy of a bacterin against *Salmonella enteritidis* infection and the effect of stress after vaccination. Avian Dis. 38:717–724.

Nakamura, M., Nagamine, N., Takahashi, T., Norimatsu, M., Suzuki, S., and Sato, S. 1995. Intratracheal infection of chickens with *Salmonella enteritidis* and the effect of feed and water deprivation. Avian Dis. 39:853–858.

Nakamura, M., Takagi, M., Takahashi, T., Suzuki, S., Sato, S., and Takehara, K. 1997. The effect of the flow of air on horizontal transmission of *Salmonella enteritidis* in chickens. Avian Dis. 41:354–360.

Rigby, C.E., and Pettit, J.R. 1979. Some factors affecting *Salmonella typhimurium* infection and shedding in chickens raised on litter. Avian Dis. 23:442–455.

Sadler, W.W., Brownell, J.R., and Fanelli, M.J. 1969. Influence of age and inoculum level on shed pattern of *Salmonella typhimurium* in chickens. Avian Dis. 13:798–803.

Shivaprasad, H.L., Timoney, J.F., Morales, S., Lucio, B., and Baker, R.C. 1990. Pathogenesis of *Salmonella enteritidis* infection in laying chickens. I. Studies on egg transmission, clinical signs, fecal shedding, and serological responses. Avian Dis. 34:548–557.

Snoeyenbos, G.H., Weinack, O.M., Soerjadi-Liem, A.S., Miller, B.M., Woodward, D.E., and Weston, C.R. 1985. Large-scale competitive exclusion trials on *Salmonella* in chickens. Avian Dis. 29:1004–1011.

Soerjadi-Liem, A.S., Drutt, J.H., Lloyd, A.B., and Cumming, R.B. 1979. Effect of environmental temperature on susceptibility of young chickens to *Salmonella typhimurium*. Aust. Vet. J. 53:413-417.

Thaxton, P., Wyatt, R.D., and Hamilton, P.B. 1971. Cold stress and *Salmonella* as a cause of early mortality in chickens. Poult. Sci. 50:1636.

Thaxton, P., Wyatt, R.D., and Hamilton, P.B. 1974. The effect of environmental temperature on paratyphoid infection in neonatal chickens. Poult. Sci. 53:88–94.

Thiagarajan, D., Saeed, A.M., and Asem, E.K. 1994. Mechanism of transovarian transmission of *Salmonella enteritidis* in laying hens. Poult. Sci. 73:89–98.

Thiagarajan, D., Saeed, A.M., Turek, J., and Asem, E.K. 1996. In vitro attachment and invasion of chicken ovarian granulosa cells by *Salmonella enteritidis* phage type 8. Infect. Immun. 64:5015–5021.

Timoney, J.F., Shivaprasad, H.L., Baker, R.C., and Rowe, B. 1989. Egg transmission after infection of hens with *Salmonella enteritidis* phage type IV. Vet. Rec. 125:600–601.

Weinack, O.M., Snoeyenbos, G.H., Soerjadi, A.S., and Smyser, C.F. 1985. Influence of temperature, social, and dietary stress on development and stability of protective microflora in chickens against S. Typhimurium. Avian Dis. 29:1177–1182.

35

Competitive Exclusion in the Control of *Salmonella enterica* Serovar Enteritidis Infection in Laying Poultry

D.E. Corrier and D.J. Nisbet

Research to control salmonella growth in poultry and reduce human exposure to foodborne salmonellosis has focused on the development of immunoprophylactic measures, antisalmonella feed additives, and microbiological strategies that prevent salmonella intestinal colonization and tissue invasion in commercial poultry flocks. Microbiological strategies to increase salmonella colonization resistance have employed the treatment of newly hatched chicks with cultures of indigenous adult intestinal flora. The increase in colonization resistance against salmonellae and other enteropathogens of humans and animals that accompanies the establishment of a stable indigenous gut microflora is well documented (Freter, 1984; Stavric and D'Aoust, 1993) and has been referred to as bacterial antagonism (Freter, 1956), bacterial interference (Dubos, 1963), the barrier effect (Ducluzeau et al., 1970), colonization resistance (Van der Waaij et al., 1971), and competitive exclusion (Loyd et al., 1977).

The competitive exclusion (CE) concept was first applied to poultry by Nurmi and Rantala (1973) and Rantala and Nurmi (1973) to control an outbreak of *Salmonella* Infantis in broiler chickens that had resulted in a human salmonellosis epidemic in Finland. They suspected that the susceptibility of newly hatched chicks to salmonella colonization was probably due to the delayed establishment of normal intestinal microflora in chicks reared by commercial mass-production methods. The intestinal tract of poultry is usually naive at hatching and requires

several weeks for a stable indigenous microflora to become established (Barnes and Impey, 1980). Nurmi and Rantala demonstrated that hatchling chicks, inoculated orally with the intestinal contents from adult birds, were protected against *S.* Infantis colonization. The procedure became known as the *Nurmi concept*. Nurmi attributed the increased resistance of treated chicks to competition between the newly established indigenous flora and the invading *S.* Infantis. Loyd and colleagues (1977) confirmed that intestinal extracts from adult birds protect chicks and turkey poults against salmonella colonization and termed the protective mechanism *competitive inhibition*. The protective effect of CE cultures in poultry has been well documented in several authoritative review articles (Pivnick and Nurmi, 1982; Mead and Impey, 1986; Bailey, 1987; Mead, 1991; Stavric and D'Aoust, 1993; Stavric and Kornegay, 1995).

Metchnikoff (1908) first proposed the idea that beneficial organisms, such as lactobacillus present in yogurt, could displace noxious organisms from the lower gut, arrest intestinal putrefaction, improve health, and prolong life. Metchnikoff's proposed mechanisms, by which beneficial organisms improve health, has failed the test of time. Indeed, the proposed mechanisms by which one bacteria species excludes or reduces the growth of another still remain speculative and varied. A number of different activities of indigenous gut flora have been proposed as mechanisms that contribute to the exclusion or the reduced growth of nonindigenous organisms. These activities have been reviewed by Rolfe (1991), Fuller (1992), and Stavric and Kornegay (1995) and include (a) competition for adhesion receptor sites on the gut epithelium, (b) competition for essential nutrients, and (c) the production of antibacterial substances such as bacteriocins and short-chain volatile fatty acids. Researchers agree that any one or all of these mechanisms may be operative at any one time and that complex interactions are likely to occur in practice (Savage, 1987; Fuller, 1992; Stavric and Kornegay, 1995).

The complexity of the gut ecosystem composed of several hundred bacterial species from different genera of facultative and obligate anaerobes, and the inability thus far to determine the contribution of the various proposed protection mechanisms, have made it difficult to select and manipulate CE cultures that are composed of defined bacterial strains (Mead, 1991; Stavric, 1992). Subsequently, CE cultures for poultry have usually been prepared from the intestinal contents or fecal droppings of healthy adult birds and are composed of an undefined mixture of normal gut bacteria. Efforts to develop defined CE cultures began early after the first Nurmi and Rantala report (1973) and were due in part to concerns about the possible transmission of human and/or avian pathogens that may be present in undefined CE cultures (Loyd et al., 1977; Stavric and D'Aoust, 1993). Although undefined cultures may be composed of a mixture of unknown or partially known bacteria strains, they can be demonstrated to be free of avian and human pathogens (Mulder and Bolder, 1991; Blankenship et al., 1993) and have an excellent safety record during both laboratory studies and in commercial poultry flocks (Stavric and D'Aoust, 1993).

Defined CE cultures developed from a single strain of bacteria or from mixtures of strains from the same genus have not provided consistent protection against salmonella challenge (Stavric and D'Aoust, 1993). Similarly, probiotic cultures, composed of 1–8 live bacterial strains and used as feed supplements to improve the microbial intestinal balance of the host, have not effectively increased resistance to salmonella colonization (Fowler and Mead, 1989). Probiotic cultures, referred to as direct-fed microbial cultures by the U.S. Food and Drug Administration (FDA), are composed of organisms that are classified by the FDA and the Association of American Feed Control officials as generally regarded as safe (GRAS) because of their common usage and safety record in feed ingredients. A total of 42 different microorganisms, mostly species of lactobacilli, are considered GRAS and can be used in probiotic cultures. Little is known about how these microorganisms associate with the gut mucosa, their beneficial physiological effect, or in what way they may antagonize the growth of nonindigenous organisms in the gut (Freter, 1992). Although most cultures of single strains or mixtures of lactobacilli have not been protective against salmonellae (Stavric, 1992), researchers recently reported that a pure culture of *Lactobacillus reuteri* decreases salmonella and *Escherichia coli* colonization in chicks and turkey poults (Edens et al., 1997).

Defined mixed CE cultures containing larger numbers of bacterial strains from different genera have proved to be more successful than cultures composed of a single strain or single genus (Stavric, 1992). Mixed cultures composed of 14 strains of bacteria developed in France (Hudault et al., 1985), or 48 strains developed in the United Kingdom (Impey et al., 1982) or 28 strains (Gleeson et al., 1989) and 50 strains (Stavric et al., 1985) developed in Canada, have provided protective efficacy against experimental salmonella challenge comparable to that of undefined mixed cultures.

In addition to the absence of a clear understanding of the mechanism(s) of pathogen exclusion and therefore of clear criteria for selecting protective bacteria strains, development of defined CE cultures has been hampered by the lack of adequate selective culture media to isolate and maintain defined mixed cultures of gut flora (Mead and Impey, 1984; Stavric, 1987). Continuous-flow culture systems were recently used for the first time to maintain normal indigenous bacteria from the ceca of adult chickens in steady-state continuous culture (Nisbet et al., 1993, 1994). In subsequent studies, continuous-flow culture was used to develop a mixed culture of cecal anaerobes that was characterized to contain 29 bacterial isolates composed of 15 strains of facultative anaerobes and 14 strains of obligate anaerobes representing 10 different genera. The culture has been reported to be effective against experimental *Salmonella* Typhimurium challenge (Corrier et al., 1995c) and against environmental salmonella challenge in commercially reared broilers (Corrier et al., 1995b). The characterized continuous-flow culture known as CF3 has been patented (Nisbet et al., 1995) and licensed to a commercial company (BioScience Division, Milk Specialties, Dundee, IL). Research on the development and use of CE cultures has been directed primarily at controlling salmonellae in commercial broiler flocks. Treatment of commercially reared broilers with CE cultures has been demonstrated to reduce the prevalence of salmonellae during large-scale field trials in Sweden (Wierup et al., 1988), the Netherlands (Goren et al., 1988), Puerto Rico (Blankenship et al., 1993; Corrier et al., 1995b), and the United States (Bailey et al., 1994). The field-trial studies have indicated that CE treatment is most effective when commercial management has adhered to strict hygienic production procedures (Stavric and D'Aoust, 1993).

During the last decade, the transmission of salmonellae to humans by contaminated eggs has become a significant public health issue on several continents (O'Brien, 1990). Reported outbreaks of human salmonella food poisoning due to *S. enterica* serovar Enteritidis (*S.* Enteritidis) began to increase in the United Kingdom and in the United States during the late 1970s. In both the United Kingdom and the United States, grade-A shell eggs were identified as the principal source of human infection (St. Louis et al., 1988; Humphrey et al., 1989). Invasive stains of *S.* Enteritidis such as phage type 4 (PT4) have been identified as the most likely source of egg contamination due to transovarian transmission and eggshell penetration (Eckroade et al., 1988; Humphrey et al., 1989). The presence of *S.* Enteritidis (phage type not reported) has been reported in environmental samples collected from broiler farms in the United States. *Salmonella* Enteritidis PT4, which is widespread in both layer and broiler flocks in several countries, has now been isolated from a layer flock in the United States (Kinde et al., 1996). The widespread appearance of *S.* Enteritidis in both layer and broiler flocks and its importance as a zoonotic disease have prompted studies to evaluate the protective effect of CE treatment against *S.* Enteritidis in both broiler and layer chickens.

Treatment of broiler chicks in Finland with a commercially produced CE product (Broilact; Orion, Turku, Finland), an undefined culture that contains a limited mixture of normal intestinal bacteria, was reported to decrease the population of *S.* Enteritidis PT4 significantly in the ceca of experimentally challenged chicks (Schneitz, 1992). During this study, newly hatched chicks were sprayed with the CE product and exposed the following day to seeder chicks that were challenged orally with 10^3 *S.* Enteritidis PT4; 12 days after challenge, the average population of salmonellae in the ceca was reduced from 6.7 $\log_{10}$ units (U)/g in control seeder chicks to 3.3 $\log_{10}$ U/g in the CE-treated seeder chicks. Pooled organ samples (liver, gallbladder, heart, and spleen) from the control groups were salmonella positive while CE treatment prevented organ invasion in treated chicks. Additionally, the transmission of *S.* Enteritidis from the experimentally infected seeder chicks to the contact chicks was prevented by treatment with the CE culture.

The effect of CE treatment in reducing the spread of *S.* Enteritidis from infected seeders to contact chicks was also observed during trials carried out in England (Mead, 1991). In these trials, newly hatched chicks were treated with an undefined CE culture and immediately exposed to seeder chicks that were challenged with 10^4 *S.* Enteritidis PT4. Both the incidence of *S.* Enteritidis–positive contact chicks and the population of *S.* Enteritidis in the ceca were reduced in the treated contact chicks compared with untreated contacts in the control group. In Mexico, the spread of *S.* Enteritidis from seeder chicks challenged with 10^4 *S.* Enteritidis PT4 to contact broiler chicks was prevented when the contacts were spray treated with Aviguard (Bayer, Mexico City, Mexico), a commercially produced, undefined CE culture (Cameron et al., 1996).

During studies in Japan, CE treatment with commercially produced CF3 culture was reported to control cecal colonization effectively in seeder chicks challenged with 10^4 *S.* Enteritidis PT4 and to prevent horizontal spread of *S.* Enteritidis to contact chicks (Sakata et al., 1997). Similarly, the beneficial effect of CE cultures in protecting contact chicks from salmonella-infected seeders was reported from studies conducted in Mexico (Nisbet et al., 1996). During repeated trials, hatchling chicks were treated with the characterized CF3 culture and exposed to seeder chicks that were challenged with 2.5×10^5 *Salmonella* Gallinarum. The spread of salmonellae from the infected seeders to CF3-treated contacts was effectively reduced. Additionally, mortality due to fowl typhoid caused by the salmonella infection was reduced from 45% or higher in untreated chicks to zero in the CF3-treated contact chicks. Significant reductions in the spread of *S.* Enteritidis PT13 from colonized seeders to CF3-treated contacts were also observed in the United States (Corrier et al., 1991, 1995a).

Treatment of leghorn chicks with an undefined CE culture was reported to reduce the population of *S.* Enteritidis PT13 in the cecal contents, decrease organ invasion, and control the spread of salmonellae from seeder to contact chicks (Corrier et al., 1991). The chicks were treated with the CE culture by oral inoculation into the crop (crop gavage) on the day of hatch and challenged orally 2 days later with either 10^6 or 10^4 *S.* Enteritidis PT13. At 21 days after challenge, the population of salmonellae in the cecal contents of the treated chicks was significantly reduced compared with untreated controls. Organ invasion was diminished in the treated chicks compared with controls but not sufficiently to be significant statistically. During this study, additional groups of chicks were provided lactose as 5% (wt/wt) of the feed ration. The dietary lactose enhanced colonization resistance in the CE-treated chicks such that the combined treatment provided better protection against *S.* Enteritidis colonization than did either CE treatment or dietary lactose alone. The results of the study indicated that although treatment with this particular undefined CE culture was beneficial, the protective effect of the culture was not great enough to warrant its use in the absence of dietary lactose supplementation.

During subsequent studies, dietary lactose supplementation was combined with treatment using a defined CE culture to control *S.* Enteritidis colonization in leghorn chicks (Corrier et al., 1994c). The defined culture, composed of 11 indigenous strains of cecal bacteria, was selected and maintained in continuous-flow culture using lactose or lactose-fermentation products as a primary carbon source. During four trials, leghorn chicks were treated with the defined CE culture by crop gavage on the day of hatch and challenged orally with 10^4 *S.* Enteritidis PT13 the following day. Treatment with the culture, without dietary lactose supplementation, diminished *S.* Enteritidis cecal and organ colonization but failed to provide consistent protection. Similarly, dietary lactose supplementation without CE treatment failed to be consistently protective. However, CE treatment combined with dietary lactose significantly reduced *S.* Enteritidis cecal and organ colonization in each of the trials. The results clearly indicated that the efficacy of the defined CE culture, composed of bacterial isolates that were selected for their ability to utilize lactose, was dependent on providing lactose in the diet of the CE-treated chicks. Although the combined treatment with the defined culture and dietary lactose was demonstrated to be highly protective against *S.* Enteritidis, the requirement for dietary lactose was considered to increase the cost of treatment for poultry producers and reduce the cost-effectiveness of the culture for potential use in commercially reared poultry.

Other studies have investigated the efficacy of different delivery methods for treating layer chicks with CE cultures (Corrier et al., 1994a,b). Undefined CE cultures were administered to leghorn chicks on the day of hatch by crop gavage, in the first drinking water, by whole-body spray, or encapsulated in alginate beads provided in feed pans. Clearly, the administration of CE cultures by crop gavage is used only as a research procedure and was included in the studies only for comparison with more practical delivery methods. The chicks were challenged by crop gavage with 10^4 S. Enteritidis PT13 two days after treatment, and S. Enteritidis cecal colonization was evaluated 7 days after challenge. During repeated trials, the incidence of S. Enteritidis cecal colonization was significantly decreased in each of the treatment groups compared with controls. The S. Enteritidis population in the cecal contents of the control groups ranged from 4.91 to 5.35 $\log_{10}$ U/g compared with 0–1.1 $\log_{10}$ U/g in the groups treated by crop gavage, with drinking water, or by whole-body spray. Provision of CE cultures encapsulated in alginate beads was less effective than the other delivery methods tested. The results further serve to demonstrate the protective effect of CE treatment against S. Enteritidis in layer chicks and that CE treatment can be effectively administered by practical delivery methods. Delivery of CE cultures by spray application (Goren et al., 1988; Corrier et al., 1995b), in the drinking water (Wierup et al., 1988; Mead, 1991), or by a combination of both methods (Blankenship et al., 1993; Bailey et al., 1994) has been used successfully to treat commercial broiler chicks during large-scale field trials.

Studies to evaluate the practical application of CE in older birds such as adult breeders or replacement laying hens have been conducted in England (Fowler and Mead, 1990; Mead, 1991) and by the Dutch Poultry Health Ministry in the Netherlands. In England, CE treatment was used in combination with antibiotic therapy to prevent salmonella reinfection in 250,000 adult breeder birds (chickens, turkeys, and ducks) in 22 field trials from 1986 to 1988. All of the flocks involved had a previous history of salmonella infection. The serovars isolated most frequently were S. Enteritidis and S. Typhimurium. During the trials, the birds were moved at about 19 weeks of age from rearing sites to laying farms. Prior to transfer, the birds received appropriate antibiotic treatment in the feed. One day after the withdrawal of antibiotics, the birds were provided CE cultures in the drinking water. The combined antibiotic–CE treatment prevented reinfection in 20 of the 22 field trials, as determined from cloacal swabs taken at monthly intervals over a 3-month period following treatment.

In the Netherlands, CE treatment was used in 32 S. Enteritidis–positive breeder flocks after medication with antibiotics. After antibiotic therapy, the birds were treated with a commercially produced, undefined CE culture (Aviguard; Bayer, Mannheim, Germany) to reestablish indigenous cecal flora. A success rate of 72% was reported after one combined antibiotic–CE treatment and 93% success was obtained after two combined treatments. Salmonella colonization status after treatment was evaluated by bacteriological culturing of the breeder flocks and progeny.

Clearly, the results of numerous studies have indicated that the early establishment of indigenous intestinal flora in newly hatched broiler or layer chicks effectively increases resistance to S. Enteritidis colonization. These studies further support the conclusions of other researchers that CE treatment increases colonization resistance against a broad variety of salmonella serovars (Mead and Barrow, 1990; Stavric and D'Aoust, 1993). Additionally, the use of CE cultures to reestablish indigenous flora in older birds after medication or other factors have disrupted the protective gut flora appears to be beneficial. As was previously suggested (Stavric and D'Aoust, 1993), further progress in the practical application of CE to reduce poultryborne salmonellae effectively will require the identification of farm management practices that optimize the protective potential of CE treatment. Because of the many stages involved in the production and processing of poultry meat and egg products, an integrated multifaceted control program will be required to assure food safety. CE has the potential to serve as a useful component in an integrated control program by helping to prevent the growth and spread of salmonellae in poultry flocks.

REFERENCES

Bailey, J.S. 1987. Factors affecting microbial competitive exclusion in poultry. Food Technol. 41:88–92.

Bailey, J.S., Cox, N.A., Stern, N.J., and Robach, M.C. 1994. Reduction of salmonellae colonization in commercial broilers with a mucosal competitive exclusion treatment. Poult. Sci. 71(Suppl. 1):46.

Barnes, E.M., and Impey, C.S. 1980. Competitive exclusion of salmonellas from the newly hatched chick. Vet. Rec. 106:61–62.

Blankenship, L.C., Bailey, J.S., Cox, N.A., Stern, N.J., Brewer, R., and Williams, O. 1993. Two-step mucosal competitive exclusion flora treatment to diminish salmonellae in commercial broiler chickens. Poult. Sci. 72:1667–1672.

Cameron, D.M., Carter, J.N., and Mansell, P. 1996. Evaluation of Aviguard against a Salmonella enteritidis infective model in broiler chickens. In: Proceedings of the 45th Western Poultry Disease Conference, Cancun, Mexico, pp. 256–259.

Corrier, D.E., Hargis, B.M., Hinton, A., Jr., Lindsey, D., Caldwell, D., Manning, J., and DeLoach, J.R. 1991. Effect of anaerobic cecal microflora and dietary lactose on colonization resistance of layer chicks to invasive Salmonella enteritidis. Avian. Dis. 35:337–343.

Corrier, D.E., Hollister, A.G., Nisbet, D.J., Scanlan, C.M., Beier, R.C., and DeLoach, J.R. 1994a. Competitive exclusion of Salmonella enteritidis in leghorn chicks: comparison of treatment by crop gavage, drinking water, spray, or lyophilized alginate beads. Avian Dis. 38:297–303.

Corrier, D.E., Nisbet, D.J., Hollister, A.G., Beier, R.C., Scanlan, C.M., Hargis, B.M., and DeLoach, J.R. 1994b. Resistance against Salmonella enteritidis cecal colonization in leghorn chicks by vent lip application of cecal bacteria culture. Poult. Sci. 73:648–652.

Corrier, D.E., Nisbet, D.J., Scanlan, C.M., Tellez, G., Hargis, B.M., and DeLoach, J.R. 1994c. Inhibition of Salmonella enteritidis cecal and organ colonization in leghorn chicks by a defined culture of cecal bacteria and dietary lactose. J. Food Prot. 56:377–381.

Corrier, D.E., Nisbet, D.J., and DeLoach, J.R. 1995a. Prevention of horizontal transmission of Salmonella enteritidis in leghorn chicks treated with a characterized culture of cecal bacteria. Poult. Sci. 74(Suppl. 1):185.

Corrier, D.E., Nisbet, D.J., Scanlan, C.M., Hollister, A.G., Caldwell, D.J., Thomas, L.A., Hargis, B.M., Tomkins, T., and DeLoach, J.R. 1995b. Treatment of commercial broiler chickens with a characterized culture of cecal bacteria to reduce salmonellae colonization. Poult. Sci. 74:1093–1101.

Corrier, D.E., Nisbet, D.J., Scanlan, C.M., Hollister, A.G., and DeLoach, J.R. 1995c. Control of *Salmonella typhimurium* colonization in broiler chicks with a continuous-flow characterized mixed culture of cecal bacteria. Poult. Sci. 74:916–924.

Dubos, R.J. 1963. Staphylococci and infection immunity. Am. J. Dis. Child. 105:643–645.

Ducluzeau, R., Bellier, M., and Raibaud, P. 1970. Transit digestif de divers inoculums bacteriens introduits per os chez des souris axeniques et holoaxeniques (conventionelles): effect antagoniste de la microflor du tractus gastro-intestinal. Zentralbl. Bakteriol. I Orig. 213:533–548.

Eckroade, R.J., Benson, C.E., and Krandel, D.C. 1988. The *Salmonella enteritidis* situation in poultry. In: Proceedings of the 92nd annual meeting of the U.S. Animal Health Association, Little Rock, AR, pp. 344–346.

Edens, F.W., Parkhurst, C.R., Casas, I.A., and Dobrogosz, W.J. 1997. Principles of ex ovo competitive exclusion and in ovo administration of *Lactobacillus reuteri*. Poult. Sci. 76:179–196.

Fowler, N.G., and Mead, G.C. 1989. Competitive exclusion of *Salmonella* in poultry. Vet. Rec. 125:512.

Fowler, N.G., and Mead, G.C. 1990. Competitive exclusion and *Salmonella enteritidis*. Vet. Rec. 126:409.

Freter, R. 1956. Experimental enteric shigella and vibrio infection in mice and guinea pigs. J. Exp. Med. 104:411–418.

Freter, R. 1984. Interdependence of mechanisms that control bacterial colonization of the large intestine. Microbiol. Ther. 14:89–96.

Freter, R. 1992. Factors affecting the microecology of the gut. In: Fuller, R., ed. Probiotics: the scientific basis. London: Chapman and Hall, pp. 111–144.

Fuller, R. 1992. Problems and prospects. In: Fuller, R., ed. Probiotics: the scientific basis. London: Chapman and Hall, pp. 377–386.

Gleeson, T.M., Stavric, S., and Blanchfield, B. 1989. Protection of chicks against *Salmonella* infection with a mixture of pure cultures of intestinal bacteria. Avian Dis. 33:636–642.

Goren, E., de Jong, W.A., Doornenbal, P., Bolder, N.M., Mulder, R.W.A.W., and Jansen, A. 1988. Reduction of *Salmonella* infection of broilers by spray application of intestinal microflora: a longitudinal study. Vet. Q. 10:249–255.

Hudault, S., Bewa, H., Bridonneau, C., and Raibaud, P. 1985. Efficacy of various bacterial suspensions derived from cecal floras of conventional chickens in reducing the population level of *Salmonella typhimurium* in gnotobiotic mice and chicken intestines. Can. J. Microbiol. 31:832–838.

Humphrey, T.J., Cruickshank, J.G., and Rowe, B. 1989. *Salmonella enteritidis* phage type 4 and hen eggs. Lancet 1:281.

Impey, C.S., Mead, G.C., and George, S.M. 1982. Competitive exclusion of salmonellas from the chick caecum using a defined mixture of bacterial isolates from the microflora of an adult bird. J. Hyg. 89:479–490.

Kinde, H., Read, D.H., Chin, R.P., Bickford, A.A., Wather, R.L., Ardans, A., Breitmeyer, R.E., Willoughby, D., Little, H.E., Kerr, D., and Gardner, I.A. 1996. *Salmonella enteritidis* phage type 4 infection in a commercial layer flock in southern California: bacteriologic and epidemiologic findings. Avian Dis. 40:665–671.

Loyd, A.B., Cumming, R.B., and Kent, R.D. 1977. Prevention of *Salmonella typhimurium* infection in poultry by pretreatment of chickens and poults with intestinal extracts. Aust. Vet. J. 53:82–87.

Mead, G.C. 1991. Developments in competitive exclusion to control *Salmonella* carriage in poultry. In: Blankenship, L.C., ed. Colonization control of human bacterial enteropathogens in poultry. San Diego, CA: Academic, pp. 91–104.

Mead, G.C., and Barrow, P.A. 1990. *Salmonella* control in poultry by competitive exclusion or immunization. Lett. Appl. Microbiol. 10:221–227.

Mead, G.C., and Impey, C.S. 1984. Control of *Salmonella* colonization in poultry flocks by defined gut-flora treatment. In: Snoeyenbos, G.H., ed. Proceedings of the international symposium on *Salmonella*. Kennett Square, PA: American Association Avian Pathologist, pp. 72–79.

Mead, G.C., and Impey, C.S. 1986. Current progress in reducing *Salmonella* colonization of poultry by competitive exclusion. J. Appl. Bacteriol. 61(Suppl.):S67–S75.

Metchnikoff, E. 1908. Prolongation of life. New York: G.P. Putnam and Sons.

Mulder, R.W.A.W., and Bolder, N.M. 1991. Experience with competitive exclusion in the Netherlands. In: Blankenship, L.C., ed. Colonization control of human bacterial enteropathogens in poultry. San Diego, CA: Academic, pp. 77–89.

Nisbet, D.J., Corrier, D.E., and DeLoach, J.R. 1993. Effect of mixed cecal microflora maintained in continuous culture and dietary lactose on *Salmonella typhimurium* colonization in broiler chicks. Avian Dis. 37:528–535.

Nisbet, D.J., Ricke, S.C., Scanlan, C.M., Corrier, D.E., Hollister, A.G., and DeLoach, J.R. 1994. Inoculation of broiler chicks with a continuous-flow derived bacterial culture facilitates early cecal bacterial colonization and increases resistance to *Salmonella typhimurium*. J. Food Prot. 57:12–15.

Nisbet, D.J., Corrier, D.E., and DeLoach, J.R. 1995. Probiotic for control of *Salmonella*. U.S. Patent 5,478,557; 26 December.

Nisbet, D.J., Tellez, G., Kogut, M.H., Corrier, D.E., Lowry, D.K., Hernandez, L., Gonzales, J., and DeLoach, J.R. 1996. Inhibition of horizontal spread of *Salmonella gallinarum* in broiler chicks by a defined competitive exclusion culture (CF3™). Poult. Sci. 75(Suppl. 1):95.

Nurmi, E., and Rantala, M. 1973. New aspects of *Salmonella* infection in broiler production. Nature 241:210–211.

O'Brien, J.D.P. 1990. Aspects of *Salmonella enteritidis* control in poultry. World Poult. Sci. J. 46:119–124.

Pivnick, H., and Nurmi, E. 1982. The Nurmi concept and its role in the control of salmonellae in poultry. In: Davies, R., ed. Developments in food microbiology, vol. 1. Essex, UK: Applied Sciences, pp. 41–70.

Rantala, M., and Nurmi, E. 1973. Prevention of the growth of *Salmonella infantis* in chickens by flora of the alimentary tract of chickens. Br. Poult. Sci. 14:627–630.

Rolfe, R.D. 1991. Population dynamics of the intestinal tract. In: Blankenship, L.C., ed. Colonization control of human bacterial enteropathogens in poultry. San Diego, CA: Academic, pp. 59–75.

Sakata, M., Aoki, F., Vollendorf, N., and DeLoach, J.R. 1997. Comparison of three competitive exclusion products' ability to increase cecal propionic acid in chickens and use of CF3™ against *Salmonella enteritidis* in Japan. Poult. Sci. 76(Suppl. 1):110.

Savage, D.C. 1987. Factors influencing biocontrol of bacterial pathogens in the intestine. Food Technol. 41:82–87.

Schneitz, C. 1992. Automated droplet application of a competitive exclusion preparation. Poult. Sci. 71:2125–2128.

Stavric, S. 1987. Microbial colonization control of chicken intestine using defined cultures. Food Technol. 41:93–98.

Stavric, S. 1992. Defined cultures and prospects. Int. J. Food Microbiol. 55:245–263.

Stavric, S., and D'Aoust, J.Y. 1993. Undefined and defined bacterial preparations for the competitive exclusion of *Salmonella* in poultry: a review. J. Food Prot. 56:173–180.

Stavric, S., Gleeson, T.M., Blanchfield, B., and Pivnick, H. 1985. Competitive exclusion of *Salmonella* from newly hatched chicks by mixtures of pure bacterial cultures isolated from fecal and cecal contents of adult birds. J. Food Prot. 48:778–783.

Stavric, S., and Kornegay, E.T. 1995. Microbial probiotics for pigs and poultry. In: Wallace, R.J., and Chesson, A., eds. Biotechnology in animal feeds and animal feeding. New York: VCH, pp. 205–231.

St. Louis, M.E., Morse, D.L., Potter, M.E., DeMelfi, T.M., Guzewick, J.J., Tauxe, R.V., and Blake, P.A. 1988. The emergence of grade A eggs as a major source of *Salmonella enteritidis* infections: new implications for the control of salmonellosis. JAMA 259:2103–2107.

Van der Waaij, D., Berghuis-de Vries, J.M., and Lekkerkerk-Van der Wees, J.E.C. 1971. Colonization resistance of the digestive tract in conventional and antibiotic-treated mice. J. Hyg. 59:405–411.

Wierup, M., Wold-Troell, M., Nurmi, E., and Hakkinen, M. 1988. Epidemiological evaluation of the *Salmonella*-controlling effect of a nationwide use of a competitive exclusion culture in poultry. Poult. Sci. 67:1026–1033.

36

Vaccination against *Salmonella enterica* Serovar Enteritidis Infection: Dilemma and Realities

K.V. Nagaraja and G. Rajashekara

SALMONELLAE AS FOODBORNE PATHOGENS

Salmonellosis is a communicable human disease and is generally associated with the consumption of foods of animal origin that may have contained viable salmonellae. Salmonellosis is also a concern for the poultry industry, because contaminated poultry can serve as a vehicle for the disease transmission.

Foodborne infections cause an estimated 6.5 million cases of human illness and 9000 deaths annually in the United States. Salmonella infection is the third most commonly reported infectious disease in the United States. In 1995, more than 42,000 culture-confirmed cases of salmonellosis were reported in the United States, a 5% increase compared with 1994. Among many salmonella serovars, *Salmonella enterica* serovar Enteritidis (*S.* Enteritidis) is an important foodborne enteric pathogen. In the last few years, *S.* Enteritidis has become the predominant clinical isolate in the United States. Among the 20 salmonella serovars most frequently reported to the Centers for Disease Control and Prevention (CDC), *S.* Enteritidis was the serovar most often reported from nonhuman sources in 1992 (CDC, 1992). During 1985–92, health departments throughout the United States reported 437 *S.* Enteritidis outbreaks, which accounted for 15,162 cases of illness, 1734 hospitalizations, and 53 deaths (CDC, 1993). Epidemiological studies have attributed the outbreaks of *S.* Enteritidis food poisoning to the consumption of contaminated egg products (St. Louis et al., 1988; Hedberg et al., 1993). In 1991, eggs were implicated as the source of infection in 31 of 104 *S.* Enteritidis outbreaks investigated in the United States (Dreesen et al., 1992). In 1994, the U.S. Department of Agriculture, Animal and Plant Health Inspection Service (APHIS), Veterinary Division, reported 38 outbreaks of *S.* Enteritidis in the United States, and eggs were implicated in 12 of the outbreaks (APHIS, 1995). Overall, *S.* Enteritidis remains the leading cause of foodborne infection in many parts of the world, causing great concern over the safety of imported food products.

CURRENT UNDERSTANDING OF THE PATHOGENESIS OF SALMONELLAE

Salmonellae are Gram-negative, non-spore-forming, facultative anaerobic bacteria that can survive in a wide variety of environmental conditions and nutritional substrates. The main route of entry of salmonella organisms during infection is believed to be the intestinal mucosa, and subsequent invasion of the organism into the epithelial cell lining is essentially the first step in establishing infection (Groisman et al., 1990). The entry of salmonellae into the epithelial cells is associated with a series of pathological changes, beginning with the appearance of an active Golgi apparatus and the production of a variety of lysosomal vesicles (Poppiel and Turnbull, 1985). After gaining entrance into the host, the bacteria either multiply in the intestine or penetrate the intestinal mucosa and enter the lymphoid tissue of the small intestine. They either produce an enterotoxin that causes diarrhea or invade and multiply within the intestinal mucosa, causing mucosal damage and fluid loss (Gorbach, 1971; Poppiel and Turnbull, 1985; Potter, 1989). Two types of toxins have been reported from salmonellae: a heat-labile enterotoxin that increases the cyclic AMP levels and a cytotoxin that inhibits protein synthesis of the host cells during salmonella infection (Groisman et al., 1990). This provides a molecular explanation for the cellular damage observed. The organism gains access to the circulation, enters the reticuloendothelial system, and multiplies within splenic and hepatic tissues. Generally, this bacteria has the ability to invade nonphagocytic cells, withstand the antibacterial action in the phagolysosomes, and survive within macrophages (Poppiel and Turnbull, 1985; Finlay and Falkow, 1989).

Even though salmonella infection rarely causes clinical disease in adult birds, a high proportion of survivors are likely to remain carriers and become asymptomatic excreters (Gordon, 1990). Such excretion rapidly increases the spread of infection in poultry flocks. The invasive nature of S. Enteritidis can result in it being present in the ovary and oviduct in a small percentage of healthy recovered birds (Anon., 1988; Cooper et al., 1994). Vertical transmission from hens to progeny or table eggs has been well documented for S. Enteritidis (Turnbull and Snoeyenbos, 1974; Poppiel and Turnbull, 1985; Baird-Parker, 1990; Nagaraja et al., 1991).

WHAT DO WE KNOW ABOUT IMMUNITY TO SALMONELLAE?

Immunity to salmonella infection has been studied extensively in mice (Lillehoj and Chung, 1991). Host responses to intestinal microbial infections involve the complex interplay of soluble factors, leukocytes, epithelial cells, and other physiological factors of the gut-associated lymphoid tissue. Following infection, macrophage-dependent antigenic activation of T and B cells initiates a series of antigen-specific and nonspecific responses involving secretory immunoglobulins, local cells, and locally produced cytokines (Lillehoj and Chung, 1991). Although humoral immunity plays a primary role in preventing salmonella bacteremia and in negating some of the noxious effects of endotoxin (Desiderio and Campbell, 1985), intracellular multiplication of salmonellae can be controlled by the presence of T-lymphocyte-mediated response (Griffiths et al., 1983; Hancock et al., 1984; Desiderio and Campbell, 1985). Antigen-specific T cells play a critical role during the development of immunity to intracellular pathogens by the release of lymphokines, which increases the number and bactericidal action of tissue macrophages (Collins et al., 1966; Collins, 1974; Groisman et al., 1990). The

support for the idea that T cells are responsible for immunity to intracellular pathogens comes from results following experimental Salmonella Typhimurium infections in mice (Collins et al., 1966; Mackaness, 1971; Collins and Carter, 1972; Cooper et al., 1989).

IS VACCINATION A FEASIBLE APPROACH TO CONTROL SALMONELLA ENTERITIDIS INFECTION?

The development of vaccines to prevent human and poultry salmonellosis has been a major challenge in the field of immunology. Through the use of vaccines, some diseases have been eliminated while the incidence of a large number of infectious diseases has diminished. Vaccines are needed because the use of antibiotics in the treatment of many bacterial infections cannot prevent serious sequelae. The evolution of drug-resistant bacteria reduces the effect of antibiotics. From the public health and economic standpoint, an ideal salmonella vaccine is one that is safe to administer, eliminates the shedding of salmonellae, and enhances the clearance of the organism from the host. A vaccine that can meet these criteria will reduce the horizontal and vertical spread of S. Enteritidis definitely in poultry flocks. However, due to the paucity of information on colonization and immunity relating to the salmonella serovars that are usually associated with food poisoning, the development of vaccines for use in poultry has been slow.

Prophylactic vaccination is also a possible method of preventing vertical transmission of salmonellae. For the large-scale use of prophylactic vaccines, they must be both safe and effective. The effectiveness of these vaccines may vary with the method of preparation. Adjuvants of many types from alum-oil emulsions to polynucleotides have been used in prophylactic vaccines with a variety of diseases. An ideal vaccine should mimic the immunological stimulation associated with natural infection, evoke minimal side effects, and be readily available, cheap, stable, and easily administered. A number of experimental studies have been reported on the use of bacterins and attenuated live cultures as vaccines in the prevention of avian salmonellosis, but they have never been performed widely under field conditions. Components extracted from salmonellae, such as ribosomes or supernatant factors or polysaccharide-protein conjugates, have also been investigated as potential candidates for new vaccines.

INACTIVATED VACCINES FOR SALMONELLAE

Experimental inactivated S. Enteritidis phage type 4 (PT4) vaccine has been examined in chickens. A single subcutaneous vaccination at 3 weeks or two vaccinations at 3 and 6 weeks provided good protection against challenge with 10^9 colony-forming units (CFU) or 10^8 CFU of virulent S. Enteritidis administered intramuscularly or intravenously (Gast et al., 1993). Oil-emulsion bacterins have been evaluated for reducing fecal shedding of *S.* Enteritidis (Gast et al., 1992, 1993; Nakamura et al., 1994).

In one experiment (Gast et al., 1993), an experimental vaccine prepared from acetone-killed *S.* Enteritidis oil emulsion and a commercially available vaccine were compared for protection of laying hens against intestinal colonization of *S.* Enteritidis following its oral administration. In this study, each vaccine was administered twice at 4-week intervals. Two weeks after the second vaccination, the hens were challenged orally with 10^8 CFU. Both vaccines significantly reduced the incidence of intestinal colonization and mean number of *S.* Enteritidis shed in the feces at 1 week after challenge. However, more than half of the vaccinated hens still shed *S.* Enteritidis (Gast et al., 1993).

In another investigation (Gast et al., 1992), acetone-killed oil-emulsion vaccine prepared from *S.* Enteritidis PT13 was given to 23- and 45-week-old hens. A second injection was given 6 weeks after the first, and, 3 weeks after the second vaccination, all hens were challenged with an oral administration of 10^9 cells of *S.* Enteritidis PT14b. In both groups of hens, *S.* Enteritidis was isolated from fewer internal organs and pools of egg contents from vaccinated hens than from unvaccinated controls. Subcutaneous inoculation at 3 weeks or at 3 and 6 weeks of age with a formalin-inactivated oil-adjuvant *S.* Enteritidis PT4 vaccine containing 10^{11} CFU/ml protected chickens against a massive experimental challenge with 10^9 CFU by either intramuscular or intravenous administration at 5 or 8 weeks of age (Timms et al., 1990).

Numerous experiments in mice with *S.* Typhimurium and *S.* Enteritidis infections have shown that inactivated parenteral vaccines failed to elicit significant cell-mediated immunity (Collins, 1969a, 1972, 1974; Choi et al., 1989). Production of poor, inconsistent protective immunity with killed vaccines may be due to the rapid destruction and elimination of the organism from the host system and also the destruction of the relevant antigens during vaccine preparation (Barrow, 1991). Inactivated vaccines, despite eliciting acceptable levels of humoral immunity, are poor inducers of the T-cell-mediated immunity (Collins, 1974; Mackaness et al., 1976; Arnon et al., 1989) required to enhance the local mucosal immune response to prevent colonization of salmonellae in the gut and curtail the subsequent systemic spread of the organism. The protective efficacy of inactivated vaccines is further limited by their low immunogenicity especially in unprimed hosts and their inability to induce cytolytic T cells (Kaeberle, 1986). Inactivated whole-cell vaccines have generally produced poor and inconsistent protection against the fecal excretion of challenged salmonellae, both in vaccinated poultry flocks and in their progeny (Truscott, 1981; Timms et al., 1990; Gast et al., 1992). Serum antibody titers are of uncertain value as indicators of the overall extent of protection against salmonellae.

LIVE VACCINES AGAINST *SALMONELLA* ENTERITIDIS

Live attenuated vaccines against salmonellosis have been more effective in reducing mortality and shedding than have killed vaccines. Live vaccines may invade host cells, and their efficacy may be due to their particular distribution within the body, as well as to their capability of stimulating cell-mediated immunity. Live attenuated vaccines confer a level of immunity that is normally seen after infection with virulent organisms (Desiderio and Campbell, 1985; Knivett and Tucker, 1991). However, live vaccines have to comply with three important criteria: the attenuation needs to be sufficient to prevent symptomatic disease, they should prevent effective colonization of the intestine, and their reversion to virulence should be negligible (Germanier and Furer, 1971).

USE OF *AROA* MUTANTS OF *SALMONELLA* ENTERITIDIS AS VACCINE CANDIDATES

The *aro*A mutants are derived from virulent *S.* Enteritidis PT4 isolated from chickens that had reduced intraperitoneal virulence by up to 6 log in a Balb/c mouse model. They did not kill 18- to 20-day-old chickens when injected intravenously and did not multiply in tissues (Cooper et al., 1992). Protection against oral and intravenous challenge with *S.* Enteritidis in 8-week-old chickens and 23-week-old laying hens was evaluated after vaccination with strain CVL30, a genetically defined *S.* Enteritidis *aro*A live vaccine (Cooper et al., 1994). Additionally, newly hatched chicks were vaccinated with 10^5 or 10^9 CFU of live *aro*A vaccine and challenged by the intravenous route with 10^8 CFU of *S.* Enteritidis at 8 weeks of age. Reduction in colonization of the spleens, livers, and ceca was seen in the vaccinated compared with unvaccinated birds. The effects of vaccination of chickens with genetically stable, double-attenuated *S.* Enteritidis live oral vaccine have been investigated (Springer and Selbitz, 1997). In that study, newly hatched chicks were vaccinated orally with live, genetically altered mutants of *S.* Enteritidis on days 2 and 16. The vaccinated birds were challenged orally with a homologous *S.* Enteritidis strain 3 weeks after the last vaccination. There was a significant reduction in colonization of challenged *S.* Enteritidis in the liver and cecum of the vaccinated birds.

TEMPERATURE-SENSITIVE MUTANTS OF *SALMONELLA* ENTERITIDIS AS VACCINE STRAINS

A temperature-sensitive mutant of *S.* Enteritidis has been examined for its efficacy against *S.* Enteritidis challenge in mice (Gherardi et al., 1993). It was shown to confer significant protection against challenge-induced local and systemic humoral immunity. The safety of vaccine strains is essential, and the inclusion of two separate mutations conferring the "Ts coaster" phenotype would be advisable because this should diminish the chance of reversion. A similar approach with *S.* Enteritidis has also been examined by others (Ohta et al., 1987). Their mutants had ultraviolet-light-induced mutations, but the one that failed to revert unfortunately did not induce the highest level of immunity.

PLASMID-CURED STRAINS OF *SALMONELLA* ENTERITIDIS AS VACCINE CANDIDATES

It has been shown that large molecular weight plasmids are associated with virulence of the organism. Plasmid-cured strains that have been made avirulent or are of reduced virulence have proved immunogenic and protective against infection. *Salmonella* Enteritidis that was cured of a 36-kDa plasmid was shown to protect mice against challenge with virulent *S.* Enteritidis (Nakamura et al., 1985). The problem of reversion to virulence still is possible even though the plasmids may be non-self-transmissible (Barrow, 1991).

New attenuated vaccines, generated by transposon mutagenesis, are becoming available for *S.* Typhimurium. By deletion of the transposon together with part of the gene into which it has been inserted, a deletion mutant can be produced that will remove the danger of reversion of the mutant to virulence.

OUTER-MEMBRANE PROTEINS FROM SALMONELLAE ARE VERY GOOD IMMUNOGENS

Interest in the development of an effective vaccine has led researchers to explore the possibility of using outer-membrane proteins (OMPs) from Gram-negative bacteria as potential vaccine candidates (Montaraz et al., 1985; Gogolewski et al., 1988). The majority of studies of salmonella OMP for potential vaccines have used mice (Kuusi et al., 1979, 1981; Natarajan et al., 1985; Lillehoj and Chung, 1991). Several studies have demonstrated that OMPs from salmonellae possess antigenic determinants for the stimulation of both humoral and cell-mediated immunity and provide long-lasting protection against salmonella infection (Kuusi et al., 1979, 1981; Vaidya et al., 1985; Bouzoubaa et al., 1987, 1989; Udhayakumar and Muthukkaruppan, 1987; Isibasi et al., 1988; Muthukkaruppan et al., 1992). The use of cellular proteins from *Salmonella* Gallinarum for prevention of typhoid infection in chickens has been reported (Bouzoubaa et al., 1987, 1989). It was concluded that cellular proteins can be used as vaccines in chickens to protect against a lethal challenge. These vaccines were capable of inducing an immune response that cleared *S.* Gallinarum from the ovary and thus reduced egg transmission.

OMPs isolated from both smooth and rough strains of *S.* Typhimurium are known to be good protective antigens in mice (Bhatnagar et al., 1982; Udhayakumar and Muthukkaruppan, 1987). It has been demonstrated that OMPs were valuable immunogens for the prevention of typhoid fever, and the cross-protection observed between *S.* Typhi and *S.* Typhimurium indicates that they share common epitopes (Kaeberle, 1986). The salmonella OMPs can induce humoral as well as cellular immunity to mediate protection (Udhayakumar and Muthukkaruppan, 1987; Banco et al., 1993).

Adjuvant OMPs from *S.* Enteritidis have been evaluated for their protective efficacy against *S.* Enteritidis infection in turkeys (Charles et al., 1994). In that study, the adjuvant vaccines prepared with OMPs of *S.* Enteritidis were either positively or negatively charged liposomes, lipid-conjugated immunostimulating complexes (ISCOMs), or mineral-oil vaccines. After vaccination, turkeys were challenge exposed with a nalidixic acid-resistant strain of *S.* Enteritidis. Results indicated a significantly higher antibody response ($p < 0.5$) to the positively charged liposomal OMP vaccine compared with the whole-cell bacterin. Shedding of *S.* Enteritidis was reduced in all vaccinated and challenge-exposed turkeys ($p < 0.001$). The tissues from 90% to 100% of birds that received a booster vaccination of the liposomal (+ or −) or ISCOM vaccine were culture negative for *S.* Enteritidis.

Cross-protection against *S.* Enteritidis by *S.* Gallinarum has been examined by many researchers. Vaccination of mice with *S.* Gallinarum is shown to produce immunity against *S.* Enteritidis (Collins, 1969b). The 9R strain of *S.* Gallinarum has been investigated for its capability to protect laying hens against experimental *S.* Enteritidis PT4 infection (Barrow, 1991). *Salmonella* Enteritidis colonization in spleen, liver, and ovary was reduced in hens given 9R *S.* Gallinarum intramuscularly.

A number of studies done at the Avian Health Research Program at the University of Minnesota have successfully demonstrated that vaccines can be used to control shedding of salmonellae (Pritchard et al., 1978; Nagaraja et al., 1981, 1982a,b, 1984a,b, 1985, 1987, 1988a,b, 1991; Poppiel and Turnbull, 1985; Pomeroy et al., 1989). In one investigation, a vaccine against *S.* Enteritidis in chickens was investigated. Experiments were conducted with whole-cell bacterin and a vaccine made from OMPs from *S.* Enteritidis. The results were encouraging. The following report presents this particular study in detail.

Materials and Methods

Forty-two-week old purebred leghorn chickens ascertained to be free from *S.* Enteritidis infection were used. Salmonella-free feed containing no antibiotics was used. Clean water was provided ad libitum.

ISOLATION OF OUTER-MEMBRANE PROTEINS

Salmonella Enteritidis was grown on tryptic soy agar in Roux flasks at 37°C for 48 h. At the end of the incubation, the bacterial cells were harvested from the flasks with 10 mM HEPES buffer (pH 7.4). The bacterial cell suspension was centrifuged at 12,000 g for 30 min. The resulting bacterial pellet was collected and resuspended in 10 mM HEPES buffer. The bacterial cells in the resuspension were disrupted by passing them through a French press at 15,000–20,000 lb/inch. Intact cells and large debris were removed by centrifugation at 4000 g for 20 min. Total membrane preparation was harvested from the super-natant by centrifugation at 100,000 g for 60 min at 4°C. The gel-like pellet was resuspended in 10 mM HEPES buffer and extracted with an equal volume of a detergent solution (2% sodium lauryl sarcosinate in 10 mM HEPES buffer, pH 7.4) overnight at 4°C. The detergent-insoluble fraction was harvested by centrifugation of the suspension at 100,000 g for 60 min at 4°C, and the pellet was resuspended in distilled water. The protein concentration of the pellet was determined by the Bradford (1976) protein assay method, and the final concentration was adjusted to 4 mg/ml.

Formalin-killed mineral-oil-adjuvant bacterin was pre-pared for use. In brief, S. Enteritidis was grown on tryptic soy agar in Roux flasks for 48 h at 37°C. Bacterial cells were harvested in normal saline. The concentration of the bacte-rial suspension was adjusted to contain 10^{11} CFU/ml. The purity of the culture was examined by inoculating brilliant-green-agar plates. The bacterial culture was killed by adding 0.3% formalin with agitation. To prepare the oil emulsion of the bacterin, equal volumes of formalin-killed aqueous bacterial suspension and mineral oil with an emulsifier (Arlacel A) were mixed well in a Waring blender to obtain a homogeneous oil emulsion of the bacterin.

EXPERIMENT

The chickens were individually wing banded and randomly distributed. They were divided into three groups designated 1, 2, and 3. Each group contained 30 birds, and all birds were ascertained to be S. Enteritidis free by cloacal swabs and serological testing a week before use. Birds in group 1 were vaccinated with OMP extracts in oil emulsion at 2 mg per bird, and birds in group 2 were vaccinated with 0.5 ml of the oil emulsion of the bacterin. Vaccinations in groups 1 and 2 were performed subcutaneously. The birds in group 3 were kept as unvaccinated controls. Each group of birds was further divided into two subgroups designated A and B. Birds in subgroup A were challenged orally at 4 weeks after vaccination with 1 ml of broth culture containing 10^7 CFU/ml of live S. Enteritidis, and birds in subgroup B were kept as vaccinated but unchallenged controls. Cloacal-swab samples were collected from all birds at weekly inter-vals until the end of the experiment. After challenge, daily

mortality was checked, and any birds found dead were cul-tured for S. Enteritidis. All birds were killed 4 weeks after challenge. All internal organs were examined for lesions, and tissues from liver, spleen, ovary, oviduct, bone marrow, and ileocecal junction were cultured for S. Enteritidis. Blood samples from all birds were collected at weekly inter-vals after vaccination and were tested by the microaggluti-nation test for the presence of antibodies to S. Enteritidis.

ANALYSIS

All culture samples from cloacal swabs and internal organs were enriched in tetrathionate broth for 24 h at 42°C, fol-lowed by streaking on brilliant-green-agar plates and incu-bating for 24 h at 37°C. Colonies resembling salmonellae were transferred to triple-sugar iron agar. Cultures showing a typical salmonella reaction were confirmed serologically.

Results

Table 36.1 shows the results of the microagglutination tests. Chickens in groups 1 and 2 vaccinated with OMP and killed bacterin, respectively, showed a positive sero-conversion. Antibody titers increased after challenge in the vaccinated birds. In general, the geometrical mean anti-body titers in birds injected with OMP vaccine were higher than in the bacterin-injected group.

Table 36.2 shows the isolation of S. Enteritidis from cloacal-swab culture. Birds in groups 1 and 2 showed a very low isolation rate from the cloacal-swab culture after chal-lenge. In the OMP-injected group, only one bird yielded S. Enteritidis. In the control unvaccinated but challenged group, a very high percentage of birds yielded S. Enteritidis in their cloacal swabs for 2 weeks after challenge.

The results of the isolation of S. Enteritidis from tissues are summarized in Table 36.3. Two birds in the OMP-vacci-nated group and three birds in the group given killed bacterin showed S. Enteritidis. In the control unvaccinated but chal-lenged group, six of 13 birds had S. Enteritidis in the tissues.

Discussion

It is evident from previous work that protein antigens are important for protection. Most of the studies on the induction

TABLE 36.1 Geometrical means of *Salmonella* Enteritidis antibody titers using microagglutination (MA) test

Group	Treatment	Subgroup[a]	MA titers on weeks after vaccination							
			1	2	3	4[b]	5	6	7	8
1	Protein (2 mg/bird)	A	1.6	4.1	5.3	3.7	7.0	4.5	4.0	3.3
		B	1.7	3.9	6.0	3.5	3.4	2.7	2.4	2.0
2	Bacterin	A	1.2	2.5	3.6	5.0	5.7	3.9	3.6	2.8
		B	1.5	2.8	3.8	4.2	3.0	2.5	2.4	2.0
3	Control	A	0.0	0.0	0.0	0.0	2.6	2.5	2.9	3.0
		B	0.0	0.0	0.0	0.0	0.0	0.0	0.0	0.0

[a]Subgroups: A, challenged birds; and B, unchallenged birds.
[b]Birds were challenged orally at 4 weeks after vaccination with live S. Enteritidis.

TABLE 36.2 Isolation of *Salmonella* Enteritidis from cloacal-swab culture

Group	Treatment	Subgroup[a]	No. positive per no. total on weeks after vaccination							
			1	2	3	4[b]	5	6	7	8
1	Protein(2 mg/bird)	A	0/15	0/15	0/15	0/15	0/15	1/15	0/15	0/15
		B	0/15	0/15	0/15	0/15	0/15	1/15	0/15	0/14
2	Bacterin	A	0/15	0/15	0/15	0/15	2/15	2/15	1/14	0/14
		B	0/15	0/15	0/15	0/15	0/15	1/15	0/15	0/15
3	Control	A	0/15	0/15	0/15	0/15	9/15	8/13	3/13	3/13
		B	0/15	0/15	0/15	0/15	0/15	1/15	0/15	0/15

[a]Subgroups: A, challenged birds; and B, unchallenged birds.
[b]Birds were challenged orally at 4 weeks after vaccination with live S. Enteritidis.

TABLE 36.3 Isolation rate of *Salmonella* Enteritidis from tissues

Group	Treatment	Subgroup[b]	No. positive tissue[a]/total tissues						Total positive[c]	Positive (%)[d]
			Liver	Spleen	Ovary	Oviduct	Bone marrow	Cecal juction		
1	Protein (2mg/bird)	A	1/15	2/15	1/15	0/15	0/15	2/15	2	13.3
		B	0/14	0/14	0/14	1/14	1/14	1/14	0	0
2	Bacterin	A	2/14	2/14	2/14	1/14	0/14	2/14	2	13.3
		B	0/15	0/15	0/15	0/15	0/15	0/15	0	0
3	Control	A	5/13	5/13	4/13	4/13	5/13	6/13	6	46.2
		B	0/15	0/15	0/15	0/15	0/15	0/15	0	0

[a]No. of isolates of S. Enteritidis.
[b]Subgroups: A: challenged birds; B: unchallenged birds.
[c]Total positive for at least one tissue.
[d]Percent positive for at least one tissue.

of protective immunity by such protein antigens have been performed with mice and rabbits. The conclusions made from these studies are that OMPs elicit an antibody response in both animals and humans and that OMPs hold much promise for safer, more useful vaccines against a number of Gram-negative bacterial infections.

In the present study, sarkosyl was used to prepare detergent-insoluble fractions from *S.* Enteritidis outer membranes. The fractions were enriched greatly with OMPs. The sarcosinate extraction procedure described in the present study is less time consuming and technically simpler. This procedure will result in very efficient porin extraction. The porins form the basis of the outer-membrane structure in Gram-negative bacteria and are very important immunogens. However, this procedure may not result in the extraction of minor protein material.

This study also demonstrated that OMP extracts at certain levels induced an immune response that cleared the organism following challenge. The results of culture of the ileocecal junction indicated the clearance of the organism following challenge in vaccinated groups.

The OMPs used in the present study are suspected to contain some lipopolysaccharide (LPS). Some LPS core types have been considered to provoke antibody production. In previous studies, however, LPS or anti-LPS antibodies in OMP preparation were considered unlikely to be responsible for the protection. The OMP preparation was found to be superior to killed bacterins in terms of protection and clearance of *S.* Enteritidis after challenge. These results support earlier findings that demonstrated the protective activity of protein extract from salmonellae. Besides the promising protective ability of the OMP preparation, it is necessary to eliminate the LPS from the preparation so as to reduce endotoxic activity.

The results of the present work are encouraging enough to justify future work on the development of a more effective and less toxic salmonella vaccine.

REFERENCES

Animal and Plant Health Inspection Service (APHIS). 1995. Veterinary services *S.* Enteritidis control prog-status report, 17 January. Washington, DC: U.S. Department of Agriculture.

Anonymous. 1988. *Salmonella enteritidis* in poultry. Vet. Rec. 15:123.

Arnon, R. Shapira, M., and Jacob, C.O. 1989. Synthetic vaccines. J. Immunol. Methods 61:261-273.

Baird-Parker, A.C. 1990. Food borne salmonellosis. Lancet 336:1231–1235.

Banco, F., Isibasi, A., Gonzalez, C.R., Ortiz, V., Paniagua, J., Arreguin, C., and Kumate, J. 1993. Human cell mediated immunity to porins from *Salmonella typhi*. Scand. J. Infect. Dis. 25:73–80.

Barrow, P.A. 1991. Immunological control of *Salmonella* in poultry. In: Blackenship, L.C., eds. Colonization control of human bacterial enteropathogens in poultry. San Diego, CA: Academic, pp. 199–217.

Bhatnagar, N., Muller, W., and Schlecht, S. 1982. Proteins from *Salmonella* R-mutants mediating protection against *Salmonella typhimurium* infection in mice. I. Preparation of proteins free from LPS using various chromatographic methods. Zentralbl. Bakteriol. Hyg. 1 Abt. Orig. A 253:88–101.

Bouzoubaa, K., Nagaraja, K.V., Kabbaj, F.Z., Newman, J.A., and Pomeroy, B.S. 1987. Use of membrane proteins from *Salmonella gallinarum* for the prevention of fowl typhoid infection in chickens. Avian Dis. 31:699–704.

Bouzoubaa, K., Nagaraja, K.V., Kabbaj, F.Z., Newman, J.A., and Pomeroy, B.S. 1989. Feasibility of using proteins from *Salmonella gallinarum* vs. 9R live vaccine for the prevention of fowl typhoid in chickens. Avian Dis. 33:385–391.

Bradford, M. 1976. A rapid and sensitive method for the quantitation of microgram quantities of protein utilizing the principle of protein-dye binding. Anal. Biochem. 72:248–254.

Centers for Disease Control and Prevention (CDC). 1992. CDC report: U.S. Animal Health Association Meeting, Louisville, Kentucky, 31 October–6 November.

Centers for Disease Control and Prevention (CDC). 1993. Outbreaks of *Salmonella enteritidis* gastroenteritis: California. MMWR 42:793–797.

Charles, S.D., Hussain, I., Choi, C., Nagaraja, K.V., and Sivanandan, V. 1994. Adjuvanted subunit vaccines for the control of *Salmonella enteritidis* infection in turkeys. Am. J. Vet. Res. 55:636–642.

Choi, K.H., Maheswaran, S.K., and Felice, L.J. 1989. Characterization of outer membrane protein–enriched extracts from *Pasteurella multocida* isolated from turkeys. Am. J. Vet. Res. 50:676–683.

Collins, F.M. 1969a. Effect of immune mouse serum on the growth of *Salmonella enteritidis* in non vaccinated mice challenged by various routes. J. Bacteriol. 97:667–675.

Collins, F.M. 1969b. Effect of specific immune mouse serum on the growth of *Salmonella enteritidis* in mice preimmunized with live or ethyl alcohol–killed vaccines. J. Bacteriol. 97:676.

Collins, F.M. 1974. Vaccines and cell mediated immunity. Bacteriol. Rev. 38:371–402.

Collins, F.M., and Carter, P.B. 1972. Comparative immunogenicity of heat-killed and living oral *Salmonella* vaccines. Infect. Immun. 6:451–458.

Collins, F.M., Mackaness, G.B., and Blanden, R.V. 1966. Infection immunity in experimental salmonellosis. J. Exp. Med. 124:601–619.

Cooper, G.L., Nicholas, R.A., and Bracewell, C.D. 1989. Serological and bacteriological investigations of chickens from flocks naturally infected with *Salmonella enteritidis*. Vet. Rec. 125:567–572.

Cooper, G.L., Venables, L.M., Nicholas, R.A.J., Cullen, G.A., and Hormaeche, C.E. 1992. Vaccination of chicken derived *Salmonella enteritidis* phage-type 4 *aro A* live oral *Salmonella* vaccine. Vaccine 10:247–254.

Cooper, G.L., Venables, L.M., Woodward, M.J., and Hormaeche, C.E. 1994. Vaccination of chickens with strain CVL30, genetically defined *Salmonella enteritidis aroA* live oral vaccine candidate. Infect. Immun. 62:4747–4754.

Desiderio, J.V., and Campbell, S.G. 1985. Immunization against experimental murine salmonellosis with liposome-associated O-antigen. Infect. Immun. 48:658–663.

Dreesen D.W., Barnhart, H.M., Burke, J.L., Chen, T., and Johnson, D.C. 1992. Frequency of *Salmonella enteritidis* and other salmonellae in the ceca of spent hens at the time of slaughter. Avian Dis. 36:247–250.

Finlay, B.B., and Falkow, S. 1989. Common themes in microbial pathogenicity. Microbiol. Rev. 53:210–230.

Gast, R.K., Stone, H.D., Holt, P.S., and Beard, C.W. 1992. Evaluation of the efficacy of an oil-emulsion bacterin for protecting chickens against *Salmonella enteritidis*. Avian Dis. 36:992–999.

Gast, R.K., Stone, H.D., and Holt, P.S. 1993. Evaluation of the efficacy of oil-emulsion bacterins for reducing fecal shedding of *Salmonella enteritidis* in laying hens. Avian Dis. 37:1085–1091.

Germanier, R., and Furer, E. 1971. Immunity in experimental salmonellosis. II. Basis for the avirulence and protective capacity of gal E. mutants of *Salmonella typhimurium*. Infect. Immun. 4:663–673.

Gherardi, M.M., Garcia, V.E., Sordelli, D.O., and Cerquetti, M.C. 1993. Protective capacity of a temperature sensitive mutant of *Salmonella enteritidis* after oral and intragastric inoculation in a murine model. Vaccine 11:19–24.

Gogolewski, R.P., Kania, S.A., Liggitt, H.D., and Corbeil, L.B. 1988. Protective ability of antibodies against 78- and 40-kilodalton outer membrane antigens of *Haemophilus somnus*. Infect. Immun. 56:2307–2316.

Gorbach, S.L. 1971. Intestinal microflora. Gastroenterology 60:1110–1129.

Gordon, R. 1990. Enterobacteriaceae. In: Jordan, F.T.W., ed. Poultry diseases. London: Bailliere Tindall, pp. 2–41.

Griffiths, E., Stevenson, P., and Joyce, P. 1983. Pathogenic *Escherichia coli* express new outer membrane proteins when growing in vivo. FEMS Microbiol. Lett. 16:95–99.

Groisman, E.A., Fields, P.I., and Heffron, H. 1990. Molecular biology of *Salmonella* pathogenesis. In: Gunsalus, I.C., Sokatch, J.R., and Ornston, L.N., eds. The bacteria: a treatise on structure and function. New York: Academic, pp. 251–272.

Hancock, F.E., Movat, W.E.C., and Speert, D.P. 1984. Quantitation and identification of antibodies to outer membrane proteins of *Pseudomonas aeruginosa* in sera of patients with cystic fibrosis. J. Infect. Dis. 149:220–226.

Hedberg, C.W., David, M.J., White, K.E., MacDonald, K.L., and Osterholm, M.T. 1993. Role of egg consumption in sporadic *Salmonella enteritidis* of phage type 4 for chickens and *Salmonella typhimurium* infections in Minnesota. J. Infect. Dis. 167:107–111.

Isibasi, A., Ortiz, V., Vargas, M., Paniagua, J., Gonzalez, C., Moreno, J., and Kumate, J. 1988. Protection against *Salmonella typhi* infection in mice after immunization with outer membrane proteins isolated from *Salmonella* typhi 9, 12, d, Vi. Infect. Immun. 56:2953–2959.

Kaeberle, M.L. 1986. Function of carriers and adjuvants in induction of immune response. In: Nervig, R.M., Gough, P.M., and Kaeberle, M.L., eds. Advances in carriers and adjuvants for veterinary biologic, 1st ed. Ames: Iowa State University Press, pp. 11–23.

Knivett, V.A., and Tucker, J.F. 1991. The evaluation of a live *Salmonella* vaccine in mice and chickens. J. Hyg. 69:233–245.

Kuusi, N., Nuriminen, M., Saxen, H., Valtonen, M., and Makela, P.H. 1979. Immunization with major outer membrane proteins in experimental salmonellosis of mice. Infect. Immun. 25:857–862.

Kuusi, N., Nuriminen, M., Saxen, H., and Makela, P.H. 1981. Immunization with outer membrane protein preparations in experimental murine salmonellosis: effect of lipopolysaccharide. Infect. Immun. 34:328–332.

Lillehoj, H.S., and Chung, K.S. 1991. Intestinal immunity and genetic factors influencing colonization of microbes in the gut. In: Blankenship, L.C., ed. Colonization control of human bacterial enteropathogens in poultry. San Diego, CA: Academic, pp. 219–241.

Mackaness, G.B. 1971. Resistance to intracellular infection. J. Infect. Dis. 123:439–445.

Mackaness, G.B., Blanden, R.V., and Collins, F.M. 1976. Host-parasite relations in mouse typhoid. J. Exp. Med. 124:573–583.

Montaraz, J.A., Novotny, P., and Ivanyi, J. 1985. Identification of a 68-kilodalton protective protein antigen from *Bordetella bronchiseptica*. Infect. Immun. 47:744–751.

Muthukkaruppan, V.R., Nandakumar, K.S., and Palanivel, V. 1992. Monoclonal antibodies against *Salmonella* porins: generation and characterization. Immunol. Lett. 33:201–206.

Nagaraja, K.V., Nivas, S., Pomeroy, B.S., Newman, J.A., and Peterson, I. 1981. *Salmonella* feasibility studies in turkeys. Minn. Turkey Res. 179:112–115.

Nagaraja, K.V., Nivas, S., Pomeroy, B.S., Newman, J.A., and Peterson, I. 1982a. A three year study of *Salmonella arizonae*-free parent turkey breeding flocks. Am. Vet. Med. Assoc. 181:284.

Nagaraja, K.V., Pomeroy, B.S., Newman, J.A., and Peterson, I. 1982b. Vaccination of turkeys with killed oil adjuvant *Salmonella san-diego* vaccine. J. Am. Vet. Med. Assoc. 181:284.

Nagaraja, K.V., Emery, D.A., Sherlock, L.F., Newman, J.A., and Pomeroy, B.S. 1984a. Control of *Salmonella* by immunization. Minn. Turkey Res. 30:61–63.

Nagaraja, K.V., Newman, J.A., and Pomeroy, B.S. 1984b. Use of oil adjuvant vaccines for the control of *Salmonella* infections in turkeys. In: Proceedings of the international symposium on *Salmonella*, Kennett Square, PA, pp. 374–375.

Nagaraja, K.V., Kumar, M.C., Newman, J.A., and Pomeroy, B.S. 1985. Control of *Salmonella arizonae* infection in turkey breeding flocks by immunization. J. Am. Vet. Med. Assoc. 187:309.

Nagaraja, K.V., Pomeroy, B.S., Ausherman, L.T., and Friendshuh, K.A. 1987. *Salmonella* control programs in Minnesota Turkey Industry. In: Proceedings of the 23rd world veterinary congress, Montreal, Canada, p. 317.

Nagaraja, K.V., Bouzoubaa, K., and Pomeroy, B.S. 1988a. Prophylactic immunization with outer membrane proteins from *Salmonella gallinarum* for the prevention of fowl typhoid. In: Proceedings of the 37th Western Poultry Disease Conference, pp. 121–122.

Nagaraja, K.V., Kim, C.J., and Pomeroy, B.S. 1988b. Outer-membrane proteins in prophylactic vaccines for salmonella. J. Am. Vet. Med. Assoc. 192:1784.

Nagaraja, K.V., Pomeroy, B.S., and Williams, J.E. 1991. Paratyphoid infections. In: Calnek, B.W., Barnes, H.J., Beard, C.W., Reid, W.M., and Yoder, H.W., eds. Diseases of poultry, 9th ed. Ames: Iowa State University Press, 99–130.

Nakamura, M., Sato, S., Ohya, T., Suzuki, S., Ikeda, S., and Koeda, T. 1985. Plasmid-cured *Salmonella enteritidis* AL1192 as a candidate for a live vaccine. Infect. Immun. 50:586–587.

Nakamura, M., Nagamine, N., Takahashi, T., Suzuki, S., and Sato, S. 1994. Evaluation of the efficacy of a bacterin against *Salmonella enteritidis* infection and the effect of stress after vaccination. Avian Dis. 38:717–724.

Natarajan, M., Udhayakumar, V., Krishnaraju, K., and Muthukkaruppan, V.R. 1985. Role of outer-membrane proteins in immunity against murine salmonellosis. 1. Antibody response to crude outer-membrane proteins of *Salmonella typhimurium*. Comp. Immunol. Microbiol. Infect. Dis. 8:9–16.

Ohta, M., Kido, N., Fuji, Y., Arakawa, Y., Komatsu, T., and Kato, T. 1987. Temperature-sensitive growth mutants as live vaccines against experimental murine salmonellosis. Microbiol. Immunol. 31:1259–1265.

Pomeroy, B.S., Nagaraja, K.V., Ausherman, L.T., Peterson, I.L., and Friendshuh, K.A. 1989. Studies on feasibility of producing *Salmonella*-free turkeys. Avian Dis. 33:1–7.

Poppiel, I., and Turnbull, P.C.B. 1985. Passage of *Salmonella enteritidis* and *Salmonella thompson* through chick ileocecal mucosa. Infect. Immun. 47:786–792.

Potter, M.E. 1989. Public health significance of poultry infections by *Salmonella*, *Campylobacter* and *Listeria*. In: Avian enteric diseases symposium, AAAP/AVMA annual meeting, pp. 1–11.

Pritchard, D.G., Nivas, S.C., York, M.D., and Pomeroy, B.S. 1978. Effects of Gal-E mutant of *Salmonella typhimurium* of experimental salmonellosis in chickens. Avian Dis. 22:502–575.

Springer, S., and Selbitz, H.J. 1997. Effects of vaccination of chickens with genetically stable, double attenuated *Salmonella enteritidis* live oral vaccine candidates. In: Proceedings of the international symposium on *Salmonella* and salmonellosis, St. Brieuc, Ploufragan, France, pp. 507–510.

St. Louis, M.E., Morse, D.L., Potter, M.E., DeMelfi, T.M., Guzewich, J.J., Tauxe, R.V., and Blake, P.A. 1988. The emergence of grade A eggs as a major source of *Salmonella enteritidis* infection. JAMA 259:2103–2107.

Timms, L.M., Marshall, R.N., and Breslin, M.F. 1990. Laboratory assessment of protection given by an experimental *S. Enteritidis* PT4 inactivated adjuvant vaccine. Vet. Rec. 22:611–614.

Truscott, R.B. 1981. Oral *Salmonella* antigens for the control of *Salmonella* in chickens. Avian Dis. 25:810–820.

Turnbull, P.C.B., and Snoeyenbos, G.H. 1974. Experimental salmonellosis in the chicken. 1. Fate and host response in alimentary canal, liver and spleen. Avian Dis. 18:153–177.

Udhayakumar, V., and Muthukkaruppan, V.R. 1987. Protective immunity induced by outer membrane proteins of *Salmonella typhimurium* in mice. Infect. Immun. 55:816–821.

Vaidya, H.C., Dietzler, D.N., and Ladenson, J.H. 1985. Inadequacy of traditional ELISA for screening hybridoma supernatants for murine monoclonal antibodies. Hybridoma 4:271–276.

37

Control of *Salmonella enterica* Serovar Enteritidis Infection in Chickens by Using Live Avirulent *Salmonella* Typhimurium Vaccine Strain

J.O. Hassan and R. Curtiss III

INTRODUCTION

Foodborne pathogens continue to plague society on a worldwide scale and appear to be increasing despite research and management efforts to remedy the problem. In the United States, 80%–90% of human salmonella transmission is by persistent infection of farm animals and subsequent contamination of meat, eggs, and dairy products. In 1989, *Salmonella enterica* serovar Typhimurium (*S.* Typhimurium), *Salmonella enterica* serovar Enteritidis (*S.* Enteritidis), *S.* Heidelberg, *S.* Hadar, and *S.* Agona accounted for 57.9% of salmonella serovars isolated from human infections and accounted for 46.5% of isolations obtained from poultry (Centers for Disease Control, 1990). Infections by *S.* Enteritidis were associated with the consumption of food containing eggs. Isolates of *S.* Enteritidis of the same phenotype were found in patients and implicated raw eggs and the ovary of hens from the farm that supplied the eggs (Telzac et al., 1990). The sharp increase in the number of food-poisoning outbreaks among humans due to *S.* Enteritidis in the United States in the past decade was associated with *S.* Enteritidis contamination of grade-A shell eggs (Shivaprasad et al., 1990; Telzac et al., 1990).

Salmonella Enteritidis isolates in the United States belong primarily to phage type 8 (PT8) and PT13a, with 48% of poultry and 64% of animal salmonella isolates in the United States being PT8 (Mason and Ebel, 1992). In Europe, human infection by *S.* Enteritidis is a major problem in many countries. In Italy, *S.* Enteritidis infection increased from 3%–4% in the mid-1980s to more than 30% in 1990 (Binkin et al., 1993). *Salmonella* Enteritidis PT4 is the predominant isolate in Germany (Schroeter et al., 1991) and Britain (Rampling et al., 1989). *Salmonella* Enteritidis PT4 was responsible for 56% of all human isolates from Britain in 1993 (Anon., 1988).

The major obstacle to salmonella control in the poultry industry is the ubiquitous presence of salmonellae. Once salmonellae reach a farm, they spread rapidly because infected chickens and rodents serve as carriers. Salmonella carriers constantly shed salmonellae and contaminate the feed and watering systems and the farm environment. In salmonella-contaminated farms, proliferation of live wild-type salmonella strains results in fecal excretion of salmonellae by infected chickens. Salmonella excretion may persist during the growth of chickens on the farm, with possible contamination of finished poultry products by salmonella strains (Todd, 1980; Green et al., 1982; Hassan et al., 1991b). *Salmonella* Enteritidis is invasive in laying hens, and the potential for its vertical transmission has been documented (Snoeyenbos et al., 1969; Hopper and Mawer, 1988; Thiagarajan et al., 1994).

Salmonella Enteritidis is also invasive in broiler chickens (Lister, 1988) and PT4 has been isolated from the muscle of raw carcasses purchased from retail outlets (Humphery, 1991).

The present methods of controlling food-poisoning-related salmonellae on farms are inadequate or too expensive to enforce. The use of antibiotics has been reduced because of complications resulting from the development of antibiotic-resistant salmonella strains (Smith and Tucker, 1975; Alper and Ames, 1978; Holmberg et al., 1984), the experimental implication of some antibiotics in enhancing salmonella excretion (Barrow et al., 1990a), and the risk of feeding consumers poultry products containing antibiotic residue. Inoculation of nonpathogenic gut flora from adult chickens into day-old chicks, a phenomenon known as *competitive exclusion,* has been shown to reduce colonization of young chicks by pathogenic organisms (Schleifer, 1985). Treatment of finished poultry products with irradiation is an emerging approach but is an expensive means of product sterilization.

The emergence of *S.* Enteritidis infection among humans as a result of egg contamination by salmonellae led to the establishment in 1990 of a task force in the United States for *S.* Enteritidis control in the poultry industry (U.S. Department of Agriculture, 1991). Poultry feed is a major source of salmonella infection for chickens, because of the use of salmonella-contaminated raw materials from rendering plants. In the United States, the Food and Drug Administration center for veterinary medicine has now focused on using microbiological and chemical standards instead of the old organoleptic criteria in the inspection of rendering plants (Mitchell and McChesney, 1991). The ultimate aim is to obtain salmonella-free feed. The attainment of a low level of salmonellae in feed and strict adherence to sanitary regulations and biosecurity on farms will definitely reduce the level of salmonellae on farms. These efforts will not lead to salmonella-free chickens because the prolific nature of salmonellae in infected chickens will obliterate all control efforts.

Therefore, there is a need for the induction of an inherent protective mechanism within chickens at the production level that will ensure a low level or elimination of salmonella contamination. The development of efficacious live vaccines has been acknowledged by the World Health Organization as part of an overall control strategy to contain salmonellae in food animals (Anon., 1994). We believe that vaccination should be a major component of the salmonella control program. Vaccination helped in the control of *Salmonella* Gallinarum (Smith, 1956), and *Salmonella* Pullorum was eliminated by identification and removal of seropositive flocks. Killed salmonella vaccines have not produced convincing levels of protection against wild-type salmonella challenge (Truscott, 1981; Barrow et al., 1990b; Gast et al., 1992, 1993). Parenteral vaccination of chickens with outer membranes of *S.* Enteritidis was better than vaccination with killed bacteria in preventing colonization of immunized chickens by wild-type *S.* Enteritidis after challenge (Nagaraja et al., 1991). Oral vaccination with live homologous salmonellae has been shown to induce protection against visceral invasion by challenge strains, with reduction in the colonization of the gastrointestinal tract (Knivett and Stevens, 1971; Pritchard et al.,

1978; Suphabphant et al., 1983; Barrow et al., 1990b; Cooper et al., 1992, 1994). Intramuscular vaccination failed to protect vaccinated chickens against intestinal colonization (Barrow et al., 1990b). Live vaccines produced better protection than killed vaccines (Collins et al., 1972; Germanier, 1972; Alper and Ames, 1978; Truscott, 1981; Alderton et al., 1991; Hassan et al., 1991a), but killed vaccines appeal more to producers and regulators because they do not pose the possible public health risks of salmonella shedders that may accompany the use of a live attenuated paratyphoid vaccine in the poultry industry. However, killed vaccines do not induce enough protection to eliminate the salmonella carrier status in chickens (Alper and Ames, 1978). Live salmonella vaccines replicate, colonize, and invade intestinal and visceral organs of inoculated chickens, thereby leading to the induction of strong immunity in these chickens (Germanier, 1972; Pritchard et al., 1978; Truscott, 1981; Barrow et al., 1984, 1990b; Cooper et al., 1990, 1992, 1994; Hassan and Curtiss, 1990, 1994a; Alderton et al., 1991; Hassan et al., 1993).

Advances in molecular genetics have led to the production of microbial pathogens with known genetic deletions that render virulent bacteria avirulent (Macrina, 1984; Goebel, 1985; Cooper et al., 1994). One such mutant is the Δcya Δcrp *S.* Typhimurium vaccine strain χ3985 (Curtiss et al., 1991). We have shown that χ3985 is avirulent, stable, and immunogenic (Curtiss and Kelly, 1987; Hassan and Curtiss, 1990; Curtiss et al., 1991; Hassan et al., 1993); that it does not enhance the development of salmonella carrier status in chickens (Hassan and Curtiss, 1994b); and that it effectively protects vaccinated chickens against challenge with homologous and heterologous virulent salmonella serovars (Hassan and Curtiss, 1994a). Oral infection of 1-day-old chickens with *S.* Typhimurium wild-type strain χ3761 induced lymphocyte depletion and immunosuppression, which facilitate the establishment of salmonella carrier status in infected chickens (Hassan and Curtiss, 1994a). This negative attribute of *S.* Typhimurium χ3761 was overcome by the deletion of the *cya crp* genes from χ3761 (Hassan and Curtiss, 1994a). Although no live vaccine is in use in the United States at present, Europe has opened up the poultry industry to the use of live salmonella vaccines (Meyer, 1991; Vielitz et al., 1992). Salmonella vaccination is now compulsory in all German poultry-breeding and poultry-rearing units with more than 250 hens. We are awaiting the approval of χ3985 for use as a live vaccine in the United States later in the year or in early 1999. This chapter presents a summary of many of our unique publications (Hassan and Curtiss, 1990, 1994a, 1996; Hassan et al., 1993, 1997) that address the control of salmonellae in the poultry industry using live avirulent χ3985.

PROPERTIES OF AVIRULENT Δcya Δcrp *SALMONELLA* TYPHIMURIUM STRAIN χ3985

Salmonella Typhimurium χ3985 is an avirulent Δcya Δcrp derivative of *S.* Typhimurium χ3761, which is highly virulent for 1-day-old chicks, with a median lethal oral dose of 2×10^3 colony-forming units (CFU). A detailed characteristic of $\chi3985$ has been described (Hassan and Curtiss, 1990).

EVALUATION OF SALMONELLA TYPHIMURIUM $\chi3985$ AS A VACCINE STRAIN

Salmonella Typhimurium $\chi3985$ was used to immunize chickens at various time points and intervals to determine whether it can induce protection against visceral and intestinal colonization of vaccinated chickens by wild-type salmonella strains. Most of our studies were conducted with specific pathogen-free (SPF) white leghorn chickens hatched in our facilities from eggs received from SPAFAS (Roanoke, IL). Chickens were maintained in biological level-2 facilities. On the day of hatch and at 3 days of age, or at 2 weeks of age, chickens were orally administered the organism to compare single versus multiple immunization with doses ranging from 10^5 to 10^8 CFU, followed by challenge with wild-type strain at 1 or 2 weeks after the last vaccination (Hassan and Curtiss, 1990; Hassan et al., 1993). Colonization of gastrointestinal tract or invasion of visceral organs by challenged salmonella strain was determined by quantifying the number of salmonellae in the organ samples. The degree of protection was determined by comparing data obtained from vaccinated chickens with those obtained from nonvaccinated chickens.

The single immunization of chickens with S. Typhimurium $\chi3985$ led to a significant reduction in fecal excretion of S. Typhimurium wild-type strain $\chi3761$ but failed to reduce cecal colonization by $\chi3761$ in vaccinated chickens (Hassan and Curtiss, 1990). However, double immunization of chickens with $\chi3985$ at 1 and 14 days of age produced an immune response that, within 3 days of the last immunization, cleared the immunizing strain from the ceca and protected vaccinated chickens effectively from cecal colonization by $\chi3761$ (Hassan and Curtiss, 1990). The inability of a single immunization to protect against cecal colonization by salmonellae despite adequate proliferation in the ceca, which is located close to the cecal tonsil and the bursa of Fabricius, demonstrates that salmonella proliferation within the cecum plays little or no role in the induction of protective immunity. We suggest that protection was initiated by the second dose of $\chi3985$ in the small intestine and the subsequent invasion of $\chi3985$ into the intestinal mucosal and splenic immune cells.

Double vaccination of chickens with 10^7 or 10^8 CFU avirulent $\chi3985$ at 1 day and 2 weeks of age precludes colonization by virulent $\chi3761$ used as the challenge strain (Hassan et al., 1993; Hassan and Curtiss, 1994b). At lower doses of 10^5 and 10^6 CFU, $\chi3985$ did not induce protection in vaccinated chickens. The level of colonization observed in nonvaccinated chickens after challenge with 10^6 $\chi3761$ was similar to (p > 0.05) and not significant from the colonization level in chickens vaccinated at 1 and 2 weeks of age with 10^5 or 10^6 CFU $\chi3985$ and challenged with 10^6 CFU $\chi3761$ (Hassan et al., 1993).

EFFICACY OF VACCINATION WITH *SALMONELLA* TYPHIMURIUM $\chi3985$ AGAINST HOMOLOGOUS AND HETEROLOGOUS SALMONELLA CHALLENGES

Salmonella Typhimurium was the most predominant salmonella serovar associated with the poultry industry until the late 1980s, when S. Enteritidis emerged in the laying industry. By the early 1990s, S. Enteritidis overtook S. Typhimurium as the predominant isolate from food poisoning in humans caused by salmonellae. *Salmonella* Enteritidis strain Δcya Δcrp was not as effective as $\chi3985$ in our vaccination experiments. The very encouraging observations with the use of $\chi3985$ led to its use in these experiments. Chickens were either immunized at 1 and 14 days of age with 10^8 CFU $\chi3985$ and challenged at 4 weeks of age with 10^6 CFU wild-type strains, or were immunized at 2 and 4 weeks of age with 10^6 CFU of $\chi3985$ and challenged at 6 weeks of age with either 10^6 or 10^8 CFU of the challenge strain (Hassan and Curtiss, 1994b). The challenge strains used were from the following serovars: group B (S. Typhimurium F98, S. Agona, S. Heidelberg, and S. Bredeney), group C (S. Albany, S. Hadar, S. Infantis, and S. Montevideo), group D (S. Enteritidis 27A PT8, Y-8P2 PT8, S. Enteritidis B6996 PT13a, 4973 PT13a, and S. Panama), and group E (S. Anatum).

Oral vaccination of chickens at 1 and 14 days of age with Δcya Δcrp S. Typhimurium $\chi3985$ induced significant protection against challenge with 10^6 CFU of wild-type by S. Typhimurium–homologous salmonella strains from group B, and solid protection against a visceral invasion by S. Agona and S. Bredeny. Oral vaccination of chickens at 2 and 4 weeks of age precludes colonization of the ileum, cecum, the bursa of Fabricius, the spleen, and the ovary by 10^6 CFU wild-type S. Enteritidis PT8 or PT13a, S. Typhimurium, or S. Anatum, and also prevented visceral invasion by 10^8 CFU of highly invasive S. Typhimurium 2921-1 or S. Enteritidis strains implicated in human salmonella outbreaks caused by egg consumption. Oral vaccination of chickens at 1 and 14 days of age induced strong protection against colonization and invasion of vaccinated chickens by homologous salmonella strains with group-B O antigens. A lower level of protection was observed against cecal colonization of vaccinated chickens by heterologous salmonella strains. The results obtained are better than those from earlier studies in which oral vaccination with S. Typhimurium F98 was used to prevent colonization of the ceca by homologous strains (Barrow et al., 1990b; Hassan et al., 1991a,b) or $\chi3985$ (Hassan and Curtiss, 1990; Curtiss et al., 1991; Hassan et al., 1993).

Double oral vaccination of chickens with Δcya Δcrp S. Typhimurium $\chi3985$ at 2 and 4 weeks of age induced stronger protection against serovars from groups B, C, D, and E used in this study. Overall, protection against serovars B was excellent, protection against serovars D and

E was good, and protection against group C serovars was marginal (Hassan et al., 1993). In vaccinated chickens, χ3985 also induced very good protection against 10^8 CFU of highly invasive *S.* Enteritidis or *S.* Typhimurium strains. Most of the *S.* Enteritidis strains used in this study are highly invasive and were implicated in human food-poisoning outbreaks that were traced to eggs, with major economic loss and public health problems (Lin et al., 1988; St. Louis et al., 1988; Telzac et al., 1990; Jones et al., 1991). Most previous investigations involving the use of live oral salmonella vaccine strains in chickens did not address cecal colonization or were not effective in preventing cecal colonization of vaccinated chickens by homologous salmonella strains (Pritchard et al., 1978; Barrow et al., 1984, 1990; Cooper et al., 1990, 1992, 1994; Alderton et al., 1991).

The induction of excellent protection against homologous salmonella serovars and significant protection against heterologous salmonella serovars induced by double oral vaccination of chickens with live avirulent χ3985 at 2 and 4 weeks of age is more effective than vaccination at 1 and 14 days of age. Comparison of results from a single vaccination at 3 days (Curtiss et al., 1991) and double vaccination with avirulent salmonellae at 1 and 14 days or 2 and 4 weeks shows that induction of protection depends on age and vaccination schedule. Double vaccination at 1 and 14 days of age or at 2 and 4 weeks of age prevented visceral invasion of wild-type salmonellae in vaccinated chickens, but double vaccination at 1 and 14 days was less effective than vaccination at 2 and 4 weeks in preventing cecal colonization. This may be related to the age at vaccination such that at 1 day of age, when chicks are less immunocompetent, vaccination efficacy may be reduced. Interference in the efficacy of primary vaccination may also prevent development of an adequate number of memory cells required for the induction of an anamnestic response to secondary vaccination. This may reduce the ability of vaccination at 1 and 14 days of age to induce cross-protection against intestinal colonization by heterologous salmonella serovars.

EFFICACY OF *SALMONELLA* TYPHIMURIUM χ3985 AS A VACCINE STRAIN IN LAYERS

Salmonella Enteritidis is invasive in laying hens, with possible vertical and horizontal transmission of salmonellae into egg. The protection of vaccinated chickens from colonization of the gastrointestinal tract and invasion of the visceral organs by *S.* Enteritidis led us to investigate the effect of vaccination on salmonella isolation from eggs laid by infected layers and the duration of induced immunity in layers. Chickens were immunized at 2 and 4 weeks of age with 10^8 CFU χ3985, and some of the vaccinated chickens were challenged with 10^6 CFU *S.* Enteritidis 27A PT8 or *S.* Typhimurium F98 at 3, 6, 9, or 12 months of age. Eggs were collected from each group for 2 weeks after challenge; after 2 weeks, the chickens were killed and tissue samples collected for salmonella isolation.

A comparison of salmonella isolation from challenged vaccinated and challenged nonvaccinated pullets and layers showed that χ3985 protected vaccinated layers against challenge with *S.* Enteritidis or *S.* Typhimurium for 11 months after vaccination when the experiment was terminated. Nonvaccinated controls displayed significant levels of colonization of visceral organs, including ovaries and oviducts, and exhibited 8%–26% salmonella isolation from yolk, egg white, or shell, whereas no salmonellae were isolated from the eggs or ovary or oviduct samples collected from vaccinated birds for 2 weeks after challenge. Vaccination at 2 and 4 weeks of age effectively protected against challenge with *S.* Enteritidis or *S.* Typhimurium during the laying season and protected layers from the reduced egg production that we observed with salmonella infection of layers. Nonvaccinated layers showed an egg production reduction from 74% to 43% when challenged with *S.* Typhimurium F98 and from 75% to 60% when challenged with *S.* Enteritidis 27A PT8. Egg production in vaccinated layers was similar to that of nonvaccinated nonchallenged layers (Hassan et al., 1997).

EFFECTS OF MATERNAL ANTIBODY ON SALMONELLA COLONIZATION AND VACCINATION EFFICACY

Significant salmonella-specific immunoglobulin G (IgG) was detectable in the egg yolk in high titers up to 30 weeks after vaccination when the experiment was terminated. Maternal antibody was detected at 3 days of age in vaccinated hens' progeny (VHP) but decreased with time and was lowest at 3 weeks of age. Maternal antibody significantly reduced the ability of *S.* Typhimurium F98 to colonize the gastrointestinal tract of infected VHP, when compared with infected SPF chicks. Vaccination of VHP at 1 and 3 weeks of age followed by challenge with *S.* Enteritidis or *S.* Typhimurium led to the isolation of a higher titer of salmonellae from the cecum and ileum of the challenged VHP when compared with vaccinated SPF chicks used as positive controls. Vaccination of VHP at 2 and 4 weeks of age induced excellent protection that precluded colonization of *S.* Enteritidis or *S.* Typhimurium wild-type challenge strain at 2 weeks after vaccination (Hassan et al., 1996).

Vaccination of hens with *S.* Typhimurium χ3985 induced salmonella-specific antibody responses that were detectable in eggs laid by the chickens. The predominant immunoglobulin isotype detected was IgG, mainly from the egg yolk. Injection of hens with 10^8 CFU of live avirulent *S.* Typhimurium χ3985 induced a prolonged antibody response that was transferred to eggs laid by the vaccinated hens throughout the first 30 weeks of egg production. VHP showed reduced colonization of both avirulent *S.* Typhimurium vaccine strain χ3985 and virulent strain F98 in the visceral organs and the intestine for up to 2–3 weeks of age. This protection can be attributed to the presence of maternal antibody. Double vaccination of hens at 16 and 18 weeks of age with live avirulent *S.* Typhimurium vaccine strain χ3985 induced salmonella-specific antibody that was passively transferred in eggs and was detected as salmonella-specific maternal intestinal IgA and serum IgG in VHP. Maternal antibody reduced salmonella colonization of chicks and did not affect the efficacy of vaccination in chickens vaccinated at 2 and 4 weeks of age (Hassan et al., 1996).

Protection was enhanced in the ileal and cecal contents of vaccinated SPF chickens compared with that in VHP that were challenged 2 weeks after immunization at 1 and 3 weeks of age. The major difference between the two groups lies in the fact that the VHP have high titers of maternal antibodies in their intestines during the first week after hatching. Maternal antibody may have reduced the efficacy of the first dose of vaccine by preventing the proliferation of χ3985 in vaccinated VHP. The organism in the first vaccination of SPF chickens effectively proliferated and induced primary immunity in vaccinated SPF chickens. A second vaccination induced stronger anamnestic response in the vaccinated SPF chickens than in the VHP, therefore inducing better protection against salmonella infection. Both vaccination of VHP and SPF chickens at 1 and 3 weeks or at 2 and 4 weeks of age was able to protect against visceral invasion by homologous salmonellae, but only vaccination of VHP and SPF chickens at 2 and 4 weeks of age was protective against both *S.* Enteritidis and *S.* Typhimurium invasion of visceral organs and intestinal colonization (Hassan et al., 1996).

Salmonella-specific maternal antibody may reduce vaccine efficacy if vaccination is carried out in the first week after hatching. The observed difference in the efficacy of vaccination at 1 and 3 weeks or at 2 and 4 weeks of age may be related to the high maternal antibody titer in the first week after hatching, the age-enhanced immunocompetence of 2-week-old chickens, and the affinity, intensity, and effectiveness of the immune responses induced by vaccination at 2 and 4 weeks of age.

Susceptibility of chicks to salmonellae is age dependent: day-of-hatch chicks with an immature immune system are very susceptible to salmonella infection (Smitha and Tucker, 1980; Barrow et al., 1987; Gast and Beard, 1989; Hassan and Curtiss, 1990). We previously demonstrated that early exposure of chicks to salmonella infection causes transient lymphocyte depletion of lymphoid organs, which enhances the development of salmonella carrier status in chickens (Hassan and Curtiss, 1994b). The presence of maternal antibody in VHP reduced salmonella colonization. Vaccination of hens with the avirulent live *S.* Typhimurium vaccine strain χ3985 reduced salmonella proliferation in VHP and subsequently reduced lymphocyte depletion, which is associated with enhanced salmonella proliferation. Reduced lymphocyte depletion prevented the development of salmonella carrier status in chickens raised in salmonella-contaminated environments. A reduction in the number of salmonella carriers in the poultry industry will reduce environmental and poultry-product contamination by salmonellae.

We reported previously that vaccination of SPF chickens at 2 and 4 weeks of age protected the vaccinated chickens from challenge with homologous and heterologous salmonella serovars (Hassan et al., 1996). We therefore conclude that a combination of hen and VHP vaccination with avirulent live *S.* Typhimurium vaccine strain χ3985 may protect the poultry industry from salmonella infection of broilers, pullets, layers, and breeders raised on salmonella-contaminated farms.

CONCLUSION

Vaccination at 3 days with χ3985 reduced fecal excretion of wild-type challenge at 4 weeks after vaccination but did not affect cecal colonization. Vaccination at 1 and 14 days, followed by wild-type challenge at 3 weeks of age, showed solid protection against small intestinal colonization but only reduced rectal colonization by 50%, with no protection against cecal colonization. A wild-type challenge at 4 weeks of age induced strong protection against colonization of the small intestine and 90% protection against cecal and rectal colonization. Vaccination at 1 and 14 days did not provide solid protection against intestinal colonization by wild-type *S.* Enteritidis challenge but did protect against ovarian invasion. Vaccination of SPF chickens and VHP at 2 and 4 weeks of age provided excellent protection against wild-type challenge with highly invasive *S.* Enteritidis 4973 (PT13a) or Y-8P2 (PT8) or 27A (PT8) and *S.* Typhimurium F98. Vaccination of chickens at 2 and 4 weeks of age induced long-lasting protection in layers and prevented the transmission of *S.* Enteritidis into eggs. Eggs hatched from immunized breeders produced progeny that did not exhibit lymphocyte depletion of the bursa of Fabricius when infected with wild-type salmonellae but displayed a robust immune response that enhanced immunization at 2 and 4 weeks of age.

The data on the χ3985 vaccine strain that were developed and evaluated by the authors in experimental investigations (Hassan and Curtiss, 1990, 1994a; Hassan et al., 1993, 1996, 1997) and summarized in this chapter support the efficacy of the described vaccine. We are confident that the observations reported here will be validated in the field once χ3985 is approved for use as a live vaccine by the U.S. Food and Drug Administration. The exemplary results of our experiments and observations lead us to conclude that, with comprehensive planning and judicious use of this avirulent live salmonella vaccine by veterinarians, salmonellae as a problem in the poultry industry can be contained in the early 21st century. We definitely deserve some relief after 100 years of salmonella menace in the poultry industry.

REFERENCES

Alderton, M.R., Faley, K.J., and Coloe, P.J. 1991. Humoral responses and salmonellosis protection in chickens given a vitamin-dependent *Salmonella typhimurium* mutant. Avian Dis. 35:435–442.

Alper, M.D., and Ames, B.N. 1978. Transport of antibiotics and metabolite analogs by systems under cyclic AMP control: positive selection of *Salmonella typhimurium cya* and *crp* mutants. J. Bacteriol. 133:149–157.

Anonymous. 1988. Recommendations for research. WHO Tech. Rep. Ser. 774:65–69.

Anonymous. 1994. Update on salmonellae infection, 18th ed. London: Public Health Laboratory Service/State Veterinary Service, Colindale.

Barrow, P.A., Smith, H.W., and Tucker, J.F. 1984. The effect of feeding diets containing avoparcin on the excretion of *Salmonella* by chickens experimentally infected with natural sources of *Salmonella* organisms. J. Hyg. 93:439–444.

Barrow, P.A., Higgins, M.B., Lovell, M.A., and Simpson, J.M. 1987. Observation of pathogenesis of experimental *Salmonella typhimurium* infection in chickens. Res. Vet. Sci. 42:194–199.

Barrow, P.A., Hassan, J.O., and Berchieri, A. 1990a. Reduction in fecal excretion of *Salmonella typhimurium* strain F98 in chickens vaccinated with live and killed *S. typhimurium* organisms. Epidemiol. Infect. 104:413–426.

Barrow, P.A., Lovell, M.A., and Berchieri, A. 1990b. Immunization of laying hens against *Salmonella enteritidis* phage type 4 with live, attenuated vaccines. Vet. Rec. 126:241–242.

Binkin, N., Scuder, G., Novaco, F., et al. 1993. Egg-related *Salmonella enteritidis*, Italy, 1991. Epidemiol. Infect. 110:227–237.

Centers for Disease Control (CDC). 1990. CDC *Salmonella* surveillance annual summary: 1989. Atlanta, GA: U.S. Department of Health and Human Services.

Collins, F.M., and Carter, P.B. 1972. Comparative immunogenicity of heat-killed and living oral *Salmonella* vaccines. Infect. Immun. 55:3035–3043.

Cooper, G.L., Nicholas, R.A.J., Cullen, G.A., and Hormaeche, C.A. 1990. Vaccination of chickens with a *Salmonella enteritidis aroA* live oral *Salmonella* vaccine. Microb. Pathog. 9:255–265.

Cooper, G.L., Venables, L.M., Nicholas, R.A.J., Cullen, G.A., and Hormaeche C.A. 1992. Vaccination of chickens with chicken-derived *Salmonella enteritidis* phage type 4 aroA oral *Salmonella* vaccine. Vaccine 10:247–254.

Cooper, G.L., Venables, L.M., Woodward, M.J., and Hormaeche, C.E. 1994. Vaccination of chickens with strain CVL30, a genetically defined *Salmonella enteritidis aroA* live oral vaccine candidate. Infect. Immun. 62:4747–4754.

Curtiss, R., and Kelly, S.M. 1987. *Salmonella typhimurium* deletion mutants lacking adenylate cyclase and cyclic AMP receptor protein are avirulent and immunogenic. Infect. Immun. 55:3035–3043.

Curtiss III, R., Porter, S.B., Munson, M., Tinge, S.A., Hassan, J.O., Gentry-Weeks, C., and Kelly, S.M. 1991. Nonrecombinant and recombinant avirulent *Salmonella* live vaccines for poultry. In: Blankenship, L.C., Bailey, J.S., Cox, N.A., Stern, N.J., and Meinersmann, R.J., eds. Colonization control of human bacterial enteropathogen in poultry. New York: Academic, pp. 169–198.

Gast, R.K., and Beard, C.W. 1989. Age related changes in the persistence and pathogenicity of *Salmonella typhimurium* in chicks. Poult. Sci. 68:1454–1460.

Gast, R.K., Stone, H.D., Holt, P.S., and Beard, C.W. 1992. Evaluation of the efficacy of an oil-emulsion bacterin for protecting chickens against *Salmonella enteritidis*. Avian Dis. 36:992–999.

Gast, R.K., Stone, H.D., and Holt, P.S. 1993. Evaluation of the efficacy of oil-emulsion bacterins for reducing fecal shedding of *Salmonella enteritidis* by laying hens. Avian Dis. 37:1085–1091.

Germanier, R. 1972. Immunity in experimental salmonellosis. III. Comparative immunization with viable and heat-inactivated cells of *Salmonella typhimurium*. Infect. Immun. 5:792–797.

Goebel, W. 1985. Genetic approaches to microbial pathogenicity. Curr. Top. Microbiol. Immunol. 118:253–277.

Green, S.S., Moran, A.B., Johnston, R.W., Uhler, P., and Chiu, J. 1982. The incidence of *Salmonella* species and serotypes in young whole chicken carcasses in 1979 as compared with 1967. Poult. Sci. 61:288–293.

Hassan, J.O., and Curtiss III, R. 1990. Control of colonization by virulent *Salmonella typhimurium* by oral immunization of chickens with avirulent Δ*cya* Δ*crp* *S. typhimurium*. Res. Microbiol. 141:839–850.

Hassan, J.O., and Curtiss III, R. 1994a. Virulent *Salmonella typhimurium* induced lymphocyte depletion and immunosuppression in chickens. Infect. Immun. 62:2027–2036.

Hassan, J.O., and Curtiss III, R. 1994b. Development and evaluation of oral vaccination program using live avirulent *Salmonella typhimurium* to protect vaccinated chickens against challenge with homologous and heterologous *Salmonella* serotypes. Infect. Immun. 62:5519–5527.

Hassan, J.O., and Curtiss III, R. 1996. Effect of vaccination of hens with an avirulent strain of *Salmonella typhimurium* on immunity of progeny challenged with wild-type *Salmonella* strains. Infect. Immun. 64:938–944.

Hassan, J.O., and Curtiss III, R. 1997. Efficacy of a live avirulent *Salmonella typhimurium* vaccine in preventing colonization and invasion of laying hens by *Salmonella typhimurium* and *Salmonella enteritidis*. Avian Dis. 41:783–791.

Hassan, J.O., Mockett, A.P.A., Catty, D., and Barrow, P.A. 1991a. Infection and reinfection of chickens with *Salmonella typhimurium*: bacteriology and immune responses. Avian Dis. 35:809–819.

Hassan, J.O., Olowoparija, S.O., and Odi, D.F. 1991b. Prevalence of *Salmonella* on a farm in Nigeria and its implication on the products of the resident poultry processing plant. In: Proceedings of the 42nd North Central Avian Disease Conference, Des Moines, IA.

Hassan, J.O., Porter, S.B., and Curtiss III, R. 1993. Effect of infective dose on humoral immune responses and colonization in chickens experimentally infected with *Salmonella typhimurium*. Avian Dis. 37:19–26.

Holmberg, S.D., Osterholm, M.T., Senger, K.A., and Cohen, M.L. 1984. Drug-resistant *Salmonella* from animal feed antimicrobials. N. Engl. J. Med. 311:617–622.

Hopper, S.A., and Mawer, S. 1988. *Salmonella enteritidis* in a commercial layer flock. Vet. Rec. 123:351.

Humphrey, T.J. 1991. Food poisoning: a change in pattern? Vet. Annu. 31:32–37.

Jones, F., Axtell, R.C., Tarver, F.R., Rives, V., Scheideler, S.E., and Wineland, M.J. 1991. Experimental factors contributing to *Salmonella* colonization of chickens. In: Blankenship, L.C.,

Bailey, J.S., Cox, N.A., Stern, N.J., and Meinersmann, R.J., eds. Colonization control of human bacterial enteropathogens in poultry. New York: Academic, pp. 3–21.

Knivett, V.A., and Stevens, W.K. 1971. The evaluation of a live *Salmonella* vaccine in mice and chickens. J. Hyg. 69:233–245.

Lin, F.-Y.C., Morris, J.G., Jr., Trump, D., Tulghman, D., Wood, P.K., Jackman, N., Isreal, E., and Libonati, J.P. 1988. Investigation of an outbreak of *Salmonella enteritidis* gastroenteritis associated with consumption of eggs in a restaurant chain in Maryland. Am. J. Epidemiol. 128:839–844.

Lister, S. 1988. *Salmonella enteritidis* infection in broilers and broiler breeders. Vet. Rec. 123:350.

Macrina, F.L. 1984. Molecular cloning of bacterial antigens and virulence determinants. Annu. Rev. Microbiol. 38:193–219.

Mason, J., and Ebel, E. 1992. APHIS *Salmonella enteritidis* control program. In: Snoeyenbos, G.H., ed. Proceedings of the symposium on the diagnosis and control of *Salmonella*. Pp. 78–109.

Meyer, H. 1991. Use of modified live vaccine in young livestock. In: Proceedings of the symposium on the diagnosis and control of *Salmonella*. San Diego, CA, pp. 43–58.

Mitchell, G.A., and McChesney, D.G. 1991. A plan for *Salmonella* control in animal feeds. In: Snoeyenbos, G.H., ed. Proceedings of the symposium on the diagnosis and control of *Salmonella*. Pp. 28–31.

Nagaraja, K.V., Kim, C.J., Kumar, M.C., and Pomeroy, B.S. 1991. Is vaccination a feasible approach for the control of *Salmonella*? In: Blankenship, L.C., Bailey, J.S., Cox, N.A., Stern, N.J., and Meinersmann, R.J., eds. Colonization control of human bacterial enteropathogens in poultry. New York: Academic, pp. 243–258.

Pritchard, D.G., Nivas, S.C., York, M.D., and Pomeroy, B.S. 1978. Effect of galE mutant of *Salmonella typhimurium* on experimental salmonellosis in chickens. Avian Dis. 22:562–575.

Rampling, A., Upson, R., Ward, L., Anderson, J., Peters, E., and Rowe, B. 1989. *Salmonella enteritidis* PT4 infection of broiler chickens: a hazard to public health. Lancet 2:436–438.

Schleifer, J.H. 1985. A review of the efficacy and mechanism of competitive exclusion for the control of *Salmonella* in poultry. World's Poultry Sci. J. 41:72–82.

Schroeter, V.A., Pietzch, O., Stienbeck, A., et al. 1991. Epidemiologische Untersuchungen zum *Salmonella enteritidis* Guschehen in der Bundesrepublik Deutschland 1990. Orig. Ubersichtsarbeit. 4:147–151.

Shivaprasad, H.L., Timoney, J.F., Morales, S., Lucio, B., and Baker, R.C. 1990. Pathogenesis of *Salmonella enteritidis* infection in laying chickens: studies on egg transmission, clinical signs, fecal shedding and serological responses. Avian Dis. 34:548–557.

Smith, H.W. 1956. The use of live vaccines in experimental *Salmonella gallinarum* infection in chickens with observation on their interference effect. J. Hyg. 75:275–292.

Smith, H.W., and Tucker, J.F. 1975. The effect of antibiotics therapy on the fecal excretion of *Salmonella typhimurium* by experimentally infected chickens. Avian Dis. 27:602–615.

Smith, H., and Tucker, J.F. 1980. The virulence of *Salmonella* strains for chickens: their excretion by infected chickens. J. Hyg. Camb. 84:479–488.

Snoeyenbos, G.H., Smyster, C.F., and Van Roekel, H. 1969. *Salmonella* infections of the ovary and peritoneum of chickens. Avian Dis. 13:668–670.

St. Louis, M.E., Morse, D.L., Potter, M.E., DeMelfi, T.M., Guzewich, J.J., Tauxe, R.V., and Blake, P.A. 1988. The emergence of grade A eggs as a source of *Salmonella enteritidis* infections. JAMA 259:2103–2107.

Suphabphant, W., York, M.D., and Pomeroy, B. 1983. Use of two vaccines (live G30D or killed RW 16) in the prevention of *Salmonella typhimurium* infection in chickens. Avian Dis. 27:602–615.

Telzac, E.E., Budnick, L.D., Zweig, M.S., Greenberg, S.B., Shayegani, M., Benson, C.E., and Shultz, S. 1990. A nosocomial outbreak of *Salmonella enteritidis* infection due to the consumption of raw eggs. N. Engl. J. Med. 323:394–397.

Thiagarajan, D., Saeed, A.M., and Asem, E.K. 1994. Mechanism of transovarian transmission of *Salmonella enteritidis* in laying hens. Poult. Sci. 73:89–98.

Todd, E.C.D. 1980. Poultry associated foodborne disease: its occurrence, cost, sources, and prevention. J. Food Prot. 43:129–139.

Truscott, R.B. 1981. Oral *Salmonella* antigens for the control of *Salmonella* in chicks. Avian Dis. 25:810–820.

U.S. Department of Agriculture, Animal and Plant Health Inspection Services. 1991. Title 9, Code of Federal Regulations, part 82: chickens affected by *Salmonella enteritidis*, final rule. Washington, DC.

Vielitz, E., Conrad, C., Vob, M., Lohren, U., Bachmeier, J., and Hahn, I. 1992. Immunization against *Salmonella* infections using live and inactivated vaccine preparations. In: World Poultry Congress, Amsterdam, pp. 435–438.

38

Immunoprophylaxis of Chicks against *Salmonella enterica* Serovar Enteritidis

B.M. Hargis, D.J. Caldwell, and M.H. Kogut

INTRODUCTION

From the perspective of the pathogen, the enteroinvasive *Salmonella enterica* serovar Enteritidis (*S.* Enteritidis) faces a series of formidable obstacles in order to effectively colonize the intestine, invade the intestinal mucosa, and enter the circulation for dissemination to internal organs. Nevertheless, many field isolates of *S.* Enteritidis are quite capable of organ invasion, resulting in disease and/or vertical transmission.

Although the immune system is one of the most important obstacles for systemic infection and organ invasion in neonatal chicks, this protective system frequently fails to protect chicks under commercial conditions. Conventional wisdom suggests that vaccination would provide a reasonably effective and convenient solution for protecting chicks against salmonellae. Indeed, traditional vaccination against salmonellae, either with killed bacterins (Gast et al., 1992, 1993) or live mutants (Hassan et al., 1993; Cooper et al., 1994; Hassen and Curtiss, 1994), has been shown to provide some protection to chickens. However, this approach has met with limited success and commercial acceptance for neonatal chicks, partly because of the necessity to revaccinate (booster) to provide effective immunity (Nagaraja et al., 1991).

EVIDENCE FOR A PROTECTIVE T-LYMPHOCYTE-DERIVED LYMPHOKINE

An alternative method for chick immunoprophylaxis against *S.* Enteritidis organ invasion involved the administration of soluble products produced by T-lymphocytes, derived from *S.* Enteritidis-immune hens, cultured in the presence of concanavalin A (Tellez et al., 1993). In these experiments, product(s) from stimulated T-lymphocytes, later named *S.* Enteritidis-immune lymphokine (SE-ILK), were intraperitoneally administered to 18-day-old leghorn chicks. Prophylactic administration reduced the ability to recover *S.* Enteritidis from internal organs by more than 60% when challenge occurred either 30 min or 6 days after treatment. In this study, the protective component(s) were determined to be greater than 10 kDa. Protection was associated with a tremendous influx of inflammatory cells into the lamina propria, causing a significant, approximately fivefold increase in the thickness of this layer of the intestine, based on morphometric analysis. Based on light microscopy, many of the inflammatory cells appeared to be heterophils.

McGruder et al. (1993) further investigated the protective properties of this lymphokine preparation. In these experiments, the investigators compared supernates from concanavalin A-stimulated T-lymphocytes or lipopolysaccharide (LPS)-stimulated monocytes derived from either *S.* Enteritidis–immune or –nonimmune hens for ability to protect chicks on day of hatch. Similar to the results reported by Tellez et al. (1993), supernates from concanavalin A-stimulated immune T-lymphocytes provided marked protection for chicks challenged with *S.* Enteritidis. Importantly, supernates of similarly cultured T-lymphocytes derived from nonimmune hens were not protective in these experiments, indicating that T-lymphocyte activation, due to the in vivo infection of the donor hens, was required for production of the protective lymphokine. That T-lymphocytes specifically produced the protective lymphokine was supported by the observation that LPS-stimulated monocyte supernates were not protective in this study, regardless of the immune status of the donor birds.

ROLE OF HETEROPHILS IN LYMPHOKINE-MEDIATED PROTECTION

Monocytes and heterophils are the primary elements of the innate cellular immune response in poultry (Powell, 1987a,b). Of these cell types, heterophils were demonstrated to be the most effective for phagocytosis and killing of *S.* Enteritidis in vitro, although opsonization of the organisms increased phagocytosis by both cell types (Stabler et al., 1994). Providing further support for the premise that heterophils are important for protection against *S.* Enteritidis infection in chicks, Kogut et al. (1993) developed a granulocytopenic chicken model. In these experiments, 5-fluorouracil (5-FU) was demonstrated to cause a profound but selective decrease in circulating polymorphonuclear cells (almost entirely heterophils). Treated granulocytopenic chicks were also demonstrated to be more susceptible to *S.* Enteritidis organ invasion than were control chicks, with susceptibility directly proportional to the observed reduction in circulating heterophils. In a subsequent study, Kogut et al. (1994b) provided further support for the importance of heterophils in protection of chicks against *S.* Enteritidis organ invasion. Using the previously established granulocytopenic chicken model (Kogut et al., 1993), 5-FU was again demonstrated to decrease numbers of circulating heterophils markedly and to reduce the minimal infectious oral dose for *S.* Enteritidis organ invasion by 150-fold. When infectious intravenous *S.* Enteritidis doses were determined, 4000-fold fewer bacteria were required for organ invasion of granulocytopenic chicks as compared with controls. Further, granulocytopenic chicks developed *S.* Enteritidis dose-dependent reductions in body weight with increased mortality and gross eye, heart, and thymus lesions consistent with clinical systemic salmonellosis. These findings suggest that reduction in heterophil numbers or effectiveness may cause subclinical salmonella infections to become clinical and confirm the importance of the heterophil in the protection of chicks from *S.* Enteritidis organ

invasion. Later, SE-ILK was demonstrated to cause a dramatic leukocytosis within 4 h of lymphokine injection (Kogut et al., 1994a). Furthermore, this leukocytosis was almost entirely accounted for by an elevation in the number of circulating heterophils, resulting in the hypothesis that SE-ILK-induced protection against *S.* Enteritidis organ invasion was heterophil mediated.

Further investigating the possible heterophil involvement in the protection against infection observed after administration of SE-ILK, Kogut et al. (1995a) evaluated the effect of the intraperitoneal administration of SE-ILK, with or without live *S.* Enteritidis, on inflammatory cell influx into the peritoneum. In this study, either SE-ILK or live *S.* Enteritidis alone significantly increased heterophil influx into the peritoneum, and the combination caused an approximate further 2.5-fold increase in heterophil influx. However, no significant effect of either the SE-ILK or live *S.* Enteritidis, alone or in combination, on macrophage accumulation was observed. Heterophil accumulation was not influenced by polymyxin B, nordihydroguaiaretic acid, or indomethacin, suggesting that neither LPS nor arachidonic acid metabolites were involved in heterophil recruitment. Importantly, the heterophil-recruiting activity of the SE-ILK was abrogated by heat treatment (100°C for 1 h), indicating that the active component is heat sensitive and further indicating that LPS was not responsible for the observed heterophil recruitment.

In another study investigating the role of heterophils in SE-ILK-mediated protection of chicks against *S.* Enteritidis organ invasion, the effects of an anti-inflammatory dose of dexamethasone were compared with SE-ILK (McGruder et al., 1995b). In these experiments, SE-ILK caused a small numerical increase in circulating heterophils, whereas dexamethasone treatment markedly and significantly increased circulating heterophil numbers by almost sevenfold. Interestingly, a synergistic increase in the dexamethasone-mediated heterophilia was observed in chicks treated with the combination of SE-ILK and dexamethasone. Dexamethasone, while causing the greatest increase in circulating heterophils, did not alter *S.* Enteritidis organ invasion frequency. Similar to previous studies, SE-ILK markedly reduced the frequency of *S.* Enteritidis organ invasion, although this response was abrogated by cotreatment with both dexamethasone and SE-ILK. Thus, dexamethasone increased circulating heterophils to a much greater extent than SE-ILK but did not protect against *S.* Enteritidis organ infection. This apparent paradox was solved when in vitro activities of heterophils, derived from control, SE-ILK-treated, or dexamethasone-treated chicks were compared. Heterophils from SE-ILK-treated chicks exhibited markedly increased adherence and in vitro salmonella killing, whereas heterophils derived from dexamethasone-treated birds were similar to controls. That heterophil adherence and chemotaxis, as well as *S.* Enteritidis phagocytosis and killing, were all significantly increased following SE-ILK administration was confirmed in an additional study (Kogut et al., 1995b). Thus, it appeared that heterophil activation was more important than absolute circulating numbers with regard to protection against *S.* Enteritidis organ invasion. Interestingly, heterophils from SE-ILK-treated chicks were more efficient killers of *Salmonella* Typhimurium, *Salmonella* Gallinarum, and *Escherichia coli*, suggesting that the spectrum of SE-ILK activity might not be limited to *S.* Enteritidis (Kogut et al., 1995b).

Because of these close associations of SE-ILK-induced heterophilia and heterophil activation with in vivo protection against *S.* Enteritidis organ invasion, it was postulated that a functional component of SE-ILK could be a colony-stimulating factor (CSF) (McGruder et al., 1996). CSFs such as granulocyte CSF (G-CSF) and granulocyte-macrophage CSF (GM-CSF) are glycoproteins with potent immunobiological activities, including myelopoiesis induction, polymorphonuclear cell priming functions, and induction of polymorphonuclear-predominated leukocytosis in the peripheral blood (Metcalf, 1985, 1986; Asano and Ono, 1987; Clark and Kamen, 1987). In these studies (McGruder et al., 1996), either SE-ILK alone or serum from SE-ILK-treated chicks caused significant increases in the number of colony-forming units (CFU) from cultured bone marrow. Following 10 days of incubation in vitro, exposure of bone marrow to SE-ILK enabled growth of granulocytic bone marrow colonies. Thus, it appears that a CSF is present in the SE-ILK. Further experiments provided convincing evidence that this factor is solely responsible for the SE-ILK-mediated protection (Kogut et al., 1997). Using a purified, monospecific, polyclonal antibody against human G-CSF, the authors demonstrated that pretreatment of SE-ILK with this antibody resulted in (a) the elimination of SE-ILK-induced heterophilia, (b) inhibition of the SE-ILK-induced protection against *S.* Enteritidis organ invasion, (c) the elimination of the heterophil influx into the peritoneum, and (d) a significant decrease in the survival of chicks challenged intraperitoneally with *S.* Enteritidis.

POTENTIAL FOR COMMERCIAL USE OF *SALMONELLA* ENTERITIDIS-IMMUNE LYMPHOKINE

Several studies have indicated that SE-ILK could be effective for prevention of systemic salmonellosis in commercial poultry. Although SE-ILK-induced prophylaxis does not reduce intestinal colonization, the protective effects on organ invasion were consistent and marked in several studies with high challenge doses of a highly invasive strain of *S.* Enteritidis as discussed above. Recently, SE-ILK was evaluated for the ability to protect chicks against a highly pathogenic isolate of *S.* Gallinarum (Kogut et al., 1996). In these experiments, SE-ILK was reported to virtually eliminate organ invasion and mortality when administered 30 min prior to oral challenge with 1×10^4 viable organisms. While challenge with very high doses of this organism (1×10^6 CFU) partially reduced the observed protection, mortality was reduced by almost 50%. Importantly, the growth rate of challenged chicks was also improved by SE-

ILK treatment. As in previous studies with *S.* Enteritidis challenge (McGruder et al., 1993), no effect of similarly prepared lymphokine from T cells derived from nonimmune donors (nonimmune lymphokine) was observed when treated chicks were challenged with *S.* Gallinarum (Kogut et al., 1996), further supporting the premise that in vivo activation of T cells is required for production of protective lymphokine.

Throughout the world, there are still many areas where commercial poultry flocks are regularly infected with highly virulent salmonella isolates such as *S.* Gallinarum (Lucio et al., 1985; Silva, 1985) and the highly virulent isolates of *S.* Enteritidis, discussed elsewhere in this book. In contemplation of the possible commercial utility of SE-ILK, the ability of the protective lymphokine to cross-protect against highly pathogenic isolates of a distinctly different serovar is perhaps important. Previous studies have indicated that heterophils from SE-ILK-treated chicks were more efficient killers of *S.* Typhimurium, *S.* Gallinarum, and *E. coli*, suggesting that the spectrum of SE-ILK activity might extend to other important enteroinvasive genera (Kogut et al., 1995b). If this hypothesis is correct, SE-ILK might be expected to improve performance, not only when challenged with highly pathogenic salmonella isolates, but also as commercial broilers are frequently challenged with a multitude of low-level enteropathogens. Furthermore, as low-virulence "paratyphoid" salmonella isolates are frequently an important production problem for turkey producers (McCapes et al., 1991), SE-ILK may find commercial utility with this species. In support of this premise, Ziprin et al. (1996) recently demonstrated that immune lymphokines could be produced by using immune T-lymphocytes from turkeys. Moreover, SE-ILK produced by chicken T-lymphocytes reduced organ infection to 10% of control levels when administered to poults immediately prior to *S.* Enteritidis challenge.

With regard to potential commercial use, the efficacy of SE-ILK is strictly limited to prophylaxis, with little or no effect resulting when the lymphokine is administered after infection (McGruder et al., 1995a). As young poultry are most susceptible to salmonella infection at or near the time of hatch, the most effective use of SE-ILK for intervention would be at the hatchery, preferably prior to hatch and potential exposure to horizontal transmission. In a previous study, McGruder et al. (1995c) demonstrated that amnionic administration of SE-ILK at 18 days of embryogenesis increased circulating levels of heterophils after hatch, increased in vitro killing of *S.* Enteritidis by heterophils, and markedly and significantly reduced *S.* Enteritidis organ invasion when chicks were challenged on the day of hatch. As embryonic vaccination of poultry is rapidly gaining commercial acceptance, this approach may prove a useful method for SE-ILK delivery. Very recently, an immortalized cell line capable of producing protective SE-ILK has been established (Kogut, patent allowed), potentially allowing for continuous production of quality-controlled SE-ILK.

Although the efficacy of SE-ILK is subject to the limitations of required parenteral administration, with efficacy restricted to prophylaxis against organ invasion and associated morbidity and mortality, this product has several important attributes. A single administration is capable of immediate, marked, and sustained protection during the critical first week of life for young poultry. Also, SE-ILK can be effectively administered by embryonic injection at the time of egg transfer from the incubator to hatching cabinets, a convenient time for embryonic manipulation. Furthermore, evidence to date suggests that SE-ILK is not serovar specific, allowing for simultaneous protection against multiple salmonella serovars and possibly other genera. With the recent generation of an immortalized cell line capable of producing protective SE-ILK, a relatively inexpensive means of preparing the lymphokine is now available. Regardless of eventual commercial acceptance and utility of SE-ILK, perhaps the most exciting aspect of this research is the demonstration that the chick immune system, provided that appropriate stimuli are administered, is capable of very rapid maturation to a highly effective barrier against salmonella organ invasion and systemic disease.

REFERENCES

Asano, S., and Ono, M. 1987. Human granulocyte colony-stimulating factor: its biological actions and clinical implication. Nippon Ketsueki Gakkai Zasshi 50:1550–1556.

Clark, S.C., and Kamen, R. 1987. The hematopoietic colony-stimulating factors. Science 236:1229–1237.

Cooper, G.L., Venables, L.M., Woodward, M.J., and Hormaeche, C.E. 1994. Vaccination of chickens with strain CVL30, a genetically defined Salmonella enteritidis aroA live oral vaccine candidate. Infect. Immun. 62:4747–4754.

Gast, R.K., Stone, H.D., Holt, P.S., and Beard, C.W. 1992. Evaluation of the efficacy of an oil emulsion bacterin for protecting chickens against Salmonella enteritidis. Avian Dis. 36:992–999.

Gast, R.K., Stone, H.D., and Holt, P.S. 1993. Evaluation of the efficacy of oil-emulsion bacterins for reducing fecal shedding of Salmonella enteritidis by laying hens. Avian Dis. 37:1085–1091.

Hassan, J.O., and Curtiss III, R. 1994. Development and evaluation of an experimental vaccination program using a live avirulent Salmonella typhimurium strain to protect immunized chickens against challenge with homologous and heterologous Salmonella serotypes. Infect. Immun. 62:5519–5527.

Hassan, J.O., Porter, S.B., and Curtiss III, R. 1993. Effect of infective dose on humoral immune responses and colonization in chickens experimentally infected with Salmonella typhimurium. Avian Dis. 37:19–26.

Kogut, M.H., Tellez, G.I., Hargis, B.M., Corrier, D.E., and DeLoach, J.R. 1993. The effect of 5-fluorouracil treatment of chicks: a cell depletion model for the study of avian polymorphonuclear leukocytes and natural host defenses. Poult. Sci. 72:1873–1880.

Kogut, M.H., McGruder, E.D., Hargis, B.M., Corrier, D.E., and DeLoach, J.R. 1994a. Dynamics of the avian inflammatory response to Salmonella-immune lymphokines: changes in avian blood leukocyte populations. Inflammation 18:373–388.

Kogut, M.H., Tellez, G.I., McGruder, E.D., Hargis, B.M., Williams, J.D., Corrier, D.E., and DeLoach, J.R. 1994b. Heterophils are decisive components in the early responses of chickens to Salmonella enteritidis infections. Microb. Pathog. 16:141–151.

Kogut, M.H., McGruder, E.D., Hargis, B.M., Corrier, D.E., and DeLoach, J.R. 1995a. Characterization of the pattern of inflammatory cell influx in chicks following the intraperitoneal administration of live Salmonella enteritidis and Salmonella enteritidis-immune lymphokines. Poult. Sci. 74:8–17.

Kogut, M.H., McGruder, E.D., Hargis, B.M., Corrier, D.E., and DeLoach, J.R. 1995b. In vivo activation of heterophil function in chickens following injection with Salmonella enteritidis-immune lymphokines. J. Leukoc. Biol. 57:56–62.

Kogut, M.H., Tellez, G., McGruder, E.D., Wong, R.A., Isibasi, A., Ortiz, V.N., Hargis, B.M., and DeLoach, J.R. 1996. Evaluation of Salmonella enteritidis-immune lymphokines on host resistance to Salmonella enterica ser. gallinarum infection in broiler chicks. Avian Pathol. 25:737–749.

Kogut, M.H., Moyes, R.B., and DeLoach, J.R. 1997. Neutralization of G-CSF inhibits ILK-induced heterophil influx: granulocyte-colony stimulating factor mediates the Salmonella enteritidis-immune lymphokine potentiation of the acute avian inflammatory response. Inflammation 21:9–25.

Lucio, B., Padron, M., and Mosqueda, A. 1985. Fowl typhoid in Mexico. In: Snoeyenbos, G.H., ed. Proceedings of an international symposium on Salmonella. Kennett Square, PA: American Association of Avian Pathologists, pp. 382–383.

McCapes, R.H., Osburn, B.I., and Reimann, H. 1991. Safety of food of animal origin: model for elimination of Salmonella contamination of turkey meat. J. Am. Vet. Med. Assoc. 199:875–880.

McGruder, E.D., Ray, P.M., Tellez, G.I., Kogut, M.H., and Hargis, B.M. 1993. Salmonella enteritidis immune leukocyte-stimulated soluble factors: effect on increased resistance to Salmonella organ invasion in day-old leghorn chicks. Poult. Sci. 72:2264–2271.

McGruder, E.D., Kogut, M.H., Corrier, D.E., DeLoach, J.R., and Hargis, B.M. 1995a. Comparison of prophylactic and therapeutic efficacy of Salmonella enteritidis-immune lymphokines against Salmonella enteritidis organ invasion in neonatal leghorn chicks. Avian Dis. 39:21–27.

McGruder, E.D., Kogut, M.H., Corrier, D.E., DeLoach, J.R., and Hargis, B.M. 1995b. Interaction of dexamethasone and Salmonella enteritidis-immune lymphokines on Salmonella enteritidis organ invasion and in vitro polymorphonuclear leukocyte function. FEMS Immunol. Med. Microbiol. 11:25–34.

McGruder, E.D., Ramirez, G.A., Kogut, M.H., Moore, R.W., Corrier, D.E., DeLoach, J.R., and Hargis, B.M. 1995c. In ovo administration of Salmonella enteritidis-immune lymphokines confers protection to neonatal chicks against Salmonella enteritidis organ infectivity. Poult. Sci. 74:18–25.

McGruder, E.D., Kogut, M.H., Corrier, D.E., DeLoach, J.R., and Hargis, B.M. 1996. Characterisation of colony-stimulating activity in the avian T cell–derived factor, Salmonella enteritidis-immune lymphokine. Res. Vet. Sci. 60:222–227.

Metcalf, D. 1985. The granulocyte-macrophage colony-stimulating factor. Science 229:16–22.

Metcalf, D. 1986. The molecular biology and functions of granulocyte-macrophage colony-stimulating factors. Blood 67:257–267.

Nagaraja, K.V., Kim, C.J., Kumar, M.C., and Pomeroy, B.S. 1991. Is vaccination a feasible approach for the control of *Salmonella*? In: Blankenship, L.C., Bailey, J.S., Cox, N.A., Stern, N.J., and Meinersmann, R.J., eds. Colonization control of human bacterial enteropathogens in poultry. New York: Academic, pp. 243–258.

Powell, P.C. 1987a. Immune mechanisms in infections of poultry. Vet. Immunol. Immunopathol. 15:87–113.

Powell, P.C. 1987b. Macrophages and other non-lymphoid cells contributing to immunity. In: Toivanen, A., and Toivanen, P., eds. Avian immunology: basis and practice, vol. 1. Boca Raton, FL: CRC, pp. 195–212.

Silva, E.N. 1985. The *Salmonella gallinarum* problem in Central and South America. In: Snoeyenbos, G.H., ed. Proceedings of the international symposium on *Salmonella*. Kennett Square, PA: American Association of Avian Pathologists, pp. 150–156.

Stabler, J.G., McCormick, T.W., Powell, K.C., and Kogut, M.H. 1994. Avian heterophils and monocytes: phagocytic and bactericidal activities against *Salmonella enteritidis*. Vet. Microbiol. 38:293–305.

Tellez, G.I., Kogut, M.H., and Hargis, B.M. 1993. Immunoprophylaxis of *Salmonella enteritidis* infection by lymphokines in leghorn chicks. Avian Dis. 37:1062–1070.

Ziprin, R.L., Kogut, M.H., McGruder, E.D., and Hargis, B.M. 1996. Efficacy of *Salmonella enteritidis* (SE)-immune lymphokines from chickens and turkeys on SE liver invasion in one-day-old chicks and turkey poults. Avian Dis. 40:186–192.

39

Methods for Isolating Salmonellae from Poultry and the Poultry Environment

W.D. Waltman

INTRODUCTION

With the report of egg-associated *Salmonella enterica* serovar Enteritidis (*S.* Enteritidis) human outbreaks in the United States (St. Louis et al., 1988; Centers for Disease Control, 1992; Morse et al., 1994) and egg- and meat-associated human outbreaks of *S.* Enteritidis in other countries in the 1980s (Rodrigue et al., 1990; North et al., 1996), there has been renewed interest in the presence of *Salmonella* in poultry. This increase and a general heightened awareness of *Salmonella* as a public health problem have resulted in increased monitoring and surveillance of poultry flocks for *Salmonella*, especially *S.* Enteritidis. This monitoring has shifted from primarily bird culturing and serological testing (especially in the United States) to sampling various environmental sources. The emphasis on culturing environmental samples poses several challenges, including (a) the numbers of *Salmonella* in these samples may be relatively low, (b) the *Salmonella* present may be "injured," and (c) a high concentration of other bacteria is typically present. To compound these challenges, many of the currently used media and methodologies were not developed specifically for isolating *Salmonella* from environmental sources.

In the United States, the National Poultry Improvement Plan (NPIP) took a leading role in monitoring poultry breeding flocks for salmonellae, especially *S.* Enteritidis. Microbiologists working within the NPIP revised the recommended isolation procedures in response to the shift toward environmental monitoring [U.S. Department of Agriculture (USDA), 1996]. As a result of these changes, Waltman and Mallinson (1995) conducted a survey of laboratories in the United

States that were involved in the isolation of salmonellae from poultry and poultry environmental samples to determine the media and methods currently in use. Their findings showed a great diversity in the procedures used by laboratories.

Earlier, the European community realized that laboratories were using widely different isolation procedures for salmonellae. They recognized the potential for discrepancies in the ability to isolate salmonellae and the impact it may have on trade between countries. A comparative study (Edel and Kampelmacher, 1968) was conducted in eight laboratories using naturally and artificially contaminated swine-feces and minced-meat samples. They found that the laboratory with the highest recovery of *Salmonella* detected only 78% of the positive samples. The lowest detection rate was 20%, and only three of the laboratories detected more than 50% of the positive samples.

In a follow-up study, Edel and Kampelmacher (1969) sent naturally and artificially inoculated samples to nine laboratories and had them use a standardized isolation procedure and their "own" laboratory procedure. The recovery rate of most of the laboratories was not improved by the use of the standardized procedure. In laboratories having poorer isolation methods, it did increase the isolation rate; in other laboratories, however, the standardized procedure did not detect as many positive samples as the "in-house" method. They warned that laboratory personnel are typically experienced in their own procedures and that any introduction of new media or methodology requires thorough training. Thus even though a superior procedure is introduced, without adequate training of the laboratory technicians, inferior results may be obtained.

The obvious need for some type of standardized methodology has been recognized and recommended by others (Salmonellosis Committee, 1970; World Health Organization, 1994), but few comparative studies have been conducted that have provided thorough-enough testing to provide the necessary answers to define optimal methodology for different types of samples.

ISOLATION METHODS

The isolation of salmonellae is a complex procedure. There are probably more media and methods available for the isolation of salmonellae than for any other single bacterium. This has resulted in confusion and conflicting reports in the literature regarding the optimal method of isolation. Several factors may contribute to the conflicting reports in the literature. These include

1. The types of samples cultured (for example, clinical, food, feed, or environmental samples). The number of salmonellae relative to other bacteria and the presence of stressed salmonellae vary significantly between sample types.
2. Whether the samples are artificially or naturally contaminated. The use of artificially inoculated samples in studies to determine optimal isolation techniques or for comparing different procedures may give different results than when naturally contaminated samples are used. The organisms used in artificial inoculation studies are laboratory adapted and may react differently than field strains.
3. The enrichment(s) and particular enrichment formulations that are used. Different formulations of enrichments (tetrathionates, for example) may perform differently.
4. The temperature for incubating the enrichment (for example, 37°C or >40°C).
5. The length of time the enrichment is incubated before plating (for example, 24 h, 48 h, or longer).
6. The types of plating media used.
7. The number of suspect colonies screened.

Additional information dealing with the theory and practice of isolating *Salmonella* may be found in several review articles (Jameson, 1962; McCoy, 1962; Fagerberg and Avens, 1976; Harvey and Price, 1979; D'Aoust, 1981; Moats, 1981; Fricker, 1987; Busse, 1995; Andrews, 1996).

Bird Culture

Generally, young birds are more susceptible to salmonellae infections than are older birds. One method of monitoring for the presence of salmonellae in poultry flocks has been culturing day-old chicks. A group of chicks are killed and three tissue pools are collected and cultured for salmonellae. The internal organs (for example, liver, heart, spleen, gallbladder) are pooled together, the yolk sacs are pooled together, and portions of the intestinal tracts are pooled

together. These tissue pools are cultured through selective enrichment (USDA, 1996).

Birds reacting in the pullorum-typhoid agglutination test or birds experiencing morbidity or mortality suggestive of salmonellosis should be cultured for salmonellae. A representative sample of birds from the flock should be brought into the laboratory and necropsied following standard procedures (Zander and Mallinson, 1991). Any abnormal or infected tissues should be inoculated directly onto selective and nonselective agar plates. Internal organs, such as liver, spleen, heart, and gallbladder, may be pooled into one container. Although the ovary and oviduct may be placed into the organ pool, pooling them in separate containers may provide additional information as to the location of *Salmonella* in the bird. A third tissue pool may consist of portions of the ceca, cecal tonsils, and intestinal tract. These tissue pools should be selectively enriched for salmonellae (USDA, 1996).

Typically, salmonellae are not difficult to isolate from acutely infected birds. It is important to culture birds before treating with any antimicrobial agents.

Egg Culture

The ability of *S.* Enteritidis to infect ovarian tissues and to be deposited into the developing egg has resulted in the increased incidence of salmonellosis in humans from the consumption of grade-A shell eggs. Normally, *S.* Enteritidis infection in layer chickens does not result in clinical disease. Therefore, it is difficult to predict or detect flocks or individual birds that may be laying infected eggs. Studies have shown that even in known infected flocks the percentage of contaminated eggs is extremely low and sporadic (Humphrey et al., 1989, 1991).

Environmental culture has become the most common method of monitoring flocks for the possible presence of *Salmonella*, but it is only an indicator. Culturing bird tissues may provide better evidence of infection, but it may require culturing a large number of birds, and it still does not prove the birds are laying contaminated eggs. The only method of directly proving that a flock is laying *S.* Enteritidis-contaminated eggs is by culturing the organism from eggs. This has proven to be difficult, because large numbers of eggs must be cultured to find the small percentage of positive eggs. Also, most contaminated eggs have less than 10 *S.* Enteritidis per egg (Humphrey et al., 1989).

Studies have shown that eggs may be pooled in groups of 10–30 (Gast, 1993b; Henzler et al., 1994). These egg pools may be allowed to incubate at 25°C or 37°C for 1–5 days (Gast, 1993b; *Salmonella* Enteritidis Pilot Project, 1995). They are then inoculated directly onto selective plating media or inoculated into preenrichment and/or selective enrichment broth. Gast (1993a) artificially inoculated pools of 10 eggs with *S.* Enteritidis and incubated them for 4 days at 25°C. He directly inoculated a novobiocin-supplemented brilliant green (BGN) agar plate, transferred 20 ml into 200 ml of tryptic soy broth (TSB) supplemented with ferrous sulfate, and transferred 20 ml into tetrathionate (TT) and Rappaport-Vassiliadis (RV) enrichment broth. After preenrichment

(PE) in TSB, the culture was transferred into TT and RV enrichment media. He found that direct plating detected only 47% of the positive egg pools, whereas direct enrichment in RV, tetrathionate brilliant green (TBG), and TSB detected 56%, 62%, and 65%, respectively. PE followed by selective enrichment in RV and TT detected 71% and 79%, respectively. Gast and Holt (1995b) found that the direct-plating procedure was not able to detect positive egg pools when they had been inoculated with <100,000 *S.* Enteritidis per 10-egg pool. They found that supplementing the egg pool with iron increased the level of growth and increased the recovery of salmonellae (Gast and Holt, 1995a). They also found that different strains of *S.* Enteritidis showed variations in the level of growth in eggs, with or without added iron. Because of the inherent lack of sensitivity, caution should be taken when attempting direct culture of eggs.

Environmental Samples

POULTRY HOUSE
Environmental monitoring of poultry houses has become a method of predicting potential salmonellae contamination of a flock (Poppe et al., 1992; *Salmonella* Enteritidis Pilot Project, 1995; USDA, 1996). It must be emphasized that environmental sampling is only an indicator and that the actual sampling of birds or eggs must be done in order to confirm the possibility of salmonellae infection.

Depending on the type of house (for example, breeder, layer, or broiler), the types and number of samples may vary. Typically, breeder houses are monitored by sampling the floor by pooled litter samples or by drag swab (boot swab), sampling the nest boxes by pooled shavings or swabs, and sampling various other dust samples. Broiler and pullet houses are sampled in much the same way, except for the nest samples. Layer houses are tested by culturing the manure pits or manure scrapers, the egg belts and elevators, walkway dust samples, and other types of dust samples. It is imperative that selective enrichment is used on all environmental samples.

HATCHERY
The hatchery provides an ideal environment for the growth and distribution of salmonellae. It is vital to maintain a constant level of sanitation and monitoring in the hatchery environment. The types of samples to be cultured depend on the type of hatchery and the stringency of the salmonellae-monitoring program that is desired. Eggs may be swabbed as they enter the hatchery to determine any potential salmonellae contamination coming into the hatchery on the eggs. Setters, hatchers, and egg-handling equipment should be routinely monitored for salmonellae by using swab samples. After the chicks hatch, fluff, hatch residue, meconium, chick papers, or even chicks may be sampled for salmonellae (Ellis et al., 1976; USDA, 1996). All samples from the hatchery should also be processed through selective enrichment.

Preenrichment

Historically, PE of samples for isolating *Salmonella* has been reserved for foods, feed, and feed ingredients. It was theorized that heating, drying, and other processes during food and feed preparation may stress *Salmonella* organisms. PE allows for the resuscitation of injured or stressed salmonellae before inoculation onto the harsh conditions of selective plating media or into selective enrichments.

A number of broth media have been used for PE (D'Aoust, 1981). The PE of choice for many years in the United States has been lactose broth (LB) (Gabis and Silliker, 1974). However, because of the severe drop in pH that may occur with some samples (Hilker, 1975; Juven et al., 1984), LB has been replaced in many laboratories by a more buffered PE media, such as buffered peptone water (BPW) (Edel and Kampelmacher, 1973; Thomason et al., 1977; Juven et al., 1984; Cox, 1988) or universal PE broth (Bailey and Cox, 1992). The buffering capacity of BPW helps reduce the decrease in pH. Also, several studies have shown that salmonellae isolation is better with BPW than with LB (Thomason et al., 1977; Thomason and Dodd, 1978; van Leusden et al., 1982; Juven et al., 1984; Fricker, 1987).

Studies have shown the benefit of PE in isolating salmonellae from various samples, including intestinal and environmental (Edel and Kampelmacher, 1973, 1974; van Schothorst and Renaud, 1983; Vassiliadis, 1983; Fricker et al., 1985; Tate et al., 1990; Schlundt and Munch, 1993).

Since the PE step increases the time required to isolate salmonellae, several studies have attempted to shorten the incubation time. D'Aoust (1981) and D'Aoust et al. (1990) found that a short PE time (3–8 h) was not effective because of the high number of false-negative samples in foods. Most protocols recommend incubating the PE media for 16 h or longer. Since the purpose of PE is to enable injured cells to resuscitate, an incubation temperature of 35°–37°C is recommended. After incubation, typically 1 ml of the PE broth is transferred into 10 ml of selective enrichment media (1:10 ratio). The exception is with RV enrichment, where 0.1 ml is transferred into 10 ml (1:100 ratio).

Selective Enrichment

PRINCIPLE
The direct inoculation of samples onto plating media, except in acute infections, is usually unsuccessful. Typically, in chronic infections, carrier animals, or environmental samples, the numbers of salmonellae are low, especially relative to the numbers of other bacteria. Therefore, these samples should be inoculated into selective enrichment media. Galton et al. (1968) found that it was difficult to isolate salmonellae without selective enrichment if the ratio of coliforms to salmonellae was as low as 10:1. Selective enrichment broths are formulated to inhibit other bacteria selectively while allowing *Salmonella* to multiply to levels that may be detected on plating media.

Several review articles have discussed the host of different selective enrichment media that have been proposed and used for isolating *Salmonella* (Jeffries, 1959; Jameson, 1962; McCoy, 1962; Greenfield and Bankier, 1969; Carlson and Snoeyenbos, 1974; Fagerberg and Avens, 1976;

Harvey and Price, 1979; D'Aoust, 1981; van Schothorst and Renaud, 1983; Vassiliadis, 1983; Patil and Parhad, 1986; Fricker, 1987). A survey of laboratories in the United States found that 17 and 13 different selective enrichment media or combinations of enrichment media were used with poultry tissue samples and environmental samples, respectively (Waltman and Mallinson, 1995). Although there are three major types of enrichment media, there are several different formulations within each type of medium.

Typically, as the number of enrichment and plating media are increased for each sample, the number of isolations of *Salmonella* will also increase. However, several factors limit the number of media that can be used, including the labor and expense involved.

TETRATHIONATE ENRICHMENT MEDIA

Mueller (1923) described an enrichment broth that contained iodine and sodium thiosulfate, which would combine to form TT. Kauffman (1930, 1935) modified the TT enrichment medium of Mueller by adding ox bile and brilliant green (BG). The inhibitory effect of TT broth is not well understood, but Palumbo and Alford (1970) postulated the toxicity was due to concentrations of thiosulfate and TT and possible inactivation of bacterial enzyme sulfhydryl groups.

Hajna and Damon (1956) modified the conventional TT enrichment by adding yeast extract, dextrose, and mannitol to encourage growth. They also decreased the bile salt concentration while increasing the sodium thiosulfate concentration. As a result, the iodine-iodide concentration was also modified. An advantage of this formulation is that the BG dye is contained in the dehydrated media and does not have to be added. TT hajna, as it is called, also is more highly buffered than conventional TT media.

The concentration of TT in TT enrichment media is a result of the combination of thiosulfate in the media and the addition of iodine (iodine/potassium-iodide) solution. Because different TT enrichment media contain differing amounts of thiosulfate, the iodine solution is also different. Laboratory personnel should be aware of the particular formulation of TT enrichment media that is used and the correct formulation of iodine to be used with it.

Reports are contradictory regarding the efficacy of TT enrichment as compared with other enrichment media. Possible reasons for this have been discussed previously. Various studies have shown that TT enrichment was superior to selenite enrichment (Sharma and Packer, 1969; Smyser et al., 1970; Snoeyenbos and Carlson, 1972; Carlson and Snoeyenbos, 1974; D'Aoust et al., 1992; Waltman et al., 1995).

Patil and Parhad (1986) compared the recovery of salmonellae when contaminated with different bacteria using selenite, TT, and RV enrichment media. They found that TT was best when coliforms were present in high numbers, but RV was best when *Pseudomonas aeruginosa* was present in high numbers. Therefore, the enrichment of choice may depend on the sample type and the background flora (Poppe et al., 1992).

SELENITE ENRICHMENT MEDIA

Leifson (1936) formulated the first selenite enrichment medium, commonly known as selenite F (SF). Selenite is reduced by bacteria, resulting in an increased pH. This increased pH reduces the toxicity of selenite. Therefore, a fermentable sugar, usually lactose that is attacked by enterococci and coliforms, is added to keep the pH in the acidic range. The mode of action of selenite is not well known, but Weiss et al. (1965) postulated two mechanisms: (a) selenite reacts with sulfhydryl groups of cellular components, and/or (b) selenium is incorporated into analogues of sulfur compounds.

North and Bartram (1953) modified SF by adding cystine (selenite-cystine), which increased the growth of salmonellae in the presence of organic material. It was also known from early studies that selenite selectivity was enhanced under reduced conditions (Leifson, 1936).

Stokes and Osborne (1955) modified SF enrichment by changing the carbohydrate source from lactose to mannitol, and adding sodium taurocholate and BG, thus producing selenite–brilliant green (SBG). They cited the deficiency of SF to inhibit *Proteus* and coliforms. They found that most salmonellae grew better in SBG and that it was more inhibitory to nonsalmonellae than was SF. They found that *Salmonella* Pullorum did not grow as well as other salmonella serovars in either media.

After Osborne and Stokes (1955) formulated SBG enrichment medium, they found it was not very effective for culturing whole egg. The addition of 10% liquid whole egg to SBG reduced its ability to suppress the growth of *Escherichia coli* and especially *Proteus*. They found that the addition of sulfapyridine (SBGS) restored the inhibitory effects of the medium.

Osborne and Stokes (1955) studied the effect of incubating the enrichment for 48 h and found that this additional incubation was detrimental to most salmonellae, except for *S.* Pullorum. They found that salmonellae die rapidly after they reach full growth and that nonsalmonellae, especially *Proteus,* increase in growth with prolonged incubation. Carlson and Snoeyenbos (1974) found that SBGS was not as good as other enrichments, because it allowed major die-offs of salmonellae between 24 and 48 h of incubation. This die-off was especially apparent when incubation was at 43°C.

Selenite enrichment media generally have a shorter shelf life than TT or RV enrichment media, because they must be made fresh daily. Selenite is reduced to selenium, a toxic heavy metal, which has been associated with reduced fertility, congenital defects, and an increase in hepatocellular carcinomas and adenomas in animals (Andrews, 1996; Goyer, 1996). Also, because selenium is considered a hazardous chemical, selenite enrichment media must be disposed of as a hazardous waste.

RAPPAPORT-VASSILIADIS ENRICHMENT MEDIA

Rappaport et al. (1956) described an enrichment media based on *Salmonella*'s ability to (a) survive relatively high osmotic pressures (achieved using magnesium chloride), (b) multiply at relatively low pH (pH 5.2), (c) survive malachite green (106 mg/liter), and (d) grow with minimal nutritional requirements (5 g peptone/liter). Later, Vassiliadis et al. (1970) modified the medium by reducing the concentration of malachite green. This modified medium is referred to as R25. Vassiliadis et al. (1976) further reduced the concentration of malachite green to 36 mg/liter, which made the medium suitable for incubation at 43°C. This medium is referred to as R10, but more commonly as RV.

The original purpose of RV enrichment was for use with fecal samples, but it has been found to be effective in isolating salmonellae from various sources (Vassiliadis et al., 1979, 1984; van Schothorst and Renaud, 1983; Fricker et al., 1985; Schlundt and Munch, 1993; June et al., 1995).

The use of RV has been shown to be most effective following PE in BPW. The optimal sample to enrichment inoculation ratio with RV is 1:100, which differs from the 1:10 inoculation ratio for TT or selenite enrichment media (Vassiliadis, 1983; Fricker et al., 1985). RV enrichment media is incubated routinely at 41.5°C for 24 h. However, Fricker et al. (1985) found that RV enrichment was most effective when incubated for 48 h.

MODIFIED SEMISOLID RAPPAPORT-VASSILIADIS ENRICHMENT MEDIA

Goossens et al. (1984) developed a semisolid medium based on the Rappaport formulation. De Smedt and Bolderdijk (1987) developed the commercially available modified semisolid Rappaport-Vassiliadis (MSRV) enrichment medium. There are several differences between MSRV and RV enrichment media. MSRV enrichment media contains more nutrients, a greater buffering capacity, decreased magnesium-chloride concentration, novobiocin, and a semisolid matrix. Like RV, MSRV is incubated at 41.5°C and follows PE in BPW.

Enrichment using MSRV media has been shown to be very effective in recovering salmonellae (Aspinall et al., 1992; Poppe et al., 1992; De Smedt and Bolderdijk, 1994; Read et al., 1994; Oggel et al., 1995). Davies and Wray (1994a) preenrich samples in BPW for 18–24 h at 37°C, and inoculate 0.2 ml of the broth into the depths of an MSRV agar plate supplemented with 20 µg/ml of novobiocin. A paper disk containing poly-H antisera is placed onto the surface of the agar at the edge of the plate. The plate is incubated at 41.5°C for 18–24 h (if negative, incubate an additional 24 h). Any growth radiating from the point of inoculation that fails to grow around the disk is subcultured onto Rambach (RAM) agar, which is incubated at 41.5°C for 18–24 h.

If MSRV enrichment media is used for isolating *S. Pullorum* or *Salmonella* Gallinarum, which are nonmotile, the growth at the point of inoculation of the MSRV plate must be subcultured onto a selective agar plate. The resulting growth must be screened for salmonellae. This may result in screening numerous negative samples.

Incubation Conditions

INCUBATION TEMPERATURE

Historically, PE cultures and samples containing low levels of bacteria (for example, internal organs, food, or feed) inoculated into selective enrichment media are incubated at 35°–37°C, whereas samples having high levels of bacteria (for example, intestinal or environmental) inoculated into selective enrichment media are incubated at temperatures ranging from 40°C to 43°C. Several studies have attempted to determine the optimal temperature for incubation but often have reported conflicting data. The possible reasons for this conflict have been discussed previously.

Early reports comparing 37°C with 43°C showed that optimum growth of *Salmonella* and other bacteria in pure culture occurred at 37°C. With naturally contaminated samples, however, the selective benefits of the higher temperatures were found to be more pronounced. Jameson (1962) suggested that, when selenite enrichment is used at 37°C, its content of selenite may be less than optimal. A fixed concentration of a selective agent that exerts a bacteriostatic effect on a competitor at 37°C may at a higher temperature exert a bactericidal effect. Thus, changing the formulation of an enrichment may change its selective properties when incubation temperatures are changed. Therefore, selective enrichment media should not be arbitrarily incubated at different temperatures without proper validation.

Harvey and Thompson (1953) first reported an increased recovery of *Salmonella* by using selenite enrichment incubated at 43°C. However, they found that incubation above 43°C inhibited certain serovars of salmonellae, specifically *S.* Typhi and *S.* Pullorum. Several studies have also shown the effectiveness of incubating at temperatures from 40°C to 43°C (Dixon, 1961; Spino, 1966; Carlson et al., 1967; Harvey and Price, 1968; Banfer, 1971; Dusch and Altwegg, 1995).

Waltman et al. (1995) compared the recovery of salmonellae at 37°C and 42°C with several enrichments using naturally contaminated environmental samples. There was no real difference in the recovery rate with TT or TBG enrichment media, but incubation of TT hajna at 42°C resulted in slightly fewer salmonellae isolations than at 37°C.

Some studies (McCoy, 1962; Carlson and Snoeyenbos, 1974; Harvey and Price, 1979) have found that incubation at higher temperatures, especially 43°C, can inhibit or even kill some salmonellae. Certainly, some enrichment media would be destructive to salmonellae at these high temperatures. Harvey and Price (1979) suggested that if salmonellae have recently left the human or animal intestinal tract, they should be easily recovered regardless of the isolation method used. However, if the organisms are sublethally injured, they may fail to multiply if inoculated directly into the relatively hostile environment of an enrichment medium. This inhibition or failure in isolation would be compounded if the enrichment media were incubated at a temperature above 37°C.

Generally, an incubation temperature of 41°–42°C is chosen to allow for slight incubator variations. Each laboratory should monitor the temperature of their incubators, especially when the higher temperatures are used. Different areas of the incubator should be checked for "hot spots," because temperatures just a few degrees higher than recommended can be destructive to *Salmonella*. Another incubation concern is the introduction of large quantities of enrichment media that may occur when batching samples. If the media is cold (perhaps refrigerated stock solutions), it may take several hours for the temperature of the enriched sample to reach the desired temperature. This is especially detrimental if the culture is plated only after 18–24 h of incubation, possibly resulting in reduced ability to detect salmonellae.

INCUBATION TIME

A survey of laboratories in the United States found that approximately 50% subculture only their selective enrichment broths to plating media after 24 h of incubation. Another 25% of laboratories reincubate and replate the selective enrichment media after 48 h (Waltman and Mallinson, 1995).

Sharma and Packer (1969) and Grunnet (1975) showed that subculture of the enrichment media to plating media before 24 h was not effective. Carlson et al. (1967) studied the population dynamics of pure cultures of S. Typhimurium in SBGS and TBG and found maximum populations were not reached until 32 h. Carlson et al. (1967) found that plating after 48 h of incubation gave the greatest number of positive samples when using meat and bone meal and litter samples. Edel and Kampelmacher (1968, 1973, 1974) also found increased recovery of salmonellae after 48 h of incubation.

Galton et al. (1968) found that subculture after two incubation periods, such as 24 and 48 h or 24 and 72 h, usually resulted in increased recovery of *Salmonella*. A major factor determining the time of appearance of positive subcultures is the number of salmonellae in the inoculum.

Grunnet (1975), isolating salmonellae from sewage, found that 60% of the samples were positive after the initial 24-h plating; after 48-, 72-, and 96-h platings, his recovery increased 23%, 11%, and 6%, respectively. Carlson et al. (1967) showed that incubation beyond 48 h did not increase the isolation of *Salmonella* but allowed overgrowth of *Salmonella* by other bacteria. Some selective enrichment cultures (for instance, SBGS), actually show a decrease in the number of *Salmonella* with increased incubation.

DELAYED SECONDARY ENRICHMENT

Delayed secondary enrichment (DSE) is the process whereby the original enrichment broth (typically TT) is left at room temperature after a 24-h incubation and subsequent plating. If the culture is negative after the initial plating, the enrichment broth is left at room temperature for 5–7 days. Then, 0.5–1.0 ml of this broth is then transferred to 10 ml of fresh enrichment broth and incubated at 37°C for 20–24 h and then plated.

The difference between DSE and studies investigating extended incubation times (which often showed decreases in salmonellae populations) is that the DSE cultures are left at room temperature, and not incubation temperatures of 37°C or greater.

Several studies have shown the increase in the isolation rate of salmonellae following DSE (Pourciau and Springer, 1978; Waltman et al., 1991, 1992; Waltman and Horne, 1993). Rigby and Pettit (1980) studied the usefulness of DSE with a range of samples, particularly environmental samples. They used a standard 24-h enrichment (direct enrichment), PE followed by selective enrichment, and DSE. From a total of 2283 samples, 9% were positive after direct enrichment, 12% were positive after PE, and 16% were positive after DSE. They found that replating the original enrichment culture after the room-temperature incubation prior to transfer increased recovery but not as much as if the transfer was made into fresh enrichment and incubated. They also studied whether there was a difference when doing DSE on direct enrichment and PE cultures. DSE of PE cultures gave a slightly higher recovery rate than did direct enrichment.

Using naturally contaminated samples, Waltman et al. (1993) compared the recovery of salmonellae after different incubation times. They found that substantially more salmonellae were isolated after DSE as compared with the 24-h or the 48-h platings. They also reported that the conventional 5-day DSE was better than a shorter 3-day DSE.

Waltman et al. (1995) compared various enrichment media and incubation temperatures with and without PE and DSE: 15%–20% more salmonellae were isolated following DSE than following direct enrichment or PE followed by selective enrichment.

Plating Media

PRINCIPLE

The enrichment process is designed to increase the number of salmonellae in the culture to a level that may be detected on plating media. Various plating media have been developed for isolating salmonellae by using the principles of selectivity and differentiation. Selectivity involves the addition of chemical agents to the plating media that selectively inhibit nonsalmonellae. The differential characteristic of plating media involves the addition of substances that result in salmonellae colonies appearing different from other bacterial colonies.

A survey of laboratories in the United States showed a tremendous diversity in the number and types of plating media used. The primary media used with tissue samples were MacConkey (MAC) (46%), xylose-lysine-tergitol 4 (XLT4) (42%), and BGN (37%) agars. From environmental samples, the primary plating media were XLT4 (50%), BGN (46%), BG (36%), and MAC (33%) agars.

The wide range of plating media in use may represent ties to clinical procedures and historical protocols. Several new media formulations have been shown to be very effective in isolating *Salmonella*. These media appear to be more effective with environmental samples, which invariably are highly contaminated with other bacteria.

It is recommended that at least two plating media be used that have different selective agents and differential characteristics, such as BGN and XLT4 (Mallinson, 1990; Waltman et al., 1995). It should be emphasized that not all salmonellae give "typical" reactions. Waltman et al. (1995) reported that 13% of salmonellae isolated, including S. Pullorum, were hydrogen sulfide (H_2S) negative on plating media. For this reason, one of the isolation plates should be predicated on some characteristic other than H_2S production; otherwise, several H_2S-negative colonies would have to be screened. There are also occasional lactose-positive or lysine-negative *Salmonella.*

Plating media, with few exceptions, are incubated at 35°–37°C. Davies and Wray (1994a) routinely incubate an RAM agar plate subcultured from MSRV medium at 42°C. Also EF-18 agar plates are routinely incubated at 42°C (Entis and Boleszczuk, 1991). MSRV medium, which is actually more of an enrichment medium in a plate format, is incubated at 41.5°C.

Plating media should be incubated for 20–24 h and observed for suspected *Salmonella* colonies. If the plates are negative, especially if *S.* Pullorum is suspected, the plates should be reincubated for another 24 h before being discarded as negative.

CHARACTERISTICS OF MEDIA

Bismuth Sulfite Agar

Bismuth sulfite (BS) agar was developed by Wilson and Blair (1927). BS agar contains BS and BG as selective agents and an H_2S indicator as differential agent. It was originally formulated for the isolation of *S.* Typhi and is somewhat unique in not utilizing the fermentation of any carbohydrate to produce a differential characteristic. For this reason, BS agar is advocated in situations where lactose-positive salmonellae may be found.

The media suffers from several disadvantages. The primary disadvantage is its instability. BS agar must be used within a few days of its preparation. Some investigators indicate the necessity of "aging" the medium (McCoy, 1962; Fagerberg and Avens, 1976). BS agar's inhibitory properties change rapidly during storage (Moats, 1981). Some reports suggest that non–*S.* Typhi grow better if BS plates are aged in the refrigerator for a few days (Cook, 1952; McCoy, 1962; Hobbs, 1963). This inhibitory effect decreased as the medium aged for 4–5 days in the refrigerator. This "aging" was also shown to be necessary for the development of characteristic *Salmonella* colonies (McCoy, 1962). McCoy states that characteristic colonies ("jet black circular center with sharp edge, surrounded by a clear translucent periphery") were observed after 18 h on aged plates but were not observed on fresh plates until around 48 h.

More commonly, the disadvantage is in distinguishing salmonellae colonies from nonsalmonellae colonies. This is especially difficult when intestinal and environmental samples are cultured that have a high level of other bacteria. When colonies are not well isolated on BS agar, the characteristic colonial morphology may not be easily seen. Monford and Thatcher (1961) and Erdman (1974) found that BS agar allowed the growth of high levels of coliforms and resulted in a large number of false-positive samples. Yamamoto et al. (1961) and Cox et al. (1972) also reported that BS agar was unsatisfactory.

Brilliant Green Agar and Modifications

BG agar was developed by Kristensen et al. (1925) and then modified by Kauffman (1935). BG dye is the selective agent, and lactose fermentation is the differential characteristic. Based on the addition of different antimicrobial agents, there have been two major modifications to BG agar. Galton et al. (1954) added sulfadiazine, and Osborne and Stokes (1955) added sulfapyridine to BG agar. The addition of sulfadiazine or sulfapyridine to BG agar (BGS) was for the inhibition of *Proteus* and pseudomonads.

Tate and Miller (1990) incorporated novobiocin into BG agar (BGN) and found that *Proteus* was completely inhibited on BGN, whereas on plain BG, or on BGS, swarming and nonswarming *Proteus* spp. were able to grow and interfere with the detection of salmonellae.

Several studies have advocated the use of BG agar (Banwart and Ayers, 1953; Taylor et al., 1958; Smyser et al., 1963, 1970; Moats and Kinner, 1974; Moats, 1981), BGS agar (Montford and Thatcher, 1961; Ellis et al., 1976), and BGN agar (Mallinson, 1990; Waltman et al., 1995).

Deoxycholate-Citrate Agar

Deoxycholate-citrate agar (DCA) was developed by Leifson (1935) and modified by Hynes (1942). The medium was formulated to isolate salmonellae and other enteric pathogens, including *Shigella*. The medium contains sodium deoxycholate and sodium citrate as selective agents and lactose fermentation as the differential characteristic. Leifson (1935) found that the selective action of sodium deoxycholate was enhanced by sodium citrate. The combination is found in both DCA and salmonella-shigella (SS) agars.

Jeffries (1959) found that *Proteus* grew well on DCA and interfered with salmonellae detection. He attempted to solve this problem by adding novobiocin, but found that incorporating 32 µg/ml of novobiocin only inhibited 50% of the *Proteus* strains tested. Late lactose fermenters and lactose-negative nonsalmonellae (for example, *Proteus* and pseudomonads) can grow on DCA. These bacteria are not easily differentiated from *Salmonella*, which results in a large number of false-positive samples (Monford and Thatcher, 1961; Fagerberg and Avens, 1976).

EF-18 Agar

EF-18 agar is predominantly used in conjunction with hydrophobic membrane filtration, but a few studies have been conducted using it as a standard plating medium from enrichment broth (Entis and Boleszczuk, 1991; Sherrod et al., 1995). EF-18 agar is highly selective, containing bile salts, crystal violet, sulfapyridine, and novobiocin as selective agents. It is also incubated at 42°C. The differential characteristics are conferred by the presence of sucrose and lysine. Typical salmonellae appear as blue-green colonies.

Hektoen Enteric Agar and Modification

King and Metzger (1968) formulated Hektoen enteric (HE) agar for the isolation of salmonellae and shigellae while inhibiting normal intestinal flora. The medium contains bile salts as the selective agent and lactose, sucrose, salicin, and an H_2S indicator as differential agents. HE agar suffers from specificity problems. Hoben et al. (1973) added novobiocin to HE agar (HEN) to suppress *Proteus* and *Citrobacter,* with good results. Others have also found that HEN agar is more sensitive and specific than HE agar (Restaino et al., 1977, 1982; Waltman et al., 1995).

MacConkey Agar

MAC agar was described by MacConkey (1905) for the selective isolation of Gram-negative enteric bacteria. The medium contains bile salts and crystal violet as selective agents. The incorporation of lactose and phenol red differentiates lactose fermentative and nonfermentative bacteria. MAC agar and other similar media, such as violet red bile, eosin-methylene blue (EMB), and Endo agar, are excellent for the isolation of enteric bacteria from clinical material. However, these media lack sufficient selectivity and differential properties for isolating salmonellae from intestinal and environmental sources. MAC agar may still be useful for the isolation of *S.* Pullorum where a less selective agar medium may be used to recover any organism that may fail to grow on the more selective agars.

Modified Lysine Iron Agar

Modified lysine iron agar (MLIA) was reported by Bailey et al. (1988), who added sodium thiosulfate and ferric ammonium citrate to Rappold and Bolderijk's (1979) modification of lysine iron agar. They took advantage of the differential capabilities of lysine iron agar and added novobiocin to suppress *Proteus* spp. They found that MLIA recovered more salmonellae from fresh and cured meats than either BGS or xylose-lysine-deoxycholate-novobiocin (XLDN) agars. Cox (1988) and Waltman et al. (1995) have reported good results with MLIA.

Novobiocin-Brilliant Green-Glycerol-Lactose Agar

Novobiocin-brilliant green-glycerol-lactose (NBGL) agar was developed by Poisson (1992). The selective agents include BG and novobiocin. The differential characteristics are conferred by lactose, glycerol, and an H_2S indicator system. Glycerol was added to help differentiate *Salmonella* from *Citrobacter*. Typical salmonellae produce colonies with black centers. Several studies have shown good sensitivity and specificity with NBGL agar (Poisson, 1992; Poisson et al., 1993; Ruiz et al., 1996).

Rambach Agar

Rambach (1990) formulated a plating medium based on the finding that salmonellae produce acid from propylene glycol. He found that 97% of nontyphi salmonellae produced bright red colonies on this medium. *Salmonella* Pullorum does not produce characteristic red colonies. Studies have shown good sensitivity and specificity with RAM agar (Monnery et al., 1994; Dusch and Altwegg, 1995; Waltman et al., 1995).

Salmonella Identification Agar

Salmonella identification (SMID) agar is a chromogenic media similar to RAM agar, but SMID can be used for isolating *S.* Typhi and *S.* Paratyphi. The differential characteristics involve fermentation of D-glucuronate and a β-galactosidase indicator. Salmonellae are typically red.

Davies and Wray (1994b) and Ruiz et al. (1996) found the sensitivity and specificity of SMID agar to be as good or better than other salmonellae isolation media.

Salmonella-Shigella Agar

SS agar was formulated to inhibit coliforms, while allowing the recovery of salmonellae and shigellae. Bile salts, sodium citrate, and BG serve as the selective agents. Lactose and an H_2S indicator are included as differential agents. Late lactose fermenters and lactose-negative nonsalmonellae, for example, *Proteus* and pseudomonads, may grow on SS agar and not be differentiated from *Salmonella*, resulting in a large number of false-positive samples (Fagerberg and Avens, 1976; Ruiz et al., 1996).

Xylose-Lysine Agar and Modifications

Xylose-lysine-deoxycholate (XLD) agar was developed by Taylor (1965). The medium incorporates sodium deoxycholate as the selective agent and lactose, sucrose, lysine, and an H_2S indicator as differential characteristics.

A major problem with XLD agar is the inability to suppress the growth of *Proteus* spp. The presence of H_2S, evidenced by black colonies, often obscures the difference in the lysine reaction of salmonellae and proteae. Several investigators have studied the incorporation of novobiocin into the XLD medium and have found increased sensitivity and specificity with XLDN agar (Restaino et al., 1977, 1982; Waltman et al., 1995).

Komatsu and Restaino (1981) studied the effect of adding novobiocin to XLD and HE agars. They cultured 182 fresh meat products by using an LB PE followed by enrichment in selenite-cystine. Each culture was plated onto XLD, XLDN, HE, HEN, and BGS agars. They found the addition of novobiocin to XLD increased the isolation from 50% to 82%, while decreasing the false-positive rate from 38% to 5%. The addition of novobiocin to HE increased the isolation from 75% to 85%, while decreasing the false-positive rate from 50% to 16%. The isolation and false-positive rate for BGS was 65% and 16%, respectively. In each case, the addition of novobiocin increased the isolation of *Salmonella* and decreased the number of false-positive cultures.

Miller and Tate (1990) and Miller et al. (1991) developed a modified formulation of XLD by substituting tergitol (Niaproof) 4 for deoxycholate. The new medium, XLT4, was found to inhibit *Proteus*, *Pseudomonas,* and *Providencia,* and many other nonsalmonellae. The medium was modified by the addition of proteose peptone, which enhanced the formation of black colonies produced by H_2S production (Miller et al. 1995).

Overview of Plating Media

Several studies have compared the effectiveness of contemporary plating media to determine the best medium or combination of media. Taylor and Schelhart (1971) studied the effectiveness of various plating media for isolating salmonellae and the relative number of false positives found on these media. From 1597 stool samples, they isolated 168, 299,

323, and 334 salmonellae on EMB, SS, HE, and XLD agars, respectively. The percentages of false-positive reactions were 20%, 54%, 62%, and 25%, respectively. Their work showed that HE and XLD agars were more sensitive than EMB and SS agars, but they lacked specificity. They found that *Campylobacter freundii*, slow lactose fermenters, and *Proteus* spp. were responsible for most of the false reactions on HE agar and *Pseudomonas* spp., *Proteus* spp., and slow lactose fermenters were the problems with XLD agar.

Moats (1978) conducted a similar study comparing the recovery of salmonellae from 75 beef and turkey samples on media with and without novobiocin added. He isolated 13, 17, 17, and 21 salmonellae on HE, HEN, XLD, and XLDN agars, respectively. The percentages of false-positive samples were 77%, 32%, 24%, and 3%, respectively. The addition of novobiocin to HE and XLD agars increased the isolation rate while dramatically decreasing the number of false positives. The decrease in false positives was due to the inhibition of *Proteus* spp. by novobiocin. Sherrod et al. (1995) compared the effectiveness of several plating media (BS, HE, XLD, EF-18, RAM, and XLT4 agars) for isolating salmonellae from high-moisture foods. They used artificially inoculated shrimp, oyster, egg-yolk, and lettuce samples. They also used naturally contaminated samples of pork sausage, chicken, turkey, and frog legs. With naturally contaminated samples, XLT4 agar was the best or second best plating media regardless of the enrichment used. The newer plating media (the EF-18, RAM, and XLT4 agars) outperformed the conventional plating media (the BS, HE, and XLD agars). However, with artificially inoculated samples, the conventional media rated better. They also compared the number of false-positive results for each plating media. Again, the newer plating had fewer false positives than the conventional plating media, particularly with the naturally contaminated samples.

Miller et al. (1991), who compared the recovery of salmonellae from drag swabs by using five plating media, found the following isolation rates: XLT4 (98%), BGN (85%), XLDN (84%), BG (71%), and XLD (30%). They also noted that salmonellae on the XLT4 plate was usually in almost pure culture and the plates with novobiocin had lower background bacteria than did the plates without novobiocin.

Mallinson (1990), in a similar study, compared eight plating media for isolating *Salmonella* from 196 drag swabs. He found the following isolation rates: XLT4 (98%), BGN (91%), BG (82%), XLDN (81%), BGS (72%), XLD (33%), HE (20%), and MAC (12%). He also found that the plating media having the highest isolation rates had the lowest false-positive reactions.

Waltman et al. (1995) have investigated the efficiency of different plating media by using naturally contaminated environmental samples. XLT4 and BGN agars were the best media, and when used in combination detected over 95% of the positive samples. The other novobiocin-containing media (HE, MLIA, and XLDN) and RAM also gave good sensitivity. XLT4, the novobiocin-containing media (BGN, HEN, XLDN, and MLIA), and RAM were also very specific.

There appears to be a relationship between sensitivity and specificity of a plating medium. Several studies, especially those that have tested media with and without novobiocin, have shown that an increase in specificity parallels an increase in sensitivity. This may be due to the inhibition of bacteria that resemble salmonellae, thus enabling the detection of salmonellae. It may also be due to a decrease in the amount of bacterial growth on a plate. The overgrowth of bacteria may hide or obscure salmonellae colonies, or the local pH reactions produced by nonsalmonellae colonies in the agar medium may alter the characteristic appearance of salmonellae, causing them to be overlooked.

SELECTION AND SCREENING OF SALMONELLAE SUSPECT COLONIES

After the enrichment broths are inoculated onto plating media and incubated, they are observed for suspect *Salmonella* colonies. It is imperative that laboratory personnel be trained in the characteristic appearance of salmonellae colonies on the respective plating media used. Depending on the selectivity of the respective plating media used, there may be almost a pure culture of *Salmonella* or there may be several species of bacteria growing on the plates from which *Salmonella* must be selected. The more selective plating media (for example, XLT4 and novobiocin-supplemented media) decrease the labor involved in screening large numbers of colonies and false-positive samples while increasing the likelihood of selecting true salmonellae colonies.

Typically, suspect *Salmonella* colonies are picked from plating media and inoculated into tubes of triple-sugar iron (TSI) agar and/or lysine iron agar (LIA). It is recommended that at least three colonies be screened from each plate. Multiple suspect colonies should be screened to ensure the detection of *Salmonella* and the possible detection of multiple serovars. After incubating the TSI and LIA tubes, isolates that give typical reactions in these media are processed further through biochemical and serological tests (Ewing, 1986).

As pointed out previously, laboratory personnel should be aware of the possibility of various atypical salmonellae, such as H_2S-negative, lactose- or sucrose-positive, or lysine-positive strains. The best method of detecting these atypical salmonellae is the use of multiple plates that have different differential characteristics.

Some poultry companies are particularly concerned with the presence of *S.* Enteritidis or *S.* Typhimurium. In many instances, the isolation of these serovars would result in the depopulation of the flock. A potential problem occurs when the environmental samples from a particular flock are positive for a *Salmonella* serovar other than these (for example, *S.* Heidelberg or *S.* Hadar). Typically, after an environment becomes contaminated with a particular serovar, subsequent sampling will also yield that serovar. To ensure that subsequent monitoring will be able to detect any new contamination with *S.* Enteritidis or *S.* Typhimurium, multiple salmonellae suspect colonies (for example, 5–10 colonies) should be screened.

Recently, a colony screening assay has been developed for detecting group-D salmonellae (Lamichhane et al., 1995). The assay is able to screen all the colonies on an isolation plate specifically for serogroup-D colonies, which can then be tested further.

CONFIRMATION METHODS

Biochemical Methods

It is important to identify the salmonellae isolates biochemically or at least screen the isolates with selected biochemical tests to ensure that the organisms are in fact *Salmonella*. This is necessary because some nonsalmonellae (for example, citrobacters and enterobacters) may cross-react with some somatic antisera. Ellis et al. (1976) and Ewing (1986) describe the characteristic and differential biochemical reactions of salmonellae, as do most diagnostic bacteriology textbooks.

Serological Methods

Salmonella may have three major types of antigens. The somatic (O) antigen is a heat-stable polysaccharide associated with the cell wall. The flagellar (H) antigen is a heat-labile protein associated with the flagella of the cell. The capsular (Vi) antigen is envelope material and typically found only on *S.* Typhi.

The somatic antigens of salmonellae are assigned Arabic numbers from 1 to 67 and are placed into serogroups based on the somatic content of an isolate (for example, serogroup B may contain somatic antigens 1, 4, 5, 12, and 27). Serogroups are designated with capital letters from A to Z and as groups 51 to 67. Each serogroup may contain dozens of serovars, which are identified by their H antigens. The H antigens are designated by lowercase letters and by numbers (Ewing, 1986).

Phage Typing

Some serovars of *Salmonella,* especially *S.* Enteritidis and *S.* Typhimurium, may be further subdivided based on their reactivity to a set of specific phages. Phage typing has been useful for epidemiological and pathogenicity studies.

REFERENCES

Andrews, W.H. 1996. Evolution of methods for the detection of *Salmonella* in foods. J. AOAC Int. 79:4–12.

Aspinall, S.T., Hindle, M.A., and Hutchinson, D.N. 1992. Improved isolation of salmonellae for feces using a semisolid Rappaport-Vassiliadis medium. Eur. J. Clin. Microbiol. Infect. Dis. 11:936–938.

Bailey, J.S., and Cox, N.A. 1992. Universal preenrichment broth for the simultaneous detection of *Salmonella* and *Listeria* in foods. J. Food Prot. 55:256–259.

Bailey, J.S., Chi, J.Y., Cox, N.A., and Johnson, R.W. 1988. Improved selective procedure for detection of salmonellae from poultry and sausage products. J. Food Prot. 51:391–396.

Banfer, J.R.J. 1971. Comparison of the isolation of salmonellae from human feces at 37°C and 43°C. Zentralbl. Bakteriol. Parasitenkd. Infectionskr. Hyg. 1 Abt. Orig. 217:35–40.

Banwart, G.J., and Ayers, J.C. 1953. Effect of various enrichment broths and selective agars upon the growth of several species of *Salmonella*. Appl. Microbiol. 1:196–201.

Busse, M. 1995. Media for *Salmonella*. Int. J. Food Microbiol. 26:117–131.

Carlson, V.L., and Snoeyenbos, G.H. 1972. Relationship of population kinetics of *Salmonella typhimurium* and cultural methodology. Am. J. Vet. Res. 33:177–184.

Carlson, V.L., and Snoeyenbos, G.H. 1974. Comparative efficacies of selenite and tetrathionate enrichment broths for the isolation of *Salmonella* serotypes. Am. J. Vet. Res. 35:711–719.

Carlson, V.L., Snoeyenbos, G.H., McKie, B.A., and Smyser, C.F. 1967. A comparison of incubation time and temperature for the isolation of *Salmonella*. Avian Dis. 11:217–225.

Centers for Disease Control. 1992. Outbreak of *Salmonella enteritidis* infection associated with consumption of raw shell eggs. MMWR 41:369–372.

Cook, C.T. 1952. Comparison of two modifications of bismuth sulphite agar for the isolation and growth of *Salmonella typhi* and *Salmonella typhimurium*. J. Pathol. Bacteriol. 64:559–566.

Cox, N.A. 1988. *Salmonella* methodology update. Poult. Sci. 67:921–927.

Cox, N.A., Davis, B.H., Kendall, J.H., Watts, A.B., and Colmer, A.R. 1972. *Salmonella* in the laying hen. 3. A comparison of various enrichment broths and plating media for the isolation of *Salmonella* from poultry feces and poultry food products. Poult. Sci. 51:1312–1316.

D'Aoust, J.Y. 1981. Update on preenrichment and selective enrichment conditions for detection of *Salmonella* in foods. J. Food Prot. 44:369–374.

D'Aoust, J.Y., Sewell, A., and Jean, A. 1990. Limited sensitivity of short (6 h) selective enrichment for detection of foodborne *Salmonella*. J. Food Prot. 53:562–565.

D'Aoust, J.Y., Sewell, A.M., and Warburton, D.W. 1992. A comparison of standard cultural methods for the detection of food-borne *Salmonella*. Int. J. Food Microbiol. 16:41–50.

Davies, R.H., and Wray, C. 1994a. Evaluation of a rapid cultural method for identification of salmonellae in naturally contaminated veterinary samples. J. Appl. Bacteriol. 77:237–241.

Davies, R.H., and Wray. C. 1994b. Evaluation of SMID agar for identification of *Salmonella* in naturally contaminated veterinary samples. Lett. Appl. Microbiol. 18:15–17.

De Smedt, J.M., and Bolderdijk, R.F. 1987. Dynamics of *Salmonella* isolation with modified semi-solid Rappaport-Vassiliadis medium. J. Food Prot. 50:658–661.

De Smedt, J.M., and Bolderdijk, R.F. 1994. *Salmonella* detection in cocoa and chocolate by motility enrichment on modified semi-solid Rappaport-Vassiliadis medium: collaborative study. J. AOAC Int. 77:365–373.

Dixon, J.M.S. 1961. Rapid isolation of salmonellae from feces. J. Clin. Pathol. 14:397–399.

Dusch, H., and Altwegg, M. 1993. Comparison of Rambach agar, SM-ID medium, and Hektoen enteric agar for primary isolation of non-typhi salmonellae from stool samples. J. Clin. Microbiol. 31:410–412.

Dusch, H., and Altwegg, M. 1995. Evaluation of five new plating media for isolation of *Salmonella* species. J. Clin. Microbiol. 33:802–804.

Edel, W., and Kampelmacher, E.H. 1968. Comparative studies on *Salmonella* isolation in eight European laboratories. Bull. WHO 39:487–491.

Edel, W., and Kampelmacher, E.H. 1969. *Salmonella* isolation in nine European laboratories using a standardized technique. Bull. WHO 41:297–306.

Edel, W., and Kampelmacher, E.H. 1973. Comparative studies on the isolation of "sub-lethally injured" salmonellae in nine European laboratories. Bull. WHO 48:167–174.

Edel, W., and Kampelmacher, E.H. 1974. Comparative studies on *Salmonella* isolations from feeds in ten laboratories. Bull. WHO 50:421–426.

Ellis, E.M., Williams, J.E., Mallinson, E.T., Snoeyenbos, G.H., and Martin, W.J. 1976. Culture methods for the detection of animal salmonellosis and arizonosis: a manual of the American Association of Veterinary Laboratory Diagnosticians. Ames: Iowa State University Press, 87 pp.

Entis, P., and Boleszczuk, P. 1991. Rapid detection of *Salmonella* in foods using EF-18 agar in conjunction with the hydrophobic grid membrane filter. J. Food Prot. 54:930–934.

Erdman, E.E. 1974. ICMSF methods studies. IV. International collaborative assay for the detection of *Salmonella* in raw meat. Can. J. Microbiol. 20:715–720.

Ewing, W.H. 1986. Edwards and Ewing's identification of Enterobacteriaceae, 4th ed. New York: Elsevier Science.

Fagerberg, D.J., and Avens, J.S. 1976. Enrichment and plating methodology for *Salmonella* detection in food: a review. J. Milk Food Technol. 39:628–646.

Fricker, C.R. 1987. The isolation of salmonellas and campylobacters: a review. J. Appl. Bacteriol. 63:99–116.

Fricker, C.R., Quail, E., McGibbon, L., and Girdwood, R.W.A. 1985. An evaluation of commercially dehydrated Rappaport-Vassiliadis medium for the isolation of salmonellae from poultry. J. Hyg. Camb. 95:337–344.

Gabis, D.A., and Silliker, J.H. 1974. ICMSF methodology studies. II. Comparison of analytical schemes for detection of *Salmonella* in high moisture foods. Can. J. Microbiol. 20:663–669.

Galton, M.M., Lowery, W.D., and Hardy, A.V. 1954. *Salmonella* in fresh and smoked pork sausage. J. Infect. Dis. 95:232–235.

Galton, M.M., Morris, G.K., and Martin, W.T. 1968. Salmonellae in foods and feeds: review of isolation methods and recommended procedures. Atlanta, GA: Centers for Disease Control; United States Department of Health, Education, and Welfare/Public Health Service.

Gast, R.K. 1993a. Recovery of *Salmonella enteritidis* from inoculated pools of egg contents. J. Food Prot. 56:21–24.

Gast, R.K. 1993b. Evaluation of direct plating for detecting *Salmonella enteritidis* in pools of egg contents [Research note]. Poult. Sci. 72:1611–1614.

Gast, R.K., and Holt, P.S. 1995a. Differences in the multiplication of *Salmonella enteritidis* in liquid whole egg: implications for detecting contaminated eggs from commercial laying flocks. Poult. Sci. 74:893–897.

Gast, R.K., and Holt, P.S. 1995b. Iron supplementation to enhance the recovery of *Salmonella enteritidis* from pools of egg contents. J. Food Prot. 58:268–272.

Goosens, H., Wauters, G., De Boeck, M., Janssens, M., and Butzler, J. 1984. Semisolid selective-motility enrichment medium for isolation of salmonellae from fecal specimens. J. Clin. Microbiol. 19:940–941.

Goyer, R.A. 1996. Toxic effects of metals. In: Klaassen, C.D., Amdur, M.O., and Doull, J., eds. Cassarett and Doull's toxicology: the basic science of poisons, 5th ed. New York: McGraw-Hill, pp. 691–736.

Greenfield, J., and Bankier, J.C. 1969. Isolation of *Salmonella* and *Arizona* using enrichment media incubated at 35°C and 43°C. Avian Dis. 13:864–871.

Grunnet, K. 1975. Development of a standard method for isolation of *Salmonella* from sewage and receiving waters. In: Salmonella in sewage and receiving waters. Copenhagen: FADL's Forlag, pp. 69–78.

Hajna, A.A., and Damon, S.R. 1956. New enrichment and plating media for the isolation of *Salmonella* and *Shigella* organisms. Appl. Microbiol. 4:341–345.

Harvey, R.W.S., and Price, T.H. 1968. Elevated temperature of incubation of enrichment media for the isolation of salmonellas from heavily contaminated materials. J. Hyg. Camb. 66:377–381.

Harvey, R.W.S., and Price, T.H. 1979. A review: principles of *Salmonella* isolation. J. Appl. Bacteriol. 46:27–56.

Harvey, R.W.S., and Thompson, S. 1953. Optimum temperature of incubation for isolation of salmonellae. Mon. Bull. Minist. Health Public Health Lab. Serv. Directed Med. Res. Counc. 12:149–150.

Henzler, D.J., Ebel, E., Sanders, J., Kradel, D., and Mason, J. 1994. *Salmonella enteritidis* in eggs from commercial chicken layer flocks implicated in human outbreaks. Avian Dis. 38:37–43.

Hilker, J.S. 1975. Enrichment serology and fluorescent antibody procedures to detect salmonellae in foods. J. Milk Food Technol. 38:227–231.

Hobbs, B.C. 1963. Techniques for the isolation of salmonellae from eggs and egg products. Ann. Inst. Pasteur (Paris) 104:621–637.

Hoben, D.A., Ashton, D.H., and Peterson, A.C. 1973. Some observations on the incorporation of novobiocin into Hektoen enteric agar for improved *Salmonella* isolation. Appl. Microbiol. 26:126–127.

Humphrey, T.J., Baskerville, A., Mawer, S., Rowe, B., and Hopper, S. 1989. *Salmonella enteritidis* phage type 4 from the contents of intact eggs: a study involving naturally infected hens. Epidemiol. Infect. 103:415–423.

Humphrey, T.J., Whitehead, A., Gawler, A.H.L., Henley, A., and Rowe, B. 1991. Numbers of *Salmonella enteritidis* in the contents of naturally contaminated hen's eggs. Epidemiol. Infect. 106:489–496.

Hynes, M. 1942. The isolation of intestinal pathogens by selective media. J. Pathol. Bacteriol. 54:193–207.

Jameson, J.E. 1962. A discussion of the dynamics of *Salmonella* enrichment. J. Hyg. Camb. 60:193–207.

Jeffries, L. 1959. Novobiocin-tetrathionate broth: a medium of improved selectivity for the isolation of salmonellae from feces. J. Clin. Pathol. 12:568–571.

June, G.A., Sherrod, P.S., Hammack, T.S., Amaguana, R.M., and Andrews, W.H. 1995. Relative effectiveness of selenite cystine broth, tetrathionate broth, and Rappaport-Vassiliadis medium for the recovery of *Salmonella* from raw flesh and other highly contaminated foods: precollaborative study. J. AOAC Int. 78:375–380.

Juven, B.J., Cox, N.A., Bailey, J.S., Thompson, J.E., Charles, O.W., and Shutze, J.V. 1984. Recovery of *Salmonella* from artificially contaminated poultry feeds in non-selective and selective broth media. J. Food Prot. 47:299–302.

Kauffman, F. 1930. Die Tecjnik der Typhenbestimmung in der Typhus-paratyphus-gruppe. Zentralbl. Bakteriol. Parasitenkd. Infektionskr. Hyg. Abt. Orig. 119:152–160.

Kauffman, F. 1935. Weitere Erfahrungen mit der kombinierten Anreicherungsverfahren fur Salmonella-Bacillen. Z. Hyg. Infektionskr. 117:26–32.

King, S., and Metzger, W.I. 1968. A new plating medium for the isolation of enteric pathogens. I. Hektoen enteric agar. Appl. Microbiol. 16:577–578.

Komatsu, K.K., and Restaino, L. 1981. Determination of the effectiveness of novobiocin added to two agar plating media for the isolation of *Salmonella* from fresh meat products. J. Food Saf. 3:183–192.

Kristensen, M., Lester, V., and Jurgens, A. 1925. Use of trypsinized casein, brom-thymol blue, brom cresol purple, phenol red and brilliant green for bacteriological nutrient media. Br. J. Exp. Pathol. 6:291–299.

Lamichhane, C.M., Joseph, S.W., Waltman, W.D., Secott, T., Odor, E.M., DeGraft-Hanson, J., Mallinson, E.T., Vo, V., and Blankford, M. 1995. Rapid detection of *Salmonella* in poultry using the colony lift immunoassay. Presented at the 16th meeting of Southern Poultry Science Society.

Leifson, E. 1935. New culture media based on sodium desoxycholate for the isolation of intestinal pathogens and for the enumeration of colon bacilli in milk and water. J. Pathol. Bacteriol. 40:581–599.

Leifson, E. 1936. New selenite enrichment media for the isolation of typhoid and paratyphoid (*Salmonella*) bacilli. Am. J. Hyg. 24:423–432.

MacConkey, A. 1905. Lactose fermenting bacteria in feces. J. Hyg. 5:333–379.

Mallinson, E.T. 1990. *Salmonella* monitoring system simplifies evaluation of farms. Poult. Digest September:46–47.

McCoy, J.H. 1962. The isolation of salmonellae. J. Appl. Bacteriol. 25:213–224.

Miller, R.G., and Tate, C.R. 1990. XLT4: a highly selective plating medium for the isolation of *Salmonella*. Md. Poultryman April:2–7.

Miller, R.G., Tate, C.R., Mallinson, E.T., and Scherrer, J.A. 1991. Xylose lysine tergitol 4: an improved selective agar medium for the isolation of *Salmonella*. Poult. Sci. 70:2429–2432.

Miller, R.G., Tate, C.R., and Mallinson, E.T. 1995. Improved XLT4 agar: small addition of peptone to promote stronger

production of hydrogen sulfide by salmonellae. J. Food Prot. 58:115–119.

Moats, W.A. 1978. Comparison of four agar plating media with and without added novobiocin for isolation of salmonellae from beef and deboned poultry meat. Appl. Environ. Microbiol. 36:747–751.

Moats, W.A. 1981. Update on *Salmonella* in foods: selective plating media and other diagnostic media. J. Food Prot. 44:375–380.

Moats, W.A., and Kinner, J.A. 1974. Factors affecting the selectivity of brilliant green–phenol red agar. Appl. Microbiol. 27:118–123.

Monford, J., and Thatcher, F.S. 1961. Comparison of four methods of isolating *Salmonella* from foods, and elaboration of a preferred procedure. J. Food Sci. 26:510–517.

Monnery, I., Freydiere, A.M., Baron, C., Rousset, A.M., Tigaud, S., Boude-Chevalier, M., de Montclos, H., and Gille, Y. 1994. Evaluation of two new chromogenic media for detection of *Salmonella* in stools. Eur. J. Clin. Microbiol. Infect. Dis. 13:257–261.

Morse, D.L., Birkhead, G.S., Guardino, J., Kondracki, S.F., and Guzewich, J.J. 1994. Outbreak and sporadic egg-associated cases of *Salmonella enteritidis*: New York's experience. Am. J. Public Health 84:859–860.

Mueller, L. 1923. Un nouveau milieu d'enrichissement pour la recherche du bacille typhique et des paratyphiques. C.R. Soc. Biol. (Paris) 89:434–437.

North, R.A.E., Duguid, J.P., and Sheard, M.A. 1996. The quality of public sector food-poisoning surveillance in England and Wales, with special reference to salmonella food poisoning. Br. Food J. 98:1–109.

North, W.R., and Bartram, M.T. 1953. The efficiency of selenite broth of different compositions in the isolation of *Salmonella*. Appl. Microbiol. 1:130–134.

Oggel, J.J., Nundy, D.C., Zebchuk, P.A., and Shaw, S.J. 1995. Reliability of the semi-solid Rappaport-Vassiliadis agar and the modified 1–2 test system for detection of *Salmonella* in poultry feeds. J. Food Prot. 58:98–101.

Osborne, W.W., and Stokes, J.L. 1955. A modified selenite brilliant-green medium for the isolation of *Salmonella* in eggs. Appl. Microbiol. 3:295–299.

Palumbo, S.A., and Alford, J.A. 1970. Inhibitory action of tetrathionate enrichment broth. Appl. Microbiol. 20:970–976.

Patil, M.D., and Parhad, N.M. 1986. Growth of salmonellas in different enrichment media. J. Appl. Bacteriol. 61:19–24.

Poisson, D.M. 1992. Novobiocin, brilliant green, glycerol, lactose agar: a new medium for the isolation of *Salmonella* strains. Res. Microbiol. 143:211–216.

Poisson, D.M., Nugier, J.P., and Rousseau, P. 1993. Study of Rambach and NBGL agar on 4037 stools of human origin and 584 veterinary samples submitted for isolation of salmonellae. Pathol. Biol. (Paris) 41:543–546.

Poppe, C., Johnson, R.P., Forsberg, C.M., and Irwin, R.J. 1992. *Salmonella enteritidis* and other salmonella in laying hens and eggs from flocks with *Salmonella* in their environment. Can. J. Vet. Res. 56:226–232.

Pourciau, S.S., and Springer, W.T. 1978. Evaluation of secondary enrichment for detecting salmonellae in bobwhite quail. Avian Dis. 22:42–45.

Rambach, A. 1990. New plate medium for facilitated differentiation of *Salmonella* spp. from *Proteus* spp., and other enteric bacteria. Appl. Environ. Microbiol. 56:301–303.

Rappaport, F., Konforti, N., and Navon, B. 1956. A new enrichment medium for certain salmonellae. J. Clin. Pathol. 9:261–266.

Rappold, H., and Bolderdijk, R.F. 1979. Modified lysine iron agar for isolation of *Salmonella* from food. Appl. Environ. Microbiol. 38:162–163.

Read, S.C., Irwin, R.J., Poppe, C., and Harris, J. 1994. A comparison of two methods for isolation of *Salmonella* from poultry litter samples. Poult. Sci. 73:1617–1621.

Restaino, L., Grauman, G.S., McCall, W.A., and Hill, W.M. 1977. Effects of varying concentrations of novobiocin incorporated into two *Salmonella* plating media on the recovery of four Enterobacteriaceae. Appl. Environ. Microbiol. 33:585–589.

Restaino, L., Komatsu, K.K., and Syracuse, M.J. 1982. A note on novobiocin in XLD and HE agars: the optimum levels required in two commercial sources of media to improve isolation of salmonellas. J. Appl. Bacteriol. 53:285–288.

Rigby, C.E., and Pettit, J.R. 1980. Delayed secondary enrichment for the isolation of salmonellae from broiler chickens and their environment. Appl. Environ. Microbiol. 40:783–786.

Rodrigue, D.C., Tauxe, R.V., and Rowe, B. 1990. International increase in *Salmonella enteritidis*: a new pandemic? Epidemiol. Infect. 105:21–27.

Ruiz, J., Nunez, M., Diaz, J., Lorente, I., Perez, J., and Gomez, J. 1996. Comparison of five plating media for isolation of *Salmonella* species from human stools. J. Clin. Microbiol. 34:686–688.

Salmonella Enteritidis Pilot Project progress report. 22 May 1995. Washington, DC: Animal and Plant Health Inspection Service, U.S. Department of Agriculture, 77 pp.

Salmonellosis Committee of the American Association of Avian Pathologists. 1970. Summary of 1970 AAAP Avian Salmonella Workshop. Avian Dis. 14:817–819.

Schlundt, J., and Munch, B. 1993. A comparison of the efficiency of Rappaport Vassiliadis, tetrathionate, and selenite broths with and without preenrichment for the isolation of *Salmonella* in animal waste biogas plants. Zentralbl. Bakteriol. 279:336–343.

Sharma, R.M., and Packer, R.A. 1969. Evaluation of culture media for isolation of salmonellae from feces. Appl. Microbiol. 18:589–595.

Sherrod, P.S., Amaguana, R.M., Andrews, W.H., June, G.A., and Hammack, T.S. 1995. Relative effectiveness of selective plating agars for recovery of *Salmonella* species for selected high-moisture foods. J. AOAC Int. 78:679–690.

Smyser, C.F., Bacharz, J., and Van Roekel, H. 1963. Detection of *Salmonella typhimurium* from artificially contaminated poultry feed and animal by-products. Avian Dis. 7:423–434.

Smyser, C.F., Snoeyenbos, G.H., and McKie, B. 1970. Isolation of salmonellae from rendered by-products and poultry litter cultured in enrichment media incubated at evaluated temperature. Avian Dis. 14:248–254.

Snoeyenbos, G.H., and Carlson, V.L. 1972. Comparative efficiency of tetrathionate and selenite enrichment broths for the isolation of *Arizona* serotypes. Avian Dis. 16:756–766.

Spino, D.F. 1966. Elevated temperature technique for isolation of *Salmonella* from streams. Appl. Microbiol. 14:1286–1288.

St. Louis, M.E., Morse, D.L., Potter, M.E., DeMelfi, T.M., Guzewich, J.J., Tauxe, R.V., and Blake, P.A. 1988. The emergence of grade A eggs as a major source of *Salmonella enteritidis* infections. JAMA 259:2103–2107.

Stokes, J.L., and Osborne, W.W. 1955. A selenite brilliant green medium for the isolation of *Salmonella*. Appl. Microbiol. 3:217–220.

Tate, C.R., and Miller, R.G. 1990. Modification of brilliant green agar by adding sodium novobiocin to increase selectivity for *Salmonella*. Md. Poultryman April:7–10.

Tate, C.R., Miller, R.G., Mallinson, E.T., Douglass, L.W., and Johnson, R.W. 1990. The isolation of salmonellae from poultry environmental samples by several enrichment procedures using plating media with and without novobiocin. Poult. Sci. 69:721–726.

Taylor, W.F. 1965. Isolation of shigellae. I. Xylose-lysine agars: new media for the isolation of enteric pathogens. Am. J. Clin. Pathol. 44:471–475.

Taylor, W.I., and Schelhart, D. 1971. Isolation of shigellae. VIII. Comparison of xylose lysine desoxycholate agar, Hektoen enteric agar, salmonella-shigella agar, and eosin methylene blue agar with stool specimens. Appl. Microbiol. 21:32–37.

Taylor, W.I., Silliker, J.H., and Andrews, H.P. 1958. Isolation of salmonellae from food samples. I. Factors affecting the choice of media for the detection and enumeration of *Salmonella*. Appl. Microbiol. 6:189–193.

Thomason, B.M., and Dodd, D.J. 1978. Enrichment procedures for isolating salmonellae from raw meat and poultry. Appl. Environ. Microbiol. 36:627–628.

Thomason, B.M., Dodd, D.J., and Cherry, W.B. 1977. Increased recovery of salmonellae from environmental samples enriched with buffered peptone water. Appl. Environ. Microbiol. 34:270–273.

U.S. Department of Agriculture (USDA). 1996. National Poultry Improvement Plan and auxiliary provisions. Washington, DC: Animal Plant Health Inspection Service, Veterinary Service, U.S. Department of Agriculture.

van Leusden, F.M., van Schothorst, M., and Beckers, H.J. 1982. The standard *Salmonella* isolation method. In: Coffy, J.E.L., Roberts, D., and Skinner, F.A., eds. Isolation and identification methods for food poisoning organisms. In: SAB Technical Series. New York: Academic, pp. 35–49.

van Schothorst, M., and Renaud, A.M. 1983. Dynamics of *Salmonella* isolation with modified Rappaport's medium (R10). J. Appl. Bacteriol. 54:209–215.

Vassiliadis, P. 1983. The Rappaport-Vassiliadis (RV) enrichment medium for the isolation of salmonellas: an overview. J. Appl. Bacteriol. 54:69–76.

Vassiliadis, P., Trichopoulos, D., Papoutsakis, G., and Politi, G. 1970. *Salmonella* isolations in abattoirs in Greece. J. Hyg. 68:601–609.

Vassiliadis, P., Pateraki, E., Papaiconomou, N., Papadakis, J.A., and Trichopoulos, D. 1976. Nouveau procede d'enrichissiment de *Salmonella*. Ann. Microbiol. [B] (Paris) 127:195–200.

Vassiliadis, P., Trichopoulos, D., Papoutsakis, G., and Pallandiou, E. 1979. A note on the comparison of two modifications of Rappaport's medium with selenite broth in the isolation of salmonellas. J. Appl. Bacteriol. 46:567–569.

Vassiliadis, P., Dalapothake, V., Mavrommati, C.H., and Trichopoulos, D. 1984. A comparison of the original Rappaport medium (R medium) and the Rappaport-Vassiliadis medium (RV medium) in the isolation of salmonellae from meat products. J. Hyg. 93:51–58.

Waltman, W.D., and Horne, A.M. 1993. Isolation of *Salmonella* from chickens reacting in the pullorum-typhoid agglutination test. Avian Dis. 37:805–810.

Waltman, W.D., and Mallinson, E.T. 1995. Isolation of *Salmonella* from poultry tissue and environmental samples: a nationwide survey. Avian Dis. 39:45–54.

Waltman, W.D., Horne, A.M., Pirkle, C., and Dickson, T.G. 1991. Use of delayed secondary enrichment for the isolation of *Salmonella* in poultry and poultry environments. Avian Dis. 35:88–92.

Waltman, W.D., Horne, A.M., Pirkle, C., and Johnson, D.C. 1992. Prevalence of *Salmonella enteritidis* in spent hens. Avian Dis. 36:251–255.

Waltman, W.D., Horne, A.M., and Pirkle, C. 1993. Influence of enrichment incubation time on the isolation of *Salmonella*. Avian Dis. 37:884–887.

Waltman, W.D., Horne, A.M., and Pirkle, C. 1995. Comparative analysis of media and methods for isolating *Salmonella* from poultry and environmental samples. In: Proceedings of the symposium on the diagnosis of *Salmonella* infections. United States Animal Health Association and American Association of Laboratory Veterinary Diagnosticians, pp. 1–14.

Weiss, K.F., Ayres, J.C., and Kraft, A.A. 1965. Inhibitory action of selenite on *E. coli, P. vulgaris, S. thompson.* J. Bacteriol. 90:857–862.

Wilson, W.J., and Blair, E.M. 1927. Use of glucose bismuth sulphite iron medium for the isolation of *B. typhosus* and *B. proteus.* J. Hyg. 26:374–391.

World Health Organization Consultation. 1994. Control of salmonella infections in animals and prevention of human food-borne *Salmonella* infections. Bull. WHO 72:831–833.

Yamamoto, R., Sadler, W.W., Adler, H.E., and Stewart, G.F. 1961. Comparison of media and methods for recovering *Salmonella typhimurium* from turkeys. Appl. Microbiol. 9:76–80.

Zander, D.V., and Mallinson, E.T. 1991. Principles of disease prevention: diagnosis and control. In: Calnek, B.W., Barnes, H.J., Beard, C.W., Reid, W.M., and Yoder, H.W., Jr., eds. Diseases of poultry, 9th ed. Ames: Iowa State University Press, pp. 3–44.

Index

ISBN 0-8138-2707-8

9 780813 827070

90000